ALLERGY AND ALLERGIC DISEASES
THE NEW MECHANISMS AND THERAPEUTICS

ALLERGY AND ALLERGIC DISEASES

THE NEW MECHANISMS AND THERAPEUTICS

Edited by

JUDAH A. DENBURG, MD

MCMASTER UNIVERSITY, HAMILTON, ONTARIO, CANADA

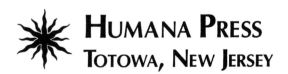

HUMANA PRESS
TOTOWA, NEW JERSEY

© 1998 Humana Press Inc.
999 Riverview Drive, Suite 208
Totowa, New Jersey 07512

For additional copies, pricing for bulk purchases, and/or information about other Humana titles, contact Humana at the above address or at any of the following numbers: Tel: 973-256-1699; Fax: 973-256-8341; E-mail: humana@humanapr.com

Due diligence has been taken by the publishers, editors, and authors of this book to assure the accuracy of the information published and to describe generally accepted practices. The contributors herein have carefully checked to ensure that the drug selections and dosages set forth in this text are accurate and in accord with the standards accepted at the time of publication. Notwithstanding, as new research, changes in government regulations, and knowledge from clinical experience relating to drug therapy and drug reactions constantly occurs, the reader is advised to check the product information provided by the manufacturer of each drug for any change in dosages or for additional warnings and contraindications. This is of utmost importance when the recommended drug herein is a new or infrequently used drug. It is the responsibility of the treating physician to determine dosages and treatment strategies for individual patients. Further it is the responsibility of the health care provider to ascertain the Food and Drug Administration status of each drug or device used in their clinical practice. The publisher, editors, and authors are not responsible for errors or omissions or for any consequences from the application of the information presented in this book and make no warranty, express or implied, with respect to the contents in this publication.

Cover illustration: Fig. 1 from Chapter 31, " Airway Remodeling and Repair," by Peter M. Hockey, Ratko Djukanović, William R. Roche, and Stephen T. Holgate.

Cover design by Patricia F. Cleary

This publication is printed on acid-free paper. ∞
ANSI Z39.48-1984 (American National Standards Institute) Permanence of Paper for Printed Library Materials.

Library of Congress Cataloging-in-Publication Data

Allergy and allergic diseases : the new mechanisms and therapeutics/edited by Judah A. Denburg
    p.   cm.
  Includes index.
  ISBN 0-89603-404-6 (alk. paper)
  1. Allergy. I. Denburg, Judah A.
  [DNLM: 1. Hypersensitivity.   WD 300 A432507 1998]
  RC584.A39 1998
  616.97—dc21
  DNLM/DLC
  for Library of Congress
                                         98-17728
                                         CIP

To my father of blessed memory, a student day and night.

PREFACE

Allergy and Allergic Diseases has been organized to provide an up-to-date, clinically relevant compilation of one of the most exciting areas of investigation in medicine today—allergic disease, especially as it pertains to the skin, airways, and bowel. With the dramatic rise in the incidence of various allergic disorders worldwide, and the coming of age of the discipline of Clinical Immunology and Allergy, the interface between basic and clinical science in this arena demands highlighting in this comprehensive new synthesis. It is with the hope of filling this evident need that *Allergy and Allergic Diseases: The New Mechanisms and Therapeutics* has been put together.

The book's content is divided into both basic and clinical sections, with emphasis on various components of the immune and inflammatory response as they relate to the development of allergic disease. Topics span the range from molecular biology to clinical symptomatology, with an effort to make this of interest to as broad a constituency as possible. This book will therefore be of substantial interest to specialists in Clinical Immunology and Allergy, scientists studying the cellular and molecular biology of inflammation and immunity, as well as internists, teachers, developers of medical school curricula, and members of industry focused on drug discovery and therapeutics. Indeed, a separate section has been added to deal with some specific issues in this latter field.

Wherever possible, figures and schematic drawings of mechanisms have been added to chapters; of necessity, some areas might be covered in more than one chapter, and we expect that this minor redundancy will result in clearer, deeper understanding among readers.

Our hope in creating *Allergy and Allergic Diseases* is that the general principles enunciated, as well as the specific lines of investigation discussed in the basic science section, will result in a work having genuine and lasting value as a standard reference resource for years to come.

Finally, this book could not have come together without the patient and indefatigable assistance of Lynne Larocque.

Judah A. Denburg

CONTENTS

CONTRIBUTORS

DIETRICH ABECK, MD • *Department of Dermatology and Allergy Biederstein, Technical University Munich, Munich, Germany*

KEN-ICHI ARAi, MD, PHD • *Department of Molecular and Developmental Biology,Institute of Medical Science, University of Tokyo, Tokyo, Japan*

PETER J. BARNES, DM, DSC, FRCP • *Department of Thoracic Medicine, Imperial School of Medicine at National Heart and Lung Institute, London, UK*

A. DEAN BEFUS, PHD • *Pulmonary Research Group, Heritage Medical Research Centre, University of Alberta, Edmonton, Alberta, Canada*

THOMAS BIEBER, MD, PHD • *Department of Dermatology, University of Bonn, Bonn, Germany*

BENGT BJÖRKSTÉN, MD • *Department of Paediatrics, University Hospital, Linköping, Sweden*

SERGIO BONINI, MD, PHD • *Immunology Office, European Academy of Allergology and Clinical Immunology, Rome, Italy*

STEFANO BONINI, MD • *Eye Clinic, University of Rome, Rome, Italy*

DAVID H. BROIDE, MBCHB • *Department of Medicine, University of California, San Diego, La Jolla, CA*

MARTIN K. CHURCH, MPHARM, PHD, DSC • *Immunopharmacology Group, Southampton General Hospital, Southampton, UK*

CHRISTOPHER J. CORRIGAN, MD, PHD • *Department of Medicine, Charing Cross and Westminster Medical School, London, UK*

RONALD DAHL, MD • *Department of Respiratory Diseases, Aarhus University Hospital, Aarhus, Denmark*

ULF DARSOW, PHD • *Department of Dermatology and Allergy Biederstein, Technical University Munich, Munich, Germany*

JAN E. DE VRIES, PHD • *Human Immunology Department, DNAX Research Institute of Molecular and Cellular Biology, Palo Alto, CA*

JUDAH A. DENBURG, MD, FRCP(C) • *Department of Medicine, McMaster University, Hamilton, Ontario, Canada*

RATKO DJUKANOVIĆ, MD, MSC, DM • *Immunopharmacology Group, University Medicine and University Pathology, Southampton University, Southampton, UK*

STEPHEN R. DURHAM, MD, FRCP • *Department of Allergy and Clinical Immunology, National Heart and Lung Institute, London, UK*

ALAN M. EDWARDS, MRCGP • *International Medical Communications–Respiratory and Allergy, Rhone-Poulenc Rorer, Leicestershire, UK*

MARIUSZ J. GIZYCKI, MD • *Lung Pathology Unit, Department of Histopathology, Royal Brompton Hospital, London, UK*

DANIEL L. HAMILOS, MD • *Washington University School of Medicine, St. Louis, MO*

ALEXIS E. HARPER, MSC • *International Medical Communications–Respiratory and Allergy, Rhone-Poulenc Rorer, Leicestershire, UK*

PETER M. HOCKEY, MBBCH, MRCP • *Immunopharmacology Group, University Medicine and University Pathology, Southampton University, Southampton, UK*

STEPHEN T. HOLGATE, MD, DSC, FRCP • *Immunopharmacology Group, University Medicine and University Pathology, Southampton University, Southampton, UK*

MARK HUMBERT, MD • *Department of Allergy and Clinical Immunology, National Heart and Lung Institute, London, UK; Service de Pneumologie et Reanimation Respiratoire, INSERM, Institut Paris Sud sur les Cytokines, Hopital Antoine Beclere, Clamart, France*

MARK D. INMAN, MD, PHD • *Department of Medicine, McMaster University, Hamilton, Ontario, Canada*

PETER K. JEFFERY, PHD • *Lung Pathology Unit, Department of Histopathology, Royal Brompton Hospital, London, UK*

ALLAN P. KAPLAN, MD • *Asthma and Allergy Center, Division of Pulmonary and Critical Care Medicine, Allergy and Clinical Immunology, Department of Medicine, Charleston Medical University of South Carolina, Charleston, SC*

DAVID M. KEMENY, BSC, PHD, MRCPATH • *Department of Immunology, King's College School of Medicine and Dentistry, London, UK*

HIROHITO KITA, MD • *Department of Immunology, Mayo Clinic and Foundation, Rochester, MN*

HIROKAZU KURATA, MD • *Department of Molecular and Developmental Biology, Institute of Medical Science, University of Tokyo, Tokyo, Japan*

PAIGE LACY, PHD • *Department of Medicine, Wellington School of Medicine, Wellington, New Zealand*

TONG-JUN LIN, PHD • *Pulmonary Research Group, Heritage Medical Research Centre, University of Alberta, Edmonton, Alberta, Canada*

PAUL A. MACARY, BSC • *Department of Immunology, King's College School of Medicine and Dentistry, London, UK*

ANGUS J. MACDONALD, PHD • *Pulmonary Research Group, Heritage Medical Research Centre, University of Alberta, Edmonton, Alberta, Canada*

DONALD W. MACGLASHAN, JR., MD, PHD • *Johns Hopkins Asthma and Allergy Center, Baltimore, MD*

DEREK M. MCKAY, PHD • *Intestinal Disease Research Programme, Department of Pathology, McMaster University, Hamilton, Ontario, Canada*

REDWAN MOQBEL, PHD, MRCPATH • *Department of Medicine, Pulmonary Research Group, Heritage Medical Research Centre, University of Alberta, Edmonton, Alberta, Canada*

NIELS MYGIND, MD • *Department of Respiratory Diseases, Aarhus University Hospital, Aarhus, Denmark*

HAROLD S. NELSON, MD • *Department of Medicine, National Jewish Center for Immunology and Respiratory Medicine, Denver, CO*

ALAN A. NORRIS, PHD • *International Medical Communications–Respiratory and Allergy, Rhone-Poulenc Rorer, Leicestershire, UK*

PAUL M. O'BYRNE, MB, FRCPI, FRCP(C), FCCP • *Asthma Research Group, Department of Medicine, McMaster University, Hamilton, Ontario, Canada*

MARY H. PERDUE, PHD • *Intestinal Disease Research Programme, Department of Pathology, McMaster University, Hamilton, Ontario, Canada*

THOMAS A. E. PLATTS-MILLS, MD, PHD, FRCP • *Asthma and Allergic Diseases Center, University of Virginia, Charlottesville, VA*

JUHA PUNNONEN, MD, PHD • *Human Immunology Department, DNAX Research Institute of Molecular and Cellular Biology, Palo Alto, CA*

D. KEN RAINEY, PHD • *International Medical Communications–Respiratory and Allergy, Rhone-Poulenc Rorer, Leicestershire, UK*

JOHANNES RING, PHD • *Department of Dermatology and Allergy Biederstein, Technical University Munich, Munich, Germany*

WILLIAM R. ROCHE, MSC, MD, FRCPATH • *Immunopharmacology Group, University Medicine and University Pathology, University of Southampton, Southampton, UK*

ANDREW V. ROGERS, BSC • *Lung Pathology Unit, Department of Histopathology, Royal Brompton Hospital, London, UK*

SERGIO ROMAGNANI, MD • *Division of Clinical Immunology and Allergy, Institute of International Medicine and Immunoallergology, University of Florence, Florence, Italy*

ANTHONY P. SAMPSON, MA, PHD • *Immunopharmacology Group, Southampton General Hospital, Southampton, UK*

ROMA SEHMI, PHD • *Department of Medicine, McMaster University, Hamilton, Ontario, Canada*

PETER VALENT, MD • *Department of Internal Medicine I, Division of Hematology, University of Vienna, Vienna, Austria*

DONATA VERCELLI, MD • *Molecular Immunoregulation Unit, DIBIT-San Raffaele Scientific Institute, Milan, Italy*

ANDREW J. WARDLAW, PHD, FRCP • *Department of Respiratory Medicine, Glenfield Hospital, Leicester, UK*

LISA M. WHEATLEY, MD • *Asthma and Allergic Diseases Center, University of Virginia, Charlottesville, VA*

FIONA L. WILLS, PHD • *Pulmonary Research Group, Heritage Medical Research Centre, University of Alberta, Edmonton, Alberta, Canada*

JUDITH A. WOODFOLK, MD • *Asthma and Allergic Diseases Center, University of Virgina, Charlottesville, VA*

I

EPIDEMIOLOGY/IgE

1

Molecular Mechanisms of Isotype Switching to IgE

Donata Vercelli, MD

CONTENTS

THE TWO-SIGNAL MODEL FOR THE INDUCTION OF IgE SYNTHESIS

During an immune response, B-lymphocytes express different immunoglobulin (Ig) heavy-chain isotypes sharing the same variable region. This phenomenon (isotype switching) allows a single B-cell clone to produce antibodies with the same fine specificity, but different effector functions. In order to switch to a particular isotype, a B-cell needs to receive two signals: signal 1 is cytokine-dependent, results in the activation of transcription at a specific region of the Ig locus, and determines isotype specificity. Signal 2 activates the recombination machinery, and leads to DNA switch recombination.

The two signals required for switching to the IgE isotype are delivered to B-cells by T-cells through a complex series of interactions. Allergen-specific B-cells capture the antigen via their surface Ig molecules, internalize it, and process it into peptides, which are then presented to T-cells in the context of major histocompatibility complex (MHC) class II molecules. Recognition of the antigen/MHC class II complex by the T-cell receptor leads to two crucial events: the secretion of lymphokines (interleukin [IL]-4 or IL-13) that provide signal 1 for IgE induction, and the expression of CD40 ligand (CD40L). Notably, CD40L is absent on resting T-cells, and it is the expression of this molecule following activation that renders T-cells fully competent to induce switching to IgE. Engagement of CD40 on B-cells by its ligand on T-cells delivers signal 2, and triggers switch recombination to IgE. Amplification circuits involving costimulatory molecules, particularly the CD28/B7 pair, then induce high-rate lymphokine secretion and IgE synthesis. In this chapter, the author discusses how the molecular events triggered in B-cells by these signals lead to IgE isotype switching.

MOLECULAR EVENTS IN THE INDUCTION OF IgE SYNTHESIS

Analysis at the DNA and RNA level provides the key to understanding the complex cell–cell interactions required to trigger IgE switching. Indeed, each of the main steps in T-/B-cell interactions described corresponds to a critical event that must occur at the gene level in order for switching to proceed. Signal 1, i.e., the cytokine IL-4 or IL-13, induces ε germline transcription, whereas CD40 engagement activates the switch recombination machinery (Fig. 1).

From: *Allergy and Allergic Diseases: The New Mechanisms and Therapeutics*
Edited by: J. A. Denburg © Humana Press Inc., Totowa, NJ

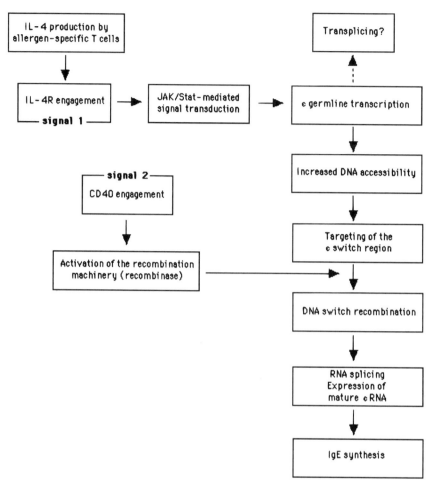

Fig. 1. Molecular events in isotype switching to IgE. IL-4 or IL-13 induce ε germline transcription and make the Sε region accessible for switch recombination. CD40 engagement activates the recombination machinery, and results in Sμ/Sε switch recombination. Intervening sequences are deleted as switch circles.

Signal 1 Induces Germline Transcription

Isotype switching results from a DNA recombination event that juxtaposes different downstream C_H genes to the expressed VDJ gene. Switching is not a random event, but is directed by cytokines in conjunction with the regulation of B-cell proliferation and differentiation *(1)*. Molecular analysis has shown that induction of isotype switching to a particular C_H gene invariably correlates with the transcriptional activation of the same gene in germline configuration. Several murine and human germline transcripts have been cloned, and share structural similarities *(2)*. The germline transcripts initiate from non-TATAA promoters a few kilobases upstream of the switch (S) region, and proceed through short exons (I_H exons) that are spliced to the first exon of the C_H gene. The region containing the germline promoter and the I_H exon is deleted during switch recombination.

Germline transcripts are unable to encode any mature protein of significant length, because the I_H exon contains multiple stop codons in all three reading frames. Therefore, these transcripts are also referred to as "sterile." Alternatively, germline transcripts are referred to as "truncated," because the I exon is usually 200–300 basepairs (bp) shorter than the VDJ exon present in mature transcripts. Although there is no significant conservation of the sequences of germline transcripts of different isotypes, their overall structure is conserved *(2)*.

Germline transcription is thought to direct switching by modulating the accessibility of a particular S region to a common recombinase. The importance of germline transcription in the regulation of isotype switching has recently been shown by gene knockout experiments. Deletion of the Iγ1 *(3)* or Iγ2b *(4)* exons and their promoter resulted in the inhibition of class switching to the corresponding genes, even though the corresponding S regions were not affected by the mutation. These results suggest that transcription in the S region is necessary to target the appropriate S region for recombination and switching. However, it is apparently not sufficient: replacement of Iε with a B-cell-specific promoter cassette containing the murine Eμ intronic enhancer and a V_H promoter, without the Iε splice donor site, resulted in only marginal switch recombination to IgE, at about 1% of the frequency induced by IL-4 *(5)*. In contrast, replacement of all known IL-4-inducible control elements in the Sγ1 region with the heterologous human metallothionein II_A promoter did not impair switch recombination to IgG1, provided that a 114-bp sequence that contains the Iγ1 splice donor site was included in the construct, thus allowing for the induction of artificial, but processed, germline transcripts *(6)*. These data indicate that artificial induction of structurally conserved, spliced germline transcripts can target switch recombination, whereas transcription in the S region as such cannot. Spliced switch transcripts (or the process of splicing) may thus have a functional role in switch recombination *(6)*. The most intriguing speculation is that germline transcripts are part of the switch recombinase machinery, providing the specificity to target distinct S regions. Alternatively, the 114-bp region that contains the Iγ1 splice donor site may also contain regulatory elements for γ1 switching unidentified to date.

Interestingly, the Iμ germline promoter is constitutively active in B-cells before and after the Sμ region sequence has undergone a primary recombination event *(7)*. Because Cμ is deleted upon switch recombination, the Iμ-containing germline transcript generated after a primary switching event is a hybrid that includes Iμ correctly spliced to the now-juxtaposed downstream C_H exon (i.e., Iμ-Cγ2b) *(7)*. These findings are consistent with a model in which simultaneous germline expression of both the 5' and 3' genes involved in a given switch recombination event is needed to target them for the process. The specificity of primary or sequential switching events comes from cytokine-induced germline transcription of the involved 3' C_H gene. Gene targeting experiments are required to understand whether continuous transcription through Iμ is required for either primary and/or sequential switching.

Germline transcripts have also been proposed to play a major role in interchromosomal RNA *trans*-splicing, whereby transcripts from rearranged VDJ exons are joined to C_H germline transcripts *(8)*. This process, which would result in heavy chain class switching in the absence of deletional DNA rearrangement in the C_H locus, has recently been shown to underlie multiple Ig isotype expression in the TG.SA transgenic mouse model *(9)*. Splenic B-cells from TG.SA mice expressed the transgenic human IgM and endogenous murine IgG simultaneously after stimulation with lipopolysaccharide (LPS) and IL-4. The B-cells bearing double isotypes expressed several mRNA species, i.e., transgenic human VDJ properly spliced to the endogenous mouse Cγ genes (*trans*-mRNA), together with the transgenic human μ RNA and germline transcripts derived from the mouse Cγ gene. No rearrangement of the transgene was detected *(10)*. It is conceivable that B-cells expressing multiple Ig isotypes might be intermediates for class switching. *Trans*-splicing involving germline transcripts might therefore be of general importance for class switching, although the role played by this mechanism in physiologic conditions is not yet clear.

ε *Germline Transcription Is Regulated By Nuclear Factors*

Nuclear factors specifically bind to relatively short (10–20 bp) DNA sequences, functionally defined as responsive elements (RE). The general paradigm for weak promoters, such as the I_H promoters, is that all slots for nuclear transcription factors need to be filled, in order for the gene to "fire." This implies a level of tight combinatorial control. Thus, the activation function of different transcription factors can operate at different limiting steps in the initiation reaction.

Because transcription through the I_H exon and the S region seems to be required to target the appropriate S region for recombination and switching, the induction of germline transcripts is a key step in determining the isotype specificity of the switching event. Different cytokines specifically induce different nuclear factors that activate transcription at the appropriate germline promoter. The specificity in the induction of transcription factors is essential for the specificity of cytokine-induced germline transcripts and isotype switching.

Expression of ε germline transcripts is regulated at the transcriptional level by nuclear factors that bind to the Iε promoter and adjacent regions. The requirements for the induction of ε germline transcripts seem to differ between mice and humans. Two signals, IL-4 (or IL-13) and LPS, are required for ε germline transcription in most murine B-cell lines, whereas the cytokine alone is sufficient in humans. A number of transcription factors have been found to bind to the ε germline promoter (Fig. 1); their roles, individually and with respect to each other, have not yet been fully characterized (Table 1).

A major IL-4 RE has been shown to bind a complex formed by a member of the C/EBP family, NF-kB p50, and the IL-4-inducible factor Stat6 (signal transducer and activator of transcription) (NF-IL-4, IL-4 NAF: *see below*) *(11)*. It has been proposed that these factors may have to interact physically in order to induce ε germline transcripts. The importance of NF-kB for the induction of murine germline transcripts has recently been confirmed by the finding that expression of germline transcripts for several isotypes, including IgE, and switching to the same isotypes, is severely impaired in NF-kB p50 knockout (KO) mice *(12)*. NF-kB seems to be essential for human ε germline transcription, as well (M. Woisetschläger, personal communication).

Stat6 *(13,14)* belongs to the newly identified family of signal transducers and activators of transcription (STAT) *(15)*. Binding of IL-4 to its receptor leads to activation by tyrosine phosphorylation of two receptor-associated cytoplasmic tyrosine kinases, Janus kinase (JAK)-3 and, to a lesser extent, JAK-1 *(16)*. These kinases are believed to rapidly induce tyrosine phosphorylation of Stat6, a latent cytoplasmic factor. The phosphorylated Stat6 homodimerizes, translocates to the nucleus, and binds to the promoter of a number of genes, contributing to the activation of transcription *(13)*. Stat6 preferentially binds dyad symmetric half-sites separated by 4 bp (TTCNNNNGAA). DNA binding specificity is localized to a region of 180 amino acids at the N-terminal side of the putative SH3 domain *(17)*. The discovery of JAKs and Stats has provided an explanation for the apparent paradox that the IL-4R, like the receptors for a number of other cytokines, lacks kinase domains, and yet couples ligand binding to tyrosine phosphorylation. Stat6 is not B-cell-specific, and is induced by IL-4 in monocytes, where it participates in the transcriptional regulation of the IL-4-inducible CD23b promoter, and possibly of the FcγR1 promoter *(18)*. Stat6 binding sites have been identified in the promoters of a number of other IL-4-responsive genes, such as Cε *(11,19,20)*, Cγ1, MHC class II *(18,20)*. The presence of homologous RE in the promoter of different genes underlies the concerted regulation of these genes by a single cytokine. Thus, the concerted modulation in the expression of ε germline transcription, CD23, and MHC class II in B-cells stimulated with IL-4 is mediated by IL-4 RE located in the promoters of these genes.

The B-lineage-specific B-cell-specific activator protein (BSAP) is essential for the IL-4-dependent induction of ε germline transcription. Deletion of the BSAP binding site has been

Table 1
Regulatory Elements in the ε Germline Promoter

Factor	Function
BSAP (B-cell lineage-specific activator protein)	Positive regulator of ε germline transcription
	Positive regulator of the CD19 promoter
	Repressor of the Ig 3′α enhancer and XBP 1 promoter
	Required for B-cell proliferation
	B-cell-specific
	Constitutively expressed
Stat6 (signal transducer and activator of transcription)	Latent cytoplasmic factor
	Induced by IL-4
	Translocates to the nucleus upon phosphorylation and dimerization
	Positive regulator of IL-4-inducible genes (CD23b, MHC class II, FcγR1)
	Required for IL-4-dependent ε germline transcription and IgE switching
	Repressor of ε germline transcription at baseline
	Non-B-cell-specific
NF-κB (nuclear factor-κB)	Involved in B-cell proliferation/differentiation
	Required for germline transcription and class switching
	Non-B-cell-specific
	Constitutively expressed

shown to severely impair the induction of ε germline promoter activity by IL-4 + LPS in murine B-cells (21), and by IL-4 alone in human B-cells (22). BSAP is the mammalian homolog of the sea urchin DNA binding protein TSAP (tissue-specific transcription activator protein), a regulator of late histone genes, and belongs to the Pax gene family of homeodomain transcription factors. It contains at the N-terminus a paired domain, which is necessary and sufficient for DNA binding, even as a monomer. BSAP is expressed in B-lymphocytes (from pro-B to mature B, but not in terminally differentiated plasma cells), the developing central nervous system (CNS), and adult testis (23). BSAP KO mice show a complete block of early B-cell differentiation (at the $B220^+/sIgM^-/CD43^+$ stage: pro–pre-BI cells) and alterations in the morphogenesis of the posterior midbrain. The role of BSAP in regulating transcription seems to be quite important, and certainly quite peculiar. BSAP interacts with DNA sequences of different composition: binding sites for BSAP have been identified in the promoter of a number of different B-cell-related genes, such as CD19, λ5, V_{preB1}, XBP 1, the tyrosine kinase *blk*, and the intronic regions of a number of Ig C_H genes (μ, γ1 γ2a, ε, α) (24,25). Interestingly, although BSAP binding increases transcription from various promoters (e.g., CD19), binding of BSAP to sites in the Ig 3′ α enhancer and XBP 1 promoter has a negative effect (25,26). Negative regulation of enhancer activity seems to be due to the ability of BSAP to suppress binding of NF-αP, a protein that positively controls enhancer activity and heavy chain transcription (26). Interestingly, BSAP is upregulated by proliferative stimuli (mitogens, cross-linking of sIgD or CD40) (27), and downregulated by OX40 ligand cross-linking (28). Indeed, recent evidence suggests that BSAP may confer CD40 responsiveness to the ε germline promoter, and may thus be involved in CD40-dependent upregulation of IL-4-induced ε germline transcription (22,29).

The minimal set of elements in the human ε germline promoter required to confer full IL-4 inducibility to a heterologous promoter has not been determined. In the mouse, a region containing the binding sites for Stat6 and a C/EBP factor seems to be sufficient to transfer

IL-4 inducibility to a minimal c-*fos* promoter *(11)*. Interestingly, the Stat6 binding site in the murine *(11)* and human ε germline promoter *(19)* shares a peculiar functional property with the site that binds the nonhistone chromosomal protein high mobility group (HMG-I)(Y) *(30)* in the mouse. Deletion or mutation of either site results in the loss of IL-4 inducibility, but in a marked increase in basal promoter activity. Thus, these elements seem to have a bifunctional activity, i.e., they are required for IL-4-induced promoter activation, but they repress the activity of the promoter in the absence of IL-4. These findings may suggest that expression of ε germline transcripts and IgE in resting B-cells is low in part because the germline promoter is kept in a state of repression that requires derepression through specific pathways.

Signal 2 Upregulates Germline Transcription and Induces DNA Switch Recombination

Although IL-4 (signal 1) is by itself sufficient for the initiation of transcription through the ε locus, switching and expression of mature Cε transcripts containing VDJ spliced to Cε1-4 require signal 2, i.e., engagement of CD40 by CD40L. The role of signal 2 in the induction of IgE switching is likely to be quite complex. In addition to triggering DNA recombination (see below), CD40/CD40L interactions are also critically involved in upregulating IL-4-induced ε germline transcription *(31,32)*. This transcriptional effect of CD40 engagement may be crucial for switching because optimal transcription through the S region may be required to target recombination. Thus, CD40 may control key events not only at the DNA, but also at the RNA level.

The DNA modifications that follow the delivery of the second signal for switching to IgE have only recently been fully characterized. According to the classical model switching occurs via loop-out and deletional recombination between highly repetitive S regions *(33)*. This was challenged in the late 1980s, at least for the IgE isotype. Indeed, it was reported that IgE could be produced by B-cells in which the immunoglobulin locus was retained in germline configuration *(34,35)*. Although that finding was probably the result of *trans*-splicing (*see* Signal 1 Induces Germline Transcription), it became important to characterize the molecular mechanisms that underlie the expression of mature VDJ-Cε mRNA in normal human B-cells. This issue was investigated using a polymerase chain reaction (PCR) that allows for amplification, cloning, and sequencing of either chimeric Sμ/Sε switch fragments (composed of the 5′ Sμ joined to the 3′ portion of the targeted Sε region) or switch circles, their reciprocal products. DNA sequencing of Sμ/Sε switch fragments amplified from IgE-producing B-cell cultures formally proved that deletional switch recombination had occurred. Most of the switch fragments represented direct joining of Sμ to Sε *(31,36,37)*. Interestingly, some switch fragments contained insertions at the Sμ/Sε junction that were derived from Sγ4 *(37)*. This finding suggested that some B-cells had undergone sequential isotype switching from IgM to IgG4 to IgE. Indeed, IL-4 has been shown to induce isotype switching to IgG4 *(38)*, as well as to IgE, and single B-cells can give rise to clones that secrete IgG4 and IgE *(39)*. More recently, analysis of switch circles has indicated that sequential switching from μ to ε can occur through γ1, as well as γ4 *(40,41)*.

Sequential switching and direct switching coexist. Sequencing of switch circles generated in B-cells triggered to switch to IgE by IL-4 and anti-CD40 mAb showed the presence of μ–γ–ε switching, and of sequential events even more complex (μ–α1–γ–ε). However, μ–ε circles representing direct switching events were also found, at high frequency *(42)*. Likewise, sequence analysis of Sμ/Sε switch fragments from B-cells of atopic dermatitis patients showed a predominance of direct Sμ/Sε joining *(43)*.

A chimeric Sμ/Sγ1 region resulting from a switching event between μ and γ1 can undergo a secondary recombination between the very 5′ end of Sμ and the very 3′ end of Sγ1. The secondary recombination essentially removes all the tandemly repeated S region sequences from the corresponding chromosome *(44)*. The mechanisms responsible for secondary recombination events in previously rearranged, chimeric S regions are still unknown. In particular, it is unclear whether secondary recombination requires retargeting of the recombinase. This would be problematic because of the deletion of the region encompassing the I_H exon and the germline promoter. Secondary recombination may, however, represent a mechanism to prevent continued switching to downstream isotypes, and ensure isotype stabilization of switched B-cells. On secondary recombination, in fact, the S sequences retained by the active Ig gene may be insufficient to serve as a substrate for further S/S recombination.

Whether sequential switching is an obligate step in vivo was investigated by examining switching to IgE in mutant mice that lacked the $S\gamma1$ region *(3)* and were therefore unable to support sequential switching via IgG1. In these mice, the frequency of switching to IgE was not affected *(45)*. These results indicated that sequential switching may merely reflect the simultaneous accessibility of two acceptor S regions for switch recombination induced by one cytokine. The apparent dominance of sequential switching observed in the generation of murine IgE-expressing cells following IL-4 stimulation may be due to the parallel activation of $S\gamma1$ and $S\varepsilon$ by IL-4, $S\gamma1$ being intrinsically more accessible to recombination with $S\mu$ *(3,45)*. Thus, the overall low frequency of IgE switching is an autonomously determined intrinsic feature of $S\varepsilon$ and its control elements. This may explain why, in the presence of saturating concentrations of IL-4 in vitro, the frequency of IgE switching reaches at most 10% of the frequency of switching to IgG1, which is also induced by IL-4.

REFERENCES

1. Coffman RL, Lebman DA, Rothman P (1993) The mechanism and regulation of immunoglobulin isotype switching. Adv Immunol 54:229.
2. Vercelli D, Geha RS (1992) Regulation of isotype switching. Curr Opin Immunol 4:794.
3. Jung S, Rajewsky K, Radbruch A (1993) Shutdown of class switch recombination by deletion of a switch region control element. Science 259:984.
4. Zhang J, Bottaro A, Li S, Stewart V, Alt FW (1993) Targeted mutation in the $I\gamma2b$ exon results in a selective $I\gamma2b$ deficiency in mice. EMBO J 12:3529.
5. Bottaro A, Lansford R, Xu L, Zhang J, Rothman P, Alt FW (1994) S region transcription *per se* promotes basal IgE class switch recombination but additional factors regulate the efficiency of the process. EMBO J 13:665.
6. Lorenz M, Jung S, Radbruch A (1995) Switch transcripts in immunoglobulin class switching. Science 267:1825.
7. Li SC, Rothman PB, Zhang J, Chan C, Hirsh D, Alt FW (1994) Expression of $I\mu$-$C\gamma$ hybrid germline transcripts subsequent to immunoglobulin heavy chain class switching. Int Immunol 6:491.
8. Durdik J, Gerstein RM, Rath S, Robbins PF, Nisonoff A, Selsing E (1989) Isotype switching by a microinjected μ immunoglobulin heavy chain gene in transgenic mice. Proc Natl Acad Sci USA 86:2346.
9. Shimizu A, Nussenzweig M, Mizuta T-R, Leder P, Honjo T (1989) Immunoglobulin double-isotype expression by trans-mRNA in a human immunoglobulin transgenic mouse. Proc Natl Acad Sci USA 86:8020.
10. Shimizu A, Nussenzweig MC, Han H, Sanchez M, Honjo T (1991) Trans-splicing as a possible molecular mechanism for the multiple isotype expression of the immunoglobulin gene. J Exp Med 173:1385.
11. Delphin S, Stavnezer J (1995) Characterization of an IL-4 responsive region in the immunoglobulin heavy chain germline ε promoter: Regulation by NF-IL-4, a C/EBP family member, and NF-kB/p50. J Exp Med 181:181.
12. Snapper CM, Zelazowski P, Rosas FR, Kehry MR, Tian M, Baltimore D, Sha WC (1996) B cells from p50/NF-κB knockout mice have selective defects in proliferation, differentiation, germ line C_H transcription, and Ig class switching. J Immunol 156:183.
13. Hou J, Schindler U, Henzel WJ, Ho TC, Brasseur M, McKnight SL (1994) An interleukin-4-induced transcription factor: IL-4 Stat. Science 265:1701.
14. Quelle FW, Shimoda K, Thierfelder W, Fischer C, Kim A, Ruben SM, Cleveland JL, Pierce JH, Keegan AD, Nealms K, Paul WE, Ihle JN (1995) Cloning of murine and human Stat6, Stat proteins that are

tyrosine phosphorylated in response to IL-4 and IL-3 but are not required for mitogenesis. Mol Cell Biol 15:3336.

15. Ivashkiv LB (1995) Cytokines and STATs: How can signals achieve specificity? Immunity 3:1.

16. Malabarba MG, Kirken RA, Rui H, Koettnitz K, Kawamura M, O'Shea JJ, Kalthoff FS, Farrar WL (1995) Activation of JAK3, but not JAK1, is critical to interleukin-4 stimulated proliferation and requires a membrane proximal region of IL-4 receptor α. J Biol Chem 270:9630.

17. Schindler U, Wu P, Rothe M, Brasseur M, McKnight SL (1995) Components of a Stat recognition code: evidence for two layers of molecular selectivity. Immunity 2:689.

18. Kotanides H, Reich NC (1993) Requirement of tyrosine phosphorylation for rapid activation of a DNA binding factor by IL-4. Science 262:1265.

19. Albrecht B, Peiritsch S, Woisetschläger M (1994) A bifunctional control element in the human IgE germline promoter involved in repression and IL-4 activation. Int Immunol 6:1143.

20. Köhler I, Rieber EP (1993) Allergy-associated Iε and Fcε receptor II (CD23b) genes activated via binding of an interleukin-4-induced transcription factor to a novel responsive element. Eur J Immunol 23:3066.

21. Liao F, Birshtein BK, Busslinger M, Rothman P (1994) The transcription factor BSAP (NF-HB) is essential for immunoglobulin germ-line ε transcription. J Immunol 152:2904.

22. Thienes CP, DeMonte L, Montecelli S, Busslinger M, Gould HJ, Vercelli D (1997) The transcription factor B-cell-specific activator protein (BSAP) enhances both IL-4 and CD40-mediated activator of the human ε germline promoter. J Immunol 158:5874.

23. Adams B, Dörfler P, Aguzzi A, Kozmik Z, Urbanek P, Maurer-Fogy I, Busslinger M (1992) Pax-5 encodes the transcription factor BSAP and is expressed in B lymphocytes, the developing CNS, and adult testis. Genes Dev 6:1589.

24. Hagman J, Grosschedl R (1994) Regulation of gene expression at early stages of B-cell differentiation. Curr Opin Immunol 6:222.

25. Reimold AM, Ponath PD, Li Y-S, Hardy RR, David CS, Strominger JL, Glimcher LH (1996) Transcription factor B cell lineage-specific activator protein regulates the gene for human X-box binding protein 1. J Exp Med 183:393.

26. Neurath MF, Max EE, Strober W (1995) Pax5 (BSAP) regulates the murine immunoglobulin 3′α enhancer by suppressing binding of NF-αP, a protein that controls heavy chain transcription. Proc Natl Acad Sci USA 92:5336.

27. Wakatsuki Y, Neurath MF, Max EE, Strober W (1994) The B cell-specific transcription factor BSAP regulates B-cell proliferation. J Exp Med 179:1099.

28. Stüber E, Neurath M, Calderhead D, Perry Fell H, Strober W (1995) Cross-linking of OX40 ligand, a member of the TNF/NGF cytokine family, induces proliferation and differentiation in murine splenic B cells. Immunity 2:507.

29. Fujita K, Jumper MD, Meek K, Lipsky PE (1995) Evidence for a CD40 response element, distinct from the IL-4 response element, in the germline ε promoter. Int Immunol 7:1529.

30. Kim J, Reeves R, Rothman P, Boothby M (1995) The non-histone chromosomal protein HMG-I(Y) contributes to repression of the immunoglobulin heavy chain germ-line ε RNA promoter. Eur J Immunol 25:798.

31. Shapira SK, Vercelli D, Jabara HH, Fu SM, Geha RS (1992) Molecular analysis of the induction of IgE synthesis in human B cells by IL-4 and engagement of CD40 antigen. J Exp Med 175:289.

32. Warren WD, Berton MT (1995) Induction of germ-line γ1 and ε Ig gene expression in murine B cells. IL-4 and the CD40 ligand-CD40 interactions provide distinct but synergistic signals. J Immunol 155:5637.

33. Max EE (1993) Immunoglobins: Molecular Genetics. In: Paul WE, ed. Fundamental Immunology. Raven, New York, p. 235.

34. MacKenzie T, Dosch HM (1989) Clonal and molecular characteristics of the human IgE-committed B cell subset. J Exp Med 169:407.

35. Chan MA, Benedict SH, Dosch H-M, Huy MF, Stein LD (1990) Expression of IgE from a nonrearranged ε locus in cloned B-lymphoblastoid cells that also express IgM. J Immunol 144:3563.

36. Shapira SK, Jabara HH, Thienes CP, Ahern DJ, Vercelli D, Gould HJ, Geha RS (1991) Deletional switch recombination occurs in IL-4 induced isotype switching to IgE expression by human B cells. Proc Natl Acad Sci USA 88:7528.

37. Jabara HH, Loh R, Ramesh N, Vercelli D, Geha RS (1993) Sequential switching from μ to ε via γ4 in human B cells stimulated with IL-4 and hydrocortisone. J Immunol 151:4528.

38. Lundgren M, Persson U, Larsson P, Magnusson C, Smith CIE, Hammarström L, Severinson E (1989) Interleukin 4 induces synthesis of IgE and IgG4 in human B cells. Eur J Immunol 19:1311.

39. Gascan H, Gauchat J-F, Aversa G, van Vlasselaer P, de Vries JE (1991) Anti-CD40 monoclonal antibodies or CD4⁺ T cell clones and IL-4 induce IgG4 and IgE switching in purified human B cells via different signaling pathways. J Immunol 147:8.

40. Fujieda S, Zhang K, Saxon A (1995) IL-4 plus CD40 monoclonal antibody induces human B cells γ subclass-specific isotype switch: switching to γ1, γ3, and γ4, but not γ2. J Immunol 155:2318.

41. Mills FC, Mitchell MP, Harindranath N, Max EE (1995) Human Ig Sγ regions and their participation in sequential switching to IgE. J Immunol 155:3021.

42. Zhang K, Mills FC, Saxon A (1994) Switch circles from IL-4-directed ε class switching from human B lymphocytes—evidence for direct, sequential and multiple step sequential switch from μ to ε Ig heavy chain gene. J Immunol 152:3427.

43. van der Stoep N, Korver W, Logtenberg T (1994) In vivo and in vitro IgE isotype switching in human B lymphocytes: evidence for a predominantly direct IgM to IgE class switch program. Eur J Immunol 24:1307.

44. Zhang K, Cheah H-K, Saxon A (1995) Secondary deletional recombination of rearranged switch region in Ig isotype-switched B cells. A mechanism for isotype stabilization. J Immunol 154:2237.

45. Jung S, Siebenkotten G, Radbruch A (1994) Frequency of Immunoglobulin E class switching is autonomously determined and independent of prior switching to other classes. J Exp Med 179:2023.

2 Cytokines and IgE Regulation

Juha Punnonen, MD, PhD,
and Jan E. de Vries, PhD

Contents

INTRODUCTION

Synthesis of allergen-specific immunoglobulin E (IgE) in vivo is a result of multiple interactions among B-cells, T-cells, and professional antigen-presenting cells (APC). B-cell activation is initiated when specific B-cells recognize the allergen by cell surface immunoglobulin (sIg). However, costimulatory molecules expressed by activated T cells in both soluble and membrane-bound forms are necessary for differentiation of B-cells into Ig-secreting plasma cells *(1)*. Activation of T helper (Th) cells requires recognition of an antigenic peptide in the context of major histocompatibility complex (MHC) class II molecules on the plasma membrane of APC, such as monocytes, dendritic cells, Langerhans cells, or primed B-cells. Professional APC can efficiently capture the antigen, and the peptide-MHC class II complexes are formed in a post-Golgi, proteolytic intracellular compartment and subsequently exported to the plasma membrane, where they are recognized by T-cell receptor (TCR) *(2)*. In addition, activated B-cells express CD80 (B7-1) and CD86 (B7-2, B70), which are the counter receptors for CD28 and which provide a costimulatory signal for T-cell activation resulting in T-cell

From: *Allergy and Allergic Diseases: The New Mechanisms and Therapeutics*
Edited by: J. A. Denburg © Humana Press Inc., Totowa, NJ

proliferation and cytokine synthesis *(3)*. Since allergen-specific T-cells from atopic individuals generally belong to the Th2-cell subset, activation of these cells also leads to production of interleukin (IL)-4 and IL-13, which, together with membrane-bound costimulatory molecules expressed by activated T-helper cells, direct B-cell differentiation into IgE-secreting plasma cells.

During humoral immune responses the first isotypes to be produced are IgM and IgD, and in order to produce Ig of other isotypes B-cells have to undergo class switching, which occurs by DNA recombination *(1,4)*. The genes for the constant regions of heavy chains are clustered at the 3' end of the Ig heavy chain locus on human chromosome 14 and on mouse chromosome 12. The human heavy chain locus comprises nine functional genes and two pseudo genes, which are arranged in the following order: 5' μ-δ-γ3-γ1-$\psi\epsilon$-α1-$\psi\gamma$-γ2-γ4-ϵ-α2 3' *(1,4)*. DNA recombination is mediated by repetitive segments known as switch regions (S) that are generally located approx 1 kb or less 5' to each heavy chain locus *(1,4–6)*. Recombination, which occurs through S–S joining, brings a specific variable region adjacent to a new heavy chain gene, and the sequences intervening the variable region and the new heavy chain are deleted in the process. Therefore, the specificity of the Ab produced does not change during isotype switching. However, the functional properties of the newly synthesized Ab may be profoundly altered, because the effector functions of immunoglobulins, such as complement fixation, Fc receptor binding, and traversal of basal membranes, are determined by the constant regions of the heavy chains, whereas the variable regions determine antigen specificity *(1)*. For example, one specific property of IgE is that it binds to high-affinity IgE receptors on mast cells and basophils, which results in activation of these cells.

Until recently, IL-4 was considered as the only cytokine capable of inducing IgE switching. This conclusion was supported by the fact that IL-4-deficient mice failed to produce IgE after nematode infections *(7)*. The discovery of IL-13, and subsequent biological characterization of this cytokine, revealed that IL-13 is another cytokine that efficiently directs human B-cells to switch to IgE production. Although IL-4 and IL-13 are the only cytokines that can induce IgE synthesis by naive B-cells, several other cytokines are known to modulate IL-4- and IL-13-induced IgE synthesis by both direct and indirect mechanisms. In this chapter we review the molecular and biological characteristics of IL-4 and IL-13, as well as the effects of other cytokines on IL-4- and IL-13-induced IgE synthesis. In addition, we discuss recently characterized IL-4 and IL-13 receptor antagonists as possible means to block IL-4- and IL-13-induced IgE synthesis in atopic individuals.

IgE SYNTHESIS IS DEPENDENT ON MEMBRANE-BOUND AND SECRETED MOLECULES EXPRESSED BY T-HELPER CELLS

Although recognition of antigen by sIg is a key event in the initial phase of B-cell activation, Ig isotype switching and differentiation of B-cells into Ig-secreting plasma cells require physical interactions of B- and T-cells. Activation of CD4+ T-helper cells results in induction and upregulation of cell surface molecules that further enhance B-cell activation initiated by antigen recognition. CD40 and its ligand (CD40L) are now considered the most important pair of molecules mediating productive T–B-cell interactions. CD40–CD40L interaction plays a crucial role also in induction of IgE synthesis (Fig. 1).

CD40 is a cell surface glycoprotein, constitutively expressed on mature B-cells, that mediates signals necessary for efficient Ig isotype switching and B-cell differentiation. It is a member of the tumor necrosis factor (TNF) receptor family, which also includes the two TNF receptors (type I and II), the low-affinity nerve growth factor receptor, and CD27, CD30, Fas antigen (CD95), and OX40 protein. The cytoplasmic region of CD40 is homologous to that of

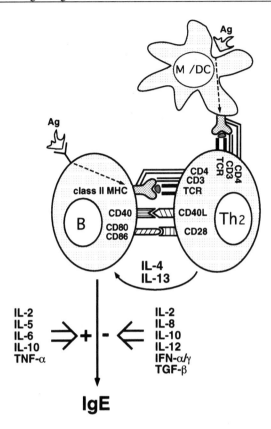

Fig. 1. A schematic model of IgE regulation. Primed B-cells, monocytes/macrophages, or dendritic cells capture the antigen/allergen and present the antigenic peptides in the context of MHC class II molecules. When the peptide/MHC class II complex is recognized by T-cell receptor on allergen-specific T-helper 2 cells, these cells become activated and start to produce IL-4 and IL-13, which direct IgE switching in the presence of costimulatory molecules, such as the ligand for CD40. This process is modulated by cytokines such as IL-2, IL-5, IL-6, IL-8, IL-10, IL-12, IFN-α, IFN-γ, TGF-β, and TNF-α. (M, monocyte/ macrophage; DC, dendritic cell; B, B-cell; Th2, T-helper 2 cell; Ag, antigen/allergen).

the p55 TNFα receptor and the Fas antigen, suggesting commonalties in the signaling pathways of these molecules (8). CD40 is not only expressed on B-cells but also on thymic epithelial cells and bone marrow-derived dendritic cells and follicular dendritic cells (9,10). Studies indicating that anti-CD40 MAbs induce B-cell activation and proliferation suggested an important function for this molecule in the regulation of B-cell activation (11). Activated T-helper cells in induction of IgE switching and IgE synthesis in vitro could be replaced by monoclonal antibodies (MAbs) specific for CD40 or transfectants expressing CD40L and exogenous IL-4 (12–14). In addition, long-term B-cell lines were established using IL-4 and anti-CD40 MAbs crosslinked to murine L-cells transfected with FcγRII (15).

The ligands for both murine and human CD40 were cloned from cDNA libraries constructed from activated T-cells (16–19). CD40L is a 33-kDa type II glycoprotein with significant homology to TNF-α and TNF-β. In contrast to activated CD4[+] T-cells, resting T-helper cells do not express CD40L and cannot give help for B-cell differentiation. Transfectants expressing CD40L or soluble recombinant CD40L induced B-cell proliferation and differentiation into IgE-secreting cells in the presence of IL-4, indicating that all the signals required for IgE switching can be delivered by CD40L and IL-4 (17–21). However, the signaling pathway through CD40 does not seem to be identical to that induced by activated CD4$^+$ T-cells *(13)*, suggesting that additional membrane-bound molecules are involved in induction of B-cell proliferation, isotype switching, and differentiation.

Mutations in the gene encoding CD40L resulting in deficient CD40L expression were shown to be the cause of hyper-IgM syndrome, an immunodeficiency characterized by very low serum levels of IgG, IgA, and IgE. The CD40L gene was mapped to the X-chromosomal location q26.3–q27.1, the same region where a gene defect in patients with X-linked hyper-IgM syndrome was localized earlier *(22–25)*. B-cells of these patients are normal, because MAbs specific for CD40 induced high levels of IgE synthesis by patients' B-cells cultured in the presence of IL-4. In contrast, T-cell clones from the majority of the patients failed to induce normal B-cell differentiation, supporting the notion that functional CD40L expression is essential for productive T–B-cell interactions. Moreover, T-cells from a subset of patients suffering from common variable immunodeficiency with low serum Ig levels were found to express suboptimal levels of CD40L *(26)*.

In addition to activated T-cells, CD40L expression was observed on human mast cells and basophils *(27)*. These cells were also able to induce IgE synthesis by human B-cells in the presence of exogenous IL-4 *(27)*. Moreover, activated mast cells are capable of producing IL-4, IL-5, and IL-13 *(28,29)*, suggesting that mast cells may play a role in the regulation of IgE synthesis in vivo. However, it remains to be determined whether mast cells are indeed capable of inducing IgE synthesis in vivo. Studies on IL-4-deficient mice suggest that this is not the case, because IgE production in these mice could be restored by administration of normal CD4$^+$ T-cells, whereas reconstitution with normal CD4$^-$ cell populations was ineffective *(30)*. These results suggest that IgE isotype switching requires productive T–B-cell interactions. This conclusion is in line with the fact that no antigen-specific receptor molecules on mast cells, which could regulate the specificity of mast cell-induced Ig synthesis, have been identified.

CD40L is not only involved in B-cell activation, but it also mediates activation signals to T-cells. Transfectants expressing CD40 enhance anti-CD3-induced T-cell activation in vitro *(31)*. In addition, antigen-specific T-cell responses are impaired in CD40L-deficient mice *(32)*, and administration of soluble CD40 to CD40-deficient mice initiates germinal-center formation *(33)*, indicating that, while providing a strong B-cell activation signal, CD40–CD40L interaction also provides a T-cell costimulatory signal, which is required for in vivo priming of CD4$^+$ T-cells and for initiation of specific T-cell responses in vivo.

Although CD40L$^-$ T-cell clones have strongly reduced capacity to provide B-cell help, some T-cell clones with defined mutations of CD40L gene could induce IgE synthesis by B-cells cultured in the presence of IL-4 *(34)*, suggesting that CD40L is probably not the only molecule capable of inducing IgE switching in the presence of cytokines. In addition, anti-CD40 MAbs and activated CD4$^+$ T-cells had synergistic effects on IL-4-dependent IgE synthesis by purified B-cells, further suggesting that membrane-bound molecules other than CD40L also contribute to the events that result in IgE switching *(13)*. As discussed in detail below, the 26-kDa membrane form of TNF-α (mTNF-α), expressed on CD4$^+$ T-cells after activation, was shown to be another molecule associated with productive T–B-cell interactions. However, IgE synthesis induced by T-cells from CD40L-deficient patients could not be blocked by neutralizing anti-TNF-α MAbs *(34)*, suggesting that additional surface-bound molecules are involved in productive T–B-cell interactions. One such pair of molecules may be CD19, which is constitutively expressed on B-cells, and its putative ligand on T-cells, because CD19-deficient mice have impaired T-cell-dependent B-cell responses *(35)*. In addition, CD22 expressed on B cells has also been demonstrated to mediate interactions with T-cells *(36)*, further demonstrating the complexity and redundancy involved in the regulation of productive T–B-cell interactions.

CYTOKINE PRODUCTION PROFILE OF ATOPIC PATIENTS

Atopic patients have been shown to have elevated production of Th2-type cytokines in vitro and in vivo (37,38). Increased Th2-cell activity is likely to be the underlying reason for increased serum IgE levels and may be the primary event leading to development of allergic diseases. A characteristic feature of Th2-type cells is production of high levels of IL-4, IL-5, and IL-13 (38–40), all of which are cytokines implicated in the pathogenesis of IgE-mediated allergies and asthma. In addition, Th2-cells produce minimal levels of or no interferon (IFN)-γ, which has been shown to antagonize many of the functions of IL-4 and IL-13, including their capacity to induce IgE production.

Early studies indicated that peripheral blood mononuclear cells (PBMC) derived from a proportion of atopic individuals spontaneously secrete IgE in vitro, indirectly suggesting ongoing IL-4 or IL-13 production by patients' T cells (41,42). In addition, T-cells and T-cell supernatants from atopic individuals, but not from healthy controls, induced IgE synthesis by normal B-cells (42), suggesting that allergen-specific T-cells secreted a soluble factor that specifically induced IgE synthesis. This activity is now known to be mediated by IL-4 and IL-13. Atopic individuals were subsequently also directly shown to produce elevated levels of IL-4 in vitro and in vivo, and neutralizing anti-IL-4 MAbs were shown to inhibit spontaneous and T-cell supernatant-induced IgE synthesis (41,43,44). Allergen challenge was also shown to induce expression of both IL-4 and IL-13 in the lungs of asthmatic patients (45,46).

Cloning of allergen-specific T-cells directly indicated that allergies are primarily mediated by Th2-cells. Allergen-specific T-cell clones derived from the skin of atopic patients produce high levels of IL-4, IL-5, and IL-13, and no or minimal levels of interferon (IFN)-γ, indicating predominantly a Th2-type cytokine production profile, whereas allergen-specific T-cells obtained from nonatopic donors generally belonged to the Th0 subset (47–51). In contrast, T-cell clones specific for tetanus toxoid and obtained from atopic patients produced high levels of IFNγ, and no or minimal levels of IL-4, indicating that these cells were of Th1 type (48). Recently, atopy was linked to genes in chromosome 5q31.1 in the area where the genes encoding IL-4 and IL-13 are located, suggesting a genetic predisposition for enhanced IL-4 and IL-13 production in atopic individuals (52).

CHARACTERISTICS OF IL-4

Human IL-4 is a protein consisting of 153 amino acids and has two potential N-glycosylation sites. Human IL-4 is only ~50% homologous to mouse IL-4, and IL-4 is species specific. The genes for human and mouse IL-4 have been mapped to chromosome's 5 and 13, respectively, in close proximity to genes encoding IL-3, IL-5, IL-9, and granulocyte macrophage-colony forming unit (GM-CSF). IL-4 is produced not only by activated T-cells, but also by basophil/mast cell lineage (29). IL-4 synthesis by T-cells is initiated after activation through T-cell receptors, whereas basophils/mast cell activation requires crosslinking of high-affinity IgE receptors (53).

IL-4 was initially identified as a B-cell stimulatory factor that costimulated proliferation of anti-IgM-activated mouse B-cells (53). Thereafter, IL-4 has been shown to stimulate Ig production and enhance expression of MHC class II molecules, sIgM, CD40, and CD23 on B-cells. However, the effects of IL-4 are not limited to the B-cell lineage. It also induces proliferation of preactivated T-cells, induces growth of mast cells, and enhances the antigen-presenting capacity and anti-tumor activity of monocytes in vitro and in vivo (54). Furthermore, IL-4 enhances expression of CD23 and MHC class II molecules on monocytes.

Because of its inhibitory effects on synthesis of proinflammatory cytokines by monocytes, IL-4 has potent anti-inflammatory effects both in vitro and in vivo *(53)*.

IL-4 induces IgE synthesis and IgE switching by B-cells (discussed below). IL-4 can also indirectly enhance IgE production, because it directs the differentiation of Th2-cells, producing high levels of IL-4, IL-5, and IL-13. Naive CD4+ T-cells produce mainly IL-2 after primary stimulation, and IL-4 and IL-12 appear to be the major factors that determine whether these cells develop into Th2- or Th1-type cells, respectively. Mice infected with *Leishmania major* and treated with neutralizing anti-IL-4 MAbs generated Th1 responses, whereas administration of anti-IFN-γ MAbs resulted in the development of a Th2 cytokine profile *(55)*. Importantly, naive human CD4+ cord blood T-cells differentiate into Th2-cells when activated by crosslinked anti-CD3 MAbs and cultured in the presence of IL-4, but in the absence of professional APC, indicating that IL-4 acts directly on precursor T-helper cells *(56)*. Stimulation of naive cord blood T-cells in the presence of IL-12 induced these cells to differentiate into Th1-cells, producing high levels of IFN-γ *(56)*.

The crucial role of IL-4 in inducing Th2-cell differentiation and Th2 responses was also demonstrated in IL-4-deficient mice, which have impaired production of Th2-type cytokines such as IL-5 and IL-13 *(57,58)*. In contrast, production of IFN-γ is elevated in these mice as compared to wild-type control mice. Interestingly, although eosinophilia is primarily induced by IL-5 *(59–61)*, peripheral blood eosinophilia in IL-4 deficient mice was reduced by up to 80 percent after infection with *Nippostrongylus brasiliensis* or *Schistosoma mansoni (58)*. Thus, IL-4 also appears to be of crucial importance also for the induction of eosinophilia by regulating the levels of IL-5 synthesis in vivo, emphasizing the role of Th2-cells in this process.

Although it is well established that IL-4 directs Th2 differentiation, the cellular source of IL-4 in primary T-cell responses remains controversial. During stimulation of naive cord blood CD4+ T-cells only IL-2 mRNA was detectable *(62)*, whereas IL-4 production appears to be restricted to CD45RO+ memory T-cells *(63,64)*. Recently it was shown that NK1.1+ T-cells, which represent a minor T-cell subset, produce high levels of IL-4 rapidly following activation, and it was suggested that they are the primary source of IL-4 in early phases of T-cell activation *(65,66)*. NK1.1+ T-cells can also provide help for IgE synthesis *(65,66)*. On the other hand, it has also been suggested that virtually every naive CD4+ T-cell primed and cultured in the absence of exogenous IL-4 can produce IL-4 in quantities that are high enough to direct Th2 development in an autocrine fashion *(67)*.

CHARACTERISTICS OF IL-13

IL-13 was first characterized as P600, a mouse protein produced by Th2-type T-cell clones. The function of IL-13 remained unknown until the human homolog was sequenced and cloned *(68,69)*. The human IL-13 gene is 66% homologous to that of the mouse and encodes a 10-kDa protein that is 58% homologous to the mouse P600. Alternative splicing results in two forms of hIL-13 consisting of 131 or 132 amino acids, respectively, the latter having an additional glutamine residue at position 98 *(68)*. No functional difference has been identified between these two forms of IL-13. Rat IL-13 was also cloned using a reverse transcriptase-polymerase chain reaction (RT-PCR) method, and the coding region of rat IL-13 displays 74% and 87% sequence identity with the coding regions of human and mouse IL-13 cDNA, respectively *(70)*.

Human IL-13 protein is only ~25% homologous to IL-4, but all residues that contribute to the hydrophobic structural core of IL-4 are conserved or have conservative replacements in the IL-13 protein, suggesting that the three-dimensional structures are similar *(71)*. In addition, the

Table 1
Summary of the Functional Properties of IL-4 and IL-13

Activity Induced or Inhibited	IL-4	IL-13
B-cell proliferation	↑↑↑	↑↑
B-cell differentiation	↑↑↑	↑↑
IgE synthesis	↑↑↑	↑↑
Germline ε transcription	↑↑↑	↑↑
sIgM, HLA-DR, and CD23 expression on B-cells	↑↑↑	↑↑
Activation of immature B-cells	↑↑	↑
Activation of pre-B-cells	↑	—
Production by Th2-cells	↑↑↑	↑↑↑
Production by Th1-cells	—	↑
Production by Th0-cells	↑	↑↑
Production by CD45RA$^+$ T-cells	—	↑↑
T-cell proliferation	↑↑	—
Th2 differentiation	↑↑↑	—
Expression of VCAM-1 on endothelial cells	↑↑↑	↑↑↑
HLA-DR and CD23 expression on monocytes	↑↑↑	↑↑↑
IFN-α and IL-12 production by monocytes	↓↓↓	↓↓↓
Proinflammatory cytokine synthesis by monocytes	↓↓↓	↓↓↓

sites that are predicted to contribute to receptor binding also share a remarkable homology between IL-4 and IL-13. The gene encoding IL-13 is located on chromosome 5 in the same region where genes encoding IL-3, IL-4, IL-5, IL-9, and GM-CSF are mapped, and it is only 12 kb 5′ to the gene encoding IL-4, suggesting that the two cytokines are results of gene duplication (72,73).

IL-13 shares many, but not all, of its biological activities with IL-4 (Table 1). Like IL-4, IL-13 modulates the phenotype of normal human B cells and induces B cell proliferation and differentiation (68,74). In addition, IL-13 upregulated the expression of CD23, CD72, sIgM, and MHC class II molecules on purified human B-cells (74). Moreover, IL-13 not only induced IgE synthesis (discussed below), but it also induced IgM and IgG synthesis by B-cells cocultured with activated CD4$^+$ T cells or anti-μ or anti-CD40 MAbs (68,74,75). Like IL-4, IL-13 inhibits IL-2-induced proliferation of chronic lymphocytic leukemia B cells (76), induces VCAM-1 expression on endothelial cells (77) and modulates the phenotype of human monocytes, and inhibits the production of proinflammatory cytokines by the cells (78). IL-13 was also shown to suppress experimental autoimmune encephalomyelitis in rats, demonstrating its anti-inflammatory properties in vivo (79).

Despite the functional similarities between IL-4 and IL-13, IL-13 did not have IL-4-like growth-promoting effects on human phytohemagglutinin (PHA)-activated T-cell blasts or activated CD4$^+$ or CD8$^+$ T-cell clones. These differential effects of IL-4 and IL-13 on T-cell function imply that IL-4 and IL-13 are likely to have clearly distinct roles in the regulation of immune responses in vivo. However, it remains to be shown whether IL-13 can indirectly affect T-cell function and T-cell differentiation through its downregulatory effects on production of monocyte-derived cytokines, such as IL-12 and IFN-α (78), which are known to direct Th1 development (80–84).

The kinetics of IL-13 production by activated T cells significantly differs from that of IL-4 production. Expression of IL-4 mRNA after polyclonal T-cell activation seems to be short-lasting. IL-4 mRNA first appears 2–4 h after activation, and after 12 h it is almost undetectable. In contrast, IL-13 mRNA can still be observed 48 h after T-cell activation, suggesting that IL-13 is produced for a significantly longer period of time after antigen-specific T-cell response *(85)*. Furthermore, the T-cell subsets producing IL-13 are different from those producing IL-4. IL-13 is not only produced by Th2-type cells, but also by Th0 and Th1 cells, and in contrast to IL-4, IL-13 is also produced by CD45RA[+] T-cells *(63,64)*. However, cells that produce IL-4 also appear to produce IL-13 when studied at the single-cell level *(64)*. These differential effects of IL-4 and IL-13 on T cells and their differential production profiles may have important consequences for the individuals role of these cytokines in the regulation of allergic inflammation and IgE synthesis in vivo.

IL-4R AND IL-13R COMPLEXES

The receptors for IL-4 and IL-13 share a common subunit, the first evidence of which came from studies indicating that a mutated form of IL-4, in which the tyrosine residue at position 124 is replaced by aspartic acid, acted an antagonist for both IL-4 and IL-13 *(71,75)*. In addition, IL-13 could partially compete for IL-4 binding to the human premyeloid cell line TF-1, which responds to both IL-4 and IL-13 *(71)*. More recent studies have shown that some MAbs specific for the 130-kDa IL-4R α-chain block the biological activities of both IL-4 and IL-13, indicating that IL-4R α-chain is shared by IL-4R and IL-13R complexes *(86)*. In addition, both IL-4 and IL-13 have been shown to induce phosphorylation of the IL-4R α-chain *(87)*, but expression of IL-4R α-chain alone on transfectants is not sufficient to provide a functional IL-4R that signals in response to IL-4 or IL-13. However, cells transfected with IL-4R α-chain can bind IL-4, but not IL-13, strongly suggesting that IL-13R complex comprises IL-4R α-chain and another IL-13 binding protein *(71)*.

A specific IL-13 binding protein (IL-13R α-chain) was recently identified by screening murine cDNA libraries for sequences homologous to members of the hemopoietin family *(88)*. Stable expression of murine IL-13R α-chain in CTLL-2 cells resulted in generation of a high-affinity IL-13 binding complex, which was also capable of transducing a proliferative signal in response to IL-13 *(88)*. Importantly, IL-4 and IL-13 were equally effective in competing for binding of ^{125}I-labeled IL-13 to these cells, supporting the conclusion that both the common γ-chain and the IL-13R α-chain can interact with the IL-4R α-chain to generate a high-affinity IL-4R complex. In addition, transfection of CTLL-2 cells with the IL-13R α-chain did not enhance affinity of IL-4 for these cells, suggesting that the common γ-chain and the IL-13R α-chain are equally effective in generating high-affinity IL-4R *(88)*.

Data obtained using cells derived from patients with X-linked severe combined immuno-deficiency (SCID) strongly support the conclusion that IL-4 can use both IL-13R and IL-4R. These patients have mutations in the gene encoding the common γ-chain, a component of receptors for IL-2, IL-4, IL-7, IL-9, and IL-15 *(89–91)*, and their T-cells are unable to respond to these cytokines, causing severe abnormalities in both T- and B-cell functions. However, it was demonstrated that B-cells derived from SCID patients strongly proliferate and produce IgE when costimulated by anti-CD40 MAbs in the presence of IL-4 or IL-13, whereas IL-2 and IL-15 were ineffective *(92)*. In addition, IL-13 was not less potent than IL-4 in inducing IgE synthesis by patients' B-cells *(92)*, suggesting that B-cells of X-linked SCID patients express a normal IL-13R complex that functions as a receptor for both IL-4 and IL-13. This conclusion is supported by recent studies directly suggesting that the common γ-chain is not a component of IL-13R complex *(93)*.

Expression of high-affinity IL-4R has been demonstrated on all cell types studied to date, but the expression of the IL-13R α-chain appears to be more cell-type-specific. Based on functional studies, IL-13R complexes are expressed on B cells, monocytes/macrophages, and endothelial cells *(74,77,94)*. An important difference in the distribution of IL-4R and IL-13R is their differential expression on human T-cells. Activated T-cells, which express high levels of IL-4R complex, do not seem to express a functional IL-13R complex, because IL-13 did not compete with IL-4 for binding to human T-cells *(71)* and, in contrast to IL-4, IL-13 failed to induce proliferation of activated T cells *(71,95)*. This conclusion is supported by recent findings indicating that transfection of CTLL-2 cells with the IL-13R α-chain renders these T cells responsive to IL-13 *(88)*.

IL-4R AND IL-13R SIGNALING PATHWAYS

Essential components of both IL-4 and IL-13 signaling pathways, as of other cytokine signaling pathways, are molecules designated signal transducers and activators of transcription (STAT) *(96)*. STAT molecules are DNA-binding proteins, which require phosphorylation to be functionally active, as originally described for IFN-α and IFN-γ signaling *(97,98)*. The cytoplasmic regions of all cytokine receptors lack motifs indicative of protein tyrosine kinase motifs, commonly present in other growth factor receptors *(96–98)*. Instead, cytokine receptors associate with protein tyrosine kinases, called Janus-family or Jak kinases (just another kinase), which are phosphorylated after ligand binding. Jak-kinases in turn phosphorylate STAT molecules, which then translocate into the nucleus and bind to specific binding sites in the DNA. To date, four Janus-family kinases, Jak1, Jak2, Jak3, and Tyk2, have been characterized. Cytokine receptors appear to associate with distinct sets of STAT and Jak proteins, partially explaining the specificity of each signaling pathway. However, cytokines with different functional activities can activate the same STAT proteins, indicating that additional, yet to be characterized, mechanisms are involved in regulating the specificity of cytokine responses.

Both IL-4 and IL-13 induce phosphorylation of STAT6 (IL-4 STAT) in human PBMC or Epstein-Barr virus (EBV)-transformed B-cell lines *(91,99,100)*. Despite these apparent similarities in the signaling pathways of IL-4 and IL-13, there clearly are also differences. IL-4, but not IL-13, induces phosphorylation of Jak3 *(101)*, which can probably be attributed to the fact that Jak3 associates with the common γ-chain, which does not appear to be a component of IL-13R complex. Jak3 can phosphorylate STAT6, because COS cells transfected with both Jak3 and STAT6 cDNAs express the phosphorylated form of STAT6 *(102)*. However, phosphorylation of Jak3 is not absolutely required for STAT6 activation, because IL-4 failed to induce phosphorylation of Jak3 in human colon carcinoma cells, whereas STAT6 was normally phosphorylated in these cells *(103)*. Induction of STAT6 phosphorylation in response to IL-4 and IL-13 has also been demonstrated in PBMC and EBV-transformed B-cell lines derived from patients with X-linked SCID, who lack a functional common γ-chain *(91,100)*, further supporting the notion that STAT6 phosphorylation in response to IL-4 or IL-13 does not require Jak3 and that IL-4 can act through a receptor lacking the common γ-chain, which is probably the IL-13R complex. IL-4 binding to human colon carcinoma cells induced phosphorylation of Jak2, instead of Jak3, a phenomenon that has not been described in T-cells *(103)*. These data further suggest that IL-4 can act through different kinds of receptors, the expression of which may vary depending on the type of target cell.

It is clear that STAT6 plays an important role in the signaling pathways resulting in IgE switching, because STAT6-deficient mice fail to produce IgE in vivo *(104)*. However, the exact role of STAT6 in this process remains to be determined, but since the germline ε promoter region contains sequences that are homologous to STAT6 binding sites *(105,106)*, it may be possible that STAT6 is necessary for induction of germline ε transcription. However,

IL-3, which does not induce IgE synthesis, also induced STAT6 activation *(99)*, indicating that STAT6 phosphorylation per se is not sufficient for induction of IgE switching.

BOTH IL-4 AND IL-13 INDUCE IgE SWITCHING AND IgE SYNTHESIS BY HUMAN B-CELLS

Early studies have shown that IL-4 induces IgG1 and IgE synthesis by lipopolysaccharide (LPS)-activated mouse B-cells *(107)*. Subsequently, IL-4 also has been shown to play a crucial role in IgE regulation in vivo. Transgenic mice overexpressing IL-4 produce highly elevated levels of IgE, and they also develop inflammatory reactions with histopathological characteristics of allergic responses *(108)*. Furthermore, neutralizing anti-IL-4 MAbs strongly inhibited IgE synthesis after nematode infections, whereas the effects on other Ig isotypes were minimal *(109)*. Initial reports on IL-4-deficient mice suggested that IgE synthesis in mice is completely dependent on IL-4, whereas IgG1 production was impaired, but not absent *(7)*. However, more recent studies have shown that mice with disrupted IL-4 gene produce significant levels of IgE and IgG1 after infection with *Plasmodium chabaudi* or *L. major*, indicating that an IL-4-independent mechanism of IgG1 and IgE switching is operational in mice *(110,111)*. Whether IL-13 accounts for this activity is presently not clear.

IL-4 also induces IgE switching and IgE synthesis by human B cells cultured in the presence of activated CD4$^+$ T-cells *(112–116)*. IgE synthesis was observed when naive sIgD$^+$ B-cells were cultured in the presence of costimulatory signals provided by activated CD4$^+$ T-cells, indicating that IL-4 acts as a switch factor. Under these culture conditions IL-4 also induces IgG4 synthesis by human B cells *(115,117)*. Moreover, IL-4 induces human IgE synthesis in SCID-hu mice transplanted with small fragments of human fetal bones and thymus (SCID-hu BM/T mice) *(118)*. In this model, human B- and T-cells and monocytes develop in the bone/thymus graft, and circulating human B- and T-cells can be detected in the periphery of the mice. These mice produce human IgM, IgG, and IgA, and approximately one-third of these mice also produce human IgE, probably in response to environmental antigens *(118)*. However, all SCID-hu BM/T mice that were human-IgE-negative produced human IgE following administration of recombinant human IL-4 *(118)*, indicating the importance of IL-4 in the regulation of human IgE synthesis in vivo.

Human B cells can also be induced to switch to IgE synthesis by IL-13 *(74)*, a phenomenon that has not been demonstrated for mouse B-cells. IL-13 induced high levels of IgE synthesis when it was added to cultures of human PBMC in the absence of any other stimuli *(74)*. IL-13-induced responses could not be blocked by neutralizing anti-IL-4 MAbs, indicating that IL-13 acted independently of IL-4. However, IL-13 is less potent than IL-4. The levels of IL-13-induced IgE synthesis were generally two to five fold lower than those induced by saturating concentrations of IL-4 *(74)*. IL-13 also induced high levels of IgG4 and IgE synthesis by sorted, highly purified sIgD$^+$ B-cells or immature fetal B-cells cultured in the presence of activated CD4$^+$ T-cells, anti-CD40 MAbs, or CD40L, indicating that IL-13-induced IgE synthesis resulted from IgE switching and not a selective outgrowth of B-cells committed to IgE synthesis *(18,74,75,94)*. IL-13 did not have any additive or synergistic effects with IL-4 when both cytokines were added at optimal concentrations *(74)*, which is in agreement with the notion that there are similarities in the signaling pathways of IL-4 and IL-13.

Serum IgE levels appear to be elevated in children with a family history of atopy already at the time of birth, and elevated cord blood IgE levels are associated with increased risk of atopy early in life *(119,120)*. Both IL-4 and IL-13 were shown to induce Ig synthesis, including IgE production, by immature B-cells derived from human fetal spleen, liver, bone marrow, or thymus (94,121–123). However, similarly to adult B-cells (74), the levels of Ig produced by fetal B-cells in response to IL-13 were significantly lower than those produced in response to IL-4 (94). IL-4- and IL-13-induced IgE synthesis was observed in immature B cells derived from fetuses as early as 16 wk after gestation (94), indicating that IgE switching machinery is operational early during fetal life.

IgE SWITCHING BY IL-4 AND IL-13 IS PRECEDED BY GERMLINE IgE HEAVY CHAIN GENE TRANSCRIPTION

Induction of IgE heavy chain class switching, like that of other isotypes, is preceded by expression of the corresponding germ-line constant heavy chain (CH) gene, which may enhance the accessibility of CH genes and their switch (S) regions to a common recombinase system (124–126). Germline IgE heavy chain (ε) gene comprises, in addition to the Cε exons, a germline exon (Iε) located 3.5 kb upstream from Cε and 5′ from Sε (127,128). The level of germline ε transcription correlates with the level of subsequent IgE synthesis in vitro and in vivo, and cytokines that modulate germline ε transcription also modulate IgE production (129–131). The crucial role of germline transcripts in the recombination events that result in class switching was demonstrated in mice lacking Iγ1 or Iγ2b exons. B-cells of these mice are unable to undergo γ1 or γ2b switching (132,133). However, transcription per se is not sufficient to direct isotype switching, suggesting that germline transcripts may be part of the switch recombinase system providing the specificity to direct switching to different isotypes (134).

Transcription of human germline ε gene is induced by IL-4 in normal human B-cells as well as in EBV-transformed B-cell lines and Burkitt's lymphoma cells (127,128,135–137). Consistent with its capacity to induce IgE synthesis, IL-13 was also shown to induce germline ε transcription in human B cells (74,138,139). However, in the absence of other stimuli, IL-13 is significantly less potent than IL-4. Anti-CD40 MAbs, which are ineffective when tested alone, strongly synergize with both IL-4 and IL-13 in inducing germline ε RNA synthesis in normal human B-cells and immature B-cells (74,138). In addition, combinations of anti-CD40 MAbs and IL-4 and IL-13 induce productive ε transcription and IgE synthesis by these cells.

Both IL-4 and IL-13 also induced germline ε transcription in human immature B cells derived from fetal spleen or bone marrow (BM) (138). Interestingly, IL-4, but not IL-13, induced germline ε RNA synthesis in sμ⁻ pre-B cells (138). Similarly, in contrast to IL-4, IL-13 did not affect the expression of CD23, CD40, or HLA-DR on pre-B-cells, suggesting differential effects of IL-4 and IL-13 on early fetal B cells (94). These distinct effects of IL-4 and IL-13 suggest that functional IL-13R is expressed at a later stage of B-cell ontogeny than IL-4R. Because IL-4 production is enhanced in atopic individuals, the capacity of IL-4 to induce germline ε transcription in human fetal immature B cells and pre-B cells suggests that commitment of B-cell precursors to IgE-producing cells may occur already during intrauterine life, and may explain increased IgE production in neonates with a family history of atopy. The differential effects of IL-4 and IL-13 on pre-B cells also suggest that IL-13, in contrast to IL-4 (123), does not regulate early B-cell maturation.

IL-4 AND IL-13-INDUCED IgE SYNTHESIS IS MODULATED BY CYTOKINES SECRETED BY T-CELLS AND MONOCYTES

Despite the fact that IL-4 and IL-13 are the only cytokines capable of inducing IgE switching, the level of IgE synthesis appears to be tightly regulated by cytokines derived from both T cells and monocytes. Cytokines that have been shown to modulate IL-4- and IL-13-induced IgE synthesis include IL-2, IL-5, IL-6, IL-8, IL-10, IL-12, IFN-α IFN-γ, TGF-β, and TNF-α

(Fig. 1). The molecular mechanisms by which these cytokines modulate the level of IgE synthesis are relatively poorly characterized, but it appears that direct effects on B cells as well as indirect effects through downregulation of helper function of T-cells or accessory cell function of monocytes are involved. IFN-α, IFN-γ, TNF-α, and TGF-β are the only cytokines that have been shown to directly affect the ε switching process by modulating the level of germline ε transcription.

IFN-α and IFN-γ

The roles of IFN-α and IFN-γ in the regulation of IL-4-dependent IgE synthesis have been intensively studied, because these cytokines have potent inhibitory effects both in vitro and in vivo. IFNs strongly block both IL-4 and IL-13-induced IgE synthesis by PBMC and B-cells cultured in the presence of activated CD4[+] T-cells and IL-4 *(94,112,113,140)*. In addition, IFN-α and IFN-γ were demonstrated to inhibit IgE synthesis in atopic patient with elevated serum IgE levels and in patients with hyper-IgE syndrome *(140–143)*. IFN-γ deficient mice also have enhanced Th2 responses, indicating the importance of IFN-γ in directing Th1 responses *(144)*.

Early studies suggested that IFN-α and IFN-γ only inhibit IgE synthesis in T-cell-dependent culture systems, and no inhibitory effects were observed when B-cells were induced to produce IgE in the absence of T cells, e.g., in the presence of anti-CD40 MAbs and IL-4 *(13,14)*. However, recently IFN-α and IFN-γ were shown to inhibit IL-4-induced germline ε transcription in purified normal mature and immature human B cells *(138,139)*. They also inhibited transcription from human germline ε promoter-reporter gene constructs transfected into Burkitt's lymphoma B-cell lines *(139)*. Similarly, IFN-γ suppressed IL-4-induced transcription in murine B-lymphoma cells transiently transfected with a 179-bp IL-4-responsive element identified in the region surrounding the initiation site of murine germline ε transcripts *(145)*. Consistent with these findings, B cells preincubated and cultured in the presence of IFN-γ produced reduced levels of IgE in response to anti-CD40 MAbs and IL-4 *(139)*, and IFN-γ inhibited IgE synthesis by purified B cells stimulated with IL-4 and EBV *(116)*.

IFN-γ has been shown to antagonize the effects of IL-4 also in several other biological assays, suggesting that IFN-induced nuclear transcription factors may block activation or binding of transcription factors induced by IL-4. This hypothesis is supported by the fact that there are similarities in the binding sites of STAT6, the germline ε promoter region, and interferon-responsive elements observed in FcγR promoter *(105,106)*. In addition, IL-4 has been shown to induce phosphorylation of STAT proteins that can bind to the same elements as IFN-induced transcription factors *(105)*. However, to date, there is no direct evidence of IFN-induced nuclear factors that bind to the germline ε promoter region, thereby preventing the effects of IL-4 and IL-13.

Transforming Growth Factor (TGF)-β

TGF-β has growth regulatory activities on essentially all cell types, and it has also been shown to have complex modulatory effects on the cells of the immune system *(146,147)*. TGF-β inhibits proliferation of both B- and T-cells, and it also suppresses development and differentiation of cytotoxic T-cells and NK-cells *(146,147)*. Furthermore, TGF-β inhibits IgM and IgG synthesis by blocking the switch from the membrane forms of μ- and γ-heavy chain mRNA to the secreted forms. However, TGF-β has been shown to direct IgA switching in both murine and human B cells *(148–150)*. It was also shown to induce germline α transcription in murine and human B cells *(149,151)*, supporting the conclusion that TGF-β can specifically induce IgA switching.

TGF-β strongly inhibits IL-4-induced germline ε RNA synthesis and IgE synthesis in vitro *(129,152)*. TGF-β also inhibited IL-4-induced germline ε RNA synthesis in fetal pre-B-cells *(138)*, supporting the conclusion that the general mechanisms regulating germline ε transcription in adult B-cells and pre-B-cells are similar, with the exception that IL-13 cannot induce germline ε RNA synthesis in pre-B-cells. However, it has to be noted that TGF-β does not just have inhibitory effects on pre-B-cells, because it can enhance human pre-B-cell maturation in vitro *(153)*.

TNF-α and TNF-β

TNF-α was originally described as cachectin because of its capacity to cause necrosis of tumors *(154)*. It is a 17-kDa protein produced at low quantities by almost all cells in the human body following activation *(155)*. TNF-α acts as an endogenous pyrogen. It induces the synthesis of several proinflammatory cytokines, stimulates, the production of acute phase proteins and induces proliferation of fibroblasts *(156)*. Because of these effects, TNF-α plays a major role in the pathogenesis of endotoxin shock *(156)*. TNF-β, also known as lymphotoxin, is a 20-kDa protein with 28% homology in its amino acid sequence with TNF-α *(157)*. TNF-α and TNF-β share many of their biological activities, because they bind to the same receptors *(158)*.

TNF-α enhances proliferation of both activated human B-cells *(159)* and T-cells *(160)*. However, TNF-α has been reported to inhibit proliferation and differentiation of EBV-stimulated B-cells *(161)*. Lymphotoxin also enhances proliferation and Ig synthesis by activated human B-cells and, like TNF-α, has been suggested to regulate B-cell function in an autocrine fashion *(162–164)*.

TNF-α is the only cytokine characterized to date that has been shown to enhance IL-4- or IL-13-induced germline ε transcription in purified human B-cells. This effect of TNF-α has been observed in normal adult B-cells, Burkitt's lymphoma cells and immature human B-cells derived from fetal BM *(129,136,138)*. Consistent with these findings, TNF-α also enhanced the levels of IgE produced in response to IL-4 *(129)*. TNF-α is also expressed as a membrane-bound form (mTNF-α), which is involved in B-T-cell interactions. Expression of mTNF-α is rapidly upregulated within 4 h following T-cell activation *(165)*. MAbs specific for mTNF-α or the p55 TNF-α receptor strongly inhibit IgE synthesis induced by activated CD4$^+$ T-cell clones or their membranes *(165)*. In addition, T-cells that were negative for CD40L and infected with HIV were shown to express high levels of mTNF-α *(166)*. These cells were capable of inducing polyclonal Ig-secretion by human B-cells, which could be inhibited by neutralizing anti-TNF-α MAbs, suggesting that mTNF-α plays a role in the polyclonal B-cell activation observed in patients infected with HIV *(166)*.

IL-2 and IL-15

IL-2 acts as a growth factor for activated B- and T-cells and it also modulates the functions of NK-cells. IL-2 is predominantly produced by Th1-like T-cell clones, and, therefore, it is considered mainly to function in delayed-type hypersensitivity reactions. However, IL-2 also has potent, direct effects on proliferation and Ig-synthesis by B-cells *(167–169)*. The complex immunoregulatory properties of IL-2 are reflected in the phenotype of IL-2-deficient mice, which have high mortality at a young age and multiple defects in their immune functions, including spontaneous development of inflammatory bowel disease *(170,171)*. IL-15 is a more recently identified cytokine produced by multiple cell types. IL-15 shares most, if not all, of its activities with IL-2, including its capacity to induce B-cell growth and differentiation *(172)*. However, assuming that IL-15 production in IL-2-deficient mice is normal, it is clear that IL-15 cannot substitute for the function of IL-2 in vivo, because these mice have multiple immunodeficiencies.

Although the effects of IL-2 on B-cells are well characterized, its role in the regulation of IgE synthesis is somewhat controversial, since both enhancing and inhibitory effects have been reported. IL-2 has been shown to synergistically enhance IL-10-induced human Ig production in the presence of anti-CD40 MAbs, but it antagonized the effects of IL-4 *(173)*. However, IL-2 was also reported to enhance IL-4-dependent IgE synthesis by purified B-cells *(174)*. On the other hand, IL-2 was shown to inhibit IL-4 dependent murine IgG1 and IgE synthesis both in vitro and in vivo *(175,176)*. Similarly, IL-2 inhibited IL-4-dependent human IgE synthesis by unfractionated human PBMC, but the effects were less significant than those of IFN-α or IFN-γ *(177,178)*. Although mice with a disrupted IL-2 gene have strongly elevated serum IgG1 levels, no specific defect in IgE regulation has been reported *(170,171)*. Thus, IL-2 is not essential in induction of IgE synthesis. However, because of its multiple effects on the immune response, IL-2 can also modulate IL-4- and IL-13-dependent IgE synthesis, but its exact effects appear to depend on the other stimuli affecting the B-cells.

IL-5

IL-5 is primarily produced by Th2-type T-cells and appears to play an important role in the pathogenesis of allergic disorders because of its ability to induce eosinophilia. IL-5 acts as an eosinophil differentiation and survival factor in both mouse and humans. Blocking IL-5 activity by neutralizing MAbs strongly inhibits pulmonary eosinophilia and hyperactivity in mouse models *(59,179)*, and IL-5-deficient mice do not develop eosinophilia *(60,61)*. These data also suggest that IL-5 antagonists may have therapeutic potential in the treatment of allergic eosinophilia.

The studies on the effects of IL-5 on B-cell function have resulted in somewhat contradictory results. IL-5 has been shown to enhance both proliferation and Ig synthesis of activated mouse B-cells *(168,180–182)*. In addition, early studies demonstrated that recombinant IL-5 also induces proliferation of activated human B-cells in vitro *(183)*. However, other studies suggested that IL-5 has no effect on proliferation of human B-cells, whereas it activated eosinphils *(184)*. IL-5 apparently is not crucial for maturation or differentiation of conventional B-cells, because Ab responses in IL-5-deficient mice are normal *(61)*. However, these mice have a developmental defect in their CD5+ B-cells indicating that IL-5 is required for normal differentiation of this B-cell subset in mice *(61)*. At suboptimal concentrations of IL-4, IL-5 was shown to enhance IgE synthesis by human B-cells in vitro *(185)*. Furthermore, a recent study suggested that the effects of IL-5 on human B-cells depend on the mode of B-cell stimulation. IL-5 significantly enhanced IgM synthesis by B-cells stimulated with *Moraxella catarrhalis (185)*. In addition, IL-5 synergized with suboptimal concentrations of IL-2, but had no effect on Ig synthesis by Staphylococcus Aureas Cowan I (SAC)-activated B-cells. Activated human B-cells also expressed IL-5 mRNA, suggesting that IL-5 may also regulate B-cell function, including IgE synthesis, by autocrine mechanisms *(186)*.

IL-6

IL-6 is a monocyte-derived cytokine that was originally described as a B-cell differentiation factor or B-cell stimulatory factor-2 because of its ability to enhance Ig levels secreted by activated B-cells *(187)*. IL-6 has also been shown to enhance IL-4-induced IgE synthesis *(174,188)*. It has also been suggested that IL-6 is an obligatory factor for human IgE synthesis, because neutralizing anti-IL-6 MAbs completely blocked IL-4-induced IgE synthesis *(189)*. However, IL-6 by itself cannot induce germline ε transcription or IgE switching by naive B-cells. Thus, it appears that IL-6 can only enhance the level of IgE produced per plasma cell, whereas the frequency of IgE-secreting cells probably does not change in response to IL-6. In addition, although IL-6 strongly enhances IgE synthesis in vitro, it does not seem to be required for IgE synthesis in vivo, because no defect in IgE synthesis has been reported in IL-6-deficient mice, although these mice have impaired capacity to produce IgA *(190)*.

IL-8

IL-8 was originally identified as a monocyte-derived neutrophil chemotactic and activating factor *(191)*. Subsequently, IL-8 was also shown to be chemotactic for T-cells and to activate basophils, resulting in enhanced histamine and leukotriene release from these cells *(192,193)*. Furthermore, IL-8 inhibits adhesion of neutrophils to cytokine-activated endothelial-cell monolayers, and it protects these cells from neutrophil-mediated damage *(194,195)*. Therefore, endothelial cell-derived IL-8 was suggested to attenuate inflammatory events occurring in the proximity of blood vessel walls *(194,195)*.

IL-8 also modulates Ig production. It inhibits IL-4-induced IgG4 and IgE synthesis by both unfractionated human PBMC and purified B-cells in vitro *(196)*. This inhibitory effect was independent of IFN-α, IFN-γ, or prostaglandin E2 *(196)*. In addition, IL-8 inhibited spontaneous IgE synthesis by PBMC derived from atopic patients *(197)*. In contrast to healthy individuals, atopic patients have detectable circulating levels of IL-8, which correlate with the severity of the disease *(198)*. The molecular mechanism by which IL-8 inhibits IgE synthesis is not known.

IL-10

IL-10 is an anti-inflammatory cytokine predominantly produced by activated monocytes. However, activated T-cells and B-cells are also capable of producing significant levels of IL-10 *(199)*. IL-10 strongly inhibits synthesis of pro-inflammatory cytokines and upregulates production of the IL-1 receptor antagonist by monocytes *(200,201)*. IL-10 prevents Ag-specific activation and proliferation of T-cells and Th0-, Th1-, and Th2-like T-cell clones by reducing the Ag-presenting capacity of monocytes, which is associated with a strong down-regulation of CD80, CD86, and class II MHC molecules on these cells *(202–206)*. Interestingly, IL-10 has a strong homology with an open reading frame in the EBV genome, BCRF1 *(207,208)*. IL-10 and the protein product of BCRF1, now designated viral(v)-IL-10, have been found to share several, but not all, of their activities.

IL-10 and v-IL-10 inhibit, in a dose-dependent fashion, spontaneous IgM, IgG, and IgA synthesis and IL-4-induced IgG4 and IgE synthesis by PBMC from healthy *(188)* or atopic individuals *(209)*. In addition, it has been shown that anti-IL-10 MAbs strongly enhance IL-4-induced IgE synthesis by PBMC, indicating that endogenous IL-10 production suppresses IgE synthesis in these cultures *(188,210)*. In contrast to its effect on unfractionated PBMC, IL-10 has strong growth- and differentiation-promoting effects on purified B-cells, and it also enhances IgE synthesis by purified B-cells cultured in the presence of anti-CD40 MAbs and IL-4 *(211,212)*.

IL-4-induced IgE synthesis in cultures of PBMC was completely monocyte-dependent. Monocyte-depleted PBMC failed to produce IgE in response to IL-4 alone, but IgE synthesis was restored after addition of autologous monocytes. However, monocytes preincubated with IL-10 or v-IL-10 failed to provide the costimulatory signals required for induction of IgE production by IL-4, indicating that the inhibitory effects of IL-10 and v-IL-10 were indirectly mediated via monocytes *(188)*. Although it is clear that IL-10 inhibited IgE synthesis indirectly, the exact mechanism of this IL-10-mediated inhibitory effect remains to be determined. We showed that the inhibitory effect of IL-10 could not be restored by exogenous IL-6 or TNF-α, suggesting that inhibition of the production of these cytokines was not the underlying mechanism *(188)*. The importance of monocytes in the regulation of IgE synthesis was also demonstrated by the observation that anti-CD14 MAbs completely blocked IL-4-induced IgE production by PBMC. However, this effect was not mediated via induced IL-10 production, because anti-CD14 MAbs also had strong inhibitory effects in the presence of neutralizing anti-IL10 MAbs, which enhanced IL-4-induced IgE production approx 10-fold *(210)*. Whether IL-10 and anti-CD14 MAbs downregulate the same accessory cell function of monocytes is presently not clear.

IL-10 also inhibited germline ε transcription in unfractionated PBMC. IL-10 strongly reduced IL-4-induced expression of both the 1.7-kb germline ε and 2.2-kb productive ε transcripts in these cultures *(188)*. The effects of IL-10 were again indirect, since IL-10 and v-IL-10 failed to modulate IL-4-induced germline ε transcription in purified B-cells. These results confirm the functional relationship between germline ε and productive ε mRNA expression and IgE synthesis *(128,129)* and indicate that IL-10 inhibits IgE production through indirect inhibition of germline ε transcription.

IL-12

IL-12 is a unique cytokine in that it is a heterodimeric glycoprotein composed of disulfide-bonded 35- and 40-kDa subunits *(213)*. It was first isolated from human B-lymphoblastoid cells and has thereafter been shown to have pleiotropic effects on immune functions. IL-12 stimulates proliferation of activated B-, T-, and natural kellin (NK) cells, enhances lytic activity of NK cells, and synergized with IL-2 in induction of lymphokine-activated killer cells *(213)*. Importantly, IL-12 can direct differentiation of naive T-cells into-Th1 cells, secreting high levels of IFN-γ. IL-12 also induces transient production of IFN-γ and inhibits the production of IL-4 by already committed Th2-type allergen-specific human $CD4^+$ T-lymphocytes *(80–82)*.

IL-12 inhibits IL-4-induced IgE synthesis by human PBMC *(214)*. IL-12 also inhibited IL-4- and IL-13-induced IgE production by $sµ^+$, $CD10^+$, and $CD19^+$ immature fetal B-cells cultured in the presence of activated $CD4^+$ T-cells *(94)*. These effects of IL-12 appear to be indirectly mediated via induction of IFN-γ production by T-cells, because no inhibitory effects were observed in T-cell independent culture systems, e.g., in the presence of anti-CD40 MAbs. In fact, IL-12 has stimulatory effects on purified B-cells, and it enhances B-cell proliferation and differentiation of activated B-cells in vitro. Furthermore, IL-12 did not affect germline ε transcription by purified human B-cells.

IL-12 also inhibits IgE synthesis in mice in vivo. The primary IgE responses to *N. brasiliensis* were effectively inhibited by administration of IL-12 as a result of general reduction in the Th2 response *(215)*. IL-12 also inhibited IgE synthesis induced by protein antigens *(216)*. The effects of IL-12 in vivo were partially or completely inhibited by neutralizing anti-IFN-γ MAbs, indicating that the inhibitory effects of IL-12 were indirectly mediated by IFN-γ *(215,216)*.

AN IL-4 MUTANT PROTEIN ACTS AS AN IL-4R AND IL-13R ANTAGONIST IN VITRO AND IN VIVO

An antagonistic IL-4 mutant protein was generated by replacing the tyrosine residue at position 124 by an aspartic acid by means of in vitro mutagenesis. This mutant protein, hIL-4.Y124D, binds with high affinity to the IL-4R α-chain without significant receptor activation *(71,217)*. Because IL-4R α-chain is shared by IL-4R and IL-13R and is required for signal transduction, hIL-4.Y124D blocks the biological activities of both IL-4 and IL-13.

hIL-4.Y124D inhibited in a dose-dependent manner IgG4 and IgE synthesis induced by optimal concentrations of IL-4 or IL-13 in vitro *(75)*. More than 90% inhibition of IgG4 and IgE synthesis was observed when hIL-4.Y124D was added at 20–50-fold excess as compared to IL-4 or IL-13. Moreover, hIL-4.Y124D effectively inhibited IL-4- and IL-13-induced B-cell proliferation and germline ε transcription *(214)*. hIL-4.Y124D had no IL-4-like agonistic activity when proliferation of purified activated B- or T-cells were studied, but it induced low levels of IgG4 and IgE synthesis at high concentrations (500 ng/mL) in cultures of unfractionated PBMC. However, a double IL-4 mutant protein, in which the arginine residue at position 121, in addition to the tyrosine at position 124, was replaced by aspartic acid (hIL-4.R121D,Y124D) did not have any detectable agonistic IL-4-like activity *(218)*.

hIL-4.Y124D also functions as an IL-4R/IL-13R antagonist in vivo. Administration of hIL-4.Y124D at 200 μg/d/mouse for 3–4 wk into SCID-hu BM/T mice, which spontaneously produced human IgE in vivo, resulted in a strong reduction in human IgE levels in the mouse sera *(118,219)*. This inhibitory effect of hIL-4.Y124D was specific for IgE, because no changes in serum IgG levels were observed. Importantly, no agonistic IL-4-like activity by hIL-4.Y124D, as judged by induction of CD23 expression on B-cells, was observed in vivo. hIL-4.Y124D strongly reduced serum IgE levels in SCID-hu BM/T mice, even when coadministered with IL-4 *(118,219)*, indicating that hIL-4.Y124D acts as an effective IL-4R/IL-13R antagonist when IL-4 is present at high concentrations, as is the case in atopic patients. Although more information about the function of hIL-4.Y124D in vivo is required, these data suggest that hIL-4.Y124D may be of therapeutic potential in the treatment of atopic patients with enhanced IgE synthesis. In contrast to anti-IL-4 MAbs or soluble IL-4R α-chain, which have been shown to inhibit IgE synthesis in animal models *(109,220)*, hIL-4.Y124D blocks the functions of both IL-4 and IL-13. Therefore, hIL-4.Y124D may be superior to these IL-4 antagonists as an approach to blocking human IgE synthesis in vivo.

Recently, a naturally occurring IL-4 antagonist that is generated through alternative splicing of IL-4 mRNA was recently described *(221)*. This variant of IL-4, called IL-4δ2, lacks one of the four exons of IL-4 and blocks the biological activity of IL-4. IL-4 and IL-4δ2 were differentially expressed in PBMC and bronchoalveolar lavage cells, suggesting that the balance between IL-4 and IL-4δ2 may play a role in the regulation of IgE synthesis in vivo *(221)*.

CONCLUDING REMARKS

IgE synthesis is tightly regulated by multiple cell surface and membrane-bound molecules expressed by B- and T-cells during immune responses. IL-4 and IL-13 are the only cytokines that have been shown to direct IgE switching in human B-cells. However, several cytokines, such as IL-2, IL-5, IL-6, IL-10, IL-12, IFN-α, IFN-γ, TNF-α, and TGF-β, modulate IL-4- and IL-13-dependent IgE synthesis, and, importantly, IFN-α, IFN-γ, and IL-12 have also been shown to inhibit IgE production in vivo, suggesting that these cytokines may have therapeutic potential in the treatment of IgE-mediated allergies. Because IL-10 inhibits proliferation of allergen-specific T-cells, production of proinflammatory cytokines by monocytes, and IgE synthesis by PBMC, IL-10 may also have potential utility in the treatment of allergic diseases.

Allergen-specific Th2-cells, which produce high levels of IL-4, IL-5, and IL-13, play a key role in the pathogenesis of allergic diseases. The mutant IL-4 protein hIL-4.Y124D and a naturally occurring splice variant of IL-4 were shown to act as IL-4 antagonists, suggesting that these proteins may be useful in antagonizing the differentiation and functions of allergen-specific Th2-cells. Indeed, hIL-4.Y124D blocked both IL-4- and IL-13-induced IgE synthesis in vitro and in vivo. The IgE molecule itself has also been targeted in order to block IgE-mediated allergic responses in vivo. Anti-IgE MAbs strongly reduced serum IgE levels in mice, and they also significantly reduced IL-4 synthesis, suggesting that IgE may indirectly regulate Th2 differentiation in vivo *(222,223)*. A humanized version of this MAb is currently in clinical trials for the treatment of allergic diseases *(224,225)*.

Although it appears that the factors regulating B-cell differentiation and IgE switching are well characterized, undoubtedly there are more molecules involved in IgE regulation to be discovered. As an example, a novel activation molecule designated signaling lymphocytic activation molecule (SLAM) was recently cloned and sequenced *(226)*. Engagement of SLAM was shown to induce high levels of IFN-γ production even in allergen-specific Th2-cells *(226)*, suggesting that SLAM may also have an important role in regulating IgE responses. Moreover, understanding of the signaling mechanisms of IL-4 and IL-13 will enable targeting the intracellular events in order to block Th2 responses and IgE production.

Despite the success of specific immunotherapy of allergic diseases in a proportion of the patients, we still lack efficient means to treat IgE-mediated allergies and reduce production of allergen-specific IgE molecules in vivo. However, the progress in our understanding of the basic mechanisms involved in IgE regulation suggests that we may soon be able to find an efficient way to block the cascade of events that results in IgE synthesis in allergic individuals.

ACKNOWLEDGMENTS

We thank Gregorio Aversa, José M. Carballido, and Benjamin G. Cocks for their contributions and JoAnn Katheiser for excellent administrative assistance.

The DNAX Research Institute of Molecular and Cellular Biology is supported by the Schering-Plough Corporation.

REFERENCES

1. Coffman RL, Lebman DA, Rothman P (1993) Mechanism and regulation of immunoglobulin isotype switching. Adv Immunol 54:229–270.
2. Germain RN (1994) MHC-dependent antigen processing and peptide presentation: providing ligands for T lymphocyte activation. Cell 76:287–299.
3. June CH, Bluestone JA, Nadler LM, Thompson CB (1994) The B7 and CD28 receptor families. Immunol Today 15:321–331.
4. Esser C, Radbruch A (1990) Immunoglobulin class switching: molecular and cellular analysis. Annu Rev Immunol 8:717–735.
5. Kataoka T, Miyata T, Honjo T (1981) Repetitive sequences in class-switch recombination regions of immunoglobulin heavy chain genes. Cell 23:357–368.
6. Yancopoulos G, DePinho R, Zimmerman R, Luzker S, Rosenberg N, Alt FW (1986) Secondary rearrangement events in pre-B cells: VhDJh replacement by a LINE-1 sequence and directed class-switching. EMBO J 5:3259–3266.
7. Kuhn R, Rajewsky K, Muller W (1991) Generation and analysis of interleukin-4 deficient mice. Science 254:707–710.
8. Itoh N, Yonehara S, Ishii A, Yonehara M, Mizushima S, Sameshima M, Hase A, Seto Y, Nagata S (1991) The polypeptide encoded by the cDNA for human cell surface antigen Fas can mediate apoptosis. Cell 66:233–243.
9. Clark EA, Ledbetter JA (1994) How B and T-cells talk to each other. Nature 367:425–428.
10. Aversa G, Punnonen J, Carballido JM, Cocks BG, De Vries JE (1994) CD40 ligand-CD40 interaction in Ig isotype switching in mature and immature human B-cells. Semin Immunol 6:295–301.
11. Clark EA, Ledbetter JA (1986) Activation of human B-cells mediated through two distinct cell surface differentiation antigens, Bp35 and Bp50. Proc Natl Acad Sci USA 83:4494–4498.
12. Jabara HH, Fu SM, Geha RS, Vercelli D (1990) CD40 and IgE: synergism between anti-CD40 monoclonal antibody and interleukin 4 in the induction of IgE synthesis by highly purified human B-cells. J Exp Med 172:1861–1864.
13. Gascan H, Gauchat JF, Aversa G, Van Vlasselaer P, de Vries JE (1991) Anti-CD40 monoclonal antibodies or CD4⁺ T-cell clones and IL-4 induce IgG4 and IgE switching in purified human B-cells via different signaling pathways. J Immunol 147:8–13.

14. Zhang K, Clark EA, Saxon A (1991) CD40 stimulation provides an IFN-gamma-independent and IL-4-dependent differentiation signal directly to human B-cells for IgE production. J Immunol 146:1836–1842.

15. Banchereau J, de Paoli P, Valle A, Garcia E, Rousset F (1991) Long-term human B-cell lines dependent on interleukin-4 and antibody to CD40. Science 251:70–72.

16. Armitage RJ, Fanslow WC, Strockbine L, Sato TA, Clifford KN, Macduff BM, Anderson DM, Gimpel SD, Davis-Smith T, Maliszewski CR, Clark EA, Smith CA, Grabstein KH, Cosman D, Spriggs MK (1992) Molecular and biological characterization of a murine ligand for CD40. Nature 357:80–82.

17. Hollenbaugh D, Grosmaire LS, Kullas CD, Chalupny NJ, Braesch-Andersen S, Noelle RJ, Stamenkovic I, Ledbetter JA, Aruffo A (1992) The human T-cell antigen gp39, a member of the TNF gene family, is a ligand for the CD40 receptor: expression of a soluble form of gp39 with B-cell co-stimulatory activity. EMBO J 11:4313–4321.

18. Cocks BG, de Waal Malefyt R, Galizzi JP, De Vries JE, Aversa G (1993) IL-13 induces proliferation and differentiation of human B-cells activated by the CD40 ligand. Int Immunol 5:657–663.

19. Spriggs MK, Armitage RJ, Strockbine L, Clifford KN, Macduff BM, Sato TA, Maliszewski CR, Fanslow WC (1992) Recombinant human CD40 ligand stimulates B-cell proliferation and immunoglobulin E secretion. J Exp Med 176:1543–1550.

20. Durandy A, Schiff C, Bonnefoy JY, Forveille M, Rousset F, Mazzei G, Milili M, Fischer A (1993) Induction by anti-CD40 antibody or soluble CD40 ligand and cytokines of IgG, IgA and IgE production by B-cells from patients with X-linked hyper IgM syndrome. Eur J Immunol 23: 2294–2299.

21. Lane P, Brocker T, Hubele S, Padovan E, Lanzavecchia A, McConnell F (1993) Soluble CD40 ligand can replace the normal T-cell-derived CD40 ligand signal to B-cells in T-cell-dependent activation. J Exp Med 177:1209–1213.

22. Fuleihan R, Ramesh N, Loh R, Jabara H, Rosen RS, Chatila T, Fu SM, Stamenkovic I, Geha RS (1993) Defective expression of the CD40 ligand in X chromosome-linked immunoglobulin deficiency with normal or elevated IgM. Proc Natl Acad Sci USA 90:2170–2173.

23. Di Santo JP, Bonnefoy JY, Gauchat JF, Fischer A, De Saint Basile G (1993) CD40 ligand mutations in x-linked immunodeficiency with hyper-IgM. Nature 361:541–543.

24. Allen RC, Armitage RJ, Conley ME, Rosenblatt H, Jenkins NA, Copeland NG, Bedell MA, Edelhoff S, Disteche CM, Simoneaux DK, Fanslow BC, Belmont J, Spriggs MK (1993) CD40 ligand gene defects responsible for X-linked hyper-IgM syndrome. Science 259:990–993.

25. Aruffo A, Farrington M, Hollenbaugh D, Li X, Milatovich A, Nonoyama S, Bajorath J, Grosmaire LS, Stenkamp R, Neubauer M (1993) The CD40 ligand, gp39, is defective in activated T-cells from patients with X-linked hyper-IgM syndrome. Cell 72:291–300.

26. Farrington M, Grosmaire LS, Nonoyama S, Fischer SH, Hollenbaugh D, Ledbetter JA, Noelle RJ, Aruffo A, Ochs HD (1994) CD40 ligand expression is defective in a subset of patients with common variable immunodeficiency. Proc Natl Acad Sci USA 91:1099–1103.

27. Gauchat JF, Henchoz S, Mazzei G, Aubry JP, Brunner T, Blasey H, Life P, Talabot D, Flores-Romo L, Thompson J, Kishi K, Butterfield J, Dahinden C, Boonefoy J-Y (1993) Induction of human IgE synthesis in B-cells by mast cells and basophils. Nature 365:340–343.

28. Burd PR, Thompson WC, Max EE, and Mills FC (1995) Activated mast cells produce interleukin 13. J Exp Med 181:1373–1380.

29. Brown MA, Pierce JH, Watson CJ, Falco J, Ihle JN, Paul WE (1987) B-cell stimulatory factor-1/ interleukin-4 mRNA is expressed by normal and transformed mast cells. Cell 50:809–818.

30. Schmitz J, Thiel A, Kuhn R, Rajewsky K, Muller W, Assenmacher M, Radbruch A (1994) Induction of interleukin 4 (IL-4) expression in T helper (Th) cells is not dependent on IL-4 from non-Th cells. J Exp Med 179:1349–1353.

31. Cayabyab M, Phillips JH, Lanier LL (1994) CD40 preferentially costimulates activation of CD4+ T-lymphocytes. J Immunol 152:1523–1531.

32. Grewai IS, Xu J, Flavell RA (1995) Impairment of antigen-specific T-cell priming in mice lacking CD40 ligand. Nature 378:617–620.

33. van Essen D, Kikutani H, Gray D (1995) CD40 ligand-transduced co-stimulation of T-cells in the development of helper function. Nature 378:620–623.

34. Life P, Gauchat JF, Schnuriger V, Estoppey S, Mazzei G, Durandy A, Fischer A, Bonnefoy JY (1994) T-cell clones from an X-linked hyperimmunoglobulin (IgM) patient induce IgE synthesis in vitro despite expression of nonfunctional CD40 ligand. J Exp Med 180:1775–1784.

35. Rickert RC, Rajewsky K, Roes J (1995) Impairment of T-cell-dependent B-cell responses and B-1 cell development in CD19-deficient mice. Nature 376:352–355.
36. Stamenkovic I, Sgroi D, Aruffo A, Sy MS, Anderson T (1991) The B-lymphocyte adhesion molecule CD22 interacts with leukocyte common antigen CD45RO on T-cells and alpha 2-6 sialyltransferase, CD75, on B-cells. Cell 66:1133–1144.
37. Kapsenberg ML, Jansen HM, Bos JD, Wierenga EA (1992) Role of type 1 and type 2 T helper cells in allergic diseases. Curr Opin Immunol 4:788–793.
38. Romagnani S (1991) Human TH1 and TH2 subsets: doubt no more. Immunol Today 12:256–257.
39. Mosmann TR and Coffman RL (1989) Heterogeneity of cytokine secretion patterns and functions of helper T-cells. Adv Immunol 46:111–147.
40. De Vries JE, Carballido JM, Sornasse T, Yssel H (1995) Antagonizing the differentiation and functions of human T helper type 2 cells. Curr Opin Immunol 7:771–778.
41. Vollenweider S, Saurat JH, Rocken M, Hauser C (1991) Evidence suggesting involvement of interleukin-4 (IL-4) production in spontaneous in vitro IgE synthesis in patients with atopic dermatitis. J Allergy Clin Immunol 87:1088–1095.
42. Saryan JA, Leung DY, Geha RS (1983) Induction of human IgE synthesis by a factor derived from T-cells of patients with hyper-IgE states. J Immunol 130:242–247.
43. Del Prete G, Maggi E, Parronchi P, Chretien I, Tiri A, Macchia D, Ricci M, Banchereau J, de Vries J, Romagnani S (1988) IL-4 is an essential factor for the IgE synthesis induced in vitro by human T-cell clones and their supernatants. J Immunol 140:4193–4198.
44. Rousset F, Robert J, Andary M, Bonnin JP, Souillet G, Chretien I, Briere F, Pene J, De Vries JE (1991) Shifts in interleukin-4 and interferon-gamma production by T-cells of patients with elevated serum IgE levels and the modulatory effects of these lymphokines on spontaneous IgE synthesis. J Allergy Clin Immunol 87:58–69.
45. Robinson DS, Hamid Q, Ying S, Tsicopoulos A, Barkans J, Bentley AM, Corrigan C, Durham SR, Kay AB (1992) Predominant TH2-like bronchoalveolar T-lymphocyte population in atopic asthma. N Engl J Med 326:298–304.
46. Huang S-K, Xiao H-Q, Kleine-Tebbe J, Paciotti G, Marsh DG, Lichtenstein LM, Liu MC (1995) IL-13 expression at the sites of allergen challenge in patients with asthma. J Immunol 155: 2688–2694.
47. Wierenga EA, Snoek M, de Groot C, Chretien I, Bos JD, Jansen HM, Kapsenberg ML (1990) Evidence for compartmentalization of functional subsets of CD2+ T-lymphocytes in atopic patients. J Immunol 144:4651–4656.
48. Parronchi P, Macchia D, Piccinni MP, Biswas P, Simonelli C, Maggi E, Ricci M, Ansari AA, Romagnani S (1991) Allergen- and bacterial antigen-specific T-cell clones established from atopic donors show a different profile of cytokine production. Proc Natl Acad Sci USA 88:4538–4542.
49. Yssel H, Johnson KE, Schneider PV, Wideman J, Terr A, Kastelein R, De Vries JE (1992) T-cell activation-inducing epitopes of the house dust mite allergen Der p I. Proliferation and lymphokine production patterns by Der p I-specific CD4+ T-cell clones. J Immunol 148:738–745.
50. van der Ploeg I, Scheynius A, Tengvall Linder M, Hagermark O, Wahlgren CF (1995) Elevated gene expression for interleukin-13 in the skin of atopic dermatitis patients (abstract). In: The 9th International Congress of Immunology, San Francisco, July 23–29.
51. Kay AB, Ying S, Varney V, Gaga M, Durham SR, Moqbel R, Wardlaw AJ, Hamid Q (1991) Messenger RNA expression of the cytokine gene cluster, interleukin 3 (IL-3), IL-4, IL-5, and granulocyte/macrophage colony-stimulating factor, in allergen-induced late-phase cutaneous reactions in atopic subjects. J Exp Med 173:775–778.
52. Marsh DG, Neely JD, Breazeale DR, Ghosh B, Freidhoff LR, Ehrlich-Kautzky E, Schou C, Krishnaswamy G, Beaty TH (1994) Linkage analysis of IL4 and other chromosome 5q31.1 markers and total serum immunoglobulin E concentrations. Science 264:1152–1156.
53. Howard MC, Miyajima A, Coffman R (1993) T-cell derived cytokines and their receptors. In: Paul WE, ed. Fundamental Immunology. Raven, New York, pp. 763–800.
54. Tepper RI, Pattengale PK, Leder P (1989) Murine interleukin-4 displays potent anti-tumor activity in vivo. Cell 57:503–512.
55. Chatelain R, Varkila K, Coffman RL (1992) IL-4 induces a Th2 response in Leishmania major-infected mice. J Immunol 148:1182–1187.
56. Sornasse T, Larenas PV, Davis KA, deVries JE, Yssel H (1996) Differentiation and stability of T helper 1 and 2 cells derived from naive human neonatal CD4+ T cells analyzed at single cell level. J Exp Med 184:473–483.

57. Kopf M, Le Gros G, Bachmann M, Lamers MC, Bluethmann H, Kohler G (1993) Disruption of the murine IL-4 gene blocks Th2 cytokine responses. Nature 362:245–248.

58. Kopf M, Le Gros G, Coyle AJ, Kosco-Vilbois M, Brombacher F (1995) Immune responses of IL-4, IL-5, IL-6 deficient mice. Immunol Rev 148:45–69.

59. Coffman RL, Seymour BW, Hudak S, Jackson J, Rennick D (1989) Antibody to interleukin-5 inhibits helminth-induced eosinophilia in mice. Science 245:308–310.

60. Foster PS, Hogan SP, Ramsay AJ, Matthaei KI, Young IG (1996) Interleukin 5 deficiency abolishes eosinophilia, airways hyperreactivity, and lung damage in a mouse asthma model. J Exp Med 183:195–201.

61. Kopf M, Brombacher F, Hodgkin PD, Ramsay AJ, Milbourne EA, Dai WJ, Ovington KS, Behm CA, Kohler G, Young IG, Matthaei KI (1996) IL-5-deficient mice have a developmental defect in CD5[+] B-1 cells and lack eosinophilia but have normal antibody and cytotoxic T-cell responses. Immunity 4:15–24.

62. Ehlers S, Smith KA (1991) Differentiation of T-cell lymphokine gene expression: the in vitro acquisition of T-cell memory. J Exp Med 173:25–36.

63. Brinkmann V, Kristofic C (1995) TCR-stimulated naive human CD4[+] 45RO[−] T-cells develop into effector cells that secrete IL-13, IL-5, and IFN-gamma, but no IL-4, and help efficient IgE production by B-cells. J Immunol 154:3078–3087.

64. Jung T, Wijdenes J, Neumann C, de Vries JE, Yssel H (1996) Interleukin-13 is produced by activated human CD45RA[+] and CD45RO[+] T-cells: modulation by interleukin-4 and interleukin-12. Eur J Immunol 26:571–577.

65. Yoshimoto T, Bendelac A, Hu-Li J, Paul WE (1995) Defective IgE production by SJL mice is linked to the absence of CD4[+], NK1.1[+] T-cells that promptly produce interleukin 4. Proc Natl Acad Sci USA 92:11,931–11,934.

66. Yoshimoto T, Bendelac A, Watson C, Hu-Li J, Paul WE (1995) Role of NK1.1[+] T-cells in a Th2 response and in immunoglobulin E production. Science 270:1845–1847.

67. Yang LP, Byun DG, Demeure CE, Vezzio N, Delespesse G (1995) Default development of cloned human naive CD4 T-cells into interleukin-4- and interleukin-5-producing effector cells. Eur J Immunol 25:3517–3520.

68. McKenzie AN, Culpepper JA, de Waal Malefyt R, Briere F, Punnonen J, Aversa G, Sato A, Dang W, Cocks BG, Menon S, de Vries JE, Banchereau J, Zurawski G (1993) Interleukin 13, a T-cell-derived cytokine that regulates human monocyte and B-cell function. Proc Natl Acad Sci USA 90:3735–3739.

69. Minty A, Chalon P, Derocq JM, Dumont X, Guillemot JC, Kaghad M, Labit C, Leplatois P, Liauzun P, Miloux B, Minty C, Casellas P, Loison G, Lupker J, Shire D, Ferrara P, Caput D (1993) Interleukin-13 is a new human lymphokine regulating inflammatory and immune responses. Nature 362:248–250.

70. Lakkis FG, Cruet EN (1993) Cloning of rat interleukin-13 (IL-13) cDNA and analysis of IL-13 gene expression in experimental glomerulonephritis. Biochem Biophys Res Commun 197:612–618.

71. Zurawski SM, Vega F Jr, Huyghe B, Zurawski G (1993) Receptors for interleukin-13 and interleukin-4 are complex and share a novel component that functions in signal transduction. EMBO J 12:2663–2670.

72. McKenzie AN, Li X, Largaespada DA, Sato A, Kaneda A, Zurawski SM, Doyle EL, Milatovich A, Francke U, Copeland NG, Jenkins NA, Zurawski G (1993) Structural comparison and chromosomal localization of the human and mouse IL-13 genes. J Immunol 150:5436–5444.

73. Smirnov DV, Smirnova MG, Korobko VG, Frolova EI (1995) Tandem arrangement of human genes for interleukin-4 and interleukin-13: resemblance in their organization. Gene 155:277–281.

74. Punnonen J, Aversa G, Cocks BG, McKenzie ANJ, Menon S, Zurawski G, de Waal Malefyt R, de Vries JE (1993) Interleukin 13 induces Interleukin 4-independent IgG4 and IgE synthesis and CD23 expression by human B-cells. Proc Natl Acad Sci USA 90:3730–3734.

75. Aversa G, Punnonen J, Cocks BG, de Waal Malefyt R, Vega FJ, Zurawski SM, Zurawski G, de Vries JE (1993) An interleukin 4 (IL-4) mutant protein inhibits both IL-4 or IL-13-induced human immunoglobulin G4 (IgG4) and IgE synthesis and B-cell proliferation: support for a common component shared by IL-4 and IL-13 receptors. J Exp Med 178:2213–2218.

76. Chaouchi N, Wallon C, Goujard C, Tertian G, Rudent A, Caput D, Ferrara P, Minty A, Vazquez A, Delfraissy J-F (1996) Interleukin-13 inhibits interleukin-2-induced proliferation and protects chronic lymphocytic leukemia B-cells from in vitro apoptosis. Blood 87:1022–1029.

77. Sironi M, Sciacca FL, Matteucci C, Conni M, Vecchi A, Bernasconi S, Minty A, Caput D, Ferrara P, Colotta F, Mantovani A (1994) Regulation of endothelial and mesothelial cell function by interleukin-13: selective induction of vascular cell adhesion molecule-1 and amplification of interleukin-6 production. Blood 84:1913–1921.

78. de Waal Malefyt R, Figdor CG, Huijbens R, Mohan-Peterson S, Bennett B, Culpepper J, Dang W, Zurawski G, de Vries JE (1993) Effects of IL-13 on phenotype, cytokine production, and cytotoxic function of human monocytes. Comparison with IL-4 and modulation by IFN-gamma or IL-10. J Immunol 151:6370–6381.

79. Cash E, Minty A, Ferrara P, Caput D, Fradelizi D, Rott O (1994) Macrophage-inactivating IL-13 suppresses experimental autoimmune encephalomyelitis in rats. J Immunol 153:4258–4267.

80. Marshall JD, Secrist H, De Kruyff RH, Wolf SF, Umetsu DT (1995) IL-12 inhibits the production of IL-4 and IL-10 in allergen-specific human CD4+ T lymphocytes. J Immunol 155:111–117.

81. Manetti R, Gerosa F, Giudizi MG, Biagiotti R, Parronchi P, Piccinni MP, Sampognaro S, Maggi E, Romagnani S, Trinchieri G (1994) Interleukin 12 induces stable priming for interferon gamma (IFN-gamma) production during differentiation of human T helper (Th) cells and transient IFN-gamma production in established Th2 cell clones. J Exp Med 179:1273–1283.

82. Yssel H, Fasler S, de Vries JE, de Waal Malefyt R (1994) IL-12 transiently induces IFN-gamma transcription and protein synthesis in human CD4+ allergen-specific Th2 T-cell clones. Int Immunol 6:1091–1096.

83. Parronchi P, De Carli M, Manetti R, Simonelli C, Sampognaro S, Piccinni MP, Macchia D, Maggi E, Del Prete G, Romagnani S (1992) IL-4 and IFN (alpha and gamma) exert opposite regulatory effects on the development of cytolytic potential by Th1 or Th2 human T-cell clones. J Immunol 149:2977–2983.

84. Demeure CE, Wu CY, Shu U, Schneider PV, Heusser C, Yssel H, Delespesse G (1994) In vitro maturation of human neonatal CD4 T lymphocytes. II. Cytokines present at priming modulate the development of lymphokine production. J Immunol 152:4775–4782.

85. de Waal Malefyt R, Abrams JS, Zurawski SM, Lecron J-C, Mohan-Peterson S, Sanjanwala B, Bennett B, Silver J, de Vries JE, Yssel H (1995) Differential regulation of IL-13 and IL-4 production by human CD8+ and CD4+ Th0, Th1 and Th2 T-cell clones and EBV-transformed B-cells. Int Immunol 7:1405–1416.

86. Zurawski SM, Chomarat P, Djossou O, Bidaud C, McKenzie ANJ, Miossec P, Banchereau J, Zurawski G (1995) The primary binding subunit of the human interleukin-4 receptor is also a component of the interleukin-13 receptor. J Biol Chem 270:13,869–13,878.

87. Smerz-Bertling C, Duschl A (1995) Both interleukin 4 and interleukin 13 induce tyrosine phosphorylation of the 140-kDa subunit of the interleukin 4 receptor. J Biol Chem 270:966–970.

88. Hilton DJ, Zhang J-G, Metcalf D, Alexander WS, Nicola NA, Willson TA (1996) Cloning and characterization of a binding subunit of the interleukin 13 receptor that is also a component of the interleukin 4 receptor. Proc Natl Acad Sci USA 93:497–501.

89. Russell SM, Keegan AD, Harada N, Nakamura Y, Noguchi M, Leland P, Friedmann MC, Miyajima A, Puri RK, Paul WE (1993) Interleukin-2 receptor gamma chain: a functional component of the interleukin-4 receptor. Science 262:1880–1883.

90. Kondo M, Takeshita T, Ishii N, Nakamura M, Watanabe S, Arai K, Sugamura K (1993) Sharing of the interleukin-2 (IL-2) receptor gamma chain between receptors for IL-2 and IL-4. Science 262:1874–1877.

91. Lin JX, Migone TS, Tsang M, Friedmann M, Weatherbee JA, Zhou L, Yamauchi A, Bloom ET, Mietz J, John S, Leonard WJ (1995) The role of shared receptor motifs and common Stat proteins in the generation of cytokine pleiotropy and redundancy by IL-2, IL-4, IL-7, IL-13, and IL-15. Immunity 2:331–339.

92. Matthews DJ, Clark PA, Herbert J, Morgan G, Armitage RJ, Kinnon C, Minty A, Grabstein KH, Caput D, Ferrara P, Callard R (1995) Function of the interleukin-2 (IL-2) receptor gamma-chain in biologic responses of X-linked severe combined immunodeficient B-cells to IL-2, IL-4, IL-13, and IL-15. Blood 85:38–42.

93. He YW, Malek TR (1995) The IL-2 receptor gamma c chain does not function as a subunit shared by the IL-4 and IL-13 receptors. Implication for the structure of the IL-4 receptor. J Immunol 155:9–12.

94. Punnonen J, de Vries JE (1994) IL-13 induces proliferation, Ig isotype switching, and Ig synthesis by immature human fetal B-cells. J Immunol 152:1094–1102.

95. Zurawski G, De Vries JE (1994) Interleukin 13, an interleukin 4-like cytokine that acts on monocytes and B-cells, but not on T-cells. Immunol Today 15: 19–26.19–26.

96. Taniguchi T (1995) Cytokine signaling through nonreceptor protein tyrosine kinases. Science 268:251–255.

97. Ihle JN, Witthuhn BA, Quelle FW, Yamamoto K, Thierfelder WE, Kreider B, Silvennoinen O (1994) Signaling by the cytokine receptor superfamily: JAKs and STATs. Trends Biochem Sci 19:222–227.

98. Darnell JE Jr, Kerr IM, Stark GR (1994) Jak-STAT pathways and transcriptional activation in response to IFNs and other extracellular signaling proteins. Science 264:1415–1421.

99. Quelle FW, Shimoda K, Thierfelder W, Fischer C, Kim A, Ruben SM, Cleveland JL, Pierce JH, Keegan AD, Nelms K (1995) Cloning of murine Stat6 and human Stat6, Stat proteins that are tyrosine phosphorylated in responses to IL-4 and IL-3 but are not required for mitogenesis. Mol Cell Biol 15:3336–3343.

100. Izuhara K, Heike T, Otsuka T, Yamaoka K, Mayumi M, Imamura T, Niho Y, Harada N (1996) Signal transduction pathway of interleukin-4 and interleukin-13 in human B-cells derived from X-linked severe combined immunodeficiency patients. J Biol Chem 271:619–622.

101. Keegan AD, Johnston JA, Tortolani PJ, McReynolds LJ, Kinzer C, O'Shea JJ, Paul WE (1995) Similarities and differences in signal transduction by interleukin 4 and interleukin 13: analysis of Janus kinase activation. Proc Natl Acad Sci USA 92:7681–7685.

102. Fenghao X, Saxon A, Nguyen A, Ke Z, Diaz-Sanchez D, Nel A (1995) Interleukin 4 activates a signal transducer and activator of transcription (Stat) protein which interacts with an interferon-gamma activation site-like sequence upstream of the I epsilon exon in a human B-cell line. Evidence for the involvement of Janus kinase 3 and interleukin-4 Stat. J Clin Invest 96:907–914.

103. Murata T, Noguchi PD, Puri RK (1995) Receptors for interleukin (IL)-4 do not associate with the common gamma chain, and IL-4 induces the phosphorylation of JAK2 tyrosine kinase in human colon carcinoma cells. J Biol Chem 270:30829–30836.

104. Kaplan MH, Schindler U, Smiley ST, Grusby MJ (1996) Stat6 is required for mediating responses to IL-4 and for the development of Th2 cells. Immunity 4:313–319.

105. Kotanides H, Reich NC (1993) Requirement of tyrosine phosphorylation for rapid activation of a DNA binding factor by IL-4. Science 262:1265–1267.

106. Hou J, Schindler U, Henzel WJ, Ho TC, Brasseur M, McKnight SL (1994) An interleukin-4-induced transcription factor: IL-4 Stat. Science 265:1701–1706.

107. Coffman RL, Ohara J, Bond MW, Carty J, Zlotnik A, Paul WE (1986) B-cell stimulatory factor-1 enhances the IgE response of lipopolysaccharide-activated B-cells. J Immunol 136:4538–4541.

108. Tepper RI, Levinson DA, Stanger BZ, Campos-Torres J, Abbas AK, Leder P (1990) IL-4 induces allergic-like inflammatory disease and alters T-cell development in transgenic mice. Cell 62:457–467.

109. Finkelman FD, Katona IM, Urban JF Jr, Snapper CM, Ohara J, Paul WE (1986) Suppression of in vivo polyclonal IgE responses by monoclonal antibody to the lymphokine B-cell stimulatory factor 1. Proc Natl Acad Sci USA 83:9675–9678.

110. von der Weid T, Kopf M, Kohler G, Langhorne J (1994) The immune response to *Plasmodium chabaudi* malaria in interleukin-4-deficient mice. Eur J Immunol 24:2285–2293.

111. Noben-Trauth N, Kropf P, Muller I (1996) Susceptibility to *Leishmania major* infection in interleukin-4-deficient mice. Science 271:987–990.

112. Pene J, Rousset F, Briere F, Chretien I, Bonnefoy JY, Spits H, Yokota T, Arai N, Arai K, Banchereau J, De Vries JE (1988) IgE production by normal human lymphocytes is induced by interleukin 4 and suppressed by interferons gamma and alpha and prostaglandin E2. Proc Natl Acad Sci USA 85:6880–6884.

113. Pene J, Rousset F, Briere F, Chretien I, Paliard X, Banchereau J, Spits H, de Vries JE (1988) IgE production by normal human B-cells induced by alloreactive T-cell clones is mediated by IL-4 and suppressed by IFN-gamma. J Immunol 141:1218–1224.

114. Vercelli D, Jabara HH, Arai K, Geha RS (1989) Induction of human IgE synthesis requires interleukin 4 and T/B-cell interactions involving the T-cell receptor/CD3 complex and MHC class II antigens. J Exp Med 169:1295–1307.

115. Gascan H, Gauchat JF, Roncarolo MG, Yssel H, Spits H, de Vries JE (1991) Human B-cell clones can be induced to proliferate and to switch to IgE and IgG4 synthesis by interleukin 4 and a signal provided by activated CD4+ T-cell clones. J Exp Med 173:747–750.

116. Thyphronitis G, Tsokos GC, June CH, Levine AD, Finkelman FD (1989) IgE secretion by Epstein-Barr virus-infected purified human B lymphocytes is stimulated by interleukin 4 and suppressed by interferon gamma. Proc Natl Acad Sci USA 86:5580–5584.

117. Lundgren M, Persson U, Larsson P, Magnusson C, Smith CI, Hammarstrom L, Severinson E (1989) Interleukin 4 induces synthesis of IgE and IgG4 in human B-cells. Eur J Immunol 19:1311–1315.

118. Carballido JM, Schols D, Namikawa R, Zurawski S, Zurawski G, Roncarolo M-G, de Vries JE (1995) IL-4 induces human B-cell maturation and IgE synthesis in SCID-hu mice: inhibition of ongoing IgE production by in vivo treatment with an IL-4/IL-13 receptor antagonist. J Immunol 155:4162–4170.

119. Michel FB, Bousquet J, Greillier P, Robinet-Levy M, Coulomb Y (1995) Comparison of cord blood immunoglobulin E concentrations and maternal allergy for the prediction of atopic diseases in infancy. J Allergy Clin Immunol 65:422–430.

120. Magnusson CG (1988) Cord serum IgE in relation to family history and as predictor of atopic disease in early infancy. Allergy 43:241–251.

121. Punnonen J, de Vries JE (1993) Characterization of a novel CD2$^+$ human thymic B-cell subset. J Immunol 151:100–110.

122. Punnonen J, Aversa GG, Vandekerckhove B, Roncarolo M-G, de Vries JE (1992) Induction of isotype switching and Ig production by CD5$^+$ and CD10$^+$ human fetal B-cells. J Immunol 148:3398–3404.

123. Punnonen J, Aversa G, de Vries JE (1993) Human pre-B cells differentiate into Ig-secreting plasma cells in the presence of interleukin-4 and activated CD4$^+$ T-cells or their membranes. Blood 82:2781–2789.

124. Lutzker S, Rothman P, Pollock R, Coffman R, Alt FW (1988) Mitogen- and IL-4-regulated expression of germ-line Ig gamma 2b transcripts: evidence for directed heavy chain class switching. Cell 53:177–184.

125. Berton MT, and Vitetta ES (1990) Interleukin 4 induces changes in the chromatin structure of the g1 switch region in resting B-cells before switch recombination. J Exp Med 172:375–388.

126. Stavnezer J, Radcliffe G, Lin YC, Nietupski J, Berggren L, Sitia R, Severinson E (1988) Immunoglobulin heavy-chain switching may be directed by prior induction of transcripts from constant region genes. Proc Natl Acad Sci USA 85:7704–7708.

127. Rothman P, Chen YY, Lutzker S, Li SC, Stewart V, Coffman R, Alt FW (1990) Structure and expression of germ line immunoglobulin heavy-chain epsilon transcripts: interleukin-4 plus lipopolysaccharide-directed switching to C epsilon. Mol Cell Biol 10:1672–1679.

128. Gauchat JF, Lebman DA, Coffman RL, Gascan H, de Vries JE (1990) Structure and expression of germline epsilon transcripts in human B-cells induced by interleukin 4 to switch to IgE production. J Exp Med 172:463–473.

129. Gauchat JF, Aversa G, Gascan H, de Vries JE (1992) Modulation of IL-4 induced germline epsilon RNA synthesis in human B-cells by tumor necrosis factor-alpha, anti-CD40 monoclonal antibodies or transforming growth factor-beta correlates with levels of IgE production. Int Immunol 4:397–406.

130. Thyphronitis G, Katona IM, Gause WC, Finkelman FD (1993) Germline and productive C epsilon gene expression during in vivo IgE responses. J Immunol 151:4128–4136.

131. Ichiki T, Takahashi W, Watanabe T (1992) The effect of cytokines and mitogens on the induction of C epsilon germline transcripts in a human Burkitt lymphoma B-cell line. Int Immunol 4:747–754.

132. Jung S, Rajewsky K, Radbruch A (1993) Shutdown of class switch recombination by deletion of a switch region control element. Science 259:984–987.

133. Zhang J, Bottaro A, Li S, Stewart V, Alt FW (1993) A selective defect in IgG2b switching as a result of targeted mutation of the I gamma 2b promoter and exon. EMBO J 12:3529–3537.

134. Lorenz M, Jung S, Radbruch A (1995) Switch transcripts in immunoglobulin class switching. Science 267:1825–1828.

135. Rothman P, Lutzker S, Cook W, Coffman R, Alt FW (1988) Mitogen plus interleukin 4 induction of C epsilon transcripts in B lymphoid cells. J Exp Med 168:2385–2389.

136. Gauchat JF, Gascan H, de Waal Malefyt R, de Vries JE (1992) Regulation of germ-line epsilon transcription and induction of epsilon switching in cloned EBV-transformed and malignant human B-cell lines by cytokines and CD4$^+$ T-cells. J Immunol 148:2291–2299.

137. Jabara HH, Schneider LC, Shapira SK, Alfieri C, Moody CT, Kieff E, Geha RS, Vercelli D (1990) Induction of germ-line and mature C epsilon transcripts in human B-cells stimulated with rIL-4 and EBV. J Immunol 145:3468–3473.

138. Punnonen J, Cocks BG, de Vries JE (1995) IL-4 induces germline IgE heavy chain gene transcription in human fetal pre-B cells: evidence for differential expression of functional IL-4 and IL-13 receptors during B-cell ontogeny. J Immunol 155:4248–4254.

139. Cocks BG, Gauchat J-F, Aversa G, Punnonen J, Jehn C-D, Zavodny P, de Vries JE. IL-4 and IL-13-induced germline ε promoter activity in human B-cells is transiently inhibited by IFN-γ and IFN-α. (submitted)

140. Pene J, Chretien I, Rousset F, Briere F, Bonnefoy JY, de Vries JE (1989) Modulation of IL-4-induced human IgE production in vitro by IFN-gamma and IL-5: the role of soluble CD23 (s-CD23). J Cell Biochem 39:253–264.

141. Souillet G, Rousset F, de Vries JE (1989) Alpha-interferon treatment of patient with hyper IgE syndrome. Lancet 1:1384.

142. Finkelman FD, Svetic A, Gresser I, Snapper C, Holmes J, Trotta PP, Katona IM, Gause WC (1991) Regulation by interferon alpha of immunoglobulin isotype selection and lymphokine production in mice. J Exp Med 174:1179–1188.

143. King CL, Gallin JI, Malech HL, Abramson SL, Nutman TB (1989) Regulation of immunoglobulin production in hyperimmunoglobulin E recurrent-infection syndrome by interferon gamma. Proc Natl Acad Sci USA 86:10,085–10,089.

144. Wang ZE, Reiner SL, Zheng S, Dalton DK, Locksley RM (1994) CD4+ effector cells default to the Th2 pathway in interferon gamma-deficient mice infected with *Leishmania major*. J Exp Med 179:1367–1371.

145. Xu L, Rothman P (1994) IFN-gamma represses epsilon germline transcription and subsequently downregulates switch recombination to epsilon. Int Immunol 6:515–521.

146. Kehrl JH, Taylor A, Kim SJ, Fauci AS (1991) Transforming growth factor-beta is a potent negative regulator of human lymphocytes. Ann NY Acad Sci 628:345–353.

147. Wahl SM (1992) Transforming growth factor beta (TGF-beta) in inflammation: a cause and a cure. J Clin Immunol 12:61–74.

148. Van Vlasselaer P, Punnonen J, de Vries JE (1992) Transforming growth factor β directs IgA switching in human B-cells. J Immunol 148:2062–2067.

149. Stavnezer J (1995) Regulation of antibody production and class switching by TGF-beta. J Immunol 155:1647–1651.

150. Defrance T, Vanbervliet B, Briere F, Durand I, Rousset F, Banchereau J (1992) Interleukin 10 and transforming growth factor beta cooperate to induce anti-CD40-activated naive human B-cells to secrete immunoglobulin A. J Exp Med 175:671–682.

151. Islam KB, Nilsson L, Sideras P, Hammarstrom L, Smith CI (1991) TGF-beta 1 induces germ-line transcripts of both IgA subclasses in human B lymphocytes. Int Immunol 3:1099–1106.

152. Wu CY, Brinkmann V, Cox D, Heusser C, Delespesse G (1992) Modulation of human IgE synthesis by transforming growth factor-beta. Clin Immunol Immunopathol 62:277–284.

153. Rehmann JA, Le Bien TW (1994) Transforming growth factor-beta regulates normal human pre-B-cell differentiation. Int Immunol 6:315–322.

154. Carswell EA, Old LJ, Kassel RL, Green S, Fiore N, Williamson B (1975) An endotoxin-induced serum factor that causes necrosis of tumors. Proc Natl Acad Sci USA 72:3666–3670.

155. Aggarwal BB, Kohr WJ, Hass PE, Moffat B, Spencer SA, Henxel WJ, Bringman TS, Nedwin GE, Goeddel DV, Harkins RN (1985) Human tumor necrosis factor. J Biol Chem 260:2345–2354.

156. Ziegler EJ (1988) Tumor necrosis factor in humans. N Engl J Med 318:1533–1534.

157. Pennica D, Nedwin GE, Hayflick JS, Seeburg PH, Derynck R, Palladino MA, Kohr WJ, Aggarwal BB, Goeddel DV (1984) Human tumor necrosis factor: precursor structure, expression and homology to lymphotoxin. Nature 312:724–729.

158. Aggarwal BB, Eessalu TE, Hass PE (1985) Characterization of receptors for human tumor necrosis factor and their regulation by gamma-interferon. Nature 318:665–667.

159. Kehrl JH, Miller A, Fauci AS (1987) Effect of tumor necrosis factor alpha on mitogen-activated human B-cells. J Exp Med 166:786–791.

160. Yokota S, Geppert TD, Lipsky PE (1988) Enhancement of antigen- and mitogen-induced human T lymphocyte proliferation by tumor necrosis factor-alpha. J Immunol 140:531–536.

161. Janssen O, Kabelitz D (1988) Tumor necrosis factor selectively inhibits activation of human B-cells by Epstein-Barr virus. J Immunol 140:125–130.

162. Kehrl JH, Alvarez-Mon M, Delsing GA, Fauci AS (1987) Lymphotoxin is an important T-cell-derived growth factor for human B-cells. Science 238:1144–1146.

163. Boussiotis VA, Nadler LM, Strominger JL, Goldfeld AE (1994) Tumor necrosis factor alpha is an autocrine growth factor for normal human B-cells. Proc Natl Acad Sci USA 91:7007–7011.

164. Worm M, Geha RS (1994) CD40 ligation induces lymphotoxin alpha gene expression in human B-cells. Int Immunol 6:1883–1890.

165. Aversa G, Punnonen J, de Vries JE (1993) The 26-kD transmembrane form of tumor necrosis factor alpha on activated CD4+ T-cell clones provides a costimulatory signal for human B-cell activation. J Exp Med 177:1575–1585.

166. Macchia D, Almerigogna F, Parronchi P, Ravina A, Maggi E, Romagnani S (1993) Membrane tumour necrosis factor-alpha is involved in the polyclonal B-cell activation induced by HIV-infected human T-cells. Nature 363:464–466.

167. Muraguchi A, Kehrl JH, Longo DL, Volkman DJ, Smith KA, Fauci AS (1985) Interleukin 2 receptors on human B-cells. Implications for the role of interleukin 2 in human B-cell function. J Exp Med 161:181–197.

168. Karasuyama H, Rolink A, Melchers F (1988) Recombinant interleukin 2 or 5, but not 3 or 4, induces maturation of resting mouse B lymphocytes and propagates proliferation of activated B-cell blasts. J Exp Med 167:1377–1390.

169. Punnonen J, Eskola J (1987) Recombinant interleukin 2 induces proliferation and differentiation of human B lymphocytes. Acta Path Microbiol Immunol Scand 95:167–172.

170. Schorle H, Holtschke T, Hunig T, Schimpl A, Horak I (1991) Development and function of T-cells in mice rendered interleukin-2 deficient by gene targeting. Nature 352:621–624.

171. Sadlack B, Merz H, Schorle H, Schimpl A, Feller AC, Horak I (1993) Ulcerative colitis-like disease in mice with a disrupted interleukin-2 gene. Cell 75:253–261.

172. Armitage RJ, Macduff BM, Eisenman J, Paxton R, Grabstein KH (1995) IL-15 has stimulatory activity for the induction of B-cell proliferation and differentiation. J Immunol 154:483–490.

173. Nonoyama S, Farrington ML, Ochs HD (1994) Effect of IL-2 on immunoglobulin production by anti-CD40-activated human B-cells: synergistic effect with IL-10 and antagonistic effect with IL-4. Clin Immunol Immunopathol 72:373–379.

174. Maggi E, Del Prete GF, Parronchi P, Tiri A, Macchia D, Biswas P, Simonelli C, Ricci M, Romagnani S (1989) Role for T-cells, IL-2 and IL-6 in the IL-4-dependent in vitro human IgE synthesis. Immunology 68:300–306.

175. Miyajima H, Hirano T, Hirose S, Karasuyama H, Okumura K, Ovary Z (1991) Suppression by IL-2 of IgE production by B-cells stimulated by IL-4. J Immunol 146:457–462.

176. Nakanishi K, Yoshimoto T, Chu CC, Matsumoto H, Hase K, Nagai N, Tanaka T, Miyasaka M, Paul WE, Shinka S (1995) IL-2 inhibits IL-4-dependent IgE and IgG1 production in vitro and in vivo. Int Immunol 7:259–268.

177. Spiegelberg HL, Falkoff RJ, O'Connor RD, Beck L (1991) Interleukin-2 inhibits the interleukin-4-induced human IgE and IgG4 secretion in vivo. Clin Exp Immunol 84:400–405.

178. Punnonen J, Punnonen K, Jansen CT, Kalimo K (1993) Interferon(IFN)-α, IFN-γ, interleukin(IL)-2, and arachidonic acid metabolites modulate IL-4 induced IgE synthesis similarly in healthy individuals and atopic dermatitis patients. Allergy 48:189–195.

179. Egan RW, Athwahl D, Chou CC, Emtage S, Jehn CH, Kung TT, Mauser PJ, Murgolo NJ, Bodmer MW (1995) Inhibition of pulmonary eosinophilia and hyperreactivity by antibodies to interleukin-5. Int Arch Allergy Immunol 107:321–322.

180. Loughnan MS, Nossal GJ (1989) Interleukins 4 and 5 control expression of IL-2 receptor on murine B-cells through independent induction of its two chains. Nature 340:76–79.

181. Kinashi T, Harada N, Severinson E, Tanabe T, Sideras P, Konishi M, Azuma C, Tominaga A, Bergstedt-Lindqvist S, Takahashi M, Matsuda F, Yaoita Y, Takatsu K, Honjo T (1986) Cloning of complementary DNA encoding T-cell replacing factor and identity with B-cell growth factor II. Nature 324:70–76.

182. Alderson MR, Pike BL, Harada N, Tominaga A, Takatsu K, Nossal GJ (1987) Recombinant T-cell replacing factor (interleukin 5) acts with antigen to promote the growth and differentiation of single hapten-specific B lymphocytes. J Immunol 139:2656–2660.

183. Azuma C, Tanabe T, Konishi T, Noma T, Matsuda F, Yaoita Y, Takatsu K, Hammarström L, Smith CIE, Severinson E, Honjo T (1986) Cloning of cDNA for human T-cell replacing factor (interleukin-5) and comparison with the murine homologue. Nucleic Acids Res 14:9149–9158.

184. Glutterbuck E, Shields JG, Gordon J, Smith SH, Boyd A, Callard RE, Campbell HD, Young IG, Sanderson CJ (1987) Recombinant human interleukin 5 is an eosinophil differentiation factor but has no activity in standard human B-cell growth factor assays. Eur J Immunol 17:1743–1750.

185. Pene J, Rousset F, Briere F, Chretien I, Wideman J, Bonnefoy JY, de Vries JE (1988) Interleukin 5 enhances interleukin 4-induced IgE production by normal human B-cells. The role of soluble CD23 antigen. Eur J Immunol 18:929–935.

186. Huston MH, Moore JP, Mettes HJ, Tavana G, Huston D (1996) Human B-cells express IL-5 receptor messenger ribonucleic acid and respond to IL-5 with enhanced IgM production after mitogenic stimulation with *Moraxella catarrhalis*. J Immunol 156:1392–1401.

187. Hirano T, Yasukawa K, Harada H, Taga T, Watanabe Y, Matsuda T, Kashiwamura S, Nakajima K, Koyama K, Iwamatsu A, Tsunasawa S, Sakiyama F, Matsui H, Takahara Y, Taniguchi T, Kishimoto T (1986) Complementary DNA for a novel human interleukin (BSF-2) that induces B lymphocytes to produce immunoglobulin. Nature 324:73–76.

188. Punnonen J, de Waal Malefyt R, van Vlasselar P, Gauchat J-F, de Vries JE (1993) IL-10 and viral

IL-10 prevent IL-4-induced IgE synthesis by inhibiting the accessory cell function of monocytes. J Immunol 151:1280–1289.

189. Vercelli D, Jabara HH, Arai K, Yokota T, Geha RS (1989) Endogenous interleukin 6 plays an obligatory role in interleukin 4-dependent human IgE synthesis. Eur J Immunol 19:1419–1424.

190. Ramsay AJ, Husband AJ, Ramshaw IA, Bao S, Matthaei KI, Koehler G, Kopf M (1994) The role of interleukin-6 in mucosal IgA antibody responses in vivo. Science 264:561–563.

191. Lindley I, Aschauer H, Seifert JM, Lam C, Brunowsky W, Kownatzki E, Thelen M, Peveri P, Dewald B, von Tscharner V, Walz A, Baggiolini M (1988) Synthesis and expression in *Escherichia coli* of the gene encoding monocyte-derived neutrophil-activating factor: biological equivalence between natural and recombinant neutrophil-activating factor. Proc Natl Acad Sci USA 85:9199–9203.

192. Larsen CG, Anderson AO, Appella E, Oppenheim JJ, Matsushima K (1989) The neutrophil-activating protein (NAP-1) is also chemotactic for T-lymphocytes. Science 243:1464–1466.

193. Dahinden CA, Kurimoto Y, De Weck AL, Lindley I, Dewald B, Baggiolini M (1989) The neutrophil-activating peptide NAF/NAP-1 induces histamine and leukotriene release by interleukin 3-primed basophils. J Exp Med 170:1787–1792.

194. Gimbrone MA Jr, Obin MS, Brock AF, Luis EA, Hass PE, Hebert CA, Yip YK, Leung DW, Lowe DG, Kohr WJ, Darbonne WC, Bechtol KB, Baker JB (1989) Endothelial interleukin-8: a novel inhibitor of leukocyte-endothelial interactions. Science 246:1601–1603.

195. Luscinskas FW, Kiely JM, Ding H, Obin MS, Hebert CA, Baker JB, Gimbrone MA Jr (1992) In vitro inhibitory effect of IL-8 and other chemoattractants on neutrophil-endothelial adhesive interactions. J Immunol 149:2163–2171.

196. Kimata H, Yoshida A, Ishioka C, Lindley I, Mikawa H (1992) Interleukin 8 (IL-8) selectively inhibits immunoglobulin E production induced by IL-4 in human B-cells. J Exp Med 176:1227–1231.

197. Kimata H, Lindley I, Furusho K (1995) Selective inhibition of spontaneous IgE and IgG4 production by interleukin-8 in atopic patients. Blood 85:3191–3198.

198. Kimata H, Lindley I (1994) Detection of plasma interleukin-8 in atopic dermatitis. Arch Dis Child 70:119–122.

199. Moore KW, O'Garra A, de Waal Malefyt R, Vieira P, Mosmann TR (1993) Interleukin-10. Annu Rev Immunol 11:165–190.

200. de Waal Malefyt R, Abrams J, Bennett B, Figdor CG, De Vries JE (1991) Interleukin 10 (IL-10) inhibits cytokine synthesis by human monocytes: an autoregulatory role of IL-10 produced by monocytes. J Exp Med 174:1209–1220.

201. Fiorentino DF, Zlotnik A, Mosmann TR, Howard M, O'Garra A (1991) IL-10 inhibits cytokine production by activated macrophages. J Immunol 147:3815–3824.

202. de Waal Malefyt R, Haanen J, Spits H, Roncarolo MG, te Velde A, Figdor C, Johnson K, Kastelein R, Yssel H, de Vries JE (1991) Interleukin 10 (IL-10) and viral IL-10 strongly reduce antigen-specific human T-cell proliferation by diminishing the antigen-presenting capacity of monocytes via downregulation of class II major histocompatibility complex expression. J Exp Med 174:915–924.

203. Ding L, Shevach EM (1992) IL-10 inhibits mitogen-induced T-cell proliferation by selectively inhibiting macrophage costimulatory function. J Immunol 148:3133–3141.

204. Taga K, Tosato G (1992) IL-10 inhibits human T-cell proliferation and IL-2 production. J Immunol 148:1143–1152.

205. Willems F, Marchant A, Delville JP, Gerard C, Delvaux A, Velu T, de Boer M, Goldman M (1994) Interleukin-10 inhibits B7 and intercellular adhesion molecule-1 expression on human monocytes. Eur J Immunol 24:1007–1009.

206. Buelens C, Willems F, Delvaux A, Pierard G, Delville JP, Velu T, Goldman M (1995) Interleukin-10 differentially regulates B7-1 (CD80) and B7-2 (CD86) expression on human peripheral blood dendritic cells. Eur J Immunol 25:2668–2672.

207. Moore KW, Vieira P, Fiorentino DF, Trounstine ML, Khan TA, Mosmann TR (1990) Homology of cytokine synthesis inhibitory factor (IL-10) to the Epstein-Barr virus gene BCRFI. Science 248:1230–1234.

208. Vieira P, de Waal-Malefyt R, Dang MN, Johnson KE, Kastelein R, Fiorentino DF, De Vries JE, Roncarolo MG, Mosmann TR, Moore KW (1991) Isolation and expression of human cytokine synthesis inhibitory factor cDNA clones: homology to Epstein-Barr virus open reading frame BCRFI. Proc Natl Acad Sci USA 88:1172–1176.

209. Bober LA, Grace MJ, Pugliese-Sivo C, Waters TA, Sullivan LM, Narula SK (1994) Human IL-10 reduces the number of IL-4-induced IgE B-cells in cultures of atopic mononuclear cells. Int. Arch. Allergy Immunol 105:26–31.

210. Jabara HH, Vercelli D (1994) Engagement of CD14 on monocytes inhibits the synthesis of human Igs, including IgE. J Immunol 153:972–978.

211. Rousset F, Garcia E, Defrance T, Peronne C, Vezzio N, Hsu DH, Kastelein R, Moore KW, Banchereau J (1992) Interleukin 10 is a potent growth and differentiation factor for activated human B lymphocytes. Proc Natl Acad Sci USA 89:1890–1893.

212. Go NF, Castle BE, Barrett R, Kastelein R, Dang W, Mosmann TR, Moore KW, Howard M (1990) Interleukin 10, a novel B-cell stimulatory factor: unresponsiveness of X chromosome-linked immuno-deficiency B-cells. J Exp Med 172:1625–1631.

213. Trinchieri G (1995) Interleukin-12: a proinflammatory cytokine with immunoregulatory functions that bridge innate resistance and antigen-specific adaptive immunity. Annu Rev Immunol 13:251–276.

214. Kiniwa M, Gately M, Gubler U, Chizzonite R, Fargeas C, Delespesse G (1992) Recombinant inter-leukin-12 suppresses the synthesis of immunoglobulin E by interleukin-4 stimulated human lympho-cytes. J Clin Invest 90:262–266.

215. Morris SC, Madden KB, Adamovicz JJ, Gause WC, Hubbard BR, Gately MK, Finkelman FD (1994) Effects of IL-12 on in vivo cytokine gene expression and Ig isotype selection. J Immunol 152:1047–1056.

216. Germann T, Bongartz M, Dlugonska H, Hess H, Schmitt E, Kolbe L, Kolsch E, Podlaski FJ, Gately MK, Rude E (1995) Interleukin-12 profoundly up-regulates the synthesis of antigen-specific complement-fixing IgG2a, IgG2b and IgG3 antibody subclasses in vivo. Eur J Immunol 25:823–829.

217. Kruse N, Tony HP, Sebald W (1992) Conversion of human interleukin-4 into a high affinity antagonist by a single amino acid replacement. EMBO J 11:3237–3244.

218. Tony HP, Shen BJ, Reusch P, Sebald W (1994) Design of human interleukin-4 antagonists inhibiting interleukin-4-dependent and interleukin-13-dependent responses in T-cells and B-cells with high effi-ciency. Eur J Biochem 225:659–665.

219. Carballido JM, Aversa G, Schols D, Punnonen J, de Vries JE (1995) Inhibition of human IgE synthesis in vitro and in SCID-hu mice by an interleukin-4 receptor antagonist. Int Arch Allergy Immunol 107:304–307.

220. Sato TA, Widmer MB, Finkelman FD, Madani H, Jacobs CA, Grabstein KH, Maliszewski CR (1993) Recombinant soluble murine IL-4 receptor can inhibit or enhance IgE responses in vivo. J Immunol 150:2717–2723.

221. Atamas SP, Choi J, Yurovsky VV, White B (1996) An alternative splice variant of human IL-4, IL-4delta2, inhibits IL-4-stimulated T-cell proliferation. J Immunol 156:435–441.

222. Haba S, Nisonoff A (1994) Role of antibody and T-cells in the long-term inhibition of IgE synthesis. Proc Natl Acad Sci USA 91:604–608.

223. Amiri P, Haak-Frendscho M, Robbins K, McKerrow JH, Stewart T, Jardieu P (1994) Anti-immuno-globulin E treatment decreases worm burden and egg production in *Schistosoma mansoni*-infected nor-mal and interferon gamma knockout mice. J Exp Med 180:43–51.

224. Presta LG, Lahr SJ, Shields RL, Porter JP, Gorman CM, Fendly BM, Jardieu PM (1993) Humanization of an antibody directed against IgE. J Immunol 151:2623–2632.

225. Jardieu P (1995) Anti-IgE therapy. Curr Opin Immunol 7:779–782.

226. Cocks BG, Chang C-CJ, Carballido JM, Yssel H, de Vries JE, Aversa G (1995) A novel receptor involved in T-cell activation. Nature 376:260–263.

3

Environmental Allergens

Thomas A. E. Platts-Mills, MD, PhD, FRCP,
Judith A. Woodfolk, MD,
and Lisa M. Wheatley, MD

CONTENTS

INTRODUCTION

When Charles Blackley proved that grass pollen grains were the cause of seasonal hay fever, he took the first steps to understanding why some plants and animals in our environment are important causes of sensitization and symptoms *(1)*. Dr. Blackley was well aware of the size of pollen grains; he knew they could fly up to at least a thousand feet, and he also demonstrated that aqueous extracts of pollen would give rise to wheal and flare skin responses. The important aspects of studies on inhaled allergens are to understand which sources produce a sufficient number of protein-carrying particles, the nature of the proteins, and the properties of the particles; in particular, whether the particles become or remain airborne and whether they release protein rapidly on contact with an aqueous milieu such as the nasal or bronchial epithelium. All inhaled allergens characterized to date have been purified from an aqueous extract of the source material. Purification of allergens using classical immunochemistry was a major undertaking, and it was difficult to formally establish the nature of the protein that had been purified. Indeed during the 1960s and 1970s many allergens were purified, but their identity was subsequently "lost." By contrast, Amb a 1 from ragweed, Fel d 1 from cat dander, and Lol p 1 from Rye grass pollen were repeatedly purified and defined both physicochemically and by producing monospecific antisera *(2–4)*. Three major scientific developments transformed the immunochemistry of allergens: first, the ability to sequence proteins; second, the invention of monoclonal antibodies (MAbs); third, the cloning and sequencing of DNA *(5–7)*. Sequencing of a protein provides a permanent definition and makes it possible to search for homology with proteins from other species. MAbs also provide a simple and effectively permanent method for defining proteins and can be used to develop sensitive specific assays for allergens *(6,8,9)*. The impact of the techniques for measurement has largely been in relation to the indoor environment because, unlike pollens and most fungal spores, it is difficult to identify microscopically the particles carrying airborne mite, cat, dog, or cockroach allergens *(10–13)*. The immunoassays

From: *Allergy and Allergic Diseases: The New Mechanisms and Therapeutics*
Edited by: J. A. Denburg © Humana Press Inc., Totowa, NJ

for indoor allergens have played a major role in defining the relationship between exposure to indoor allergens and disease, and also in developing techniques for allergen avoidance (14–19).

Understanding the particles that carry allergens is essential because this is the only significant way in which proteins can become airborne. It is very unusual for a naturally occurring aerosol to contain sufficient protein to be immunogenic, and there is no evidence that free protein molecules can become airborne in significant quantities. The particles that become airborne range from ≤ 1–35 μm in diameter. At one end of this size range are particles of animal dander or the spores of fungi such as *Aspergillus* and *Penicillium*. At the large end of the range are ragweed pollen, mite fecal particles, and the spores of *Alternaria* (Fig. 1A,B). It is very important to appreciate that a large pollen grain ~30 μm in diameter may be 1000–10,000 times larger in volume than the small fungal spores that are so numerous in outdoor air. The fecal particles of *D. pteronyssinus* have been estimated to contain 0.2 ng of Der p 1 (20). If a spore of *Penicillium* contained the same concentration of allergen, the comparable value would be 0.1 pg.

For many years it was assumed that the proteins that gave rise to immediate hypersensitivity, often referred to as atopens, were a distinct type of protein. However, studies in mice have shown that any soluble protein can give rise to IgE antibody production if the immunization protocol involves repeated low-dose injections without a bacterial adjuvant. Thus, it seems likely that the characteristic that distinguishes allergens is the form in which patients are exposed. By far the most common form of exposure is repeated inhalation of particles through the nose or mouth. Thus the essence of an allergen is that it becomes airborne in a form that will deliver soluble proteins to the respiratory tract and thus to the draining lymph nodes. Particles only stay on the nasal mucosa for a few minutes before they are passed posteriorly by ciliary action and swallowed. This implies that an ideal allergen should be a foreign protein that is rapidly soluble and small enough to pass through the epithelial basement membrane, i.e., ≤ 60 kDa. Once in the subepithelial layer, it is assumed that foreign proteins are taken up by IA positive dendritic cells and that the antigens are transported to the local lymph nodes by these cells. The immune response that occurs, which is characterized by T_H2 cells, IgE antibodies, and eosinophils, is now well understood (*see* Chapter 11).

SOURCES OF ALLERGENS

Outdoor

POLLEN

Most wind-pollinated plants produce enough pollen grains to become a cause of seasonal hay fever, provided there are sufficient plants in the area. Pollen grains are gametes; after landing on the pistil they have to release protein in order to trigger the formation of a pollen tube. Thus, pollen grains are designed to deliver recognition proteins and, in keeping with this, they all have pores. Some of the known allergens are thought to be involved in recognition, but the function of the other pollen allergens is not known. In general, pollen grains have a strong cuticle, which prevents them from breaking up. Whole pollen grains have been identified in the lungs, in very old glacial ice cores, and as fossils. However, it has been recently suggested that grass pollen grains can be disrupted by rain and as a result, release multiple small starch grains. This phenomenon has been related to the epidemics of asthma occurring at the time of severe thunderstorms in Australia and England. However, it has not yet been shown that significant grass pollen allergens become airborne in the form of these starch granules. In general, the quantity of airborne pollen grains is reduced by rain. It seems equally likely that the effect of thunderstorms on asthma is caused by inhalation of water, which can provoke bronchospasm in bronchially reactive patients, or by the effects of rapid changes in barometric pressure. It is often stated that plants release pollen in the morning; however, the actual trigger is the rapid decrease in relative humidity that occurs shortly after the sun rises, provided the weather is fair. Thus, pollen counts are highest when there have been several days of fine weather. The detailed morphology of pollen grains and their seasons have been documented in many excellent manuals *(21,22)*. A skilled person can accurately describe the number of pollen grains of each species that are airborne. The pollen count is a reasonable prediction of the severity of symptoms of hay fever and in certain localities (e.g., grass pollen in northern California and Oregon) may also predict asthma symptoms among allergic individuals *(23,24)*.

Fungi

The best recognized form of exposure to fungi is as fungal spores; however detailed microscopic examination of plates or sampler rods will identify many hyphae and other particles that could be of fungal origin *(22)*. Furthermore, many fungi do not form spores under conditions that are common indoors. Thus, fungal spore counts only give partial information about exposure. In addition, spores have a much wider range of sizes than pollen grains and have a very different biological role. Spores are designed to withstand extremes of dry or cold and to germinate when the conditions are optimal for fungal growth. Thus rapid release of proteins is not part of their modus operandi. At present it is clear that many patients become allergic to fungal allergens and report symptoms during spring, summer, or fall. However, for most fungi a clear dose response relationship between exposure and symptoms has been elusive *(25)*. The only exception for airborne allergens is *Alternaria*, for which an association with asthma has been shown in some areas *(25–27)*. Furthermore, increased severity of asthma has been reported in *Alternaria*-sensitive patients during that period of the year when *Alternaria* antigens are airborne *(26)*. The fungal extracts that are widely used for skin testing are predominantly fungi imperfecti; that is, they generally reproduce asexually and do not produce large fruiting bodies or mushrooms. The mushrooms or basidiomycetes produce very large numbers of small spores that become airborne. In New Orleans and other areas, skin sensitivity to *Basidiomycete* extracts is common; however, it has not been convincingly shown that sensitive patients have increased symptoms at times of high exposure *(27)*. Indeed for most indoor and outdoor fungi, the currently available methods of measuring exposure correlate poorly with either sensitization or symptoms *(22,28)*.

The genus *Aspergillus* was given its name by the monk who first identified these fungi, because the sporing heads look like the aspergillum that is used to disperse holy water in Catholic Church services. The sporing heads are designed to release large numbers of spores. The individual species can only be identified if they form sporing bodies; neither the mycelia nor the spores are easily distinguished from other species of *Aspergillus* or *Penicillium*. Thus, at present the available methods of measuring airborne *Aspergillus* depend on culture and are not quantitative. Using an immunoassay for the *A. fumigatus* allergen Asp f 1, it was possible to demonstrate airborne antigen during disturbance of leaf mold outdoors and also in house dust *(29)*. The spores contain very little Asp f 1 and the gene for Asp f 1 is only expressed after germination. Thus, the spores are unlikely to release any antigen unless they germinate, a process that requires several hours. A major problem in studying fungi is the relatively small number of allergens that have been purified *(30)*. At present it is difficult to measure exposure or to standardize reagents used for serology or skin tests. As a result, our understanding of the role of airborne molds in asthma or rhinitis is limited.

Indoor (Table 1)

MITES

The allergenicity of house dust was first recognized in 1920, and strong associations were reported with asthma *(31)* and atopic dermatitis *(32)*. During the 1920s and 1930s, several

Table 1
Indoor Sources of Environmental Allergens

Dust mites

Dermatophagoides pteronyssinus
Dermatophagoides farinae
Euroglyphys maynei
Blomia tropicalis

Storage mites
Lepidoglyphus destructor
Tarsonimidae

Insects
Cockroaches
Blattella germanica (German)
Periplanetta americana (American)
Blatta orientalis (Oriental)

Other
Crickets, flies, beetles, fleas, moths,
midges

Fungi
Inside
Multiple species including
Penicillium, Aspergillus, Cladosporium
(growing on surfaces or rotting wood)
Outside
Entry with incoming air
Multiple species, *Alternaria*

Mammals

Cats (*Felis domesticus*)
Dogs (*Canis familiaris*)
Rabbits, ferrets
Rodents
Pets: Mice, gerbils, guinea pigs,
chinchilla, etc.
Pests: Mice (*Mus musculus*[a])
and (*Rattus rattus*)

Pollens
Derived from outside

Sundry
Horse hair in furniture, kapok
Food dropped by inhabitants
Spiders, silverfish, etc.

[a]Many small rodents become indoor pests, including many different species of mice.

sources of allergens in house dust were identified, including a range of domestic animals, horse hair in furniture, and insects. However, it was generally recognized that extracts made from some house dust samples could give very strong skin tests on allergic patients, even when there was no obvious source of allergens. This led to a search for the source of the house dust atopen. The presence of mites in a mattress was first described by Dekker in 1931, who speculated on their role as allergens. In 1967, Spieksma and Voorhorst *(33)* demonstrated that dust mites were the main source of allergens in house dust in the Netherlands. They also showed that mites were not present in dust from the high-altitude sanitarium in Davos, Switzerland, and, most important, they developed a technique for growing mites in culture. This made it possible to produce dust mite extracts and to skin test large numbers of patients. Following their work, studies from England, Australia, and Japan established that mite allergy was extremely common among asthmatic patients living in humid areas *(34–36)*.

Dust mites are eight-legged relatives of spiders, ticks, and chiggers one-third of a millimeter in length (Fig. 2A,B; Table 2). They reproduce by copulation, a fact that was first documented by Van Leeuwenhoek circa 1650. The fertile females can lay up to one egg per day. The eggs, which are 100 µm in length, hatch in 11 d and the immature forms mature over 20–30 d

Table 2
Classification of Arthropods

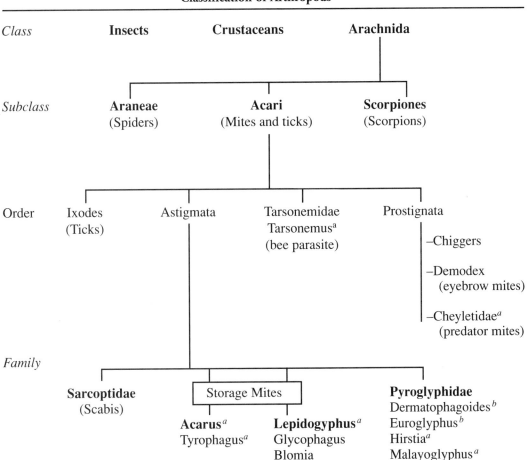

| Class | **Insects** | **Crustaceans** | **Arachnida** |

Subclass: **Araneae** (Spiders) — **Acari** (Mites and ticks) — **Scorpiones** (Scorpions)

Order: Ixodes (Ticks) — Astigmata — Tarsonemidae Tarsonemus[a] (bee parasite) — Prostignata
     –Chiggers
     –Demodex (eyebrow mites)
     –Cheyletidae[a] (predator mites)

Family:
Sarcoptidae (Scabis)   Storage Mites   **Pyroglyphidae**
     Acarus[a]   **Lepidogyphus**[a]   Dermatophagoides[b]
     Tyrophagus[a]   Glycophagus   Euroglyphus[b]
             Blomia   Hirstia[a]
                      Malayoglyphus[a]

[a] All mites found in house dust are collectively referred to as domestic mites.
[b] The term "dust miles" is generally restricted *Dermatophagoides, Euroglyphus.*

depending on conditions *(37–39)*. Mites produce up to 15 fecal pellets/d. Estimates based either on the number of mites present or on the quantity of allergen that can be extracted from dust suggested that house dust could contain 5000–500,000 fecal pellets/gm. At 0.2 ng/fecal particle this represents 1–100 µg Der p 1 (or Der f 1)/g of dust. The fecal particles range in size from 10–35 µm in diameter and release allergen very rapidly, i.e., 90% within 2 min *(20)*.

DOMESTIC ANIMALS

The most easily identified source of allergens in house dust is our friend *Felis domesticus*. The importance of this allergen is obvious to many patients. Indeed a positive history of symptoms (i.e., rhinitis, conjunctivitis, or wheezing) on exposure to cats is a very reliable indicator that a patient is atopic, i.e., that they will have positive skin tests to cat and other extracts. It is also obvious to these patients that they can develop symptoms by contact with a cat, or simply by entering a house that has a cat, whether the animal is present in the room or not. When cat allergen was first purified in 1974, Ohman and his colleagues *(4)* suggested that the allergen, Fe1 d 1, might be derived from saliva and that this was a source of allergen on the fur. More recently it was shown that the allergen accumulates rapidly on shaved skin even when the cat is prevented from licking the skin *(40)*. When Fe1 d 1 was sequenced and cloned, it was possible to demonstrate expression of the gene for this allergen in the sebaceous glands of the skin. It is now clear that cat allergen is primarily produced in the skin *(9,41)*. Commercial extracts are made by either washing cats or extracting the pelts. These two approaches produce extracts with a different distribution of proteins; the pelt extracts have a higher proportion of serum proteins, including cat albumin, relative to the major allergen, Fe1 d 1. Direct assay of washings from cat hair demonstrated the presence of 20–1,000 µg Fe1 d 1/g. This allergen must be coated on the hairs or on small particles of dander stuck on the hair. At present the nature of the particles that become airborne is not clear, but they appear to range in size from 20 to ≤ 1 µm in diameter. Some particles are visible on cat hair (Fig. 3A) and can be visualized using the micro-ochterlony technique (Fig. 3B). Dog allergen has not been as fully studied as cat allergen. The properties of Can f 1 in terms of distribution in houses and airborne appear to be similar to those of cat allergen *(42)*. In particular, dog allergen has been found airborne in undisturbed conditions, can be reduced by air filtration, and can be obtained by washing dogs *(43)*.

RODENTS

Many different rodents come into contact with humans, and they are very potent sources of allergens. The major allergens that have been defined are predominantly found in urine. As a consequence, litter represents an important source of exposure. This is true for both laboratory animals and pet rodents. Many rodents, particularly the males, develop heavy proteinuria; male rat urine may contain more than 1 mg of allergen/mL *(44)*. Disturbance of litter can produce very high levels of airborne allergen. This, however, depends on how wet the litter is. As litter dries out, the allergen that becomes airborne on disturbance dramatically increases *(45)*. Controlling exposure to allergen in an animal house can be achieved by using different forms of litter and arranging the airflow so that the air crossing the cages travels away from personnel. A large number of scientists and people working in animal houses become allergic, and many suffer from severe symptoms, including rhinitis, asthma, and, occasionally, anaphylaxis *(46)*. Anaphylaxis following a rat bite or acute episodes of asthma on entering an animal house are a sufficiently common problem to justify keeping injectable adrenaline available in animal houses.

COCKROACHES

Cockroaches were first recognized as a source of allergens in 1960 by Bernton and Brown *(47)*. Subsequently many authors recognized that patients with asthma living in cities were commonly sensitized to this insect. Provisional identification of allergens was reported by Twarog et al. *(48)* in 1976; however, the definition of those proteins was subsequently "lost". In the 1980s a series of clinic and emergency room studies established an association between sensitization to cockroach allergens and acute asthma *(49,50)*. Furthermore, it was clear that this risk was restricted to areas where significant cockroach allergen was found in the houses *(51,52)*. More recently, the National Cooperative Inner City Asthma Study has confirmed that sensitization and exposure to cockroach allergens are a major factor in the severity of asthma among children and adolescents from low-income families in North America *(53)*.

There are many species of cockroaches, and they are common pests in houses in many parts of the world. In origin they are tropical, and they only flourish if buildings are heated year round (i.e., hospitals, zoos, and apartment blocks) or the climate is sufficiently hot for cockroaches to live outside (e.g., the southern half of the United States). Prevention of cockroach

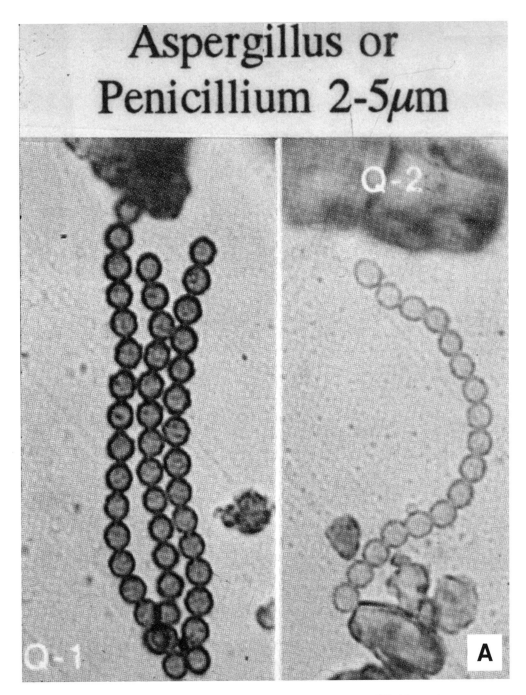

Fig. 1.(A) Aspergillus and Penicillium spores approx 2–5 µ diameter. **(B)** Alternaria spores approx 10 × 20 µ. (Figures from "Sampling and Identifying Allergenic Pollens and Molds." E. Grant Smith. Courtesy of Blewstone Press, Texas.)

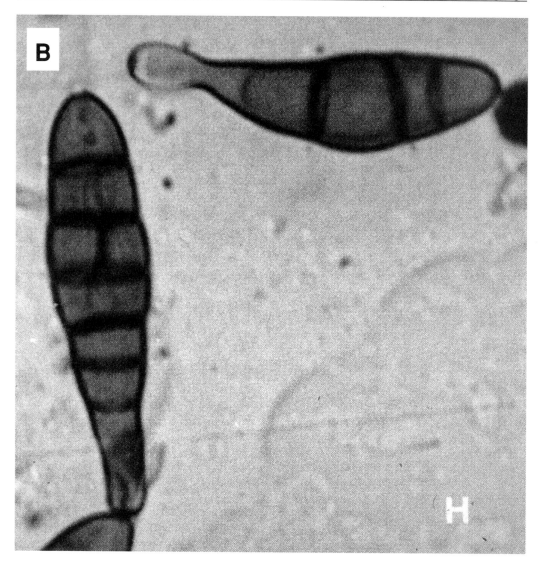

infestation requires obsessional control of food sources and regular use of bait poisons. Several different allergens have now been identified, and it is probable that cockroach allergens derive from several sources (i.e., saliva, fecal material, and debris from dead bodies). Certainly, significant allergens can be obtained from washing roaches or from the frass that accumulates at the bottom of the jars in which roaches are kept in the laboratory. Although sensitization to cockroaches is strongly associated with asthma, patients are generally not aware of being allergic to them. In particular, allergic patients do not report acute symptoms on entering a house that is infested with roaches. In keeping with this, cockroach allergens are not airborne in undisturbed conditions. During vacuum cleaning, cockroach allergens become airborne *(13)*. Preliminary studies suggest that the particles are relatively large, i.e., > 10 μm in diameter, and the implication is that, like dust mite particles, they will fall rapidly *(13,54,55)*.

(text continues on page 53)

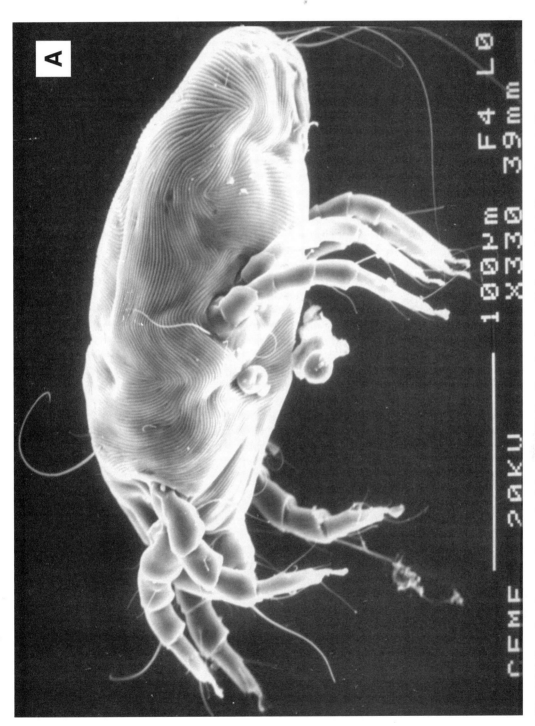

Fig. 2. (A) Scanning electron micrograph of dust mite. (B) Detail to show legs with foot pads that allow mites to hold on to surfaces. (Figures courtesy of J. Vaughan and B. Sheppard.)

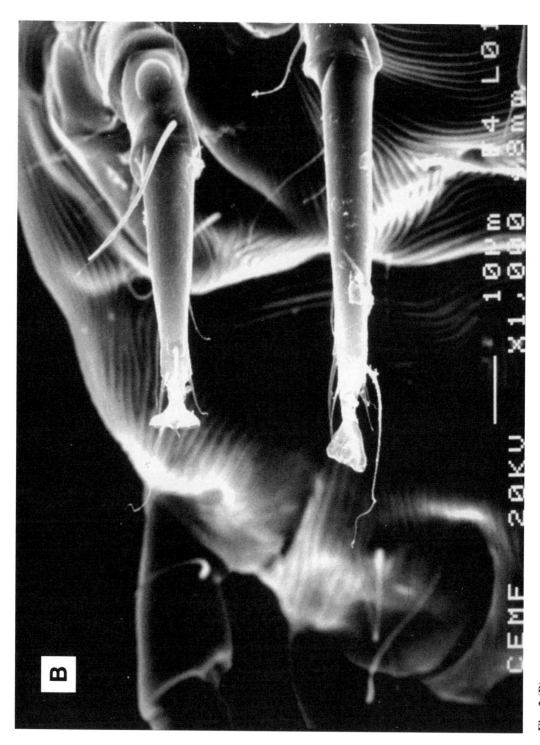

Fig. 2.(B)

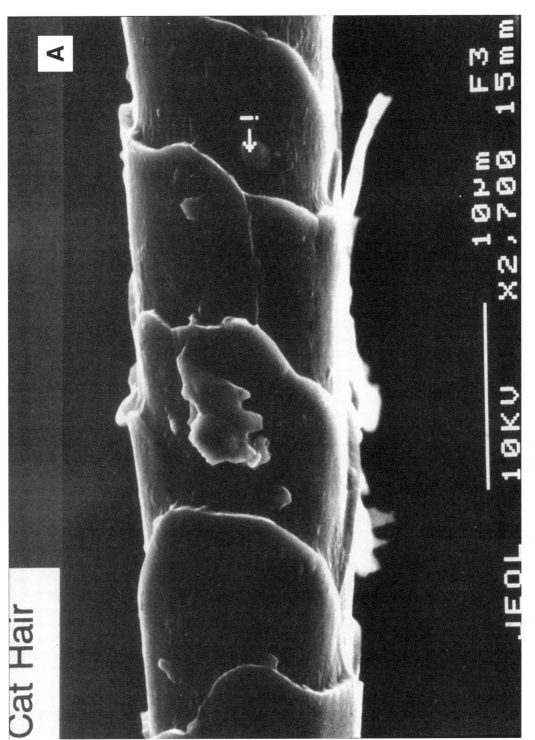

Fig. 3.(A) Cat hair showing shaft ~10 μm diameter and adherent fragments of dander. (Courtesy of Dr. J. Woodfolk, Virginia.)

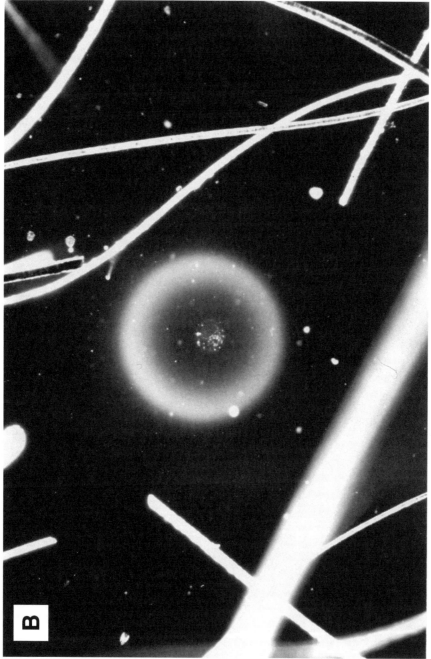

Fig. 3.(B) Micro-ochterlony technique with cat hairs and fragments of dander. (Courtesy of Dr. E. Tovey, Sydney University.)

SPIDERS, MOTHS, SILVERFISH

Houses contain many different arthropods and, inevitably, they all contribute proteins to house dust that could become allergens *(39)*. In some cases this is obvious because a closely related insect has been shown to be a source of allergens. Thus, crickets are close relatives of grasshoppers and locusts, which are very potent causes of sensitization in a laboratory setting. Moths have been shown to be a source of allergen in Japan and in an experimental setting. Although it is inevitable that many different species contribute to the allergenicity of house dust, in most cases there are insufficient studies to demonstrate their importance epidemiologically, and the immunochemistry of the allergens has not been studied.

PURIFIED ALLERGENS

Allergens have been purified from many different sources and, not surprisingly, they represent a diverse collection of proteins. By 1980, it was already clear that inhalant allergens had common physical properties *(56)*. They are rapidly soluble in aqueous solution and are rather homogeneous in size: 15–50 kDa, and they are immunologically foreign. The size appears to reflect some simple physical characteristics of the nasal epithelium. The basement membrane is only permeable to molecules < 60 kDa, and proteins < 15 kDa would be expected to pass rapidly into the blood stream. The implication is that the size of the major allergens reflects those proteins that would be most likely be presented to the local lymph nodes. Many allergens have now been purified, sequenced, and cloned (Tables 3 and 4). The first full sequence of an inhaled allergen was reported by Mole in 1975 (Amb a 5) *(5)*. In most cases the biological roles of these proteins have not been established; however, their function may be apparent from sequence homology with known proteins from other species. No common chemical characteristics of allergens have become obvious, although many of the proteins have sequence homology with known enzymes (*see* Tables 3 and 4). It has been known for 30 yr that allergen extracts have enzymic activity. More recently, enzymic activity has been demonstrated with purified allergens *(57)*. It has also been proposed that enzymic activity is relevant to allergenicity. There are some aspects of this question that are susceptible to experimental investigation. Is it likely that these proteins are enzymically active under conditions in the nasal epithelium where that property could influence the immune response to them? Secondly, what aspect of the immune response would be affected by the enzymic activity? In evaluating the possible local effects of allergens it is essential to know what concentration of the protein is present. Several estimates of exposure to allergens have suggested that 5–50 ng of allergen is inhaled per day. Clearly, diluting 5 ng into the human respiratory tract or circulation would result in a very low concentration. On the other hand, the calculated concentration of Lol p 1 in a Rye grass pollen, or of Der p 1 in a mite fecal particle is ~10 mg/mL. Thus, there may well be a sufficient local concentration at the site of deposition of a particle for these enzymes to be active. It has been demonstrated that Der p 1, which has strong homology to cysteine proteases, can cleave CD23 on the surface of B cells, and it was speculated that the activity could increase its immunogenicity *(58)*. At present we could conclude:

1. Many allergens have sequence homology with known enzymes and some have been shown to have enzymic activity in the laboratory *(57,59–61)*.
2. Several important allergens (e.g., Fel d 1, Der p 2, and Bla g 4) have no sequence homology with enzymes and no enzymic activity *(9,41,62–65)*.
3. It remains to be proved that allergens have enzymic activity in vivo.
4. The view that enzymic activity could be an important property of allergens remains a hypothesis.

Table 3
Properties of Purified Indoor Allergens

Source and Allergens		Molecular weight, kDa	Sequence	Status[a]	Function	MAbs[b]	Assay
House Dust Mite							
Group 1[b]	Der p 1	25	cDNA	M	Cysteine	++	ELISA
	Der f 1	25	cDNA	M	protease	++	ELISA
	Eur m 1	25	Nucleotide	—		+	—
Group 2	Der p 2	14	cDNA	M	Unknown	++	ELISA
	Der f 2	14	n-terminal	M		++	ELISA
Group 3	Der p 3	29	n-terminal	—	Serine	—	RIA[a]
	Der f 3	29	terminal	—	proteases	++	RIA[a]
Blomia							
tropicalis	Blo t 5	14	cDNA	M	Unknown	—	RIA
Cat—(*Felis domesticus*)							
Fel d 1		35	cDNA	M	Unknown	++	ELISA
Albumin		68	—	—	—	+	RIA[a]
Dog—(*Canis familiaris*)							
Can f 1		27	cDNA	M	Unknown	++	ELISA[a]
Cockroach							
Blatella germanica							
Bla g 1		20–25	—	—	Unknown	+	ELISA[a]
Bla g 2		36	cDNA	M	—	++	ELISA
Bla g 4		21	cDNA	M		++	ELISA
Bla g 5		23	cDNA	M	Gluathione transferase		
Periplanetta americana							
Per a 1		20–25	—	?	Unknown	—	—
Rodents							
Mus musculus		19	Protein	?	Alpha-2U-	+	ELISA[a]
Rattus norvegicus		19	cDNA	M	globulin	+	RIA[a]
Fungi							
Aspergillus, Asp f 1			cDNA	M		++	RIA
Alternaria, Alt a 1			cDNA	M		+	RIA

[a]M, major allergens, i.e., ≥50% of allergic subjects react with the allergen.
[b]++, more than one epitope has been defined; +, one MAG only.
[c]Groups 1, 2, and 3 include both Der p 1 and Der f 1, and so on.

The ability to clone proteins has had several consequences in relation to studying allergens. Sequencing more allergens has confirmed that they are a diverse group of proteins with no common properties from the point of view of sequence. Some of the earliest proteins that were expressed in vitro had very poor ability to bind IgE antibodies (e.g., Der p 1) *(7)*. However, many recombinant proteins have normal or near normal tertiary structure as judged by skin test reactivity or in vitro binding studies. Currently, tertiary structure of several allergens (e.g.,

Table 4
Properties of Purified Pollen and Fungal Allergens

Source	Allergen	Molecular Weight, kDa	Sequence	Status	Function
Grasses					
Lolium perenne	Lol p 1	27	cDNA	M	Unknown
	Lol p 2	11	cDNA	M	Unknown
	Lol p 3	11	cDNA	M	Unknown
	Lol p 10	12	cDNA	—	Cytochrome C
Phleum pratense	Phl p 5	15	cDNA	M	Ribonuclease?
Poa pratense	Poa p 10	12	—	—	Cytochrome
Trees					
Betula verrucosa	Bet v 1	17	cDNA	M	Unknown
Alnus incana	Aln i 1	17	—	M	Unknown
Weeds					
Ambrosia atemisifolia	Amb a 1	37	cDNA/P	M	Unknown
(ragweed)	Amb a 2	38	—	—	Unknown
	Amb a 5	5	cDNA/P	M	Recognition protein
Salsola pestifer (Russian thistle)	Sol p 1	39	—	M	Unknown
Parietaria	Par j 1	—	—	—	—
Fungi					
Alternaria alternata	Alt a 1	30	Protein	M	—

Der p 2 and Bet v 1) is being investigated using NMR and X-ray crystallography *(66,67)*. The tertiary structure will allow rational prediction of antibody binding sites and site-directed mutagenesis to produce molecules in which binding to IgE antibodies is reduced. Mutagenesis directed at disulfide bonds on Der p 2 has already been used to produce molecules with 100-fold less skin reactivity *(68)*. Recombinant technology will also make it possible to produce large quantities of these proteins. These molecules could be used to standardize extracts, in cocktails as skin test reagents, or in a mutagenesized form for immunotherapy. The use of such allergens for standardization will depend on establishing that the recombinant is not an immunologically distinct isoform *(69)*. There is a real possibility that MAbs (but not poly-clonal antisera) will identify one isoform selectively. Thus, using a recombinant in conjunction with monoclonal antibody-based assay, requires establishing that the cloned molecule is representative of "wild-type" antigen.

Recombinant technology could contribute to new forms of immunotherapy by providing consistent supplies of antigen and by producing mutants or large peptides (i.e., ≥40 amino acids in length). Currently peptides from Fel d 1 and from Amb a 1 (which are ~26 amino acids and are synthesized) are being used in clinical trials with injections of up to 750 µg/dose. The results so far demonstrate significant effects but are not as dramatic as many had hoped *(70)*. Future work on designing modified recombinant molecules would best be based on ter-tiary structure. However, tertiary structure of molecules larger than 20 kDa may be difficult to obtain, since this is currently the maximum size for NMR, and crystallizing larger proteins remains a hit-and-miss experiment.

CONCLUSIONS

All mammals have a very advanced immune system that plays a major role in survival by rapidly reacting to infectious organisms. These immune responses can be of very different types, but helminth parasites give rise to a complex response including IgE antibodies, eosinophils, and T-cells of the T_H2 phenotype. Recent evidence in animals has confirmed that the type of immune response may be critical for successful elimination of an infection. The immune response to *Leishmania* has to be T_H1 in type; by contrast, successful elimination of parasites requires a T_H2 response *(71–73)*. Allergens induce a response that includes most of the features of the response to helminth parasites. Increased understanding of the proteins involved has not revealed any special biochemical properties that would explain this response. On the other hand, it is clear that natural exposure to environmental allergens represents repeated low-dose exposure and that an immunization regime of this kind can induce a similar response in mice. Natural exposure to pollen, mite, cat, dog, or cockroach allergens represents > 1 µg/d. The logical conclusion is that allergic patients are those individuals who are capable of responding to low doses of soluble proteins. In turn, the key characteristic of inhalant allergens is that they become airborne in a form that will deliver soluble proteins to the nasal mucosa.

The properties of particles that become airborne are governed by simple rules. Particles over 50 µm in diameter will fall so rapidly that they are unlikely to be inhaled. Particles of ~20 µm will take >10 min to fall in still air, while particles <5 µm in diameter may remain airborne for prolonged periods. In a wind, large particles such as pollen grains 20–35 µm in diameter may remain airborne for days and travel hundreds of miles. The volume of these particles is given by the formula $4/3 \ \pi r^3$, and this governs the quantity of protein they are likely to carry. A single pollen grain of 20 µm would carry 1000 times the quantity of protein found in a 2-µm fungal spore. These characteristics mean that there is a fairly restricted range of particles that are likely to be relevant to allergic disease (1–35 µm). These sizes are also highly relevant to particles entering the lung: inhaling 100 mite fecal particles, as few as 5% of which enter the bronchi, would deliver 100 times more protein than breathing in 1000 fungal spores of 2 µm as many as 40% of which could enter the bronchi *(74,75)*. In addition to their size, the particles that become airborne differ in other properties, particularly the nature of their external layer. The cuticle of a pollen grain has pores, the peritrophic membrane surrounding a mite fecal particle will allow free passage of proteins, and, by contrast, the outer layer of most fungal spores is designed to resist desiccation and is not permeable. Exposure to fungal proteins may occur after germination of the spore (as is thought to occur with *A. fumigatus*) or from particles such as hyphae. What is clear is that the properties of the airborne particles are just as important as the nature of the protein.

Over the last 10 yr there has been a very rapid expansion of knowledge about the proteins that cause allergic disease. This means that the major allergens are defined both by sequence data and by specific MAbs. The sequence data have confirmed that the allergens represent a very diverse group of proteins in keeping with the very wide range of sources. For several allergens, it has been possible to synthesize overlapping peptides and to define the peptides that are recognized by T cells and also to begin to identify the sites that react with antibodies. However, most of the sites that bind antibodies (B-cell epitopes) are dependent on the conformation of the molecule and cannot be defined using peptides. Current work should provide tertiary structure for some allergens and make it possible both to define epitopes that bind to IgE antibodies and to create mutagenized recombinants that have these epitopes modified.

Almost any foreign protein that is soluble, has a mol wt between 15 and 60 kDa and is delivered regularly to the nasal epithelium can become an allergen. Whether the increase in allergic disease, and particularly asthma, can be attributed to increased exposure to allergens or reflects a change in susceptibility has not been resolved. What is clear is that the investigation, diagnosis, and management of allergic disease is dependent on determination of sensitization and accurate measurement of exposure to both indoor and outdoor allergens. It is also clear that we spend an inordinate amount of time indoors and that many patients benefit from reducing exposure to allergens in their houses *(15)*. The advances that have occurred over the last 10 yr have made it possible to quantitatively study the relationship between exposure and sensitization, to design avoidance regimes, and to develop new strategies for immunotherapy. Many different allergen-specific approaches are being developed to manage allergic disease. On the one hand, T-cell peptides are being tested for immunotherapy, and mutagenized recombinant molecules are being designed that could be used in immunotherapy. On the other hand, aggressive physical measures to decrease exposure to relevant indoor allergens are now an important part of managing perennial rhinitis, asthma, and atopic dermatitis.

ACKNOWLEDGMENT

This work was supported by NIH Grants AI-20565, AI-30840, and AI-34607.

REFERENCES

1. Blackley CH (1959) Experimental research in the causes and nature of catarrhus aestivus (hay fever or hay asthma). Dawson, London.
2. King TP, Norman PS (1962) Isolation studies of allergens from ragweed pollen. Biochem 1:709–720.
3. Marsh DG (1975) Allergens and the genetics of allergy. In: Sela M, ed. The Antigens. Academic, New York, pp, 271–360.
4. Ohman JL, Lowell FC, Bloch KJ. (1974) Allergens of mammalian origin. III. Properties of a major feline allergen. J Immunol 113:1668–1676.
5. Mole LE, Goodfriend L, Lapkoff CB, Kehoe JM, Capra JD. (1975) The amino acid sequence of ragweed pollen allergen Ra5. Biochemistry 14:1216–1220.
6. Chapman MD, Sutherland WM, Platts-Mills TAE. (1984) Recognition of two *Dermatophagoides pteronyssinus*-specific epitopes on antigen P1 by using monoclonal antibodies: binding to each epitope can be inhibited by serum from dust mite-allergic patients. J Immunol 133:2488–2495.
7. Chua KY, Stewart GA, Thomas WR, Simpson RJ, Dilworth RJ, Plozza TM, Turner KJ. (1988) Sequence analysis of cDNA coding for a major house dust mite allergen, Der p I: Homology with cysteine proteases. J Exp Med 167:175–182.
8. Luczynska CM, Arruda LK, Platts-Mills TAE, Miller JD, Lopez M, Chapman MD. (1989) A two-site monoclonal antibody ELIZA for the quantitation of the major *Dermatophagoides* spp. allergens, *Der p* I and *Der f* I. J Immunol Meth 118:227–235.
9. Chapman MD, Aalberse RC, Brown MJ, Platts-Mills TAE. (1988) Monoclonal antibodies to the major feline allergen *Fel d* I. II. Single step affinity purification of *Fel d* I, N-terminal sequence analysis, and development of a sensitive two-site immunoassay to assess *Fel d* I exposure. J Immunol 140:812–818.
10. Tovey ER, Chapman MD, Wells CW, Platts-Mills TAE. (1981) The distribution of dust mite allergen in the houses of patients with asthma. Amer Rev Resp Dis 124:630–635.
11. Findlay S, Stosky E, Lietermann K, Hemady Z, Ohman JL. (1983) Allergens detected in association with airborne particles capable of penetrating into the peripheral lung. Am Rev Respir Dis 128:1008–1012.
12. Luczynska CM, Li Y, Chapman MD, Platts-Mills TAE. (1990) Airborne concentrations and particle size distribution of allergen derived from domestic cats (*Felis domesticus*): Measurements using cascade impactor, liquid impinger and a two site monoclonal antibody assay for *Fel d* I. Am Rev Resp Dis 141:361–367.
13. Mollet JA, Vailes LD, Avner DB, Perzanowski MS, Arruda LK, Chapman MD, Platts-Mills TAE. (1997) Evaluation of German cockroach (Orthoptera: *Blattelidae*) allergen and seasonal variation in low-income housing. J Med Entomol 34:307–311.

14. Platts-Mills TAE, Chapman MD. (1987) Dust mites: immunology, allergic disease, and environmental control [Review]. J Allergy Clin Immunol 80:755–775.
15. Platts-Mills TAE, Thomas WR, Aalberse RC, Vervloet D, Chapman MD (1992) Dust mite allergens and asthma: Report of a 2nd international workshop. J Allergy Clin Immunol 89:1046–1060.
16. Peat JK, Salome CM, Woolcock AJ (1990) Longitudinal changes in atopy during a 4 year period: relation to bronchial hyperresponsiveness and respiratory symptoms in a population sample of Australian schoolchildren. J Allergy Clin Immunol 85:65–74.
17. Lau S, Falkenhorst G, Weber A, Werthman I, Lind P, Bucttner-Goetz P, Wahn U (1989) High mite-allergen exposure increases the risk of sensitization in atopic children and young adults. J Allergy Clin Immunol 84:718–725.
18. Kuehr J, Frischer T, Meinert R, Barth R, Forster J, Schraub S, Urbanek R, Karmaus W (1994) Mite allergen exposure is a risk for the incidence of specific sensitization. J Allergy Clin Immunol 94:44–52.
19. Sporik RB, Holgate ST, Platts-Mills TAE, Cogswell J (1990) Exposure to house dust mite allergen (*Der p* I) and the development of asthma in childhood: A prospective study. N Eng J Med 323: 502–507.
20. Tovey ER, Chapman MD, Platts-Mills TAE (1981) Mite faeces are a major source of house dust allergens. Nature 289:592–593.
21. Lewis WH, Vinay P, Zenger VE, eds. (1983) Airborne and Allergenic Pollen of North America. The Johns Hopkins University, Baltimore.
22. Solomon WR, Mathews KP (1988) Aerobiology and inhalant allergens. In: Middleton E, ed. Allergy Principles and Practice. Mosby, St. Louis, pp. 312–372.
23. Norman PS, Marsh DG, Lichtenstein LM (1979) Long term immunotherapy with ragweed allergen and allergoid. J Allergy Clin Immunol 63:166.
24. Reid MJ, Moss RB, Hsu YP, Kwasnicki JM, Commerford TM, Nelson BL (1986) Seasonal asthma in northern California: allergic causes and efficacy of immunotherapy. J Allergy Clin Immunol 78:590–600.
25. Strachan DP, Flannigan B, McCabe EM, McGarry F (1990) Quantification of airborne moulds in the homes of children with wheeze. Thorax 45:382–387.
26. O'Holleren MT, Yuninger JW, Offord KP, Somers MJ, O'Connell EJ, Ballard DJ, Sachs MI (1991) Exposure to an aeroallergen as a possible precipitating factor in respiratory arrest in young patients with asthma. N Eng J Med 324:359–363.
27. Lehrer SR, Lopez M, Butcher BT, Olson J, Reed M, Salvaggio JE (1986) Basidiomycete mycelia and spore-allergen extracts: skin test reactivity in adults with symptoms of respiratory allergy. J Allergy Clin Immunol 78:478–485.
28. Neas LM, Dockery DW, Burge H, Koutrakis P, Speizer FE (1996) Fungus spores, air pollutants and other determinants of peak expiratory flow rate in children. Am J Epidemiol 143:797–807.
29. Sporik RB, Arruda LK, Woodfolk J, Chapman MD, Platts-Mills TAE (1993) Environmental exposure to *Aspergillus fumigatus* (*Asp f* I). Clin Exp Allergy 23:326–331.
30. Deards MJ, Montague AE (1991) Purification and characterization of a major allergen of *Alternaria alternata*. Mol Immunol 28:409–15.
31. Kern RA (1921) Dust sensitization in bronchial asthma. Med Clin N Am 5:751–758.
32. Tuft LA (1949) Importance of inhalant allergen in atopic dermatitis. J Invest Derm 12:211–219.
33. Voorhorst R, Spieksma FThM, Varekamp H, Leupen MJ, Lyklema AW (1967) The house dust mite (*Dermatophagoides pteronyssinus*) and the allergens it produces: Identity with the house dust allergen. J Allergy 39:325–339.
34. Smith JM, Disney ME, Williams JD, Goels ZA (1969) Clinical significance of skin reactions to mite extracts in children with asthma. Brit Med J 1:723–726.
35. Clarke CW, Aldons PW (1979) The nature of asthma in Brisbane. Clin Allergy 9:147.
36. Miyamoto T, Oshima S, Ishizaka T, Sato S (1968) Allergic identity between the common floor mite (*Dermatophagoides farinae*, Hughes 1961) and house dust as a causative agent in bronchial asthma. J Allergy Clin Immunol 42:14–28.
37. Arlian LG (1989) Biology and ecology of house dust mites, *Dermatophagoides* spp. and *Euroglyphus* spp. Imm All Clinics N A 9:339–356.
38. Wharton GW (1976) House dust mites [Review]. J Med Entomol 12:577–621.
39. Van Bronswijk JEMH (1981) House dust biology. NIB Publishers, Zoelmond.

40. Charpin C, Mata P, Charpin D, Lavaut MN, Allasia C, Vervloet D (1991) Fel d I allergen distribution in cat fur and skin. J Allergy Clin Immunol 88:77.

41. Morgenstern J, Griffith I, Bauer A, Bond J, Rogers B, Chapman MD, Kuo M (1991) Determination of the amino acid sequence of *Fel d* I, the major allergen of the domestic cat: protein sequence analysis and cDNA cloning. Proc Natl Acad Sci USA 88:9690–9694.

42. Ingram JM, Sporik R, Rose G, Honsinger R, Chapman MD, Platts-Mills TAE (1995) Quantitative assessment of exposure to dog (Can f I) and cat (Fel d I) allergens: Relationship to sensitization and asthma among children living in Los Alamos, NM. J Allergy Clin Immunol 96:449–56.

43. Custovic A, Green R, Fletcher A, Smith A, Pickering CAC, Chapman MD, Woodcock AA (1997) Aerodynamic properties of the major dog allergen. Can f 1: Distribution in homes, concentration and particle size of allergens in the air. Amer J Resp Crit Care Med 155:94–98.

44. Longbottom JL (1983) Characterization of allergens from the urines of experimental animals. In: Kerr JW, Ganderston MA, eds. Proceedings of the XI International Congress of Allergology and Clinical Immunology. Macmillan, London, p. 525.

45. Platts-Mills TAE, Heymann PW, Longbottom JL, Wilkins SR (1986) Airborne allergens associated with asthma: particle sizes carrying dust mite and rat allergens measured with a cascade impactor. J Allergy Clin Immunol 77:850–857.

46. Hesford JD, Platts-Mills TAE, Edlich RF (1995) Anaphylaxis after laboratory rat bite: an occupational hazard. J Emerg Med 13:765–768.

47. Bernton HS, Brown H (1964) Insect allergy: preliminary studies of the cockroach. J Allergy Clin Immunol 35:506–513.

48. Twarog FJ, Picone FJ, Strunk RS, So J, Colten HR (1976) Immediate hypersensitivity to cockroach: isolation and purification of the major antigens. J Allergy Clin Immunol 59:154–160.

49. Pollart SM, Chapman MD, Fiocco GP, Rose G, Platts-Mills TAE (1989) Epidemiology of acute asthma: IgE antibodies to common inhalant allergens as a risk factor for emergency room visits. J Allergy Clin Immunol 83:875–882.

50. Hulett AC, Dockhorn RJ (1979) House dust mite (*D. farinae*) and cockroach allergy in a midwestern population. Ann Allergy 42:160–165.

51. Gelber LE, Seltzer LH, Bouzoukis JK, Pollart SM, Chapman MD, Platts-Mills TAE (1993) Sensitization and exposure to indoor allergens as risk factors for asthma among patients presenting to hospital. Amer Rev Resp Dis 147:573–578.

52. Call RS, Smith TF, Morris E, Chapman MD, Platts-Mills TAE (1992) Risk factors for asthma in inner city children. J Pediatr 121:862–866.

53. Rosenstreich DL (1996) Relationship between sensitization, allergen levels and asthma morbidity in inner city children. Am J Resp Crit Care Med 153:255A.

54. Pollart S, Smith TF, Morris EC, Gelber LE, Platts-Mills TAE, Chapman MD (1991) Environmental exposure to cockroach allergens: Analysis with monoclonal antibody-based enzyme immunoassays. J Allergy Clin Immunol 87:505–510.

55. De Blay F, Kassel O, Chapman MD, Ott M, Verot A, Pauli G (1992) Mise en evidence des allergenes majeurs des blattes par test ELISA dans la poussiere domestique. La Press Med 21:1685.

56. Platts-Mills TAE (1982) Type I or immediate hypersensitivity: Hay fever and asthma. In: Lachmann PJ, Peters DK, eds. Clinical Aspects of Immunology. Blackford, Oxford, 579–686.

57. Stewart GA, Thompson PJ (1996) The biochemistry of common aeroallergens. Clin Exp Allergy 26:1020–1044.

58. Hewitt CRA, Brown AP, Hart BJ, Pritchard DI (1995) A major house dust allergen disrupts the Immunoglobulin E network by selectively cleaving CD23: innate protection by antiproteases. J Exp Med 182:1537–44.

59. Chapman MD, Platts-Mills TAE (1980) Purification and characterization of the major allergen from *Dermatophagoides pteronyssinus*-antigen P1. J Immunol 125:587–592.

60. Arruda LK, Vailes LD, Hayden ML, Benjamin DC, Chapman MD (1995) Molecular cloning of cockroach allergen, Bla g 4, identifies ligand binding proteins (or calycins) as a cause of IgE antibody responses. J Biol Chem 270:31,196–31,201.

61. Arruda LK, Vailes LD, Platts-Mills TAE, Hayden ML, Chapman MD (1997) Induction of IgE antibody responses by glutathione S-transferase from the German cockroach (blattella germanica). J Biol Chem 33:20,907–20,912.

62. Heymann PW, Chapman MD, Aalberse RC, Fox JW, Platts-Mills TAE (1989) Antigenic and structural analysis of Group II allergens (*Der f* II and *Der p* II) from house dust mites (Dermatophagoides spp). J Allergy Clin Immunol 83:1055–1067.

63. Chua KY, Dilworth RJ, Thomas WR (1990) Expression of *Dermatophagoides pteronyssinus* allergen *Der p* II in *Escherichia coli* and binding studies with human IgE. Int Arch Allergy Appl Immunol 91:124–129.

64. Arruda LK, Vailes LD, Hayden ML, Benjamin DC, Chapman MD. Molecular cloning of cockroach allergens, Bla g 4, identifies ligand binding proteins (or calycins) as a cause of IgE antibody responses. J Biol Chem 270:31196–31201.

65. Ansari AA, Shenbagamurthi P, Marsh DG (1989) Complete primary structure of a *Lolium perenne* pollen allergen, Lol p III: Comparison with known Lol p I and Lol p II sequences. Biochem 28:8665–70.

66. Mueller G, Smith AM, Williams DC, Hakkaart GAJ, Aalberse RC, Chapman MD, Rule GS, Benjamin DC (1997) Expression and secondary structure determination by NMR methods of the major house-dust-mite allergen Der p 2. J Biol Chem 272:26,893–26,898.

67. Fedorov AA, Ball T, Valenta R, Almo SC (1997) X-ray crystal structures of birch pollen profilin and Phl p 2. Int Arch Immunol 113:109–113.

68. Smith AM, Chapman MD (1996) Reduction in IgE binding to allergen variants generated by site-directed mutagenesis: contribution of disulfide bonds to the antigenic structure of the major house dust mite allergen, Der p 2. Mol Immunol 33:399–405.

69. Chua KY, Huang CH, Shen HD, Thomas WR (1996) Analysis of sequence polymorphism of a major mite allergen, Der p 2. Clin Exp Allergy 26:829–837.

70. Norman PS, Ohman JL, Long AA, Creticos PS, Gefter ML, Shaked Z, Wood RA, Eggleston PA, Lichtenstein LM, Jones NH, Nicodemus CF (1995) Follow on study of the first clinical trial with T cell defined peptides from cat allergen Fel d 1. J Allergy Clin Immunol 95:259.

71. Urban JR Jr, Madden KB, Svetic A, Cheever A, Trotta PP, Gause WC, Katona IM, Finkelman FD (1992) The importance of T_H2 cytokines in protective immunity to nematodes. Immunol Rev 127:205–20.

72. Alfonso LCC, Scharton TM, Viera LQ, Wysocka M, Trinchieri G, Scott P (1994) The adjuvant effect of interleukin-12 in a vaccine against *Leishmania major*. Science 263:235.

73. Abbas Abul K, Murphy KM, Sher A (1996) Functional diversity of helper T-lymphocytes. Nature 383:787–793.

74. Svartengren M, Falk R, Linnman L, Philipson K, Camner P (1987) Deposition of large particles in human lung. Experimental Lung Research 12:75–88.

75. Task Group on Lung Dynamics (1966) Deposition and retention models for internal dosimetry of the human respiratory tract. Health Phys 12:173–207.

4

Ontogeny of Allergy

Bengt Björkstén, MD

INTRODUCTION

Sensitization, as proven by the demonstration of low levels of immunoglobin E (IgE) antibodies directed against environmental allergens, appears to be part of the normal immune response *(1)*. In most instances these antibodies are only temporary, as the continuing IgE antibody formation is rapidly suppressed. But when genetically predisposed individuals are exposed to an allergen at a time when the regulation of the immune system is immature, then higher levels of IgE antiIbodies, lasting for a long time, may appear. The more susceptible to sensitization the individual is, the lower is the allergen dose needed for this to occur. The fact that an individual is sensitized does not, however, necessarily mean that clinical symptoms, i.e., allergic disease, will develop. It is not known which factors decide what allergic manifestations will appear in an atopic individual, e.g., whether he or she will suffer from atopic dermatitis, asthma, hay fever, gastrointestinal allergy, or several of them.\It is likely, however, that the selection of a target organ is also at least partially under genetic control.

Sensitivity to allergens and manifest disease are thus the end results of an interaction between genetically determined susceptibility to atopy, exposure to allergen, and exposure to adjuvant factors. In this chapter the ontogeny of allergy will be discussed, including the impact of certain factors that may either enhance or reduce the likelihood of sensitization and trigger clinical disease in sensitized individuals (Table 1).

CLINICAL ASPECTS

The Atopic March

The clinical manifestations of allergy vary with age. Dermatitis, appearing on the face and trunk during the first months of life, is often the initial clinical manifestation of the "atopic

From: *Allergy and Allergic Diseases: The New Mechanisms and Therapeutics*
Edited by: J. A. Denburg © Humana Press Inc., Totowa, NJ

Table 1
Factors Possibly Affecting the Development of Sensitization to Allergens and Manifestations of Allergic Disease

Genetic susceptibility
Prenatal
   Maternal medication
   Maternal tobacco smoking
   Maternal immunity?
Infancy and early childhood
   Exposure to tobacco smoke
   Exposure to other air pollutants, e.g., from industry and traffic
   Poorly ventilated homes
   Exposure to chemical compounds, e.g., pesticides, consumer products, building material
   Early formula feeding
   High-level exposure to allergens
   Certain infections, e.g., RSV
Lack of tolerance induction, e.g., few infections, altered intestinal microbial flora?

march." It may be associated with food allergy, gastrointestinal symptoms, and sometimes even systemic manifestations. Although wheezing in conjunction with respiratory infections is commonly encountered in infancy and usually is not a sign of atopy, in the atopic child it may be a forerunner of asthma. If an IgE-mediated allergy is verified, the offending allergen is usually a food, e.g., egg or cow's milk protein.

Infantile eczema usually resolves after infancy, sometimes to recur after 2–3 yr, then as flexural dermatitis, i.e., with a localization similar to that in adults. At this age, it may also become obvious that the wheezing infant has now developed clinically manifest asthma. For unknown reasons most children become clinically tolerant to foods, and IgE-mediated food allergy is therefore relatively uncommon after 4 yr. Instead, clinically manifest allergy to inhalant allergens becomes increasingly common after this age.

The next step in the "atopic march" is the development of allergic rhinoconjunctivitis, with an increasing prevalence from about 5 yr of age, although in a few children the manifestations may appear earlier in life. The prevalence of atopic manifestations often decreases during puberty, often to recur, however, in early adulthood, reaching a peak prevalence in the late 20s.

Sensitization in Early Life

It is thus obvious that the likelihood of developing an allergic disease is not constant over time, even if the general propensity is genetically determined. Not only clinical symptomatology but also the risk of sensitization is affected by the precise time and the conditions under which exposure to allergens takes place. With regard to sensitization, there seems to be a period in early life during which an infant is particularly susceptible to sensitization (1,2). This could partly explain the observation in several, but not all, studies indicating that early weaning to cow's milk formula may be associated with an increased risk for allergic disease (reviewed in refs. 3 and 4).

The increased likelihood for sensitization after exposure to allergens in early infancy appears to be true also for inhalant allergens, even if the clinical symptoms of allergy may not become obvious for many years. In a large epidemiological study comprising 40,000 individuals, a Finnish team observed a significantly higher prevalence of allergy to birch and grass pollen in 10-yr-old children who were born in the spring than in children who were born at other times of the year (5). Subsequently the authors reported that the risk of pollen allergy, as diagnosed at 10 yr of age, was affected not only by the month of birth, but also by the intensity of the pollen season during the year they were born *(6)*. The intensity of the first pollen season even had a stronger impact than the intensity of the pollen season when the symptoms first appeared. A similar increase in grass allergy has been reported in British children born in the spring *(7)* and for the prevalence of ragweed allergy in Americans born during the peak ragweed season in the late summer *(8)*. Similar to the apparent effects of early exposure to pollen, early contacts with animal epithelia and house dust appear to influence the incidence of allergy. Thus, children born in the autumn, i.e., before the main indoor season, seem to be more prone to sensitization to indoor allergens than babies born at other times of the year *(9,10)*.

In a Swedish study it was observed, however, that the relationship between season of birth and allergy development was limited to children with elevated IgE levels in the cord blood, i.e., with a congenital propensity for allergy *(11)*, again supporting the concept that manifestations of disease are the result of an interaction between environmental and genetic factors. These observations in pollen-, dander-, and mite-sensitive individuals could indicate that early exposure to an allergen increases the risk for allergy or alternatively the presence of seasonal variations in the transfer of maternal immunity to seasonal allergens.

Variations in the Propensity to Sensitization

Variations in individual susceptibility to sensitization over time may also partly be explained by the presence or absence of respiratory tract infection. The role of infections in the respiratory tract as risk factors for the development of childhood allergic disease and asthma is complex, however. It is well established that infections may trigger and aggravate asthma in already sensitized individuals and that infections increase bronchial hyperreactivity. On the other hand, recent data indicate that recurrent infections during the time period when primary immune responses to inhaled allergens occur, i.e., usually in early childhood, may in fact prevent sensitization. The presence or absence of infections may thus explain variations in susceptibility to disease manifestations in the individual over time. The role of infections in relation to sensitization is discussed in more detail below.

There are also other environmental factors that may affect the likelihood for sensitization at a certain time. Animal studies and clinical observations have indicated that stress alters the immune response, as measured by various laboratory tests of inflammatory responses, immunoglobulin production, and cell-mediated immunity *(12,13)*. Clinical studies also indicate that stress may cause reduced resistance to infections *(14,15)*. While it is well established that psychological factors influence the severity of asthmatic symptoms and allergic reactions in affected patients, little is known regarding a possible adjuvant effect on sensitization.

EPIDEMIOLOGICAL ASPECTS

Epidemiological studies show that there are large regional differences in the prevalence of asthma and allergies both in children and in adults *(16–19)*. With the exception of a few isolated groups of people, the reported differences between populations are not genetically determined. Rather, they seem to be explained by differences in living conditions. Factors associated with "Western lifestyle" appear to have resulted in a large increase in the prevalence of allergic disorders over the past few decades *(20–23)*. The increase seems so far to be largely limited to children and young adults under 35 yr of age, i.e., to cohorts born after about 1960 (Fig. 1). It is likely that environmental factors that are encountered in early childhood are of particular significance and that the increasing prevalence seen in young adults is a result of a cohort effect.

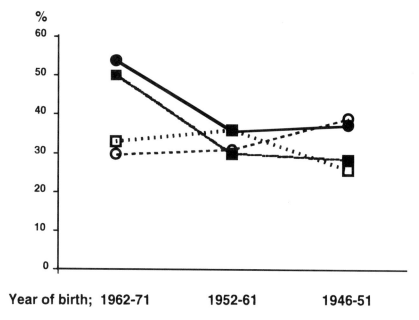

Fig. 1. Prevalence of circulating IgE antibodies and positive skin prick tests to inhaled allergens in Eastern and Western Germany after the reunification of the country, in relation to year of birth (data from ref. *23*). West: ■, skin prick test; ●, radioallergosorbent test. East: □, skin prick test; ○, RAST.

The regional differences are not caused by genetic factors. This statement is supported by the results from studies in genetically similar populations living under different conditions in the same country and studies comparing migrants with those who remained in their community of origin. Thus, the prevalence of allergic disease in developing countries seems to be higher in people living under privileged conditions than among the poor. More than 20 yr ago Morrison Smith observed that the prevalence of asthma was low in children migrating to Britain from the West Indies with their parents *(7)*. Interestingly, the prevalence of asthma in the younger children in these families, who were born in Britain, was similar to that of the native British children. A South African study yielded similar results, in that children of the Xhosa tribe who were born in a rural area had much less asthma and other allergies than Xhosa children raised in Cape Town *(24)*. The influence of living conditions on childhood asthma has also been noted among Tokelauans living in their home environment in the Pacific and in New Zealand, with a much lower prevalence of disease among the former *(25)*.

Environmental differences in the prevalence of allergy are also recorded between urban and rural areas in industrialized countries. As an example, two recent Swedish studies showed that the relative risk for a positive skin prick test is 70% higher among 11-yr-old children living in a moderately polluted town in Northern Sweden than among children living in the neighboring countryside *(26,27)*.

Understanding of the role of environmental factors has become complicated by some recent observations. Air pollution is a major problem in many formerly socialist countries in Central and Eastern Europe. Yet, the prevalence of atopy among children is much lower than in western Europe. As an example, the prevalence of positive skin prick tests in Leipzig in Eastern Germany is less than half of that among children of the same age living in Munich in Western Germany *(28,29)*. Similarly, atopic sensitization is much lower in Konin in Central Poland and in Estonia than in Northern Sweden, despite generally less environmental pollution in the latter

Table 2
Prevalence of Positive Skin Tests and Airway Symptoms Among 11–12-yr-old School Children in Five Regions Around the Baltic Sea and the Levels of Certain Common Air Pollutants[a]

	Sweden		Poland	Estonia	
	Urban	Rural	Konin	Tallinn	Tartu
≥1 positive skin prick test, %	24.2	35.3	13.7	14.3	8.1
Odds ratio[b]	1	1.71	0.49	0.46	0.28
Cough >2 wk, %	5.7	12.0	15.1	18.8	13.8
Respiratory infection >6/yr, %	6.3	8.0	14.0	10.4	10.5
Wheeze, %	.3	11.6	10.4	9.4	5.8
Asthma diagnosed, %	6.7	9.5	2.9	3.2	2.5
SO_2, $\mu g/m^3$ mean	1.9	2.3	17.1	6	?
Range	0.8–3.9	1.0–14.7	4.3–70.9	?	
NO, $\mu g/m^3$, mean	8.4	19.0	17.5	?	?
Range	1.0–34.8	1.3–66.9	3.9–25.9		
Particles, $\mu g/m^3$, mean	4.9	4.4	32.3	?	?
Range	0–11.2	0–21.2	4.9–99.0		

[a]Data from refs. 27 and 30.

[b]? = not determined.

[c]Odds ratio for a positive skin prick test among children in Tallinn (industrialized city) was 1.81 as compared to Tartu (university town).

region (Table 2) *(29–31)*. The low prevalence of atopy was not associated with less respiratory disease in Estonia and Poland, however. Thus, the responses to questionnaires given to 2600 11-yr-old children revealed that symptoms of bronchial hyperreactivity and wheezing were similar to or higher than in Sweden, although the diagnosis "asthma" was much more common in Sweden. The relative influence of known risk factors such as exposure to tobacco smoke, living in a town with air pollution, and a family history of allergy was similar in the three countries. As demonstrated in Fig. 1, the high prevalence of allergy in industrialized countries with a market economy, as opposed to that in the formerly socialist countries in Eastern Europe, seems to be limited to the population born around 1960 or later *(23)*.

The studies in formerly socialistic countries of Eastern and Central Europe strongly indicate that other factors connected with "Western lifestyle" are important for the development of allergy and that these factors have become particularly significant over the last 35 yr. It is not known what these factors are, since the differences cannot be explained by any of the recognized risk factors that are discussed in more detail below.

THE CLINICAL IMMUNOLOGY OF ALLERGY

General Aspects

The analysis of allergen-specific T-cell responses in atopic and nonatopic adult humans has provided proof that allergen-specific T-helper memory cells responsive to the major inhalant allergens occur with comparable frequency in both symptomatic atopic and nonsymptomatic normal subjects *(33)*. The respective T-cell cytokine profiles differed markedly between these groups, however, being polarized toward the murine equivalent of T-helper-1 (Th-1, IL-2 and interferon γ [IFNγ]) in normals versus Th-2 (IL-4 and IL-5) in atopics *(34)*. While it is clear that the murine Th-1/2 paradigm cannot be extrapolated to man without reservation, it has nevertheless proved to be a useful experimental framework for studies in the human system. Thus, recent developments on basic and clinical immunology and the results of several epidemiological studies have given rise to a model for IgE immunoregulation, namely, that the magnitude of the IgE component of antigen-specific immune responses to persistent allergens is ultimately determined by the relative balance between antigen-specific Th-1 and Th-2 cells that become established in relevant T-memory populations (35).

Animal experiments show that repeated inhalation of an allergen by immunologically naive rat pups usually results in a transient low-level IgE antibody response. Susceptibility to this form of tolerance induction is genetically determined (35), but it can be markedly influenced by a range of environmental factors. The T-cell responses in rat pups of a strain with the normal low propensity to IgE antibody formation, "low responders," were mostly of the Th-1 type, while the Th-2 phenotype dominated in pups of an IgE high-responder strain, indicating that the propensity for a certain-type of immune response was genetically determined (Fig. 2). The ultimate expression of Th profiles was, however, influenced by environmental factors. Thus, the Th-2 responses in the high-responder rat pups could be suppressed by exposure to infections and microbial adjuvants concomitantly with the allergen or by high antigen doses. A switch toward Th-2 responses could be induced in pups of the low-responder strain by simultaneously exposing them to allergen and air pollutants, e.g., tobacco smoke.

It is important to note that it was only possible to induce tolerance in animals via inhalation or ingestion against antigens to which the animals were immunologically naive, i.e., once stable immunological memory is established in the Th-2 population and persistent IgE responses develop, further exposure to the relevant antigens only boosts ongoing responses. Additionally, this form of tolerance is preferentially directed against IgE, as the animals typically manifest IgG responses against the same allergens (36).

The efficiency of this "immune deviation" process is determined to a significant extent by genetic factors, as revealed in dose response studies demonstrating 1000- to 10,000-fold differences between animal strains in the threshold exposure levels of aerosolized antigen required for selective suppression of IgE antibody production—the latter occurs in low-IgE-responder strains at (inhaled) antigen doses in the low nanogram range, whereas repeated exposure to doses in the high microgram range is required to elicit similar effects in animals expressing the high-IgE-responder phenotype (37).

Primary Immune Responses to Allergens

The data accumulating on cytokine regulation of IgE synthesis in humans are broadly consistent with the major predictions from the animal models. There are indications that blood mononuclear cells from infants with a family history of allergy have a lower capacity to produce IFN-γ, which would support a less efficient induction of Th-1-type responses (38–40). Furthermore, infants who develop allergic disease during their first 18 mo of life have elevated serum levels of IL-4, which is the major cytokine of Th-2-type cells (41).

The early responses to both food and inhalant allergens are dominated by IL-4. This finding does not prove the initiation of Th-2-skewed immunity but may simply reflect the contribution of naive T-cells undergoing primary stimulation, that may trigger a "default" IL-4 response (42).

The kinetics of humoral antibody responses to food antigens and inhalant allergens in infants and young children lend further support to the clinical relevance of the studies in animals. Thus, IgG antibodies to ubiquitous environmental antigens appear very early in life and remain detectable in serum from the majority of both atopics and normals throughout life (43,44). The picture for IgE antibodies is markedly different, however. Prospective analysis of serum IgE

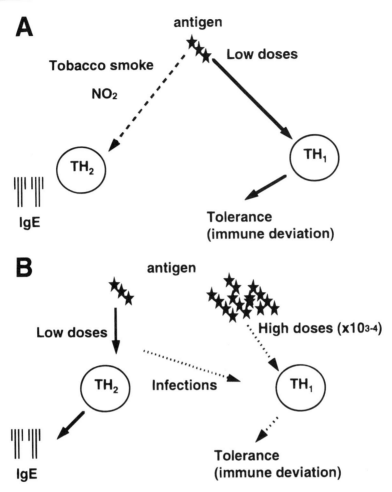

Fig. 2. Primary immune responses to an inhaled antigen in rat pups with a low (**A**) and high (**B**) propensity for IgE antibody formation. The tendency toward a Th1- or Th2-type response is modified by environmental factors, e.g., exposure to high doses of antigen, concurrent infection, and exposure to air pollutants.

levels to environmental allergens in individual children indicates that antibodies to foods are commonly detected both in atopic and nonatopic infants during the first year of life, although the magnitude of the response is higher and of longer duration in the former (Fig. 3) *(45,46).* In virtually all children, these initial IgE responses to foods are terminated spontaneously by age 2–4 yr, leaving intact IgG responses to the same antigens *(47).* In support of these findings, transient skin test reactivity to food allergens is also common during this period *(48).*

The hallmark of the primary immune response of both normal and atopic children to mucosally delivered allergens is thus transient IgE antibody production, which in most cases spontaneously terminates with continued exposure, with the concomitant preservation of low IgG antibody responses. This closely parallels the immune deviation process described above, as the normal response of experimental animals to inhaled antigens.

The pattern for IgE responses to ingested and inhaled allergens differs in at least two significant respects. First, the latter responses usually do not appear until after 1 yr of age, i.e., at a higher age than the IgE responses to foods. Second, whereas IgE responses against foods

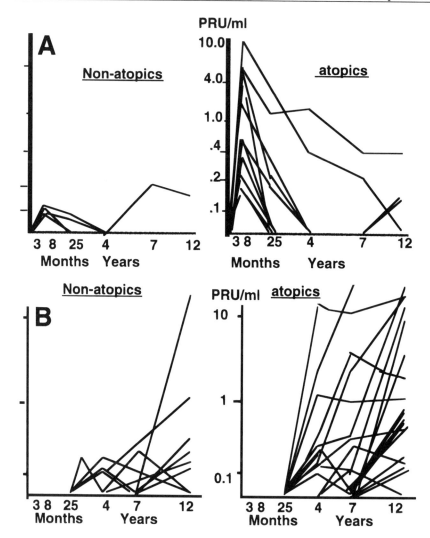

Fig. 3. (**A**) IgE antibodies to egg; (**B**) IgE antibodies to pollen. Appearance of IgE antibodies to ingested and inhaled allergens in atopic and nonatopic individuals (data from ref. *46*).

usually do not persist beyond early childhood, a much larger proportion of children continue to produce IgE antibodies against one or more inhalant allergens into adulthood. Immune responses to both groups of allergens appear to be induced very early in life, in some cases even during fetal life *(49)*.

It appears increasingly likely that one of the key elements of perinatal immune function may be perinatal T-cell cytokine production. Possibly, the kinetics of postnatal maturation of immune competence may be slower in children who are genetically at high risk (HR) for atopy than in their low-risk (LR) counterparts. Thus, in a study performed on children between the ages of 2 and 4 yr, a markedly reduced frequency of immunocompetent T-cell precursors was detected in the blood of MR children, and cloned T-cells from this group demonstrated lower production of IL-4 and (particularly) IFN-γ *(50)*.

During the early postnatal period, this cellular network is poorly developed in experimental animals with respect to both cell density and major histocompatibility complex (MHC) class I expression *(51)* and capacity to respond to inductive cytokine signals *(52)*. The kinetics of postnatal maturation of this network are accelerated by inflammatory stimuli, proceeding most rapidly at sites in the airways of maximal contact with inhaled particulates, in particular, the nasal turbinates. It has not yet been determined whether the human airway dendritic cell network displays a similar ontogenic profile, but on the basis of experience with other organ systems, this seems likely. If so, environmental factors that regulate the development of the dendritic cells may accordingly dictate quantitative and qualitative aspects of inhalant allergen signaling to the central immune system during early postnatal life.

PRENATAL FACTORS

Intrauterine Sensitization

Maternal IgE is not supposed to cross the human placenta *(53,54)*. The human fetus seems capable of producing IgE antibodies, since such antibodies have been demonstrated in in vitro studies of fetal lung and liver tissues and they have also been isolated in amniotic fluid *(53,55)*. Under normal circumstances this production is limited, as the IgE levels in cord blood are usually very low, often even below the detection level of a sensitive assay *(56)*. But elevated levels of cord blood IgE, i.e., above about 0.8 kU/L, do occur in some newborns. Such elevated levels are associated with an increased risk for development of allergic disease during infancy and childhood (summarized in ref. *57*). In some cases these antibodies may indicate intrauterine sensitization, since low levels of IgE antibodies against cow's milk can be detected in some cord blood samples *(58–60)*. Furthermore, positive skin prick tests have been elicited in newborns to penicillin, helminths, cow's milk, and grass pollen *(58,61,62)*. It is possible that the fetus is not completely protected from allergenic material and may be sensitized *in utero* although this is only rarely associated with allergic manifestations. This possibility is indicated by the observation that proteins digested by pregnant rats can be isolated both in serum and in the amniotic fluid of their pups *(63)*. In humans, food allergens are often present in the serum of adults after ingestion of milk and egg *(64)*, but so far there is no documentation of food allergens in the fetal circulation.

An even more likely explanation for the presence of elevated S-IgE levels in some atopic infants already at birth, however, could be that they are a consequence of nonspecific, spontaneous IgE synthesis, perhaps lack of suppression. This notion would be supported by the negative outcome of prospective studies of manipulation of the maternal diet during pregnancy *(65,66)*.

Transplacental transfer of maternal anti-idiotypic antibodies is yet another possible explanation for the occasional finding of IgE antibodies in cord blood. Such maternal IgG antibodies directed against the antigen-specific parts of other antibodies have a structure similar to the antigen and can replace it as an immunological stimulus. As a consequence, anti-idiotypic antibodies would have the capacity to stimulate fetal antibody formation. This has been demonstrated as a possible mechanism for transfer of immunity to polio virus and certain strains of *E. coli* from mother to baby *(67,68)*. It has been suggested that the IgE synthesis in a newborn baby may be stimulated by a similar mechanism *(69)*. Very recently allergen-specific T-cell responses have been demonstrated by fetal *(49)* as well as by cord blood lymphocytes *(39,70)*, including responses to both food and inhalant allergens. It is not known whether these responses indicate "sensitization" in the sense that they are the forerunners of allergy or whether they are part of the normal maturation of the immune system.

Maternal Immunity

The fetus is protected from various external influences by the placental barrier. This barrier is selective and, for example, maternal IgG antibodies pass through it *(71,72)*. Immunity to various infectious agents is thus transferred to the fetus. It is also known that IgG antibodies to food antigens are present in cord blood at a higher concentration than in corresponding maternal blood *(73)*.

Less is known about the role of transplacental transfer of maternal immunity for the development of allergy in the infant, and the possible influence of maternal immunity on the early immune responses to allergens is unknown. We have very recently demonstrated the presence of IgG subclass antibodies to an inhalant allergen, namely, birch, in the cord blood *(73a)*. The levels were lower in infants born shortly before the pollen season as compared to other seasons. These variations were most pronounced in the babies of allergic mothers. If confirmed, the observations could support an alternative explanation for the epidemiological observations of seasonal variations in the risk for sensitization to pollen early in life, i.e., low levels of (protective?) IgG antibodies at the time of primary exposure rather than the exposure itself.

There are several ways by which transplacentally transferred immunity by maternal IgG antibodies in theory could protect the baby. One possibility could be that to prevent mucosal absorption of allergen, alternatively, high levels of IgG antibodies could possibly modify the neonatal immune response. By increasing the maternal intake of, for example, milk and egg during pregnancy it is possible to increase maternal antibody concentrations to these foods and by decreasing the intake there is a corresponding decrease in antibody concentration *(73,74)*. There are preliminary indications that maternal IgG antibodies against various foods may protect the infant from sensitization *(75)*. In two more recent and larger studies, however, there was no relationship between maternal IgG antibody levels to foods and protection against allergy *(73,74)*.

Another possibility was indicated by a recent study reporting that elevated levels of IgG anti-IgE antibodies in the cord blood were associated with less allergy during the first 18 mo of life *(76)*. This was particularly obvious in babies with a strong family history of allergy. This finding and reported individual variations in the composition of human milk *(see* below) would indicate that maternal immunity may be an important environmental factor influencing the risk for allergic manifestations in her child, even many years later. It is also possible that reports of a stronger influence of genetics when atopy is inherited from the maternal, rather than paternal, side *(77)* is not explained by genetic factors but by an early environmental influence exerted by the mother.

The immunological milieu at the fetal/maternal interface in experimental animals appears naturally skewed toward Th-2, which may represent an evolutionary adaptation for protection of the placenta against the deleterious effects of Th-1 cytokines *(78)*; of further interest is the finding that this Th-2 bias persists for variable periods into infancy *(79)*. It is possible that the immunostimulating effects of the normal gastrointestinal flora during infancy provide adjuvant signals that facilitate the establishment of a normal (adult-equivalent) Th-1/Th-2 balance.

The fact that foods are the dominating allergens in infants, as well as the possibility of prenatal induction of IgE antibody formation, has prompted studies of maternal dietary restriction during pregnancy as a means to prevent the development of IgE antibodies and allergy in babies. Some of these studies are, however, difficult to evaluate, since the maternal diet was not limited to pregnancy, but continued into the lactation period.

Two prospective studies that were limited to studying the effects of dietary manipulation during pregnancy both failed to reveal any protective effect. In one of the studies, pregnant women with a family history of allergy were randomly assigned to an unrestricted diet or to an elimination diet during the last trimester of pregnancy *(66,74)*. Allergenic foods such as cow's milk, egg, fish, and peanuts were excluded in the intervention group. In another prospective study of similarly selected mothers, the participants either had a diet low in these foods or had a diet with increased amounts of milk and eggs, namely, at least one liter of milk and one egg daily *(80)*. In contrast to the effect of dietary manipulation of breast-feeding mothers, none of the diets during pregnancy was associated with a reduced risk for food allergy or of other symptoms of atopic disease in their babies. Thus, neither avoidance of certain allergenic foods nor increased amounts of them in order to stimulate IgG antibody formation had any appreciable effects on clinical symptoms.

The studies indicate that dietary manipulation of the mothers during pregnancy is not associated with less allergy in their babies, unless continued into the lactation period. Consequently, no dietary restrictions should be imposed on pregnant women as a means for allergy prevention in the baby.

Other Pre- and Perinatal Factors

There is little doubt that maternal smoking during pregnancy is a health hazard for the baby, including growth retardation *(81)*. Studies of the possible role of this habit for the development of allergy and asthma in the baby are difficult to interpret, since very few mothers who smoke during pregnancy quit when the baby is born. It is therefore difficult to confirm whether the increased prevalence of allergy and asthma is a consequence of maternal smoking during pregnancy, smoke exposure of the infant postpartum, or both. As summarized in *(81)*, there is some evidence, however, that maternal tobacco smoking during pregnancy may increase the risk for childhood allergy and wheezing disorder.

There are also indications that certain medications to pregnant women may affect the rate of allergy in their children. Observations include a possible increase in neonatal IgE concentration in babies of mothers treated with the beta-blocking agent metoprolol *(82)*. Intrauterine exposure to metoprolol tended to be associated with an increased incidence of atopic disease during the first years of life, as compared to children of placebo-treated mothers.

Perinatal stress factors are associated with respiratory problems during the first years of life. It has also been suggested that they could increase the risk of sensitization to allergens. These studies (summarized in ref. *1*) were all retrospective, however, and they did not control for various other possibilities. In a recent Swedish study, prematurity was a moderate risk factor for hospitalization in early childhood due to wheezing, but no relationship to allergy was discussed *(83)*.

In conclusion, although much remains to be studied, it is reasonable to assume that maternal immunity, health, and medication, at least during the final part of pregnancy, all may have consequences for the incidence of respiratory disease and allergy in their babies, at least during early childhood. Whether prenatal factors may also affect the prevalence of allergy later in life remains to be studied.

INFANT FEEDING

Early weaning to cow's milk formulas has been associated with an increased rate of allergic disease. The data are conflicting, however, because there are many studies in which prolonged breast feeding is not protective against allergy (summarized in refs. *3* and *4*). The explanation for the apparently conflicting results seems to lie in the selection of patients for the studies, in the necessity for other dietary precautions, and in how the outcome was assessed. Studies showing a protective effect of prolonged exclusive breast feeding have included infants with a genetic propensity to allergy, rather than an unselected group of infants. Also, the breast feeding in these cases was associated with an avoidance of other foods, e.g., juices and solid foods. Thus, late introduction of foreign foods, i.e., after 6 mo of life, appears to lower the frequency of infants producing IgE antibodies to cow's milk and to be associated with less allergic symptoms, as compared to introduction of cow's milk products before that age *(84)*. It is also possible that any long-term effects are limited to respiratory disease rather than to allergy itself *(85)*.

Since poor breast-feeding is associated with early introduction of formula and solid foods, it is not fully understood to what extent development of allergy is a consequence of exposure to foreign allergenic foods and to what extent it is a consequence of not receiving breast milk, which contains many components that may modify the immune responses of the infant (reviewed in ref. *3*). There are therefore several possible explanations for a protective role of breast milk against allergy, including low content of allergens, protection against intestinal and respiratory infections, passive transfer of immunity from the mother by secretory IgA antibodies, and transfer of components that stimulate the maturation of the infantile immune system *(86)*. It is well established that human milk may contain food antigens such as cow's milk proteins and egg if these items are ingested by the mother (summarized in refs. *3* and *87*). This may sensitize the breast-fed baby. The small amounts of allergens that may be present in breast milk can, thus, be sufficient to cause increased sensitization in a genetically predisposed infant—and to evoke allergic symptoms during lactation.

Passive transfer of immunity is another possibility by which human milk is protective, as reported in one study where high levels in breast milk of IgA antibodies against cow's milk protein were associated with less allergic symptoms in the babies *(88)*. This observation could not be confirmed in a larger, prospectively done study *(74)*.

Several recent studies indicate that human milk may exert a regulatory role on infant immunity. Observations include an early stimulation of IgA antibody synthesis in breast-fed infants *(86,89,90)* and transfer of cell-mediated immunity *(91,92)* and cytokines *(93,94)*. The precise relation between breast feeding and infant allergy is thus not fully understood. It is reasonable to assume that any protective effects of breast feeding may vary with the individual mothers since both their diet and their immune status appear to play a role. An allergy-preventing effect of human milk seems, however, to be limited to babies with a genetically determined increased risk for allergic disease *(4)*. This lends further support to the notion that environmental factors associated with an increased rate of allergic disease in children are mainly operative in individuals with a genetic propensity for allergic sensitization and disease.

NONSPECIFIC ENVIRONMENTAL FACTORS

It is well established that various environmental factors may enhance sensitization and also trigger an allergic reaction in a sensitized individual (Table 1). Although allergy to most of the compounds listed in Table 1 is rare, they do play a role both in enhancing sensitization to allergens and in eliciting and aggravating clinical symptoms. Even if all the factors discussed in this section were added, however, this would only explain a small part of the regional differences in the prevalence of allergy, and it would certainly not explain the increasing prevalence in many countries.

Air Pollution

Air pollution such as ozone, SO_2, and NO_2 may all enhance sensitization, at least in experimental animals *(95–99)*. Data is less clear cut in humans, but in an epidemiological survey of 5300 children in Sweden, bronchial hyperreactivity and pollen allergy were both more common in children living near a moderately air-polluting paper factory than in children living in a forested unindustrialized area about 40 km away from the factory *(100)*. If the parents smoked at home, then the prevalence of bronchial hyperreactivity and allergy was further increased, indicating a synergistic effect between the two pollutants. An observation that allergy to Japanese cedar was more common in people living near a motorway than in less polluted areas would also support the concept that pollution is associated with an increased risk for sensitization *(101)*.

Differences in pollution could also possibly explain the lower prevalence of allergic manifestations in rural than in nearby urban areas in Western Europe, discussed above *(26,27)*. A similar difference in allergy prevalence between polluted and less polluted areas was also noted in former Soviet-occupied Estonia (Table 2). Thus, the prevalence of at least one positive skin prick test was significantly higher in Tallinn, an industrialized coastal city with considerable pollution, than in Tartu, which is an inland university town.

Exposure to Tobacco Smoke

Tobacco smoke is the major indoor air pollutant. Tobacco smoke is strongly associated with allergic sensitization, asthma, and other respiratory diseases. Increased serum IgE levels and an increased prevalence of positive skin tests toward occupational allergens have been shown in multiple studies (reviewed in ref. *81*). Thus, smokers are sensitized more easily to occupational allergens than nonsmokers who are exposed to the allergens to a similar degree *(102)*.

The effect of tobacco smoke is, however, not limited to active smoking. Infants and young children are particularly susceptible to the adjuvant effects of tobacco smoke as trigger of sensitization and wheezing. Children of parents who smoke at home have a significantly earlier onset of allergy and wheezy bronchitis than children of nonsmoking parents *(81,83)*.

The effect of tobacco smoke on sensitization to allergens may be explained by a local effect on the airways or by a direct effect on the immune system. The former notion is supported by the finding that smoking rats exposed to antigen in aerosol develop higher IgE responses than subcutaneously immunized animals and nonsmoking aerosol-immunized controls *(103)*.

In conclusion, passive smoking is by far the best identified risk factor for the development of allergic disease, particularly in early childhood; this is independent of how "allergy" is defined. There is little doubt that exposure to tobacco smoke is the most important environmental risk factor for childhood allergy and respiratory disease that has been identified so far. The long-time effects of childhood exposure to tobacco smoke are unknown.

Housing

Most children in Europe and North America spend at least 90% of their time indoors. It is therefore likely that the indoor environment is even more important than geographical and other macro environmental factors. Modern well-insulated buildings with poor ventilation represent a definite risk factor for allergic sensitization (summarized in ref. *104*). Many new compounds are used in modern buildings, e.g., plastic material, synthetic paints, and chemical substances, with unknown effects on human health. Combined with efficient insulation and reduced ventilation, this has created a new indoor climate. In temperate climates, energy crises and increased interest in energy-conserving measures have resulted in changed building standards, particularly, better insulation and reduced ventilation. This in turn has resulted in more "sick buildings," characterized by damage due to dampness, indoor mold growth, and the presence of various symptoms among people dwelling in the houses. At least one well-documented consequence of this is a much increased prevalence of sensitivity to house dust mite allergens in regions with a temperate climate *(105–108)*. Sensitivity to these allergens used to be rare in a climate with cold and dry winters but the creation of a warm and humid "subtropical" indoor climate has changed this.

In an epidemiological survey, it was found that homes with damage due to dampness were associated with a higher incidence of atopic disease and/or bronchial hyperreactivity in the children *(108)*. In children living in houses with damage by dampness and whose parents in addition smoked at home, there was a marked increase in allergic asthma and bronchial hyper-reactivity, as compared with children exposed to only one of these factors *(100)*. The effects of the living conditions were most marked for children with a family history of asthma. This supports the notion that the environmental influences mainly play a particular role in individuals with a genetic susceptibility to allergic disease.

Much more has to be learned about the role of the indoor climate for sensitization and triggering of allergic manifestations, e.g., the role of molds and other micro-organisms. It is, however, reasonable to conclude that a search for environmental factors influencing the development of asthma and allergy should be directed toward factors affecting the indoor climate.

Infections

The role of infections, notably in the respiratory tract, as risk factors for the development of childhood allergic disease is complex. An infection induces an inflammatory reaction in the respiratory mucosa, which in turn modifies the local immune response. They may also possibly alter the immune defense and act as adjuvants or as allergens. Furthermore, it is common knowledge that infections may trigger clinical symptoms in already sensitized individuals and that infections increase bronchial hyperreactivity. Earlier animal experiments support the clinical observations, showing an enhanced IgE production after allergen exposure and concomitant viral infection *(109)*.

Epidemiological studies of the relation between infections and manifestation of allergic disease are, however, complicated by the fact that symptoms like a runny nose, wheezing, and cough may all be caused by either an infection or an allergic reaction and that the etiology of the symptoms is therefore not always easily identified.

As already discussed, experimental studies indicate that microbial stimuli may exert significant systemic effects that influence the outcome of T-cell responses to inhalant allergens *(2)*. Evidence from a variety of sources indicates that the principal drive for maturation of the adaptive immune system from the functionally deficient fetal phenotype into the adult-equivalent immunocompetent phenotype is confrontation with the microbial environment, particularly gastrointestinal tract commensals and pathogens, giving rise to the suggestion *(35)* that variations in public health and hygiene practices (particularly as they relate to infants) may contribute to the marked differences in allergy prevalence that are being documented in different socioeconomic groups.

Certain infectious agents, e.g., respiratory syncytial virus (RSV), Epstein-Barr virus, and *Bordetella pertussis*, seem to be of particular interest. The mechanisms are probably different, however. Bronchiolitis caused by RSV in early infancy has been associated with the development of atopy and asthma. The mechanism may be that the G-protein of RSV can directly stimulate Th2-like cells, thus enhancing IgE antibody formation and other components of the allergic inflammation *(110)*.

The relationship between bronchiolitis caused by RSV during the first 6 mo of life and the development of asthma was recently studied prospectively in 47 infants *(111)*. For each child two matched controls were selected, making a study population of 140 participating in the follow-up at 3 yr. Asthma, defined as three episodes of bronchial obstruction verified by a physician, was found in 11 of the 47 children with RSV bronchiolitis (23%) and in only 1 of the 93 controls. A positive test for IgE antibodies against a mixture of allergens was recorded in 32% of the RSV children and 9% of the controls ($p = 0.02$). Of particular interest was the observation that among the former children, six of 11 with a family history of allergy developed asthma, as compared to only 5 of 36 without this family history. Thus, the risk for asthma after RSV bronchiolitis was much higher in infants with a genetic propensity to allergy.

Bordetella pertussis is of particular interest, because it is a well-established adjuvant for the induction of IgE antibody formation in experimental animals *(112)*. Furthermore, whooping cough is associated with bronchial hyperreactivity for several months *(113)*. It has also been shown that IgE antibodies to pertussis toxin appear after an infection *(114)* and after immunization against pertussis *(115,116)*. The latter observation has raised the question about a possible role of vaccinations as a risk factor for allergic disease. This notion is further strengthened by the fact that aluminum, which is used as an adjuvant in many vaccines, is also one of the most potent adjuvants for IgE antibody synthesis in animals *(112)*. In a large Swedish clinical trial of three pertussis vaccines comprising 10,000 children, however, there was no relationship between vaccination and the appearance of allergic manifestations up to 3 yr of age *(117)*. Furthermore, IgE antibody response to pertussis toxin after immunization appears to be related more to the content of aluminum than to the antigen *(116)*.

There are also IgE antibody responses to tetanus and diphtheria toxoid *(118)*, but these responses do not appear to be associated with allergic disease *(119)*. Infections with Epstein-Barr virus may be associated with atopic disease *(120)*. This is possibly explained by the general stimulatory effect on B-cells that is exerted by the virus.

Understanding of the interaction between infections and sensitization has become more complicated recently, however, in the light of experimental studies and epidemiological observations. As already discussed, rat pups who are protected against infections are more easily sensitized to inhaled allergens than pups exposed to various microbial agents *(35)*. The data from the recent animal experiments are supported by the results of epidemiological studies. In a British study an inverse relationship between many respiratory-tract infections and atopy was observed *(121)*. An inverse relationship between the number of siblings *(29)*, particularly older siblings *(122)*, and atopy has also been reported, indicating that many infections during the first year of life could protect against sensitization. Very recently it was observed that the prevalence of positive skin prick tests may be lower in tuberculin-positive than in tuberculin-negative children *(122a)*, indicating that bacterial infections and vaccinations early in life may possibly enhance the down-regulation of IgE antibody formation to allergens encountered at the time of infection. An alternative explanation is that because the atopic genotype is associated with a skewed immune response toward Th2-like immunity, atopic children would have a diminished cell-mediated reaction to tuberculin after immunization. Reports of less atopy among school children in the former socialist countries of Eastern Europe *(27,30,31,123,124)* lend support to the relevance of these findings.

Based on these experimental and clinical findings, Holt *(2,125)* suggested that improvements in public health and general living standards in the developed countries over the last 2–3 generations have progressively reduced the level of exposure of infants and young children to the natural microbial environment. According to this hypothesis, lowered microbial stimulation has resulted in a delayed postnatal development of immune competence, resulting in a prolonged period during which the immune system is at risk of generating a Th-2-type immune response with IgE antibody formation and stimulation of mast-cell and eosinophil proliferation.

Others

As previously discussed, stress appears to alter the immune response, as measured by various laboratory tests of inflammatory responses *(12–15)*. It is also clinically well-established that psychological factors influence the severity of asthmatic symptoms and allergic reactions in affected patients. For example, dysfunctional patterns of interaction and relations are more common in the families of children with severe asthma than in families of children with another severe chronic disease, namely, diabetes mellitus *(126,127)*. Patterns of low flexibility ("rigidity") and too much closeness ("enmeshment") dominated among the dysfunctional families. Family therapy to such families reduced the severity of the asthma in the affected children.

A recent prospective study addressed the question of whether disturbed family interaction is a primary finding or a consequence of disease. The study included the families of 100 infants with a strong family history of allergy *(128)*. The entire family participated in a standardized family test when the children were 3 and 18 mo old, assessing the ability to adjust to demands of the situation ("adaptability") and the balance between emotional closeness and distance ("cohesion"). An unbalanced family interplay was common at 3 mo (37%) but it was not predictive of respiratory illness. At 18 mo a dysfunctional interaction was significantly more common in families of children with eczema and obstructive symptoms than in families of healthy children. The study indicates that a dysfunctional family interaction is the result, rather than a cause, of recurrent wheezing in infancy. Further studies are needed to clarify the role of psychological factors for variations in individual susceptibility to allergic manifestations over time.

As already discussed, the prevalence of allergy in the former socialist countries in Central and Eastern Europe is much lower than in Western Europe, despite the fact that air pollution is often higher in the former. The studies strongly indicate that other factors connected with Western lifestyle are more important than air pollution for the development of allergy, although the latter also plays an obvious role. The fact that the differences in the prevalence of sensitivity to inhaled allergens between Eastern and Western Germany are limited to populations who were born after about 1960 *(23,32)* would indicate that they are caused by factors encountered early in life.

The living conditions in the former socialist countries of Europe are, in many respects, similar to those that prevailed in Western Europe 30–40 yr ago, including type of air pollution, panorama of childhood infections and immunizations, building standards, and food. The low prevalence of allergy in these countries supports the general feeling that the prevalence of allergy has increased substantially in the West over the past decades. The nature of the factors associated with the environment and/or changing living conditions is unknown. In all the studies, however, there was an inverse relation between sensitization and manifestations of allergy, on the one hand, and crowded dwellings and the number of respiratory infections among children, on the other. In currently ongoing studies, differences in the intestinal flora, dietary habits, and infections in early childhood, as well as other factors related to lifestyle, are being studied as possible explanations for the different outcome of exposure to ubiquitous inhalant allergens in Western industrialized countries and other parts of the world.

PRIMARY PREVENTION OF ALLERGY

The clinical observations that poor breast-feeding, early weaning to cow's milk-based formulas, and exposure to high levels of allergens early in life appear to be risk factors for sensitization and allergic manifestations later in life have prompted studies of the possible effects of allergy prevention *(129–132)*. The results of these studies indicate only a marginal protective effect against sensitivity to the particular allergens that were avoided. From the current knowledge of the kinetics of the primary immune responses it is not reasonable to expect a general allergy-preventive effect through avoidance of certain allergens, but merely a possible prevention of delayed sensitization to that particular allergen. The most important allergy-preventive measures are therefore not the avoidance of specific allergens but the avoidance of adjuvant factors. Exposure to tobacco smoke is by far the most significant risk

Table 3
Currently Recommended Measures for the Prevention of Childhood Allergy

During pregnancy
  No tobacco smoking
  Avoidance of certain medications, i.e., corticosteroids, beta-receptor blocking
    agents
  Elimination of pets
In infancy and early childhood
  No exposure to tobacco smoke
  Good indoor climate
  Reduction of air pollution
  Reduction of levels of house dust mites
  Elimination of pets

factor that has been identified so far. Other significant risk factors include living in poorly ventilated houses and exposure to high levels of outdoor air polutants such as NO_2. Current recommendations of allergy prevention are summarized in Table 3.

CONCLUDING REMARKS

A number of environmental factors may increase the risk for sensitization in early childhood and the subsequent development of allergic disease. Environmental factors may operate already during fetal life, e.g., maternal health and medication. After birth, the first months of life appear to be a period during which babies are particularly susceptible to sensitization, although the clinical manifestations of respiratory allergy may not appear until several years later. Infants with a genetic propensity to develop allergy and atopic disease seem particularly susceptible to various environmental influences. There are distinct differences in the early immune responses to allergens in atopic and nonatopic infants. It is possible that the apparent increase in the prevalence of atopic disease in many countries over the past decades is caused by unknown changes in lifestyle operating in early life. Even if all the known factors that may influence the incidence of allergic disease are added, however, this can only explain a fraction of the regional differences and changes over time in the prevalence of allergy. In order to implement effective prevention of allergy it is necessary to identify these environmental factors and the infants who are at risk early in life and then to support their families and encourage them to take allergy-preventive measures.

REFERENCES

1. Björkstén B (1994) Risk factors in early childhood for the development of atopic diseases. Allergy 49:400–407.
2. Holt P (1995) Postnatal maturation of immune competence during infancy and childhood. Pediatr Allergy Immunol 6:59–70.
3. Duchén K, Björkstén B (1991) Sensitization via the breast milk. In: Mestecky J, ed. Immunology of Milk and the Neonate. Plenum, New York, pp. 427–436.
4. Björkstén B (1983) Does breast feeding prevent the development of allergy? Immunol Today 4:215–217.
5. Björkstén F, Suoniemi I, Koski V (1980) Neonatal birch-pollen contact and subsequent allergy to birch pollen. Clin Allergy 10:585–591.
6. Björkstén F, Suoniemi I (1981) Time and intensity of first pollen contacts and risk of subsequent pollen allergies. Acta Med Scand 209:299–303.
7. Morrison Smith J (1973) Skin tests and atopic allergy in children. Clin Allergy 3:269–275.

8. Settipane R, Hagy G (1979) Effect of atmospheric pollen on the newborn. Rhode Island Med J 62:477–482.

9. Morrison-Smith J, Springett VH (1979) Atopic disease and month of birth. Clin Allergy 9:153–157.

10. Suoniemi I, Björkstén F, Haahtela T (1981) Dependence of immediate hypersensitivity in the adolescent period on factors encountered in infancy. Allergy 36:263–268.

11. Croner S, Kjellman N-IM (1986) Predictors of atopic disease: cord blood IgE and month of birth. Allergy 41:68–70.

12. Husband A, King M, Brown R (1987) Behaviorally conditioned modification of T cell subset ratios in rats. Immunol Lett 14:91–94.

13. King M, Husband A, Kusnecov A (1987) Behavioral conditioning of the immune system: From laboratory to clinical application. In: Sheppard J, ed. Advances in Behavioral Medicine. Cumberland College of Health Sciences, Sydney, Vol. 4, pp. 110–117.

14. Anonymous. (1987) Depression, stress and immunity. Lancet 1:1467–1468.

15. Jemmott JI, Borysenko J, Borysenko M, et al. (1983) Academic stress, power motivation, and decrease in secretion rate of salivary secretory immunoglobulin A. Lancet 1:1400–1412.

16. European Community Respiratory Health Survey. (1996) Variations in the prevalence of respiratory symptoms, selfreported asthma attacks, and use of asthma medication in the European Community Respiratory Health Survey (ECRHS). Eur Respir J 9:687–695.

17. Burney P. (1993) Epidemiology of asthma. Allergy 48:17–21.

18. Pearce N, Weiland S, Keil U, et al. (1993) Self-reported prevalence of asthma symptoms in children in Australia, England, Germany and New Zealand: an international comparison using the ISAAC protocol. Eur Respir J 6:1455–1461.

19. Åberg N (1989) Asthma and allergic rhinitis in Swedish conscripts. Clin Exp Allergy 19:59–63.

20. Barbee R, Kaltenborn W, Lebowitz M, Burrows B (1987) Longitudinal changes in allergen skin test reactivity in a community population sample. J Allergy Clin Immunol 79:16–24.

21. Burney P, Chinn S, Rona R. (1990) Has the prevalence of asthma increased in children? Evidence from the national study of health and growth 1973–86. Br Med J 300:1306–1310.

22. Burr M, Butland B, King S, Vaughan-Williams E (1989) Changes in asthma prevalence: Two surveys fifteen years apart. Arch Dis Child 64:1452–1456.

23. Wichmann H (1995) Environment, life-style and allergy: the German answer. Allergo J 4:315–316.

24. van Niekerk C, Weinberg E, Shore S, Heese HdV, van Schalkwyk D (1979) Prevalence of asthma: a comparative study of urban and rural Xhosa children. Clin Allergy 9:319–324.

25. Waite D, Eyles E, Tonkin S, O'Donnell T (1980) Asthma prevalence in Tokelauan children in two environments. Clin Allergy 10:71–75.

26. Bråbäck L, Kälvesten L (1991) Urban living as a risk factor for atopic sensitization in Swedish schoolchildren. Pediatr Allergy Immunol 2:14–19.

27. Bråbäck L, Breborowicz A, Dreborg S, Knutsson A, Pieklik H, Björkstén B (1994) Atopic sensitization and respiratory symptoms among Polish and Swedish schoolchildren. Clin Exper Allergy 24:826–835.

28. von Mutius E, Sherrill D, Fritzsch C, Martinez F, Lebowitz M (1995) Air pollution and upper respiratory symptoms in children from East Germany. Eur Respir J 8:723–728.

29. von Mutius E, Martinez FD, Fritzsch C, Nicolai T, Roell G, Thiemann HH (1994) Prevalence of asthma and atopy in two areas of West and East Germany. Am J Respir Crit Care Med 149:358–364.

30. Riikjärv M, Julge K, Vasar M, Bråbäck L, Knutsson A, Björkstén B (1995) The prevalence of atopic sensitization and respiratory symptoms among Estonian school children. Clin Exp Allergy 25:1198–1204.

31. Bråbäck L, Breborowicz A, Julge K, Knutsson A, Riikjärv M-A, Vasar M, Björkstén B (1995) Risk factors for respiratory symptoms and atopic sensitization in the Baltic area. Arch Dis Child 72:487–493.

32. Jögi R, Jansson C, Björnsson E, Boman G, Björkstén B (1996) The prevalence of athmatic respiratory symptoms among adults in an Estonian and Swedish university town. Allergy 51:331–336.

33. Halvorsen R; Bosnes V, Thorsby E (1986) T cell responses to a *Dermatophagoides farinae* allergen preparation in allergics and healthy controls. Int Arch Allergy Appl Immunol 80:62–69.

34. Wierenga EA, Snoek M, Jansen HM, Bos JD, van LR, Kapsenberg ML (1991) Human atopen-specific types 1 and 2 T helper cell clones. J Immunol 147:2942–2949.

35. Holt P (1995) Environmental factors and primary t-cell sensitization to inhalant allergens in infancy: reappraisal of the role of infections and air pollution. Pediatr Allergy Immunol 6:1–10.

36. McMenamin C, Holt PG (1993) The natural immune response to inhaled soluble protein antigens involves major histocompatibility complex (MHC) class I-restricted CD8+ T cell-mediated but MHC

class II-restricted CD4+ T cell-dependent immune deviation resulting in selective suppression of IgE production. J Exp Med 178:889–899.

37. Sedgwick J, Holt P (1984) Suppression of IgE responses in inbred rats by repeated respiratory tract exposure to antigen: responder phenotype influences isotype specificity of induced tolerance. Eur J Immunol 14:893–897.

38. Rinas U, Horneff G, Wahn V (1993) Interferon-gamma production by cord-blood mononuclear cells is reduced in newborns with a family history of atopic disease and is independent from cord blood IgE-levels. Pediatr Allergy Immunol 4:60–64.

39. Warner JA, Miles EA, Jones AC, Quint DJ, Colwell BM, Warner JO (1994) Is deficiency of interferon gamma production by allergen triggered cord blood cells a predictor of atopic eczema? Clin Exp Allergy 24:423–430.

40. Tang M, Kemp A, Thorburn J, Hill D (1994) Reduced interferon-gamma secretion in neonates and subsequent atopy. Lancet 344:983–985.

41. Björkstén B, Borres M, Einarsson R (1995) Interleukin-4, soluble CD23, and interferon-g levels in serum during the first 18 months of life. Int Arch Allergy Immunol 107:34–36.

42. Wu CY, Demeure CE, Gately M, Podlaski F, Yssel H, Kiniwa M, Delespesse G (1994) In vitro maturation of human neonatal CD4 T lymphocytes. I. Induction of IL-4-producing cells after long-term culture in the presence of IL-4 plus either IL-2 or IL-12. J Immunol 152:1141–1153.

43. Kemeny DM, Urbanek R, Ewan P, McHugh S, Richards D, Patel S, Lessof MH (1989) The subclass of IgG antibody in allergic disease: II. The IgG subclass of antibodies produced following natural exposure to dust mite and grass pollen in atopic and non-atopic individuals. Clin Exp Allergy 19:545–549.

44. Kemeny DM, Price JF, Richardson V, Richards D, Lessof MH (1991) The IgE and IgG subclass antibody response to foods in babies during the first year of life and their relationship to feeding regimen and the development of food allergy. J Allergy Clin Immunol 87:920–992.

45. Hattevig G, Kjellman B, Johansson SGO, Björkstén B (1984) Clinical symptoms and IgE responses to common food proteins in atopic and healthy children. Clin Allergy 14:551–559.

46. Hattevig G, Kjellman B, Björkstén B (1993) Appearance of IgE antibodies to ingested and inhaled allergens during first 12 years of life in atopic and non-atopic children. Pediatr Allergy Immunol 4:182–189.

47. Duchén K, Einarsson R, Grodzinsky E, Hattevig G, Björkstén B (1997) The development of IgG-1 and IgG-4 antibodies against beta-lactoglobulin and ovalbumin in healthy and atopic girls. Ann Allergy 78:363–368.

48. Van Asperen PP, Kemp AS, Mellis CM (1984) Skin test reactivity and clinical allergen sensitivity in infancy. J Allergy Clin Immunol 73:381–386.

49. Jones AC, Miles EA, Warner JO, Colwell BM, Bryant TN, Warner JA (1996) Fetal peripheral blood mononuclear cell proliferative responses to mitogenic and allergenic stimuli during gestation. Pediatr Allergy Immunol 7:109–116.

50. Holt PG, Clough JB, Holt BJ, et al. (1992) Genetic risk for atopy is associated with delayed postnatal maturation of T-cell competence. Clin Exp Allergy 22:1093–1099.

51. Nelson D, McMenamin C, Wilkes L, Holt PG (1991) Postnatal development of respiratory mucosal immune function in the rat: Regulation of IgE responses to inhaled allergen. Pediatr Allergy Immunol 4:170–177.

52. Nelson DJ, McMenamin C, McWilliam AS, Brenan M, Holt PG (1994) Development of the airway intraepithelial dendritic cell network in the rat from class II MHC (Ia) negative precursors: differential regulation of Ia expression at different levels of the respiratory tract. J Exp Med 179:203–212.

53. Madani G, Heiner DC (1989) Antibody transmission from mother to fetus. Curr Opin Immunol 1:1157–1164.

54. Miller DL, Hirvonen T, Gitlin D (1973) Synthesis of IgE by human conceptus. J Allergy Clin Immunol 52:182–188.

55. Rognum TO, Thrane S, Stoltenberg L, Vege A, Brandtzaeg P (1992) Development of intestinal mucosal immunity in fetal life and the first postnatal months. Pediatr Res 32:145–149.

56. Delespesse G, Sarfati M, Lang G, Sehon A (1983) Prenatal and neonatal synthesis of IgE. Monogr Allergy 18:83–95.

57. Kjellman N-IM (1994) IgE determinations in neonates is not suitable for general screening. Pediatr Allergy Immunol 5:1–4.

58. Businco L, Marchetti F, Pellegrini G, Perlini R (1983) Predictive value of cord blood IgE levels in 'at-risk' newborn babies and influence of type of feeding. Clin Allergy 13:503–508.

59. Høst A, Halken S (1990) A prospective study of cow milk allergy in Danish infants during the first 3 years of life. Allergy 45:587–596.

60. Høst A, Husby S, Gjesing B, Larsen J, Løwenstein H (1992) Prospective estimation of IgG, IgG subclass and IgE antibodies to dietary proteins in infants with cow milk allergy. Allergy 47:218–229.

61. Levin S, Altman Y, Sela M (1971) Penicillin and dinitrophenyl antibodies in newborn and mothers detected with chemically modified bacteriophage. Pediatr Res 5:87–88.

62. Weil G, Hussain R, Kumaraswami V, Tripathy S, Phillips K, Oliesen E (1983) Prenatal allergic sensitization to helminth antigen in offspring of parasite-infected mothers. J Clin Invest 71:1124–1129.

63. Dahl GMK, Telemo E, Wesström BR, Jacobsson I, Lindberg T, Karlsson BW (1984) The passage of orally fed protein from mother to foetus in the rat. Comp Biochem Physiol 74:199–201.

64. Husby S, Schultz Larsen F, Petersen PH (1987) Genetic influence on the serum levels of naturally occurring human IgG antibodies to dietary antigens. Quantitative assessment from a twin study. J Immunogenet 14:131–142.

65. Zeiger R, Heller S, Mellon M, Helsey J, Hamburger R, Sampson H (1992) Genetic and environmental factors affecting the development of atopy through age 4 in children of atopic parents: A prospective randomized study of food allergen avoidance. Pediatr Allergy Immunol 3:110–127.

66. Fälth-Magnusson K, Kjellman N-IM (1992) Allergy prevention by maternal elimination diet during late pregnancy—a 5-year follow-up of a randomized study. J Allergy Clin Immunol 89:709–713.

67. Mellander L, Carlsson B, Hanson L-Å (1986) Secretory IgA and IgM antibodies to E. coli and poliovirus type I antigens occur in amniotic fluid, meconium and saliva from newborns. Clin Exp Immunol 63:555–561.

68. Hahn ZM, Carlsson B, Björkander J, Osterhaus AD, Mellander L, Hanson LÅ (1992) Presence of non-maternal antibodies in newborns of mothers with antibody deficiencies. Pediatr Res 32:150–154.

69. Kimpen J, Callaert H, Embrechts P, Bosmans E (1989) Influence of sex and gestational age on cord blood IgE. Acta Paediatr Scand 78:233–238.

70. Piccinni MP, Mecacci F, Sampognaro S, Manetti R, Parronchi P, Maggi E, Romagnini S (1993) Aeroallergen sensitization can occur during fetal life. Int Arch Allergy Immunol 102:301–303.

71. Bramwell F (1970) The transmission of antibodies. In: Bramwell F, ed. The transmission of immunity from the mother to the young. North-Holland, Amsterdam, pp. 242–250.

72. Amstey MS (1991) The potential for maternal immunization to protect against neonatal infections. Semin Perinatol 15:206–209.

73. Lilja G, Dannaeus A, Fälth-Magnusson K, Graff Lonnevig V, Johansson SGO, Kjellman N-IM, Öman H (1988) Immune response of the atopic woman and foetus: effects of high- and low-dose food allergen intake during late pregnancy. Clin Allergy 18:131–142.

73a. Jenmalm M, Björkstén B (1998) Maternal influence on IgG subclass antibodies to Beta 1 during the first 18 months of life detected with a sensitive ELISA, in press.

74. Fälth-Magnusson K, Öman H, Kjellman N-IM (1987) Maternal abstention from cow milk and egg in allergy risk pregnancies. Effect on antibody production in the mother and the newborn. Allergy 42:64–73.

75. Dannaeus A, Johansson S, Foucard T (1978) Clinical and immunological aspects of food allergy in childhood II. Development of allergic symptoms and humoral immune response to foods in infants of atopic mothers during the first 24 months of life. Acta Paediatr Scand 67:497–504.

76. Vassella C, Odelram H, Kjellman N-I, Borres M, Vanto T, Björkstén B (1994) High anti-IgE levels at birth are associated with a reduced allergy incidence in early childhood. Clin Exp Allergy 24:771–777.

77. Cookson W, Young R, Sanford A, Moffatt MF, Shirakawa T, Sharp PA, Faux JA, Julier C, Le Souef P, Nakamura V (1992) Maternal inheritance of atopic IgE responsiveness on chromosome 11q. Lancet 340:381–384.

78. Wegmann T, Lin H, Guilbert L, Mosmann TR (1993) Bidirectional cytokine interactions in the maternal-fetal relationship: is successful pregnancy a Th2 phenomenon? Immunol Today 14:353–356.

79. Chen N, Field EH (1995) Enhanced type 2 and diminished type 1 cytokines in neonatal tolerance. Transplantation 60:1187–1193.

80. Lilja G, Dannaeus A, Foucard T, Graff-Lonnevig V, Johansson S, Öman H (1989) Effects of maternal diet during late pregnancy and lactation on the development of atopic diseases in infants up to eighteen months of age—in vivo results. Clin Exp Allergy 19:473–479.

81. Halken S, Høst A, Nilsson L, Taudorf E (1995) Passive smoking as a risk factor for development of obstructive respiratory disease and allergic sensitization. Allergy 50:97–105.

82. Björkstén B, Finnström O, Wichman K (1988) Intrauterine exposure to the beta-adrenergic receptor-blocking agent metoprolol and allergy. Int Arch Allergy Appl Immunol 87:59–62.

83. Rylander E, Pershagen G, Eriksson M, Nordvall L (1993) Parental smoking and other risk factors for wheezing bronchitis in children. Eur J Epidemiol 9:517–526.

84. Kajosaari M, Saarinen UM (1983) Prophylaxis of atopic disease by six months total solid food elimination. Acta Pædiatr Scand 72:411–441.

85. Saarinen U (1995) Breastfeeding as prophylaxis against atopic disease: prospective follow-up study until 17 years old. Lancet 346:1065–1069.

86. Koutras AK, Vigorita VJ (1989) Fecal secretory immunoglobulin A in breast milk versus formula feeding in early infancy. J Pediatr Gastroenterol Nutr 9(1):58–61.

87. Goldman A (1986) Immunologic system in human milk. J Pediatric Gastroenterol Nutr 5:343–345.

88. Machtinger S, Moss R (1986) Cow's milk allergy in breast-fed infants: The role of allergen and maternal secretory IgA antibody. J Allergy Clin Immunol 77:341–347.

89. Prentice A (1987) Breast feeding increases concentrations of IgA in infants' urine. Archives Disease Childhood 62:792–795.

90. Robinson G (1991) Identification of a secretory IgA receptor on breast-milk macrophages: Evidence for specific activation via these receptors. Pediatric Res 29:429–434.

91. Pittard W, Bill K (1979) Immunoregulation by breast milk cells. Cell Immunol 42:437–414.

92. Schlesinger J, Covelli HD (1977) Evidence for transmission of lymphocyte responses to tuberculin by breast-feeding. Lancet 529–532.

93. Shiba T, Minagawa T, Mito K, Nakane A, Suga K, Hanjo T, Nakao T (1987) Effect of breast feeding on responses of systemic interferon and virus-specific lymphocyte transformation in infants with respiratory syncytial virus infection. J Med Virol 21:7–14.

94. Delespesse G (1986) Presence of IgE suppressive factors in human colostrum. Eur J Immunol 16:1005–1008.

95. Osebold J, Chung Zee Y, Gershwin L (1988) Enhancement of allergic lung sensitization in mice by ozone inhalation. Proc Soc Exp Biol Med 188:259–264.

96. Holt P, McMenamin C, Nelson D (1990) Primary sensitization to inhalant allergens during infancy. Pediatr Allergy Immunol 1:3–13.

97. Holt P, McMenamin C (1989) Defense against allergic sensitization in the healthy lung: the role of inhalation tolerance. Clin Exp Allergy 19:255–262.

98. Holt P (1987) Immune and inflammatory function in cigarette smokers. Thorax 42:241–249.

99. Nilsson L, Björkstén B (1993) Factors which promote or prevent allergy. In: Dukor P, Hansson L, eds. Monographs in Allergy. S. Karger AG, Basel, Vol. 31, pp. 190–210.

100. Andrae S, Axelson O, Björkstén B, Fredriksson M, Kjellman N-IM (1988) Symptoms of bronchial hyperreactivity and asthma in relation to environmental factors. Arch Dis Child 63:473–478.

101. Ishizaki T, Koizumi K, Ikemori R, Ishyama Y, Kushibiki E (1987) Studies of prevalence of Japanese cedar pollinosis among the residents in a densely cultivated area. Ann Allergy 58:265–270.

102. Zetterström O, Osterman K, Machado L, Johansson SGO (1981) Another smoking hazard: raised serum IgE concentration and increased risk of occupational allergy. Brit Med J 283:1215–1217.

103. Zetterström O, Nordvall SL, Björkstén B, Ahlstedt S, Stelander M (1985) Increased IgE antibody responses in rats exposed to tobacco smoke. J Allergy Clin Immunol 75:594–598.

104. Munir A, Björkstén B (1992) Indoor air pollution and allergic sensitization. In: Knöppel H, Wolkoff P, eds. Chemical Microbiological Health and Comfort. ECSC, EEC, Brussels, pp. 181–199.

105. Dekker C, Dales R, Bartlett S, Brunekreef B, Zwanenburg H (1991) Childhood asthma and the indoor environment. Chest 100(4):922–926.

106. Munir AKM, Björkstén B, Einarsson R, Ekstrand-Tobin A, Warner A, Kjellman N-IM (1995) Mite allergens in relation to home conditions of asthmatic children from three climatic regions. Allergy 50:55–64.

107. Wickman M, Nordvall SL, Pershagen G (1992) Risk factors in early childhood for sensitization to airborne allergens. Pediatr Allergy Immunol 3:128–133.

108. Wickman M (1993) Residential characteristics and allergic sensitization in children especially to mites [Dissertation]. Karolinska Institutet, Stockholm.

109. Frick OL, Brooks DL (1983) Immunoglobulin E antibodies to pollens augmented in dogs by virus vaccines. Am J Vet Res 44:440–445.

110. Alwan WH, Kozlowska K, Openshaw PJ (1994) Distinct types of lung disease caused by functional subsets of antiviral T cells. J Exp Med 179:81–89.

111. Sigurs N, Bjarnason R, Sigurbergsson F, Kjellman B, Björkstén B (1995) Asthma and IgE antibodies after respiratory syncytial virus bronchiolitis: a prospective cohort study with matched controls. Pediatrics 95:500–550.

112. Pauwels R, van der Straeten M, Platteu B, Bazin H (1983) The non-specific enhancement of allergy In vitro effects of *Bordetella pertussis* vaccine on IgE synthesis. Allergy 38:239–246.

113. Sen D, Arora S, Gupta S, Sanyal R (1974) Studies of adrenergic mechanisms in relation to histamine sensitivity in children immunized with *Bordetella pertussis* vaccine. J Allergy Clin Immunol 54:25–31.

114. Hedenskog S, Björkstén B, Blennow M, Granström G, Granström M (1989) Immunoglobulin E response to pertussis toxin in whooping cough and after immunization with a whole-cell and an acellular pertussis vaccine. Int Arch Allergy Appl Immunol 89:156–161.

115. Blennow M, Granström M, Björkstén B (1990) Immunoglobulin E response to pertussis toxin after vaccination with acellular pertussis vaccine. In: Manclark CR, ed. Proceedings of the Sixth International Symposium on Pertussis. Department of Health and Human Services, United States Public Health Service, Bethesda, Maryland, pp. 184–188.

116. Duchén K, Granström M, Hedenskog S, Blennow M, Björkstén B (1996) Immunoglobulin E and G responses to pertusis toxin in children immunised with adsorbed and non-adsorbed whole-cell pertussis vaccines. Pediatr Allergy Imunol 7:in press.

117. Nilson L, Kjellman N-IM, Storsaeter J, Gustafsson L, Olin P (1996) Lack of association between pertussis vaccination and symptoms of asthma and allergy. JAMA 275:760.

118. Mark A, Björkstén B, Granström M (1995) Immunoglobulin E responses to diphteria and tetanus toxoids after booster with aluminium-adsorbed and fluid DT vaccines. Vaccine 13:669–673.

119. Mark A, Björkstén B, Granström M (1997) Immunoglobulin E and G antibodies two years after a booster dose of an aluminium-adsorbed and a fluid DT vaccine in relation to atopy. Vaccine in press.

120. Strannegård I-L, Strannegård Ö (1981) Epstein-Barr virus antibody in children with atopic disease. Int Arch Allergy Appl Immunol 64:314–319.

121. Strachan D (1989) Hay fever, hygiene and household size. Br Med J 289:1259–1260.

122. Strachan D (1995) Epidemiology of hay fever: towards a community diagnosis. Clin Exp Allergy 25:296–303.

122a. Shirakawa T, Eramoto T, Shimagu S, Hopkins J (1997) The inverse association between tuberculin responses and atopic disorders. Science 275:77–79.

123. von Mutius E, Fritzsch C, Weiland SK, Röll G, Magnussen H (1992) Prevalence of asthma and allergic disorders among schoolchildren in united Germany: a descriptive comparison. Br Med J 305:1395–1399.

124. Vasar M, Bråbäck L, Julge K, Knutsson A, Riikjärv M-A, Björkstén B (1996) Pediatr Allergy Immunol 7:in press.

125. Holt PG (1994) A potential vaccine strategy for asthma and allied atopic diseases during early child hood. Lancet 344:456–458.

126. Gustafsson PA, Kjellman N-IM, Cederblad M (1986) Family therapy in the treatment of severe child hood asthma. J Psychosom Res 30:369–374.

127. Gustafsson PA, Kjellman N-IM, Ludvigsson J, Cederblad M (1987) Asthma and family interaction. Arch Dis Child 62:258–263.

128. Gustafsson PA, Björkstén B, Kjellman N-IM (1994) Family dysfunction in asthma—A prospective study of illness development. J Pediatrics 125:493–498.

129. Hattevig G, Kjellman B, Sigurs N, Björkstén B, Kjellman N-IM (1989) Effect of maternal avoidance of eggs, cow's milk and fish during lactation upon allergic manifestations in infants. Clin Exp Allergy 19:27–32.

130. Zeiger RS, Heller S, Mellon MH, Helsey JF, Hamburger RN, Sampson HA (1992) Genetic and environmental factors affecting the development of atopy through age 4 in children of atopic parents: a prospective randomized study of food allergen avoidance. Pediatr Allergy Immunol 3:110–127.

131. Arshad SH, Matthews S, Gant C, Hide DW (1992) Effect of allergen avoidance on development of allergic disorders in infancy. Lancet 339:1493–1497.

II INFLAMMATION: *CELLULAR ASPECTS*

5

The Role of the Bone Marrow in Allergic Disease

Mark D. Inman, MD, PhD, *Roma Sehmi,* PhD,
Paul M. O'Byrne, MB,
and Judah A. Denburg, MD, FRCP(C)

CONTENTS

INTRODUCTION

A current understanding of the pathogenesis of allergen-induced airway diseases is presented in several chapters in this book. These events are schematically summarized in Fig. 1. The development of airway inflammation occurs in response to the multiple actions of mediators released primarily from mast cells and T-helper 2 (Th2) cells, including autocrine upregulation and recruitment of inflammatory cells via target cell priming, adhesion molecule activation, chemotaxis, target cell activation, and decreased apoptosis. All of these well-recognized mechanisms are concerned with the movement of cells or activation of cells in the airway. Little attention has been paid to the source of these inflammatory cells as a mechanism in allergic inflammation.

Several pro-inflammatory mediators released during allergen-induced airway responses also have hemopoietic activity. This raises the possibility that mediators released in the airway following allergen exposure, in addition to recruiting and activating inflammatory cells, act on the bone marrow to increase cell production in a true endocrine manner. In this chapter, we will outline the mechanisms and control of hemopoiesis in the marrow, as well as review

From: *Allergy and Allergic Diseases: The New Mechanisms and Therapeutics*
Edited by: J. A. Denburg © Humana Press Inc., Totowa, NJ

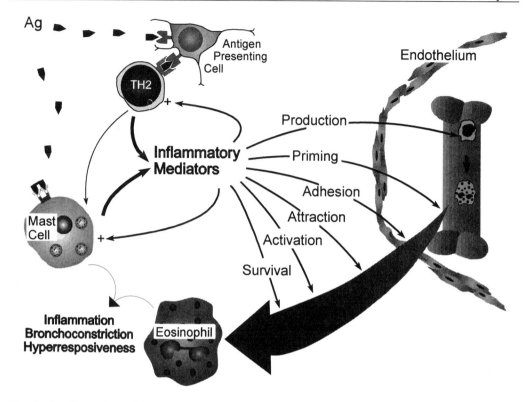

Fig. 1. An illustration of the events occurring in allergen-induced airway inflammation. The role of inflammatory mediators in the priming, adhesion, attraction, activation, and survival of inflammatory cells is well recognized. Evidence reviewed here indicates an additional role is the increased production of inflammatory cells by the bone marrow.

recent evidence that allergen exposure results in a hemopoietic message being sent from the lung to the marrow. We will also discuss the potential importance of this mechanism as a site for therapeutic intervention by existing and potential antiallergic/antiasthma drugs.

PROGENITORS AND MODELS OF DIFFERENTIATION

Pluripotent stem cells (PPSC) in bone marrow can give rise to myeloid, lymphoid, erythroid, or megakaryocytic cell lines *(1–3)* (*see* Chapter 17) (Fig. 2). PPSCs can either differentiate along these lineage-specific pathways or replicate to maintain the permanent pool. The choice between replication and differentiation appears to be stochastic, or random, in nature *(4–6)*. Differentiation progresses in a manner such that successive progenitor cells become increasingly lineage-restricted, presumably as a result of selective deletion or addition of specific programs for lineage commitment *(3)*. Terminal differentiation of oligo- or unipotential progenitors finally gives rise to specific cells that may themselves exhibit considerable interlineage heterogeneity.

The processes by which different cell lines are selected are not completely understood. Considerable evidence exists to support the concept that lineage commitment is also stochastic *(3)*. This is supported by studies where single pluripotent stem cells have produced multi-

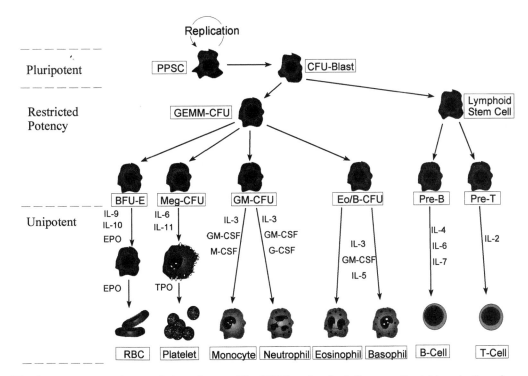

Fig. 2. Bone marrow hemopoietic pathways. The PPSC under the influence of cytokines in the micro-environment is responsible for the production of all blood cells. It is possible that cytokines generated at sites of allergic inflammation may stimulate lineage-specific hemopoiesis in a true endocrine manner.

lineage daughter cells in homogeneous support media in both murine *(7,8)* and human *(9,10)* in vitro cultures. Furthermore, it also appears that there is stochastic regulation of differentiation in in vitro cultures at each stage of lineage selection until unipotential daughter cells are achieved *(11)*. There is also evidence to suggest that lineage commitment can be regulated by local concentrations of cytokines, which can influence lineage selection by either suppressing or supporting apoptosis *(11,12)*; this suggests that lineage regulation might occur through increased survival of selected lines and programmed loss of nonselected lines. Therefore, even though the determination of lineage is, by and large, stochastic, stem cells may be directed or "forced" along specific differential lines by cytokine actions *(13)*. It is possible that a hybrid of these two proposals exists. In this system, stochastic processes determine preferred differentiation patterns in each cell, which may be reinforced or overridden, depending upon exposure to the appropriate pattern of growth factors. Whether the proportion of cells that is directed to each cell lineage stochastically has any influence on the final proportion of mature cells or whether this proportion is determined entirely by the cytokine microenvironment is not known.

It is likely that early progenitors pass through several intermediate and later stages of differentiation and that this process is complemented and regulated by specific groups of cytokines, each acting at different stages of differentiation on specific receptors and through unique signaling pathways (*see* Chapter 17). If, during this process, daughter cells emerge that are not supported by the local microenvironment, then these cells will undergo apoptosis.

HEMOPOIETIC CYTOKINES
AND INFLAMMATORY CELL DIFFERENTIATION

As introduced above, determination of which differentiation lineages are emphasized in the bone marrow depends to a large extent on local concentrations of hemopoietic cytokines. As this topic is covered extensively in Chapter 17, we will provide only a brief overview here. Regulation of myeloid cell production is complex and poorly understood. Unlike the regulation of erythropoiesis (where erythropoietin appears to act exclusively and specifically [14]), myeloid hemopoietic cytokines are active on more than one cell line, and each cell line is regulated by more than one hemopoietic factor. Furthermore, interactions between hemopoietic cytokines make the specific effects of each difficult to study.

Hemopoietic Cytokines and Their Receptors

There are multiple hemopoietic cytokines that can act on multiple cytokine receptors. These receptors are classed in two distinct groups (1) according to whether or not they contain tyrosine kinase receptors. Tyrosine kinase positive receptors bind macrophage-colony stimulating factor (M-CSF) (15) and stem cell factor (SCF) (16). Tyrosine kinase negative receptors include receptors for interleukin (IL)-2 (17), IL-3 (18,19), IL-4 (20), IL-5 (18,21), IL-6 (22), IL-7 (23), IL-11 (24), granulocyte-colony stimulating factor (G-CSF) (25), granulocyte/macrophage-colony stimulating factor (GM-CSF) (18,25), and leukemia inhibitory factor (LIF) (26).

Having several groups of hemopoietic cytokines and receptors with, to a large extent, redundant actions may seem unnecessarily complex, but this may in fact allow for subtlety in the system (1) through synergy, costimulation (1), and transactivation (27). Thus, it might not be the concentrations of individual cytokines that determine lineage selection, but rather the presence of given combinations of cytokines. For example, gp-130 (26) is a common receptor for IL-6, LIF, tumor necrosis factor (TNF)α, and IL-11 (and partially for IL-12 and G-CSF), which may allow progenitors at a given stage of differentiation to respond differently to a variety of inputs, depending on the microenvironment.

Many hemopoietic cytokines act on early pluripotent stem cells, promoting cell division and maturation (IL-1,-3,-6,-11,-12, G-CSF, GM-CSF, LIF, SCF) (1,3,28). Commitment to intermediate-stage granulocyte progenitors is influenced by factors such as G-CSF, GM-CSF, and IL-3 in particular. Additionally, these and other cytokines can act on more restricted cell lines, promoting cell survival, or on unipotent lineages, promoting terminal differentiation. As is clear from the preceding discussions, the multiple redundancies and potential interactions make a complete understanding of this system unlikely. However, recent research in this area has revealed important relationships between individual or groups of cytokines and the promotion of specific inflammatory cell lineages.

Basophil-Eosinophil Differentiation

It is not surprising, given that eosinophils and basophils share a common late-stage progenitor designated Eo/B-CFU (Eo/B-colony-forming unit) (29), to find that there are also common cytokines regulating hemopoiesis of both cell lines. Commitment to eosinophil and basophil lineages appears to be regulated to a large extent by the actions of IL-5, IL-3, and GM-CSF at late stages of myeloid progenitor differentiation (30,31). Binding sites for IL-3, IL-5, and GM-CSF have been located on mature basophils and eosinophils (32,33). Studies to demonstrate that these receptors are present on progenitors at various stages of lineage commitment or are altered in expression during allergic inflammation are much needed. While there is some evidence that IL-3 acting alone can support eosinophil/basophil lineage differentiation *(33)*, this cytokine has widespread hemopoietic activity (hence the name multi-CSF). IL-5, on the other hand, seems to act specifically on eosinophils in its hemopoietic capacity and can also produce eosinophil maturation acting alone *(30,31)*. In studies of transgenic mice overexpressing IL-5, there is marked circulating and tissue eosinophilia *(30)*. Despite these high levels of potentially harmful cells, there is no evidence of eosinophil-associated inflammatory disease in these mice, indicating that production and recruitment without subsequent local activation are not sufficient to produce cytotoxic effects.

Given that the cytokines responsible for eosinophil maturation, IL-3, IL-5, and GM-CSF, are produced at local sites of allergen-induced inflammation *(34–36)*, it seems quite likely that part of these cytokines' effects might be to promote cell production, thus contributing to the tissue and circulating eosinophilia observed following local allergen exposure *(35,37)*.

Granulocyte-Macrophage Differentiation

Increased production of neutrophils and monocytes, as evidenced by expansion of the granulocyte/macrophage progenitors (GM-CFU), can be achieved by the actions of IL-3, GM-CSF, and G-CSF *(38–40)*. Unlike IL-5 in its role in Eo/B-CFU production, there does not seem to be a cytokine with actions specific for GM-CFU expansion. These cytokines, which appear to be important in the maturation of GM-CFU, are also increased at local sites of allergen-induced inflammation *(34–36,41)*. Thus, although the role of the neutrophil in allergic inflammation is less clear than that of the eosinophil, increased production, stimulated by raised levels of hemopoietic cytokines, may play a role in the neutrophilic component of inflammation observed following allergen challenge *(42)*.

Mastopoiesis

While the origins of mast cells are controversial, it is clear from in vivo and in vitro studies of rodent systems that mast cells can be derived from the same pluripotent stem cells as other granulocytes *(43,44)*. However, it is not clear at which stage the mast cell progenitor becomes committed, nor at which sites the various stages of differentiation occur. While initial studies reported that mast cells appeared to derive from a lymphoid progenitor *(45)*, recent studies indicate that a circulating myeloid progenitor in the same lineage as granulocyte/macrophage is more likely *(46)*. There is evidence that SCF is the key cytokine that promotes mast cell production. The Sl/Sl^d mutant mouse, which is unable to produce SCF, is mast-cell-deficient *(47)*, as are W locus mutated rodents, which lack functional c-*kit*, the SCF receptor *(47–49)*. Additionally, IL-3 has been shown to support mast cell differentiation from human bone marrow *(48)*. As with eosinophils and neutrophils, it seems likely that allergic inflammation with ongoing release of hemopoietic cytokines, including SCF and IL-3, may contribute to increased production of mast cells.

The studies reviewed here have provided indirect evidence that links known hemopoietic cytokine gene expression and production at sites of allergic inflammation to the increased production of the inflammatory cells observed in tissue and circulation.

QUANTIFICATION OF PROGENITORS

Much of the recent work in our laboratory has focused on measuring hemopoietic progenitors associated with various allergic/asthmatic states or allergen challenges. These studies require the use of assays to measure the quantity of lineage-specific progenitors. Colony assays are useful for measuring the sensitivity of samples to respond in vitro to added hemopoietic cytokines. Quantification of cells expressing various surface markers using flow cytometry (fluorescence-activated cell sorter [FACS] and magnet-activated cell separation [MACS]) provides a means of identifying the absolute numbers of progenitors at various stages of development.

Colony Assays

Due to a lack of surface markers specific for the different stages of each cell line, most studies of hemopoietic progenitors have depended on colony assays. This assay, first developed independently by Pluznik and Sachs (50) and Bradley and Metcalf (51), is based on the culture of a sample of cells with suspected lineage-specific hemopoietic progenitors in media containing supporting hemopoietic mediators for that cell line. The lineage-specific colonies for a given number of cultured cells quantified after a standard period of time are, by definition, colony-forming units (CFU). Thus, the assay may be used to evaluate either the progenitor content of the cell sample (under conditions of standardized hemopoietic support media) or the hemopoietic properties of a new or uncharacterized hemopoietic mediator. This assay method has played a crucial role in the characterization of all of the hemopoietic cytokines discussed in this chapter. Its drawbacks are the length of time required to grow colonies (1 wk or more) and the assumption that colony growth under artificial in vitro conditions truly reflects the number of lineage-specific progenitors in vivo. While this assay is still widely used, these inherent drawbacks make the quantification of progenitor cells based on specific surface markers an attractive alternative.

Surface Marker Assays

The advent of flow cytometric analyses has facilitated the use of antibodies directed against specific cell-surface antigens as a rapid and highly reproducible means of marker analysis and cell sorting of progenitors in both human and animal systems. Surface marker expression by progenitors at differential stages of hemopoietic cell lineages is illustrated in Fig. 3. The markers of greatest interest include CD34 antigen, which is a monomeric O-sialylated glycophosphoprotein (105–120 kDa) whose expression within the hemopoietic system is restricted to developmentally early lymphohematopoietic stem and progenitor cells (52–54). Single-cell cloning experiments have revealed that $CD34^+$ cells coexpress varying levels of distinct surface markers at specific differentiation stages in the hemopoietic pathway (55). The earliest progenitors bear $CD34^{high}$, Thy-1/CDw90 (56), and A83/CDw109 (57) antigens and later acquire c-*kit* (the proto-oncogene cell product that binds SCF) (58), $CD38^{low}$ (59), and HLA-DR^{low} (60). Myeloid-lineage committed progenitors are characterized as $CD34^{low}$ $CD33^{high}$ cells (61), while B-lineage and T-lineage precursors bear $CD34^{low}$ $CD19^{high}$ cells and $CD34^{low}$ $CD7^{high}$, respectively (62,63).

Although the action of cytokines on early hemopoietic progenitors has been extensively investigated, little is known about the expression of cytokine receptors on these cells and their regulatory mechanisms. Recent studies on human bone marrow and peripheral blood cells have shown that high levels of the α-subunit of IL-3 receptor (IL-3R) are expressed on primitive $CD34^+$ progenitors and that this is attenuated as the cells become myeloid-lineage committed ($CD34^+$ $CD33^+$) (64). Conversely, expression of the α-subunit of GM-CSF receptor (GMR), undetectable on $CD34^+CD33^-$ cells, is upregulated on $CD34^+CD33^{low/high}$ cells (64). Several early acting cytokines, including G-CSF, IL-1, and INF-γ, upregulate the expression of IL-3Rα-subunit on $CD34^+$ cells, in vitro (64,65). Augmented expression of IL-5 receptor α-subunit mRNA has been detected on a subline of AML14 cell line that spontaneously differentiates to eosinophil myelocytes (66). Treatment with all-trans retinoic acid, which causes a switch in the differentiative program of the cells toward neutrophils, caused a downregulation IL-5 receptor α-subunit mRNA, suggesting a lineage-specific association of IL-5 receptor expression and development of eosinophils (66).

Studies of progenitor cell surface markers in allergic disease have shown a close correlation between $CD34^+$ cell numbers and total colony-forming units (Eo/B and GM-CFU) in cul-

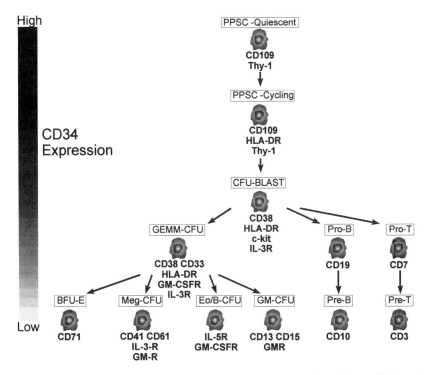

Fig. 3. Surface marker expression at differentiation stages in hemopoietic cell lines. Cell sorting based on surface marker expression allows enumeration of progenitor numbers.

tures of progenitor cells with IL-5 and GM-CSF *(67)*. These data indicate that enumeration of CD34[+] cells is predictive of the colony-forming capacity of a biological sample and may be a useful alternative tool to colony assays for enumerating progenitor cells. However, investigation of the expression of receptors for lineage-specific cytokines such as IL-5 may provide greater insight into the phenotype of eosinophil/basophil progenitor cells and the role of these cells in the development of allergic inflammation.

EVIDENCE OF INCREASED PROGENITOR ACTIVITY IN ALLERGIC INFLAMMATION

The growing evidence that hemopoietic cytokines play a major role in allergic disease supports the hypothesis that a fundamentally important aspect of allergy may be the stimulation of inflammatory cell progenitors, which would then contribute to the disease through the increased production of effector inflammatory cells *(68–70)*. Since this was first proposed, considerable evidence has been collected from both animal models and human patients, demonstrating that activation of specific progenitor cells does indeed occur in allergic disease and may well contribute to the severity of the disease. This evidence, presented in the following sections, is summarized in Table 1.

Increased Circulating Progenitors in Asthma/Allergy

The first observations that allergic disease is associated with higher inflammatory cell progenitors were made on colony assays of human blood from atopic and nonatopic individuals. Atopics demonstrated greater numbers of Eo/B-CFU than controls *(68,69)*. Initial findings

Table 1
Summary of Findings Indicating Increased Hemopoietic Activity
Associated with Allergic Inflammation or Asthma

Model	Evidence
Atopics	↑ Circulating Eo/B-CFU *(68,69)*
Compared to normal controls	↑ Circulating CD34⁺ cells *(67)*
During allergen season	Fluctuating Eo/B-CFU *(69,71)*
	Circulating Eo/B-CFU inversely correlate with tissue eosinophils and metachromatic cells *(69,71)*
Asthmatics	↑ Circulating Eo/B-CFU *(72)*
During exacerbation	
Following allergen challenge	↑ Circulating Eo/B-CFU *(73)*
	↑ Circulating CD34⁺ cells *(74)*
	↑ Bone marrow Eo/B-CFU and GM-CFU *(75)*
	↑ Bone marrow CD34⁺ cells *(76)*
Dogs	↑ Bone marrow GM-CFU *(77,78)*
Following allergen challenge	↑ Serum hemopoietic activity *(79)*
Mice	↑ Circulating and bone marrow eosinophils *(80)*
Following allergen challenge	

suggested that patients with current seasonal allergic rhinitis had lower numbers of Eo/B-CFU than those with quiescent disease, suggesting that progenitors could contribute to inflammation by trafficking to tissues *(69,71)*. However, subsequent studies have shown that the numbers of Eo/B-CFU responsive to GM-CSF are lower during seasonal allergic rhinitis, while total Eo/B-CFU are actually higher in season than out of season *(72)*. Colony assays from the peripheral blood of asthmatic patients studied at the time of an acute exacerbation of their disease grew significantly more Eo/B-CFU than assays performed following the resolution of the exacerbation *(73)*. Using flow cytometric analyses, significantly greater numbers of CD34⁺ hemopoietic progenitor cells were detected in the circulation of atopic subjects compared with normal controls *(67)*. Interestingly within the group of asymptomatic atopics, the highest levels of CD34⁺ cell numbers were detected in subjects who were skin prick test positive for house-dust mite and mold allergens, suggesting that continual exposure to low levels of these allergens may have contributed to mild subclinical inflammation resulting in the elevation of blood progenitor numbers.

The link between disease severity and progenitor numbers was further investigated by observing the effect of allergen challenge both in vitro and in vivo on the progenitor numbers in peripheral blood. Greater numbers of Eo/B-CFU were grown from the peripheral blood of atopic individuals when antigen-stimulated lymphomononuclear cell conditioned medium was included in the colony assay, indicating the generation of a hemopoietic signal following in vitro allergen exposure *(68)*. Evidence that these mechanisms are active in vivo was obtained when patients with allergic rhinitis were shown to have fluctuating numbers of Eo/B-CFU during seasonal exposure to allergen *(69,72)*, indicating a link between disease severity and hemopoietic activity. The magnitude of increases in circulating progenitor numbers was correlated with the systemic and nasal metachromatic cell infiltration and eosinophilia observed during natural allergen exposure *(69,71,74,75)*. These findings were followed by observations of allergic asthmatics during allergen-inhalation challenge. Subjects who developed late asthmatic responses following allergen challenge demonstrated significant increases in eosinophils, basophils, and Eo/B-CFU 24 h following allergen. Again, the link between disease severity and hemopoietic activity was evident since the increase in Eo/B-CFU was significantly negatively correlated with the degree of airway hyperresponsiveness measured at the same time. Individuals who did not develop late asthmatic responses or airway hyperresponsiveness did not demonstrate increases in Eo/B-CFU. Similar observations concerning antigen-specific, T-cell-generated hemopoietic signals for both in vivo and in vitro basophil production were made in guinea pig models of albumin or tick-induced basophilia (76,77).

We have recently attempted to confirm these studies using surface marker assays. We found that in subjects who developed late asthmatic responses following allergen inhalation, significant increases in blood CD34+ hemopoietic progenitors were detected 24 h postallergen. In contrast, individuals who only developed an isolated early asthmatic response to allergen challenge did not demonstrate increases in the numbers of circulating CD34+ cells (78).

These studies based on peripheral blood measurements clearly indicate increased progenitor numbers associated with allergic disease and, more importantly, correlated with the activity and severity of the disease.

Increased Bone Marrow Progenitors in Asthma/Allergy

The above studies demonstrated changes in circulating progenitors associated with allergic disease and asthma; these changes were interpreted as reflecting events taking place in the marrow. This assumption is supported by the following studies, involving colony and surface marker measurements from bone marrow aspirates.

The first studies of bone marrow response to allergen challenge were performed using a dog model of inhaled allergen-induced airway hyperresponsiveness/inflammation. This model is similar to human disease, in that the inhaled allergen (*Ascaris suum*) is associated with immediate bronchoconstriction and delayed airway hyperresponsiveness. However, unlike some human asthmatics, dogs never develop late bronchoconstrictor responses and the only inflammatory cell observed to increase in the postallergen lavage is the neutrophil (79). Studies using this model have clearly demonstrated that bone marrow myeloid progenitor cell (i.e., GM-CFU) numbers are increased following allergen challenge. Bone marrow aspirates from dogs who develop allergen-induced airway hyperresponsiveness have higher numbers of GM-CFU 24 h following allergen than following diluent challenge (79). This was not the case for dogs that were skin test positive to *Ascaris suum* but failed to develop allergen-induced hyperresponsiveness or inflammation (80). Because of the lack of available dog antibodies, it has not been possible to date to confirm these studies using surface marker assays.

To our knowledge, progenitor assays have not yet been applied to other animal models of allergic disease; interestingly, murine models of nematode or viral induced inflammation have demonstrated increases in circulating or local levels of mast cell progenitors (81,82). There is also recent evidence, using a murine model of allergen inhalation challenge, suggesting that bone marrow production of eosinophils is increased as early as 3 h following allergen inhalation (83). In this study, increased numbers of mature eosinophils were observed in the bone marrow, preceding circulating and airway lavage eosinophilia.

In accordance with these findings in animal models, we have recently demonstrated that atopy itself or allergen challenge in human atopic asthmatics is also associated with higher numbers of bone marrow progenitors. Initially, comparisons were made of surface marker levels between atopic and normal controls. Analyses of bone marrow samples from patients undergoing thoracotomy for cardiac surgery demonstrated significantly greater numbers of CD34+ progenitor cells in atopics compared with nonatopics (67). Following these observations, we studied human bone marrow progenitors from atopic asthmatics in response to allergen inhalation challenge. As with the dogs, allergen inhalation in individuals who develop late asthmatic responses, airway hyperresponsiveness, and airway eosinophilia was associated with significant increases in Eo/B-CFU and GM-CFU in colony assays *(84)*. These findings were supported by surface marker data from the same subjects, in that there was an increase in bone marrow CD34[+] cells 24 h following allergen challenge *(85)*.

Thus, it is clear that human allergic airway disease is associated with increased progenitor levels, both in circulation and in the bone marrow. These observations suggest that allergen exposure results in the production of a signal or signals that stimulate the production of specific inflammatory cells through the increased production or survival of lineage-specific progenitors.

Signaling Between Lung and Bone Marrow

Following the observations that allergic disease is associated with increased bone marrow inflammatory progenitors, we performed studies to demonstrate the presence of a hemopoietic signal in the blood following allergen exposure.

To demonstrate this hemopoietic signal, serum samples obtained from dogs following allergen exposure were used to stimulate naive bone marrow obtained from the same dog prior to allergen exposure *(80)*. Serum taken 20 min and 2 h after allergen inhalation produced significant increases in GM-CFU numbers in assays with G-CSF in the support medium, but not with GM-CSF or SCF. Serum taken 24 h after allergen inhalation produced significant increases in GM-CFU with either G-CSF, GM-CSF, or SCF in the support medium. The increase in GM-CFU numbers was similar in magnitude to that observed in postallergen bone marrow samples. Thus, these studies clearly demonstrated the presence of hemopoietic factor(s) following allergen and that these factors may be acting on select (likely more mature) progenitors as early as 20 min after allergen exposure.

Obviously, studies need to be performed to characterize and identify the hemopoietic signal(s) present following allergen exposure and to demonstrate it in human disease. The most likely explanation for the nature of the signal is that it is one or more of the many proinflammatory and hemopoietic cytokines released in association with allergen exposure. There is evidence that IL-3, IL-4, IL-5, IL-8, G-CSF, GM-CSF, M-CSF, SCF, TNFα, TGFβ, and others are expressed or produced by mast cells, lymphocytes, epithelial cells, and fibroblasts of chronically inflamed or allergen-exposed airways of patients with nasal polyposis, allergic rhinitis, and asthma *(34,86–92)*. Since many of these cytokines are involved in the stimulation or inhibition of specific hemopoietic lineages, it seems possible that an endocrine effect of one or more cytokines on the bone marrow may be important in allergic disease.

Evidence exists supporting a true endocrine effect of hemopoietic cytokines, indicating that they may be generated at sites distant from the bone marrow, achieving their effects after traveling through the circulation. Indeed, ip or iv injections of the hemopoietic cytokines LIF, IL-6, or IL-11 into mice produce increases in megakaryocytopoiesis *(93–95)*. This "endocrine" effect of hemopoietic cytokines has also been observed in the myeloid lineage, in that iv GM-CSF, G-CSF, or IL-3 in humans produce increases in both bone marrow myeloid progenitors and circulating eosinophils *(38)*. It has also been shown in monkeys that iv or subcutaneous IL-3 primes progenitors so that subsequent iv GM-CSF results in marked increases in circulating eosinophils, neutrophils, and basophils *(96,97)*. Recent work by Collins et al. *(98)* has demonstrated that the chemokine eotaxin given intradermally to guinea pigs does not produce local eosinophilia unless IL-5 is simultaneously administered intravenously, in which case increases in eosinophils are seen locally, systemically, and in the bone marrow. These findings are the first to show that a specific cytokine can result in increased production, trafficking, and local accumulation of an inflammatory cell. Similar increases in circulating and local eosinophils have recently been reported by Xing et al. *(99)*, utilizing an adenovirus to generate transient overexpression of GM-CSF in the rat airway. These studies demonstrate that hemopoietic cytokines, known to be increased following allergen challenge, may exert endocrine effects on the marrow, resulting in the increased release and, possibly, production of inflammatory cells, which are also appearing at local sites of inflammation. Whether these or other cytokines are responsible for increased hemopoietic activity observed following allergen challenge remains to be investigated.

Of equal importance to the identification of the allergen-induced hemopoietic factor(s) is the understanding of the importance of the resulting increased inflammatory-cell production to the ongoing pathology at the site of allergen exposure. Although it is possible that the increased production of specific inflammatory cells is primary and a prerequisite for the development of local inflammation, a more attractive hypothesis is that the increased inflammatory-cell production is secondary to ongoing chronic inflammation. In either case, blocking hemopoietic stimulation may be of therapeutic benefit in allergic inflammatory diseases.

Does Allergic Disease Depend on Intrinsic Properties of the Bone Marrow?

In the studies presented above, there is no evidence to suggest that the response of the bone marrow to the allergen-induced hemopoietic signal depends on an intrinsic property of the marrow. Indeed, we have recently shown that serum taken from dogs at the time of allergen-induced airway hyperresponsiveness is capable of stimulating increased GM-CFU formation from the marrow of dogs that do not develop either airway or bone marrow responses following allergen inhalation (100). These results could be interpreted as evidence that the role of the bone marrow in allergic disease is supportive, i.e., that the marrow is responding in an entirely appropriate way to the signals that have been generated by the airway, in keeping with the hypothesis that the origin of the disease resides in the airway. However, evidence obtained from patients undergoing bone marrow transplant suggests that an important determinant of atopic disease may well reside in the bone marrow. In a study of 12 recipients of bone marrow grafts from atopic donors, nine recipients developed new positive skin test responses to standard allergens, and/or asthma (101). It is quite likely that in some recipients, the new allergic sensitivity was owing to passive sensitization following the transfer of an allergen-specific B-cell clone (101). However, these studies raise the possibility that the predisposition toward allergic inflammation is resident in the pluripotent stem cells in the bone marrow. This concept is supported by recent evidence obtained from mice with genetic predisposition to airway hyperresponsiveness (102). When marrow is transplanted from these mice into normal mice, a significant component of the airway hyperresponsiveness is also transferred, implicating genetically determined intrinsic properties of the bone marrow in the development of airway pathology. If this were the case in human allergic disease, then long-term suppression of specific lineages may prove beneficial in the management of allergic/asthmatic patients. Further study is needed to determine whether the bone marrow, the airway, or both are necessary for the development of allergic airway disease.

PROGENITORS AS A POTENTIAL THERAPEUTIC TARGET IN ASTHMA/ALLERGY

In the previous section we raised the concept that treatment of allergic inflammatory diseases could involve prevention of allergen-induced increases in inflammatory cell production. In this section we review the evidence that known antiallergy/asthma drugs may exert some of their effect by this mechanism.

We have shown that patients undergoing exacerbation of their asthma demonstrate high numbers of circulating eosinophils, basophils, and Eo/B-CFU. When these subjects were treated for 2 wk with inhaled beclomethasone, the decrease in asthma symptoms was associated with decreases in circulating cells and progenitors *(73)*. Following these observations, we treated dogs known to develop allergen-induced hyperresponsiveness with inhaled budesonide prior to inhaled allergen challenge. Inhaled budesonide treatment had no effect on baseline GM-CFU numbers, but completely blocked the allergen-induced increase in GM-CFU and attenuated the allergen-induced airway hyperresponsiveness *(79)*. The explanation given at the time of these studies was that glucocorticosteroid treatment blocked the production of proinflammatory and hemopoietic cytokines, thus preventing the stimulation of the bone marrow *(73,79)*. However, both of these studies raised the possibility that there is a systemic effect of the steroid that "protects" the marrow from the allergen/asthma-induced hemopoietic effect.

We have recently investigated whether known anti-allergy/asthma drugs can protect the bone marrow from the effect of the allergen-induced serum hemopoietic factor *(103)*. We added budesonide (10^{-7} M) or PGE_2 (10^{-6} M) to naive bone marrow before adding postallergen serum. While budesonide and PGE_2 had no effect on baseline GM-CFU numbers, both treatments completely prevented the postallergen serum from stimulating an increase in GM-CFU numbers. Although it is well known that steroid treatment reduces the production of proinflammatory cytokines at the site of allergic inflammation *(104,105)*, it is possible that effects on the bone marrow and inflammatory-cell production are also important. This might explain why oral steroids with high systemic availability are necessary for the treatment of severe chronic disease or acute severe exacerbations.

The mechanism by which these drugs exert their "protective" effect on the bone marrow has not yet been investigated. A direct blocking of the hemopoietic effect of the serum factor or prevention of production of hemopoietic cytokines by the marrow in response to the serum factor both seem plausible explanations.

If the release of the hemopoietic signal and subsequent increased inflammatory-cell production represent important events in the pathogenesis of acute or chronic inflammation, then specific blocking agents of or antibodies to hemopoietic signal(s) will be therapeutically useful. This may explain in part why treatment with antibodies to IL-5 in animal models blocks allergen-induced local and systemic eosinophilia and airway hyperresponsiveness for periods lasting up to 6 mo *(106–110)*.

Further research is required to determine whether specific blocking of allergen-mediated increased inflammatory-cell production will be effective ultimately in reducing local inflammation and disease symptoms. If this turns out to be the case, it may both confirm the importance of hemopoietic mechanisms as the target of therapy as well as indicate further sites for intervention, including hemopoietic cytokine blocking agents (synthesis blockers, antibodies, receptor antagonists) and agents to block adhesion molecules required for movement of progenitors or mature cells out of bone marrow into circulation.

SUMMARY

Several studies have begun to address the role of the bone marrow in allergic inflammation. The findings of these studies are summarized in Fig. 4. There is clear evidence that allergic airway inflammation is accompanied by increased circulating and bone marrow inflammatory progenitor cells and that this effect is mediated by a hemopoietic signal, present in circulation following allergen exposure. Ongoing research in this area is directed at identifying the relevant hemopoietic signal(s) and determining the importance of the increased inflammatory-cell production/release in both acute and chronic allergic-type inflammation. A more complete understanding of these fundamental concepts may provide the basis for the development of novel therapeutic interventions in allergy and asthma (Fig. 5).

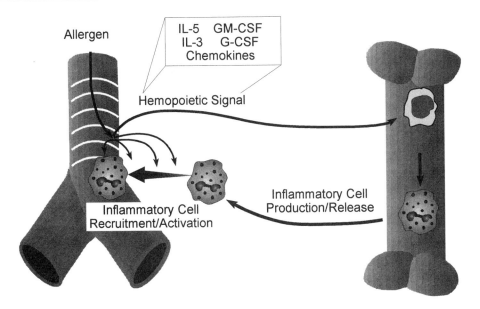

Fig. 4. The evidence presented in this chapter indicates that allergen-induced airway disease is associated with the production of serum signal(s) that have lineage-specific hemopoietic properties. The importance of the resulting inflammatory-cell production/release in the ensuing inflammatory-cell recruitment/activation is not known. Further research in this area is supported by the likelihood that one or more of these sites may prove to be an effective point for therapeutic intervention.

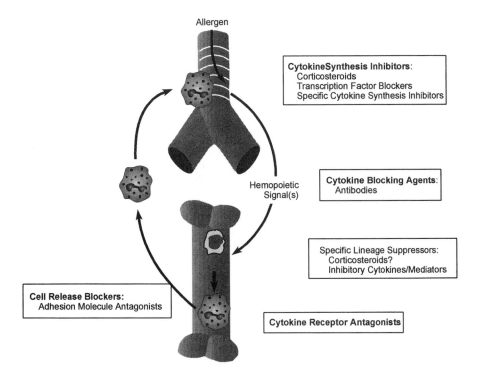

Fig. 5. Sites at which known and potential antiallergy/asthma drugs may act through the inhibition of increased inflammatory-cell production or release into circulation.

REFERENCES

1. Metcalf D (1993) Hematopoietic regulators: redundancy or subtlety. Blood 81:3515–3523.
2. Lord BI, Dexter TM (1992) Growth Factors in Haemopoiesis. Bailliere Tindall, London.
3. Ogawa M (1993) Differential and proliferation of hematopoietic stem cells. Blood, 81:2844–2853.
4. Till JE, McCullogh EA, Siminovitch L (1964) A stochastic model of stem cell proliferation, based on growth of spleen colony-forming cells. Proc Natl Acad Sci USA 51:29.
5. Humphries RK, Eaves AC, Eaves CJ (1981) Self-renewal of hemopoietic stem cells during mixed colony formation in vitro. Proc Natl Acad Sci USA 78:3629–3633.
6. Nakahata T, Gross AJ, Ogawa M (1982) A stochastic model of self-renewal and commitment to differentiation of the primitive hemopoietic stem cells in culture. J Cell Physiol 113:455–458.
7. Suda T, Suda J, Ogawa M (1983) Single-cell origin of mouse hemopoietic colonies expressing multiple lineages in variable combinations. Proc Natl Acad Sci USA 80:6689–6693.
8. Suda T, Suda J, Ogawa M (1984) Disparate differentiation in mouse hemopoietic colonies derived from paired colonies. Proc Natl Acad Sci USA 81:2520–2524.
9. Leary AG, Ogawa M, Strauss LC, Civin CI (1984) Single cell origin of multilineage colonies in culture: Evidence that differentiation of multipotent progenitors and restriction of proliferative potential of monopotent progenitors are stochastic processes. J Clin Invest 74:2193–2197.
10. Leary AG, Strauss LC, Civin CI, Ogawa M (1985) Disparate differentiation in hemopoietic colonies derived from human paired progenitors. Blood 66:327–332.
11. Fairburn LJ, Cowling GJ, Reipert BM, Dexter TM (1993) Suppression of apoptosis allows differentiation and development of a multipotent hemopoietic cell line in the absence of added growth factors. Cell 74:823–832.
12. Koury MJ (1992) Programmed cell death (apoptosis) in hemopoiesis. Exp Hematol 20:391–394.
13. Just U, Stocking C, Spooner E, Dexter TM, Osterag W (1991) Expression of the GM-CSF gene after retroviral transfer in hematopoietic stem cell lines induces synchronous granulocyte-macrophage differentiation. Cell 64:1163–1173.
14. Spivak JL (1986) The mechanism of action of erythropoietin. Int J Cell Cloning 4:139–166.
15. Sherr CJ (1990) Colony stimulating factor-1 receptor. Blood 75:1–12.
16. Yarden Y, Kuang W, Yang-Feng T, Coussens L, Munemitsu S, Dull TJ, Chen E, Schlessinger J, Francke U, Ullrich A (1987) Human proto-oncogene c-*kit*: a new surface receptor tyrosine kinase for an unidentified ligand. EMBO J 6:3341–3351.
17. Cosman D, Ceretti DP, Larsen A, Park L, March C, Domer S, Gillis S, Urdahl D (1986) Cloning and expression of human interleukin 2 receptor. Nature 312:768–771.
18. Miyajima A, Mui AL, Ogorochi T, Sakamaki K (1993) Receptors for granulocyte-macrophage colony stimulating factor, interleukin-3 and interleukin-5. Blood 82:1960–1974.
19. Kitamura T, Sato N, Arai K, Miyajima A (1991) Expression cloning of the human IL-3 receptor cDNA reveals a shared beta subunit for the human IL-3 and GM-CSF receptors. Cell 66:1165–1174.
20. Harada N, Castle BE, Gorman DM, Itoh N, Shreurs J, Barret RL, Howard M, Miyajima A (1990) Expression cloning of a cDNA encoding the murine interleukin-4 receptor based on ligand binding. Proc Natl Acad Sci USA 87:857–861.
21. Takaki S, Tominaga A, Hitoshi Y, Mita S, Sonoda E, Yamaguchi N, Takutsu K (1990) Molecular cloning and expression of the murine interleukin-5 receptor. EMBO J 9:4367–4374.
22. Yamasaki K, Taga T, Hirata Y, Yawata H, Kawanishi Y, Seed B, Taniguchi T, Hirano T, Kishimoto T (1988) Cloning and expression of the human interleukin-6 (BSF-2/IFN beta 2) receptor. Science 241:825–828.
23. Goodwin RG, Friend D, Ziegler SF, Jerzy, R Falk, BA, Gimpel S, Cosman D, Dower SK, March CJ, Namen AE, Park LS (1990) Cloning of the human and murine interleukin-7 receptors: demonstration of a soluble form and homology to a new receptor super-family. Cell 60:941–951.
24. Yang YC, Yin T (1992) Interleukin-11 and its receptor. Biofactors 4:15–21.
25. Fukanuga R, Ishizaka-Ikeda E, Seto Y, Ngata S (1990) Expression cloning of a receptor for murine granulocyte colony-stimulating factor. Cell 61:341–350.
26. Gearing DP, Thut CJ, VandenBos T, Gimpel SD, Delaney PB, King JA, Price V, Cosman D, Beckmann MP (1991) Leukemia inhibitory factor receptor is structurally related to IL-6 signal transducer, gp 130. EMBO J 10:2839–2848.
27. Vadas MA, Lopez AF, Gamble JR, Elliot MJ (1991) Role of colony stimulating factors in leukocyte responses to inflammation and infection. Curr Opin Immunol 3:97–104.

28. Smith LJ, Rubin AE, Patterson R (1988) Mechanisms of platelet activating factor-induced broncho-constriction in humans. Am Rev Resp Disease 137:1015–1019.

29. Denburg JA, Telizyn S, Messner H, Jamal BLN, Ackerman SJ, Gleich GJ, Bienenstock J (1985) Heterogeneity of human peripheral blood eosinophil type colonies: evidence for a common basophil-eosinophil progenitor. Blood 66:312–318.

30. Sanderson CJ, Warren DJ, Strath M (1985) Identification of a lymphokine that stimulates oesinophil differentiation in vitro. Its relationship to interleukin-3, and functional properties of eosinophils produced in culture. J Exp Med 162:60–74.

31. Clutterbuck EJ, Sanderson CJ (1988) Human eosinophil hematopoiesis studied in vitro by means of murine eosinophil differentiation factor (IL-5): production of fucntionally active eosinophils from normal human bone marrow. Blood 71:646–651.

32. Denburg JA (1992) Basophil and mast cell lineages in vitro and in vivo. Blood 79:846–860.

33. Valent P, Ashman LK, Hinterberger W, Eckersberger F, Majdic O, Lechner K, Bettelheim P (1989) Mast cell typing: demonstration of a distinct hematopoietic cell type and evidence for immunophenotypic relationship to mononuclear phagocytes. Blood 73:1778–1785.

34. Durham SR, Sun Ying, Varney VA, Jacobson MR, Sudderick RM, Mackay IS, Kay AB, Hamid QA (1992) Cytokine messenger RNA expression for IL-3, IL-4, IL-5 and GM-CSF in the nasal mucosa after local allergen provocation: relationship to tissue eosinophilia. J Immunol 148:2390–2394.

35. Woolley KL, Adelroth E, Woolley MJ, Ellis R, Jordana M, O'Byrne PM (1995) Effects of allergen challenge on eosinophils, eosinophil cationic protein and granulocyte-macrophage colony stimulating factor in mild asthma. Am J Resp Crit Care Med 151:1915–1924.

36. Sousa AR, Poston RN, Lane SJ, Nakhosteen JA, Lee TH (1993) Detection of GM-CSF in asthmatic bronchial epithelium and decrease by inhaled corticosteroids. Am Rev Resp Disease 147:1557–1561.

37. Resnick MB, Weller PF (1993) Mechanisms of eosinophil recruitment. Am J Resp Cell Mol Biol 8:349–355.

38. Hansen PB, Knudsen H, Gaarsdal E, Jensen L, Ralfkiaer E, Johnsen HE (1995) Short-term in vivo priming of bone marrow haematopoiesis with rhG-CSF, rhGM-CSF or rhIL-3 before marrow harvest expands myelopoiesis but does not improve engraftment capability. Bone Marrow Transpl 16:373–379.

39. Metcalf D (1980) Clonal analysis of proliferation and differentiation of paired daughter cells: action of granulocyte-macrophage colony stimulating factor on granulocyte-macrophage precursors. Proc Natl Acad Sci USA 77:5327–5330.

40. Metcalf D (1991) Lineage commitment of hemopoietic progenitor cells in developing blast cell colonies: Influences of colony stimulating factors. Proc Natl Acad Sci USA 88:11,310–11,314.

41. McDermott C, Fenwick B (1992) Neutrophil activity associated with increased neutrophil acyloxyacyl hydrolase activity during inflammation in cattle. Am J Vet Res, 53:803–807.

42. Azzawi MB, Bradley B, Jeffery PK, Frew AJ, Wardlaw AJ, Knowles G, Assoufi B, Collins JV, Durham S, Kay AB (1990) Identification of activated T lymphocytes and eosinophils in bronchial biopsies in stable atopic asthmatics. Am Rev Resp Disease 142:1407–1413.

43. Kitamura Y, Yokoyama M, Matsuda H, Ohno T, Mori KJ (1981) Spleen colony-forming cell as common precursor for tissue mast cells and granulocytes. Nature 291:159–160.

44. Kitamura Y, Go S, Hatanaka K (1978) Decrease of mast cells in W/W^v mice and their increase by bone marrow transplantation. Blood 52:447–452.

45. Ginsburg H, Lagunoff D (1967) The in vitro differentiation of mast cells. Cultures of cells from immunized mouse lymph nodes and thoracic duct lymph on fibrous monolayers. J Cell Biol 35:685–697.

46. Agis H, Willheim M, Sperr WR, Wilfing A, Boltz-Nitulescu G, Geissler K (1993) Identification of the circulating mast cell progenitor as a c-kit^+, CD43$^+$, CD14$^+$, CD17$^-$, LY$^-$, colony forming cell. Blood 82(Suppl):102a (abstract).

47. Jarboe DL, Huff TF (1989) The mast cell-committed progenitor II. W/W^v do not make mast cell committed progenitors and SI/SId fibroblasts do not support development of normal mast cell committed progenitors. J Immunol 142:2418–2423.

48. Kirshenbaum AS, Goff JP, Dreskin SC, Irani A, Schwartz LB, Metcalf DD (1989) IL-3 dependent growth of basophil-like and mast-cell-like cells from human bone marrow. J Immunol 142: 2424–2429.

49. Tei H, Kasugai T, Tsujimura T, Adachi S, Furitsu T, Tohya K, Kimura M, Zsebo KM, Newlands GF, Miller HR, Kanakura Y, Kitamura Y (1994) Characterization of cultured mast cells derived from W^s/W^s mast cell deficient rats with a small deletion at tyrosine kinase domain of c-kit. Blood 83:916–925.

50. Pluznik DH, Saks SL (1965) The cloning of normal "mast" cells in tissue culture. J Cell Comp Physiol 66:319–324.

51. Bradley TR, Metcalf D (1966) The growth of mouse bone-marrow cells in vitro. Austral J Exp Biol Biolog Sci 44:287–289.

52. Civin CI, Strauss LC, Brovall C, Schwartz JF Shaper JH (1984) Antigenic analysis of hemopoietic progenitor cell surface antigen defined by a monoclonal antibody raised against KG-1a cells. J Immunol 133:157–165.

53. Katz F, Tindle RW, Sutherland DR, Greaves MD (1985) Identification of a membrane glycoprotein associated with hemopoietic progenitor cells. Leukemia Res 9:191–198.

54. Sutherland DR, Eating A (1992) The CD34 antigen: Structure, biology and potential clinical applications. J Hemotherapy 1:115–129.

55. Civin CI, Trischman MJ, Fackler I, Bernstein I, Buhring H, Campos L, Greaves MF, Kamoun M, Katz D, Lansdorp P, Look T, Seed B, Sutherland DR, Tindle R, Uchanska-Zeigler B (1989) Summary of CD34 cluster workshop section. In: W. Knapp, (ed.), Leukocyte typing. Oxford University Press, Oxford, pp. 818–825.

56. Baum CM, Weissman IL, Tsukamoto A, Buckle A, Penult B (1992) Isolation of a candidate human hematopoietic stem cell population. Proc Natl Acad Sci USA 89:2804–2808.

57. Murray LJ, Bruno E, Yeo EL, Tsukamoto A, Hoffman R, Sutherland DR (1994) CDw109 antibody 8A3 identifies a minor subset of CD34$^+$ foetal bone marrow cells that includes multilineage and megakaryocyte progenitor cells as well as hemopoietic stem cells. Blood 84(Suppl):327 (abstract)

58. Stobl H, Takimoto M, Majdic P, Hocker P, Knaff W (1992) Antigenic analysis of human hemopoietic progenitor cells expressing the growth factor c-*kit*. Br J Haematol 82:287–294.

59. Hao Q, Shah AJ, Thiemann FT, Smogorzewska EM, Crooks, GM (1995) A functional comparison of CD34$^+$, CD38$^-$ cells in cord blood and bone marrow. Blood 86:3745–3753.

60. Sealand S, Duvert V, Caux C, Pandrau D, Favre C, Valle A, Durand I, Charbord P, deVries J, Banchereau (1992) Distribution of surface-membrane molecules on bone marrow and cord blood CD34$^+$ hemopoietic cells. Exp Hematol 20:24–33.

61. Pierelli L, Teopili L, Menichella G, Rumi C, Paolinin A, Lovino S, Puggioni PL, Bruno B (1993) Further investigations on the expression of HLA-DR, CD33 and CD13 surface antigens on purified bone marrow and peripheral blood CD34$^+$ hemopoietic progenitor cells. Br J Haematol 84:24–30.

62. Ryan D, Kossover S, Mitchell S, Frantz C, Hennessy L, Cohen H (1986) Subpopulations of common acute leukemia antigen-positive lymphoid cells in normal bone marrow identified by hemopoietic differentiation antigens. Blood 68:417–425.

63. Mossalayi MD, Dalloul AH, Betho JM, Lecron JC, Goube de Laforest P, Depre P (1990) In vitro differentiation and proliferation of purified human thymic and bone marrow CD7$^-$ CD2$^-$ T-cell precursors. Exp Hematol 18:326–331.

64. Kurata H, Arai K, Yokata T, Arai, K (1995) Differential expression of granulocyte macrophage-colony stimulating factor and IL-3 receptor subunits on human CD34$^+$ cells and leukemic cell lines. J Allergy Clin Immunol 96:1083–1099.

65. Sato N, Caux C, Kitamura T, Watanabe Y, Arai K, Banchereau J, Myajima A (1993) Expression and factor-dependent modulation of the interleukin-3 receptor subunits on human hematopoietic cells. Blood 82:752–761.

66. Paul CC, Mahrer S, Marshall T, Elbert T, Wong I, Ackerman SJ, Baumgarten C (1995) Changing the differentiation program of hematopoietic cells: Retinoic acid-induced shift of eosinohil-committed cells to neutrophils. Blood 86:3737–3744.

67. Sehmi R, Howie K, Sutherland DR, Schragge W, O'Byrne PM, Denburg JA (1996) Increased levels of CD34$^+$ hemopoietic progenitor cells in atopic subjects. Am J Resp Cell Mol Biol 15:645–654.

68. Denburg JA, Telizyn S, Belda A, Dolovich J, Bienenstock J (1985) Increased numbers of circulating basophil progenitors in atopic patients. J Allergy Clin Immunol 76:466–472.

69. Otsuka H, Dolovich J, Befus D, Telizyn S, Bienenstock J, Denburg, JA (1986) Basophilic cell progenitors, nasal metachromatic cells, and peripheral blood basophils in ragweed-allergic patients. J Allergy Clin Immunol 78:365–371.

70. Denburg JA, Dolovich J, Harnish D (1989) Basophil mast cell and eosinophil growth and differentiation factors in human allergic disease. Clin Exp Allergy 19:249–254.

71. Otsuka H, Dolovich J, Befus D, Bienenstock J, Denburg JA (1986) Peripheral blood basophils, basophil progenitors, and nasal metachromatic cells in allergic rhinitis. Am Rev Resp Disease 133:757–762.

72. Linden M, Svensson C, Andersson M, Greiff L, Andersson E, Denburg JA, Seidegard J, Persson CGA (1994) Increased numbers of circulating leukocyte progenitors in patients with allergic rhinitis during natural allergen exposure. Am J Resp Crit Care Med 149:A602 (abstract)

73. Gibson PG, Dolovich J, Girgis-Girbado A, Morris M, Anderson M, Hargreave FE, Denburg JA (1990) The inflammatory response in asthma exacerbation: changes in circulating eosinophils, basophils and their progenitors. Clin Exp Allergy 20:661–668.

74. Taylor IK, O'Shaughnessy KM, Fuller RW, Dollery CT (1991) Effect of a cysteinyl leukotriene receptor antagonist, ICI-219, on allergen-induced bronchoconstriction and airway hyperreactivity in atopic subjects. Lancet 337:690–694.

75. Gelb AF, Tashkin DP, Epstein JD, Gong H, Zamel N (1985) Exercise-induced bronchoconstriction in asthma. Chest 87:196–201.

76. Denburg JA, Davison M, Bienenstock J (1980) Basophil production: Stimulation by factors derived from guinea pig splenic T-lymphocytes. J Clin Invest 65:390–399.

77. Denburg JA, Askenase P, Brown SJ, Bienenstock J (1986) Serum basophil-stimulating activity in the guinea-pig during induction of basophilic responses to ovalbumin and tick feeding. Immunology 58:405–410.

78. Sehmi R, Wood LJ, Watson RM, Inman MD, O'Byrne PM, Denburg JA (1996) Increases in circulating CD34+ hemopoietic progenitors in allergen induced late asthmatic responses. J Allergy Clin Immunol 97:277 (abstract)

79. Woolley MJ, Denburg JA, Ellis R, Dahlback M, O'Byrne PM (1994) Allergen-induced changes in bone marrow progenitors and airway responsiveness in dogs and the effect of inhaled budesonide on these parameters. Am J Resp Cell Mol Biol 11:600–606.

80. Inman MD, Denburg JA, Ellis R, Dahlback M, O'Byrne PM (1996) Allergen-induced increase in bone marrow progenitors in airway hyperresponsive dogs: Regulation by a serum hemopoietic factor. Am J Resp Cell Mol Biol 15:305–311.

81. Kasugai T, Tei H, Okada M, Hirota S, Morimoto M, Yamada M, Nakama A, Arizono N, Kitamura Y (1995) Infection with *Nippostrongulus brasiliensis* induces invasion of mast cell precursors from peripheral blood to small intestine. Blood 85:1334–1340.

82. Sorden SD, Castleman WL (1995) Virus-induced increases in mast cells in brown Norway rats are associated with both local mast cell proliferation and increases in blood mast cell precursors. Lab Invest 73:197–204.

83. Ohwawara Y, Lei X, Stampfli X, Xing Z, Jordana M (1996) Cytokine and eosinophil responses in peripheral blood and bone marrow in a murine model of allergen-induced airways eosinophilic inflammation. Am J Resp Crit Care Med 153:A140 (abstract).

84. Wood LJ, Inman MD, Watson RM, Denburg JA, O'Byrne PM (1996) Changes in bone marrow progenitor cells following allergen challenge in mild asthmatic subjects. Am J Resp Crit Care Med 153:A250 (abstract)

85. Sehmi R, Wood LJ, Inman MD, Watson RM, O'Byrne PM, Lopez AF, Denburg JA (1996) Increases in bone marrow derived CD34+ hemopoietic progenitor cells expressing the alpha-subunit of IL-3 receptors following allergen challenge in mild asthmatics. Am J Resp Crit Care Med 153:A880 (abstract)

86. Denburg JA, Dolovich J, Ohtoshi T, Cox G, Gauldie J, Jordana M (1990) The microenvironmental differentiation hypothesis of airway inflammation. Am J Rhinol 4:29–32.

87. Jordana M, Vancheri C, Ohtoshi T, Harnish D, Gauldie J, Dolovich J, Denburg JA (1989) Hemopoietic function of the microenvironment in chronic airway inflammation. Agents Actions (suppl) 28:85–95.

88. Kim YK, Nakagawa N, Nakano K, Sulakvelidze I, Dolovich J, Denburg JA (1996) Immunolocalization of stem cell factor in inflamed nasal tissue. J Allergy Clin Immunol 97:282 (abstract).

89. Ohnishi M, Ruhno J, Bienenstock J, Dolovich J, Denburg JA (1989) Hematopoietic growth factor production by cultured cells of human nasal polyp epithelial scrapings: kinetics, cell source and relationship to clinical status. J Allergy Clin Immunol 83:1091–1100.

90. Nonaka M, Nonaka R, Woolley KL, Adelroth E, Miura K, Okhawara Y, Glibetic M, Nakono K, O'Byrne PM, Dolovich J, Jordana M (1995) Distinct immunohistochemical localization of IL-4 in human inflamed airway tissues. IL-4 is localized to eosinophils *in vivo* and released by peripheral blood eosinophils. J Immunol 155:3234–3244.

91. Broide DH, Paine MM, Firestein GS (1992) Eosinophils express interleukin 5 and granulocyte-macrophage colony stimulating factor mRNA at sites of allergic inflammation in asthmatics. J Allergy Clin Immunol 90:1414–1424.

92. Corrigan CJ, Hamid Q, North J, Barkans J, Moqbel R, Durham S, Kay AB (1995) Peripheral blood CD4, but not CD8 T lymphocytes in patients with exacerbation of asthma transcribe messenger RNA encoding cytokines which prolong eosinophil survival in the context of a Th2-type pattern: effect of glucocorticoid therapy. Am J Resp Cell Mol Biol 12:567–578.

93. Metcalf D, Nicola NA, Gearing DP (1990) Effects of injected leukemia inhibitory factor on hematopoietic and other tissues in mice. Blood 76:50–56.

94. Ishibashi T, Kimura H, Shikama Y, Uchida T, Kariyone S, Hirano T, Kishimoto T, Akiyama Y (1989) Interleukin-6 is a potent thrombopoietic factor in vivo in mice. Blood 74:1241–1244.

95. Neben TY, Loebelenz J, Hayes L, McCarthy K, Stoudemire J, Schaub R, Goldman SJ (1993) Recombinant human interleukin-11 stimulates megakaryocytopoiesis and increases in peripheral platelets in normal and splenectomized mice. Blood 81:901–908.

96. Mayer P, Valent P, Schmidt G, Liehl E, Bettelheim P (1989) The in vivo effects of recombinant human interleukin-3: Demonstration of basophil differentiation factor, histamine producing activity, and priming of GM-CSF responsive progenitors in nonhuman primates. Blood 74:613–621.

97. Donahue RE, Seehra J, Metzger M, Lefebvre D, Rock B, Carbone S, Nathan DG, Garnick M, Sehgal PK, Laston D, LaVallie E, McCoy J, Schendel PF, Norton C, Turner K, Yang Y, Clark SC (1988) Human IL-3 and GM-CSF act synergistically in stimulating hematopoiesis in primates. Science 241:1820–1823.

98. Collins PD, Marleau S, Griffiths-Johnson DA, Jose PJ, Williams TJ (1995) Cooperation between interleukin-5 and the chemokine eotaxin to induce eosinophil accumulation in vivo. J Exp Med 182:1169–1174.

99. Xing Z, Ohkawara Y, Jordana M, Graham FL, Gauldie J (1996) Transfer of granulocyte-macrophage colony-stimulating factor gene to rat lung induces eosinophilia, monocytosis and fibrotic reactions. J Clin Invest 97:1102–1110.

100. Inman MD, Ellis R, Wattie J, Lane CG, Dahlback M, Denburg JA, O'Byrne PM (1996) Increased bone marrow growth after allergen challenge in dogs depends on a serum factor. J Allergy Clin Immunol 97:297 (abstract).

101. Agosti JM, Sprenger JD, Lum LG, Witherspoon RP, Fisher LD, Storb R, Henderson WR (1988) Transfer of allergen-specific IgE mediated hypersensitivity with allogenic bone marrow transplantation. N Engl J Med 319:1623–1628.

102. De Sanctis GT, Itoh A, Qin S, Green FYH, Grobholz JK, Maki T, Martin TR, Drazen JM (1996) Bone marrow transplantation partially confers genetically determined hyperreactivity in inbred mice. Am J Resp Crit Care Med 153:A769 (abstract).

103. Metzger WJ, Zavala D, Richerson HB, Moseley P, Iwamota P, Monick M, Sjoerdsma K, Hunnunghake GK (1987) Local allergen challenge and bronchoalveolar lavage of allergic asthmatic lungs. Am Rev Resp Disease 135:433–440.

104. Barnes PJ, Adcock I (1993) Anti-inflammatory actions of steroids: molecular mechanisms. TiPS Revs 14:436–441.

105. Taylor IK, Shaw RJ (1993) The mechanism of action of corticosteroids in asthma. Resp Med 87:261–277.

106. Mauser PJ, Pitman AM, Fernandez X, Foran SK, Adams III GK, Kreutner W, Egan RW, Chapman RW (1995) Effects of an antibody to interleukin-5 in a monkey model of asthma. Am J Resp Crit Care Med 152:467–472.

107. Gulbenkian AR, Egan RW, Fernandez X, Jones H, Kreutner W, Kung T, Payvandi F, Sullivan L, Zurcher JA, Watnick AS (1992) Interleukin-5 modulates eosinophil accumulation in allergic guinea pig lung. Am Rev Resp Disease 146:263–265.

108. Kung TT, Stelts DM, Zurcher JA, Adams III GK, Egan RW, Kreutner W, Watnick AS, Jones H, Chapman RW (1995) Involvement of IL-5 in a murine model of allergic pulmonary inflammation: prophylactic and therapeutic effect of an IL-5 antibody. Am J Resp Cell Mol Biol 13:360–365.

109. Mauser PJ, Pitman A, Fernandez X, Zurcher JA, Kung T, Watnick AS, Egan RW, Kreutner W, Adams III GK (1993) Inhibitory effect of the TRFK-5 anti-IL-5 antibody in a guinea pig model of asthma. Am Rev Resp Disease 148:1623–1627.

110. Egan RW, Athwahl D, Chou C, Emtage S, Jehn C, Kung TT, Mauser PJ, Murgolo NJ, Bodmer MW (1995) Inhibition of pulmonary eosinophilia and hyperreactivity by antibodies to interleukin-5. Int Arch Allergy Immunol 107:321–322.

111. Gibson PG, Manning PJ, O'Byrne PM, Girgis-Girbado A, Dolovich J, Denburg JA, Hargreave FE (1991) Allergen-induced asthmatic responses. Relationship between increases in airway responsiveness and increases in circulating eosinophils, basophils and their progenitors. Am Rev Resp Disease 143:331–335.

6

The Role of Mast Cells in Inflammation and Homeostasis

Angus J. MacDonald, PhD, Fiona L. Wills, PhD, Tong-Jun Lin, PhD, and A. Dean Befus, PhD

CONTENTS

INTRODUCTION
PROGENITOR CELLS AND MAST CELL DEVELOPMENT
HETEROGENEITY
MAST CELL ACTIVATION AND FUNCTIONAL REGULATION
THE EFFECTS OF MAST CELLS ON THEIR MACROENVIRONMENT
CONCLUSIONS
REFERENCES

INTRODUCTION

The mast cell (MC) is a major effector of inflammation. Therefore, understanding its regulation and interplay with other cells is imperative to the management of inflammatory disease. MC populations are heterogeneous with distinct phenotypes tailored by the microenvironment to required functions: they are influenced by mediators produced by T- and B-lymphocytes, stromal, and inflammatory cells, and in turn can modulate the environment through production of cytokines and other molecules. This heterogeneity is best exemplified in the rat, where two highly divergent phenotypes, the connective tissue mast cell (CTMC) and the mucosal mast cell (MMC), have been well characterized and demonstrate many functional and morphological differences. The location of MC adjacent to blood vessels, smooth muscle, mucosal surfaces, and nerve endings *(1,2)* puts them in an ideal setting to effect regulatory functions by releasing their mediators (e.g., biogenic amines, arachidonic acid metabolites, proteoglycans, proteinases, cytokines, etc.) in controlled amounts. These same mediators, however, released in large amounts under conditions of inflammation, can deleteriously affect other cells and tissues. To elucidate the function of the MC, its contributions to acute and chronic inflammatory conditions such as rheumatoid arthritis, fibrosis, host defenses to parasitic infection, tissue remodelling, and allergic diseases, including asthma, conjunctivitis, rhinitis, and urticaria, in addition to the complexity of its roles in homeostasis and immunoregulation must be addressed *(2–4)*. Most recently the MC has also been implicated in defense against bacterial pathogens, through release of prestored mediators, resulting in the recruitment of other leukocytes to the site of infection *(5,6)*. This review addresses what is known about the functions of various MC subtypes in the underlying process of inflammation common to these pathophysiologic conditions.

From: *Allergy and Allergic Diseases: The New Mechanisms and Therapeutics*
Edited by: J. A. Denburg © Humana Press Inc., Totowa, NJ

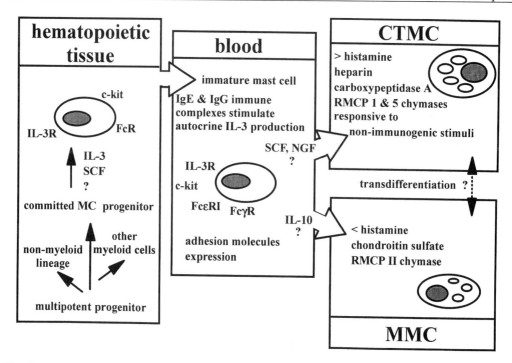

Fig. 1. Rodent mast cell maturation. Schematic diagram of the maturation process of mast cells in rats and mice. The precursors are derived from multipotent progenitors prior to differentiation into non-myeloid or granulocyte lineage. Final differentiation occurs in the peripheral tissue, where microenvironmental conditions determine ultimate phenotype. CTMC predominate in serosal tissue, and MMC predominate at mucosal sites.

An understanding of the pharmacology and biochemistry of the regulation of MC is the first step toward being able to control MC function. To date, treatment of inflammatory processes that involve a significant MC component utilize drugs whose actions are not fully understood, e.g., steroids and disodium cromoglycate (DSCG). This ignorance precludes the use of rational approaches to intervene in detrimental inflammatory functions of the MC while not impairing its essential homeostatic functions. Since the MC is constantly modulating its properties in response to the external environment, predicting how it will react when exposed to specific stimuli must be based on an understanding of the factors that contribute to the development of selective MC phenotypes and their characteristics. Thus current research attempts to understand: the origins and development of MC progenitors; the factors that cause it to differentiate into a mature MC; surface molecule expression, which determines where the cell localizes; the composition of the MC, which determines its function; and the influence of the MC on its environment. This information must be collated with knowledge of the regulation of MC function by different stimuli in its environment so that the role of the MC in inflammatory disease may be understood and controlled as appropriate.

PROGENITOR CELLS AND MAST CELL DEVELOPMENT

Mature MC are identified by their high-affinity IgE receptors, location in tissues, and metachromatic granules containing, among other mediators, histamine, proteinases, cytokines, and proteoglycans. Figure 1 outlines the general maturation scheme of MC in the rat. In rodents, MC originate from pluripotent stem cells *(7)*. Mapping MC development from stem cell to mature cell, however, is encumbered by the lack of knowledge about surface markers of MC precursors. It appears that most MC precursors exit the bone marrow before they are granulated and morphologically identifiable as MC. These progenitors develop in peripheral tissues in response to a myriad of factors that induce selective expression of genes, leading to the broad range of MC phenotypes observed.

Recently it has been shown in mice that Thy-1^{lo} c-kit^{hi} precursor cells isolated from fetal blood are committed to MC development (8). The best characterized growth factors for rodent MC are stem cell factor (SCF) and interleukin-3 (IL-3) (9,10). In in vitro systems, these cytokines do not independently support MC proliferation and development from purified c-kit^+ cells in bone marrow, mesenteric lymph node, or the peritoneal cavity. Either an unpurified cell population to provide accessory cells, conditioned media containing undefined mixtures of T-cell-derived growth factors, or a layer of feeder stromal cells is required (11). Fibroblasts produce SCF, which promotes both the survival and proliferation of peritoneal mast cells (PMC) (12). However, SCF alone cannot stimulate clonal growth of early MC progenitors (13). IL-3 promotes mouse CTMC survival, but alone does not induce proliferation of CTMC (14). It has also been shown in rats that SCF can promote the survival and proliferation of both CTMC and bone-marrow-derived mast cells (BMMC), while IL-3 stimulates BMMC, though less effectively than SCF, but does not have an independent effect on survival and proliferation of CTMC (15). Thus, in rodents, both SCF and IL-3 influence MC development coordinately with other cytokines, and the effect of the cytokine is dependent on the stage of differentiation and the cell type. For reviews of the importance of IL-3 and SCF in MC development see refs. 10 and 16.

The T-cell-derived cytokines IL-4, IL-9, and IL-10 synergize with IL-3 to increase murine MC growth (10,13,17). IL-4 added to IL-3 dependent cultures induces some MC colonies to proliferate (18), as does IgE crosslinking (19). Using mesenteric lymph nodes from mice, IL-4 was most effective for enhancing SCF-dependent MMC proliferation, while IL-10 was a late-acting cofactor for expression of selected MC phenotype, notably the MMC proteinases (13). IL-9 is able to potentiate proliferation of mouse BMMC induced by IL-3 alone or in conjunction with IL-4, and on its own can aid survival but not proliferation of immature murine BMMC cultures. After several weeks in culture, however, IL-9 is able to induce proliferation independently (20).

In humans the role of SCF in MC development has been confirmed. In contrast to murine systems, however, studies indicate that the IL-3 receptor is not expressed on human lung MC or the cell line HMC-1, and no evidence has been found that this cytokine plays a role in human MC development (17,21,22). Furthermore, IL-4 inhibits the production of tryptase and histamine in human fetal liver MC progenitors cultured with SCF, an effect associated with downregulation of c-kit expression (23). As the fetal-liver-derived MC mature in culture they become less affected by IL-4 as determined by proliferation or tryptase expression, although they are still dependent on SCF for survival. To date, no effect of IL-9 or IL-10 has been shown on human MC (22).

Nerve growth factor (NGF) is another factor produced by fibroblasts that promotes survival of rat PMC, but does not induce their proliferation (10,24). Horigome et al. (24) suggest that NGF may upregulate autocrine production of MC survival factors. Although NGF alone is not able to support MC colony formation from rat bone marrow cultures, addition of NGF to suboptimal concentrations of IL-3 greatly increases the number of MC colonies produced. These MC contained more heparin and histamine than those cultured in the absence of NGF, indicating NGF favors differentiation of the CTMC phenotype (25).

Several other factors have been identified that inhibit MC growth or differentiation. Transforming growth factor (TGF)-β1, a known antagonist of mitogenic activity in some systems, inhibits proliferation of IL-3-dependent mouse BMMC, but does not affect β-hexosaminidase or leukotriene C_4 release, or histamine or proteoglycan content in this immature MC phenotype *(26)*. In contrast, using mature CTMC, TGF-β1 has been shown to downregulate histamine release and tumor necrosis factor (TNF) α-dependent cytotoxicity by rat PMC *(27)*. Culture of mouse bone marrow cells in the presence of interferon (IFN) γ significantly reduced the proliferation rate of committed MC precursors and the number of MC observed. Unfortunately, it was not established whether the effect of IFNγ was directly on the MC progenitor or mediated through other cells in the bone marrow culture *(28)*. No growth inhibition was observed on mature MC. Granulocyte-macrophage colony stimulating factor (GM-CSF) has also been shown to inhibit differentiation of IL-3-dependent MC in the mouse *(10)*. Recently, the divergent effects of cytokines on mast cell development with respect to differentiation stage has been emphasized with the observation that IFNγ is able to potentiate mast cell induction from mouse splenocytes, while IL-4 had an inhibitory effect when added during the first 4 d of culture *(29)*. These are in contrast to previous reports *(18,28)* and suggest that the effects of specific cytokines may vary within days of mast cell culture and each phase of development and that such effects cannot be generalized for overall mast cell growth requirements.

The final stages of MC development do not occur until the cell is resident in the tissue *(10)*. The factors determining the tissue destination of the MC precursor are poorly understood. However, MC are known to express adhesion molecules such as very late activation antigen-4 (VLA-4), intercellular adhesion molecule-1 (ICAM-1), and lymphocyte Peyer's patch adhesion molecule-1 (LPAM-1), which likely mediate adhesion to the endothelium *(10)*. MC and their precursors can bind to laminin and fibronectin among other extracellular matrix (ECM) proteins following activation by phorbol 12-myristate 13-acetate (PMA) or, more physiologically relevant, by surface IgE crosslinkage or following exposure to SCF. Using competition studies, this binding has been shown to result from VLA-2, -4, -5, -6, and vitronectin receptor integrins *(30)* on the MC, the expression of which can be regulated by the activating factors that stimulate adhesion *(31,32)*. During allergic disease, such as rhinitis and conjunctivitis, the number of MC at the site of inflammation increases. It is not known whether this results from local proliferation, recruitment from other sites, or an increase in the activity of MC development in the hematopoietic tissue. Not only do the factors contributing to this increase need to be understood, but in addition, these MC are not identical to those present in normal tissue. Little is known about their phenotypic differences, but they respond to stimuli at lower concentrations than MC isolated from healthy tissue *(3)*. Thus, even for the acute effects of MC activation, the role of these cells in inflammation needs to be more fully understood.

Cell Death

Because MC can proliferate during inflammation, and their products cause wide-ranging effects, it is important that the number of MC be strictly controlled. Cell death, one mechanism of control, can occur in two fashions. The first is necrosis in which the plasma membrane integrity is lost, which results in loss of the ability to control osmolality, causing the cell to swell and rupture, releasing its contents into the environment. Alternatively, the process of apoptosis can occur, in which the cell breaks up into apoptotic bodies that maintain their osmotic integrity and do not spill their intracellular contents. In the latter case, no inflammatory reaction ensues and the apoptotic bodies can then be removed by phagocytic cells *(33)*. It is believed that cell death in MC involves, at least in part, apoptosis, especially since release of the contents of the cell through necrosis would lead to further tissue damage. While the regulatory mechanism is not fully understood, in vitro and in vivo findings show that MC undergo apoptosis when deprived of SCF or IL-3, and that this process can be reversed by supplying

SCF *(34,35)*. TGF-β1 prevents SCF-mediated rescue from apoptosis of IL-3-deprived MC *(36)*. MC also produce TGF-β1, which can downregulate their function *(27)*, suggesting autocrine, as well as external control of apoptosis.

Corticosteroids are widely used as anti-inflammatory agents, although the complete range of their effects is not fully understood. It has been shown, however, that MMC numbers in the intestine of rats are diminished substantially by corticosteroids, and pretreatment of corticosteroids can prevent systemic anaphylaxis in sensitized rats *(37,38)*. This decrease in number of MMC is not accompanied by release into the blood of MC mediators, and it has been shown that macrophages engulf whole MC without release of the cellular contents *(38)*. Although it has been shown in vitro that corticosteroids can inhibit mediator release, it has not been shown that they can affect cell survival *(39,40)*. An indirect action of corticosteroids on MC through inhibition of T-cell cytokine production has been postulated; however, their similar effects in athymic nude rats *(38)* would indicate that this cannot be the complete explanation. Further complications arise from the fact that this phenomenon of decreased MMC number and proteinase release following corticosteroid treatment does not occur in mice *(41)*. Thus, the integration of cytokine signals, which determines MC differentiation/proliferation/death, is complex and remains incompletely understood.

HETEROGENEITY

MC can express a spectrum of phenotypes as a result of environmental conditions such as the milieu of cytokines, other cells, and ECM. This diversity is manifested by variation in mediator content and responsiveness to stimuli among MC populations. In rodents, the division of MC into two divergent subtypes, CTMC and MMC, is an oversimplification since phenotype may vary greatly depending on the cell's environment. It is, however, a useful tool to understand the factors that lead to phenotypic differences. To date, the most obvious indicator of MC phenotype in rodents and humans is their serine proteinase content (see Fig. 1). In the rat, CTMC, of which PMC is the prototype, selectively express different chymases than MMC, as will be discussed in Neutral Proteinases *(42)*. In addition, PMC express carboxypeptidase A and contain substantially more histamine than MMC *(43,44)*. The content of proteoglycans and other mediators, and responses to individual stimuli, also varies between these two types. For instance, MMC stimulation is restricted to crosslinking of surface IgE, which is the familiar cause of allergy, substance P, and calcium ionophores such as A23187. In contrast, CTMC can also be stimulated by many nonimmunologic stimuli, including several neuropeptides, in addition to substance P, compound 48/80, and basic peptides *(3,44)*.

MC can be cultured from bone marrow supplemented with T-cell conditioned media. In mice, these cells share many morphological and histochemical characteristics with MMC *(1)*, although they appear morphologically immature and demonstrate considerable heterogeneity in their proteinase content *(45)*. These cells can be grown on a fibroblast feeder layer, resulting in the acquisition of CTMC-like characteristics, including increased histamine content and storage of heparin proteoglycan *(46)*. In the mouse, NGF has also been shown to support differentiation to CTMC, though not independently of other cytokines *(25)*. This indicates that in the mouse both MMC and CTMC can be derived from these cultured BMMC and that either the precursors for multiple phenotypes are present in this population or the phenotype of mouse BMMC is not fixed *(2)*. Using mouse BMMC proteinases as indicators of phenotype, SCF favors the development of CTMC, while IL-3 maintains a more immature MC *(47)*. Transdifferentiation between phenotypes, both from MMC to CTMC and the reverse, has been demonstrated in the mouse *(48)*.

In the rat, BMMC grown in conditioned medium from mesenteric lymph nodes (containing T-cell-derived factors) resemble a more homogeneous mucosal-like MC population compared to the mouse, and although SCF/fibroblast feeder layers will support survival and proliferation, they do not induce differentiation into CTMC *(15,49)*. Since rat BMMC are more homogeneous in their proteinase phenotype than those cultured from mouse bone marrow *(15,45,50)*, their more uniform MMC-like phenotype may indicate that they have differentiated beyond containing precursors capable of forming either CTMC or MMC, and explain their inability to transdifferentiate under conditions that induce mouse BMMC to become more CTMC-like. Alternatively, rat, unlike mouse, BMMC may require additional differentiation stimuli not provided by the fibroblast layer or exogenously added SCF, for the CTMC phenotype to be expressed. These species differences leave the relationship between the subtypes of mast cells undefined and controversial.

In humans, also, there is more than one MC subtype; the MC can be broadly divided into tryptase-containing cells at the mucosa and those that contain tryptase, chymase, and carboxypeptidase A in connective-tissue locations *(4)*. In a given tissue of any species, more than one subtype of mast cell will be present, and the ability to purify specific types is dependent on its relative abundance. It has proven more difficult to obtain a pure population of individual human MC subtypes than in the rodent system *(51)*. In the rat, highly purified populations of CTMC can be isolated from the peritoneal cavity, or MMC from the intestine following infection with the nematode parasite, *Nippostrongylus brasiliensis*, making study of the variation between phenotypes possible. However similar purifications are less easily obtained from human tissues, and in the mouse the intestinal MMC population has not been isolated. The importance of understanding the heterogeneity between subtypes is underlined by the differential susceptibility of CTMC and MMC to drugs such as DSCG and theophylline and to cytokines such as IFNγ, where these agents are active on rat PMC, but not always on intestinal MMC *(44)*. Thus, understanding the basis and extent of MC heterogeneity becomes important in targeting drug action or in the development of new therapeutic agents. The difficulty in purifying human MC subtypes means that little is known about the variation between phenotypes, while for laboratory rodents these differences will be further outlined in the following sections.

MAST CELL ACTIVATION AND FUNCTIONAL REGULATION

Mast Cell Activation

All MC subpopulations bear high-affinity receptors for IgE (FcεRI, 10^4–10^6/cell), although there are differences in the number and molecular mass of these receptors. Crosslinking of FcεRI induces a series of biochemical events including phosphorylation and dephosphorylation of β and γ chains of FcεRI itself and other signal transduction proteins, activation of tyrosine and serine/threonine kinases and phosphatases, activation of G proteins, and regulation of adenyl cyclases, phospholipase C, phospholipase A_2, and various ion channels *(52)*. Since DSCG and theophylline significantly inhibit antigen (Ag)-induced histamine secretion by rat CTMC, but not MMC *(53)*, distinct intracellular signal transduction pathways may be involved in FcεRI-mediated MC activation in CTMC and MMC. FcεRI-mediated activation results in the release of both preformed and newly synthesized mediators.

Regulated secretion by MC can also be induced by other mast cell surface receptors, such as SCF receptors (c-*kit*) *(16)*, NGF receptors *(54)*, and many others, or by secretagogues, such as compound 48/80 and calcium ionophore, which directly activate components of intracellular signal transduction pathways. The list of secretagogues that activate MC is long and likely to be incomplete. However, caution should be used when making generalizations about secretagogue-induced MC activation. MC from different sites and species are functionally heterogeneous, not only in FcεRI-mediated intracellular signal transduction pathways and in their distinct responses to different pharmacologic modulators (DSCG, theophylline), but also in their responses to various stimuli for mediator secretion. Some secretagogues such as compound 48/80, vasoactive intestinal peptide (VIP), endorphins, and somatostatin are potent stimuli for rat PMC but not for rat MMC *(55)*. Moreover, theophylline significantly inhibits antigen-induced histamine secretion from human intestinal MC *(56)*, but does not affect histamine release from rat intestinal MMC *(53)*. Thus, mast cell heterogeneity encompasses distinct activation and regulation properties between MC subpopulations and species.

Mast-Cell-Derived Mediators

MC are important in inflammation not only because they are effector cells that produce a spectrum of powerful multifunctional mediators, but also because MC-derived mediators recruit and activate other effector cells. These include neutrophils, eosinophils, monocytes/macrophages, and lymphocytes, which produce a broad spectrum of mediators to amplify and regulate the inflammatory response. Furthermore, as one defining component of MC heterogeneity, the range and amounts of mediators produced vary dramatically in different MC populations.

PREFORMED MEDIATORS

Amines. Histamine is a well-known MC mediator that is synthesized in the Golgi apparatus by decarboxylation of histidine and stored in MC granules at about 100 mM concentration *(57)*. Rat PMC (i.e., CTMC type) contain 10–30 pg histamine/cell, whereas MMC contain appreciably less (1–3 pg/cell) *(58)*. MC isolated from human lung, skin, lymphoid tissue, and small intestine contain 3–8 pg histamine/cell *(59)*. The wide-ranging biological effects of histamine are mediated by its interaction with H_1, H_2, and H_3 receptors. Once released, histamine has a short half-life and is rapidly catabolized by methylation (70%) and oxidation (30%) *(60)*. Histamine is the only major biogenic amine in human MC, whereas serotonin derived from tryptophan is found in both rodent CTMC (approx 1 pg/cell) and MMC *(61,62)*.

Neutral Proteinases. Neutral proteinases are the dominant protein components of secretory granules in rodent and human MC representing at least 20 to 50% of the entire cellular proteins *(63)*. Marked heterogeneity in MC proteinase expression has been identified in different MC subpopulations and between species. In rats, PMC (CTMC subtype) express multiple differentially glycosylated forms of two chymases, rat MC proteinase (RMCP)-1 (24–30 pg/cell; analogous to mouse MC proteinase-4) and MC proteinase-5, MC carboxypeptidase A (20–25 pg/cell), and small amounts of MC tryptase (0.5 pg/cell) *(64,65)*. By contrast, rat MMC express only the chymase RMCP-2 (26 pg/cell) *(64,66,67)*. In mice, the identified proteinases include six chymases (MMCP-1, -2, -3, -4, -5′, -5), MC carboxypeptidase A, and two tryptases (MMCP-6 and -7) *(68)*. The mRNA for MMCP-1 and -2 are exclusively found in MMC, whereas mRNA for MMCP-3, -4, -5, and -6, and carboxypeptidase A are present in CTMC. In humans, MC tryptase is the principal enzyme accounting for trypsin-like activity. Tryptase is stored within the secretory granules in association with heparin proteoglycan and released in parallel with histamine during degranulation. The predominant MC in human lung and intestinal mucosa are designated as MC_T, because tryptase is their only demonstrable proteinase (10 pg/cell) *(69)*. By contrast, MC that predominate in the skin are designated as MC_{TC} because they contain both tryptase (35 pg/cell) and chymase (4.5 pg/cell) *(69)*. Unlike MC_T , MC_{TC} also contain other neutral proteinases such as carboxypeptidase (34.5 kDa, 5–20 pg/cell) and a cathepsin G-like proteinase (30 kDa). The findings of neuropeptide degradation, generation of angiotensin II, stimulation of fibroblast proliferation, high-molecular-weight kininogen destruction, and basement membrane degradation by tryptase and chymase in vitro, in addition to the inhibition of allergen-induced airway and cutaneous responses by tryptase inhibitors in vivo *(70,71)*, indicate the great potential biologic activities of neutral proteinases *(4)*.

Acid Hydrolases. Unlike neutral proteinases, which perform best near neutral pH, acid hydrolases have their optimal activity at an acidic pH, which prevails at sites of inflammatory processes. Many acid hydrolases, such as β-hexosaminidase, β-glucuronidase, β-D-galactosidase, and arylsulfatase A, are found in MC granules and are released after stimulation. Although the precise function of these acid hydrolases is not known, they are likely to work in concert with neutral proteinases in the degradation of glycoproteins and proteoglycans *(4)*.

Proteoglycans. Proteoglycans are composed of a single-chain protein covalently linked with multiple glycosaminoglycan side chains that bind to histamine, neutral proteinases, and acid hydrolases at the acidic pH inside secretory granules of MC. Besides their wide variety of biological functions as extracellular mediators, such as anticoagulant and anticomplementary effects and modulation of neutral proteinases, proteoglycans appear to facilitate uptake, packaging, and regulation of preformed mediators *(4)*. Two proteoglycans, heparin (3–8 pg/cell) and chondroitin sulfate E, are found in both types of human MC (MC_{TC} and MC_T) *(72)*. By contrast, in rats, heparin predominates in CTMC (28 pg/cell) but not in MMC, and chondroitin E and di B are dominant in MMC but not in CTMC *(73,74)*.

Enzymes Involved in Free-Radical Metabolism. Rat and human MC contain both superoxide dismutase and peroxidase, which may be involved in the metabolism of reactive oxygen intermediates (ROI) and lipid-derived mediators *(75,76)*. Nitric oxide (NO) synthases (NOS) are found in MC, which may contribute significantly to MC functional regulation *(77–79)*.

Newly Generated Mediators

Lipid-Derived Mediators. MC-derived lipid mediators contribute significantly to the development of inflammation and can be divided into two classes, arachidonic acid (AA) metabolites (eicosanoids) and the 2-acetylated phospholipids structurally related to platelet-activating factor (PAF). In activated MC, AA, which accounts for 5–30% of total fatty acids, is liberated from phospholipids by a series of enzymes including phospholipase A_2 (PLA_2), PLC, and PLD and then further metabolized by cyclooxygenase (COS) and lipoxygenase (LO) to release prostaglandins (PG), thromboxanes (TX), leukotrienes (LT), and 5-, 12-HETEs (hydroxy-eicosatetraenoic acids). The most abundant COS product in human MC is PGD_2 (50–100 ng/10^6 MC), whereas the most abundant LO product is LTC_4 *(57)*. PAF, which also interacts with AA metabolism and free-radical generation, is produced by several inflammatory cells, including MC *(80,81)*. MC-derived PGD_2, LTC_4 and PAF together with other COS products (TXB_2, 6-keto-PGF_2, PGF2α and PGE_2) and LO products (LTB_4, D_4, E_4, 5-HETE and 12-HETE) possess a broad spectrum of biologic actions with potent effects on recruitment and activation of inflammatory effector and target cells.

Free Radicals. MC-derived free radicals include nitrogen radicals (NO) and ROI (superoxide anion, hydrogen peroxide, and hydroxyl radicals). Rat and human MC contain NOS *(77,78)* and constitutively produce NO *(82)*. Interestingly, NO inhibits histamine and PAF release and potentiates TNFα production in an autocrine manner *(82,83)*, whereas ROI stimulate histamine release from MC *(84)*.

Mast Cell-Derived Cytokines

The list of cytokines produced by MC is growing steadily. Cytokine mRNAs and proteins identified in freshly isolated rodent MC and human tissue MC include IL-1, -3, -4, -5, -6, -8, TNFα, TGFβ, NGF, IFNγ, macrophage inflammatory protein (MIP)-2, basic fibroblast growth factor (bFGF), and leukemia inhibitory factor (LIF) *(85)*. Interestingly, our recent experiments show that freshly isolated rat PMC also express mRNAs for IL-10 *(86)* and IL-13 *(85)*, both of which have significant effects on MC development. Several β-chemokines (I-309, MCP-1, MIP-1α, MIP-1β, and regulated upon activation, normal T expressed, and presumably secreted (RANTES)) are also found in MC lines *(87)*. Although marked MC heterogeneity has been identified both within and between species, including mediator content and responsiveness to stimuli (see Heterogeneity), the heterogeneity in the cytokine content of MC subpopulations is incompletely known. Bradding et al. *(88)* have shown that a high proportion of MC_{TC} from human skin are positive for IL-4, IL-5 and IL-6, whereas only a low proportion (15%) of MC_T express IL-4. Additional studies are required to clarify where (MC subpopulations derived from different tissues) and when (physiological and pathological MC activation) these cytokines are produced by MC and how they are regulated. Such knowledge may help to identify the importance of MC cytokines in health and disease.

Given the wide variety of MC-derived cytokines, their broad spectrum of biological effects, and the multiple non-MC sources of these cytokines (none of these cytokines is specifically produced by MC), it is difficult to assess the importance of MC in the biological effects of these cytokines. One approach has been to study the role of MC-derived cytokines in mice (W/W^v and Sl/Sl^d) that are genetically deficient in MC. It has been established in W/W^v mice that immune complex *(89)* and bacterial infection-induced *(5,6)* recruitment of leukocytes into the mouse peritoneal cavity in vivo is dependent on MC-derived TNFα. In addition, increased type-I collagen production by dermal fibroblasts is dependent on MC-derived TNFα and TGFβ *(90)*. These MC-deficient animal models together with specific cytokine knockout mice will continue to provide valuable information about MC function and the effects of MC-derived cytokines.

Regulation of Mast Cell Function

CYTOKINES

Cytokines not only play a central role in MC development, but also significantly modulate MC functions (Table 1). However, caution should be applied when making generalizations about the actions of cytokines on MC functions. The marked heterogeneity of MC extends to differential regulation of MC functions by cytokines. For example, although interferons inhibit TNF-α production by both rat PMC and MMC and inhibit histamine release from PMC, they do not inhibit histamine release from intestinal MMC *(91)*. In addition, SCF, which is an important growth and differentiation factor for MC, significantly potentiates antigen-induced histamine secretion from MC of several species, including rat CTMC *(16)* and BMMC mediator release following anti-IgE stimulation *(92)*, but it does not affect antigen-induced histamine secretion from rat intestinal MMC (T.-J. Lin and A. D. Befus, unpublished data). Moreover, the same cytokine may regulate distinct MC mediators differently. For example, SCF potentiates histamine secretion from rat PMC through protein-synthesis-independent short-term and protein-synthesis-dependent long-term mechanisms, but does not alter the antigen-induced release of TNF-α *(93)*. IL-10 inhibits both TNFα and NO production by MC, but at medium to high concentrations potentiates antigen-induced histamine release from rat PMC *(85)*. The differential regulation of mediator secretion from PMC and MMC by cytokines (IFN and SCF) and antiallergic drugs (DSCG and theophylline) emphasizes the functional heterogeneity of MC. The distinct regulation of different MC mediators (histamine and TNFα) by the same cytokine (SCF or IL-10) indicates multiple mechanisms involved in mediator secretion. The distinction between the secretory and regulatory mechanisms of different mast cell mediators has important implications for the design of strategies to control MC-related diseases in selected tissues.

Table 1
Mast Cell Functional Modulation by Cytokines[a]

Cytokine	Mast cell type	Effect on mast cell function	Reference
SCF	mouse, rat, human MC	↑ histamine, 5-HT, LTC$_4$, PGD$_2$ synthesis and release	16, 93
	rat, mouse BMMC	↑ RMCP-2, β-hexosaminidase, LTC$_4$, PGD$_2$ release	92, 94
	HMC-1	↑ chemotaxis	95
NGF	rat PMC	↑ histamine, 5-HT release	54, 96
TGFβ1	rat PMC	↑ chemotaxis	97
	mouse, rat PMC	↓ α-IgE, 48/80-induced 5-HT, histamine, TNFα release	27, 98
	mouse BMMC	↑ Ag-induced adhesion to laminin	99
GM-CSF	mouse BMMC	↑ Ag presentation	100
	MC/9 mast cell line	↑ phosphatidylinositol 3-kinase activity	101
IFNγ	mouse BMMC	↓ Ag presentation	100
	mouse, rat PMC	↓ histamine, 5-HT, TNFα release	89, 102, 103
	rat MC line (RCMC)	↑ mRNA for Fcε1α	104
IFNα/β	rat PMC	↓ TNFα release, IgE-dependent histamine release	91, 102, 105
RANTES	human MC, mouse BMMC	↑ chemotaxis	106, 107
MCP-1	mouse BMMC	↑ chemotaxis	107
	mouse MC in vivo	↑ degranulation	108
MIP-1α	mouse MC in vivo	↑ degranulation	108
ET	mouse PMC, BMMC	↑ histamine, LTC$_4$ release	109–112
PDGF-AB	mouse BMMC	↑ chemotaxis	113
VEGF	mouse BMMC	↑ chemotaxis	113
bFGF	mouse BMMC	↑ chemotaxis	113
PD-ECGF	mouse BMMC	↑ histamine release, chemotaxis	113
relaxin	rat, guinea pig PMC	↓ A23187, 48/80, Ag-induced histamine release	114
IL-1b	human adenoidal MC	↑ histamine release	115
	rat PMC	↑ resting and A23187-induced NO release	80
	rat PMC	↓ A23187-induced PAF release	80
	human lung MC	↑ Ag-induced LTC$_4$, PGD$_2$ release	116
IL-2	rat PMC	↓ 48/80-induced histamine release	117
IL-3	mouse PMC	↑ histamine release, chemotaxis	118, 119
	mouse BMMC	↑ IgE-dependent LTC$_4$ production	120
	mouse BMMC	↓ IL-10-induced MMCP-2 expression	121
IL-4	mouse PMC and in vivo	↑ IgE-dependent histamine, 5-HT, LT release	102, 122
	mouse BMMC	↑ ET-induced histamine, 5-HT synthesis and release	123
	HMC-1	↑ ionomycin-induced IL-3, -4, -8, GM-CSF production	124, 125
	HMC-1	↓ c-*kit* expression	126
	mouse BMMC	↑ Ag presentation	100

Table 1 *(Continued)*

Cytokine	Mast cell type	Effect on mast cell function	Reference
	mouse BMMC	↓ IL-9, -10-induced MMCP-1, -2; SCF-induced MMCP-4	127
IL-5	MC/9 MC line	↑ phosphatidylinositol 3-kinase, MAP kinase activity	101, 128
IL-9	MC line, mouse BMMC	↑ MMCP-1,-2, granzyme B, IL-6 production	127, 129, 130
IL-10	mouse BMMC	↑ MMCP-1, -2, PGD$_2$, LTC$_4$ production	121, 127, 131–133
	rat PMC	↑ Ag-induced histamine release	86
rat PMC, mouse BMMC		↓ TNFα, IL-6 production	86, 134, 135
	rat PMC	↓ NO production	86

*[a]*Cytokines that stimulate mast cell development include SCF, IL-3, -4, -9, -10, -13, NGF, and GM-CSF. Those that inhibit mast cell development include IFNγ and TGFβ.

ANTI-ALLERGIC AND ANTI-INFLAMMATORY DRUGS

Drugs that inhibit the secretion of MC mediators include sulfasalazine, DSCG, nedocromil sodium, β$_2$-adrenergic receptor agonists (salbutamol, salmeterol, and isoproterenol), cyclosporine A, FK506, corticosteroids (dexamethasone), and prostaglandins (PGE$_1$, E$_2$, and misoprostol). Regulation of cytokine production and mediator secretion from MC is considered to be one of the important actions of these drugs in the treatment of allergic diseases. Bissonnette et al. *(136)*, Wershil et al. *(137)*, and Williams et al. *(138)* have demonstrated that anti-inflammatory drugs such as sulfasalazine, dexamethasone, and cyclosporin A inhibit MC-mediated inflammation by multiple mechanisms, including suppression of the expression of MC TNFα mRNA, diminution of the production of MC TNFα protein, competitive inhibition of soluble TNFα, and reduction of the responsiveness of target cells to TNFα. These observations indicate that therapies that target the release of cytokine from MC may be useful in the control of allergic and inflammatory disorders.

NEUROPEPTIDES

A growing number of neuropeptides that possess regulatory effects on MC function have been identified. Together with the close anatomical association of MC and nerves, these observations emphasize the significance of neuro-immune-system interaction. Peptides that activate MC include substance P, somatostatin, neurotensin, VIP, neurokinin A, calcitonin gene-related peptide (CGRP), neuropeptide Y, β endorphin, α neoendorphin, corticostatins (defensins), dynorphin, kallidin, ACTH, and luteinizing hormone-releasing hormone *(55,139)*. The reduction of MC-mediated TNFα-dependent cytotoxicity following decentralization of rat superior cervical ganglia and inhibition of antigen-induced MC degranulation by sympathetic stimulation through β-adrenoreceptors indicate the physiological roles of neurogenic regulation on MC function *(140,141)*. The modulation of MC secretion by neuropeptides has extensive physiologic implications that deserve further study.

THE EFFECTS OF MAST CELLS ON THEIR MACROENVIRONMENT

As illustrated in the previous section, MC are a rich source of biologically active mediators that, undoubtedly play a pivotal role in the pathophysiological changes of IgE-mediated aller-

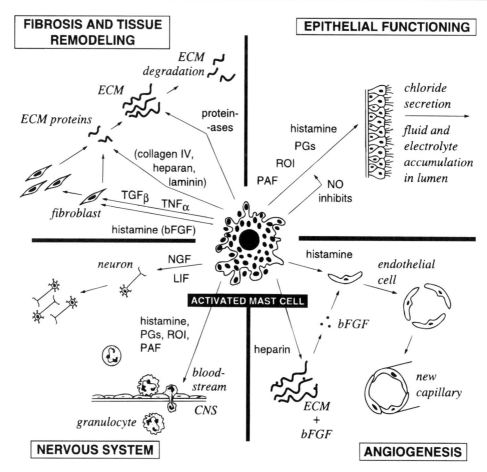

Fig. 2. The influence of mast cells on their macroenvironment. bFGF, basic fibroblast growth factor; CNS, central nervous system; ECM, extracellular matrix; LIF, leukemia inhibitory factor; NGF, nerve growth factor; NO, nitric oxide; PAF, platelet-activating factor; PGs, prostaglandins; ROI, reactive oxygen intermediates; TGFβ, transforming growth factor-β; TNFα, tumor necrosis factor-α. The use of brackets indicates a postulated effect, i.e., no experimental evidence to date.

gic inflammation. Following exposure to allergen, sensitized individuals can exhibit symptoms such as bronchospasm, rhinorrhea, and the cutaneous wheal and flare response *(4)*. Because of their capacity to secrete cytokines and growth factors over many hours or days following stimulation, MC contribute to vascular and epithelial changes, tissue remodeling, and fibrosis associated with chronic inflammation (Fig. 2). Thus, in addition to its more familiar role in acute allergic reactions, the MC has been implicated in fibrotic disease, angiogenesis in tumors, atherosclerosis, neuro-degenerative diseases, and arthritis *(142–146)*.

The remainder of this chapter will focus on the ways in which MC may influence their macroenvironment leading to homeostasis or, if inappropriately regulated, pathological conditions. Findings of MC activation (e.g., ultrastructural evidence of MC degranulation or elevated concentrations of MC-associated mediators) in various inflammatory conditions and other biological responses are not conclusive evidence that MC are necessary for such responses. Neither should the absence of "typical" MC-granule-associated mediators such as histamine or proteinases exclude the participation of MC in a particular biological response. For example, IL-6 production by rat PMC is induced by bacterial lipopolysaccharide without concomitant histamine release *(147)*. The availability of profoundly MC-deficient strains of mice such as W/W^v and Sl/Sl^d has enabled the specific role of the MC in homeostasis and pathology to be examined *(148)*.

Mast Cell Involvement in Fibrosis and Tissue Remodeling

Fibrosis is a normal part of the inflammatory process and is necessary to limit spread of the lesion and to initiate tissue repair and remodeling. It has been postulated that MC have an important role in enhanced collagen synthesis by fibroblasts and/or their increased proliferation *(142)*. Fibrosis occurs in chronic allergic disorders such as atopic dermatitis. In asthma, there is subepithelial thickening as a result of accumulation of collagen *(149)*. Other fibrotic conditions associated with MC activation include chronic graft-versus-host disease, scleroderma, idiopathic pulmonary fibrosis *(142)*, Crohn's disease *(150,151)*, and myocardial fibrosis in post-transplant hearts *(152)*. In all of these conditions, whether IgE- or non-IgE-mediated, there are increased numbers of MC and/or evidence of MC degranulation. Studies in vitro where MC products stimulated fibroblast proliferation also suggest a direct role for MC in fibrosis *(153)*.

There is obviously strong evidence of a temporal association between mastocytosis and fibrosis, but is the relationship causal, i.e., would fibrosis proceed in the absence of MC? Conflicting results have been obtained in experimental models of fibrosis when MC-deficient W/W^v and MC-sufficient mice were compared. Tight-skin mice develop an inherited fibrotic disease with many similarities to human scleroderma. Selective interbreeding between these animals and W/W^v mice resulted in MC deficient animals that developed a less pronounced skin fibrosis than their MC-sufficient littermates *(154)*. In contrast, the presence of MC was not necessary for the full expression of bleomycin-induced pulmonary fibrosis *(155)*. Clearly, the requirement for MC is not absolute for all fibrotic responses. Nevertheless, these cells are likely to be important contributors to fibrogenesis. In support of this, human systemic mastocytosis is associated with significant fibrosis in liver and bone marrow *(156)*.

There is increasing evidence from in vitro studies that MC contribute to fibrosis and tissue remodeling by effects on fibroblasts and production of ECM proteins. Mouse BMMC, mastocytoma cell lines, and rat CTMC all increased proliferation of fibroblasts. BMMC required the presence of IL-3, whereas unstimulated CTMC were fibrogenic *(46)*. When CTMC were repeatedly activated with compound 48/80 (perhaps analogous to chronic non-IgE-mediated stimulation of MC in fibrotic lesions) fibroblast proliferation and collagen secretion were markedly enhanced over that induced by nontreated CTMC *(153)*. Potential fibrogenic products of MC include bFGF, recently shown to be expressed by human skin MC *(157)*, and TGFβ and TNFα, both secreted following IgE-mediated activation of mouse skin and peritoneal MC. Both TGFβ and TNFα induced increased levels of collagen gene expression by mouse skin fibroblasts *(90)*. The possibility that MC may contribute to tissue repair and/or the overproduction of basement membrane components seen in fibrotic conditions was raised by the demonstration that rodent MC lines, BMMC, and RBL cells express both mRNA and protein of collagen IV, laminin, and heparan sulfate proteoglycan *(158)*.

The degradation of ECM proteins is a prerequisite for the tissue remodeling process, by permitting cells to migrate through tissues and cross epithelial basal lamina. Both of the major proteinases of human MC, chymase and tryptase, can degrade ECM glycoproteins. Chymase causes proteolysis of basal lamina components, including collagen IV and V, laminin, fibronectin, and elastin *(159)*, and tryptase degrades fibronectin in the ECM of human fibroblasts *(160)*. MC may contribute to inappropriate ECM proteolysis in the lesions of rheumatoid arthritis *(161)*, and MC hyperplasia has been frequently reported in rheumatoid synovia, especially at sites of cartilage erosion *(146)*. The ability of lysates of purified human synovial MC to degrade ECM glycoproteins in vitro *(162)* lends support to the view that MC at sites of chronic activation may cause structural damage and be involved in tissue remodeling.

Mast Cells and Angiogenesis

The formation of new capillaries is essential for embryonic development and wound healing and is a feature of chronic inflammation. Angiogenesis, however, also facilitates the growth of solid tumors and contributes to the pathophysiology of psoriasis and rheumatoid arthritis *(143)*. The close anatomical association between MC and newly forming vasculature suggests a possible angiogenic role for these cells and there is now good evidence that MC products facilitate this process *(143)*. For example, histamine is mitogenic for human microvascular endothelial cells in vitro *(163)*. Using the mesenteric window assay, activation of CTMC by compound 48/80 induced an angiogenic response in normal rats and mice; both endogenous MC histamine and systemically administered heparin were angiogenic *(143)*. The mode of action of heparin in angiogenesis is not clear but may be related to its ability to displace bFGF (a potent angiogenic as well as fibrogenic factor) from ECM proteins *(164)*. Moreover, human MC in a variety of tissues express collagen VIII, which is believed to provide a framework for the assembly of endothelial cells in the formation of new blood vessels *(165)*.

MC accumulate around solid tumors and are often seen in a degranulated state. Solid tumors greater than 2 mm in diameter are dependent on angiogenesis for growth and it is known that tumors secrete angiogenic factors *(143)*. Some of these are chemotactic for MC, especially TGFβ-1 which is the most potent MC chemotactic factor yet described *(97)*. Thus MC, attracted by chemotactic factors from tumor cells, may be activated and contribute to tumor-associated angiogenesis via histamine-, heparin-, and bFGF-mediated mechanisms. Tumor angiogenesis proceeds, although at a reduced level, in *W/W*[v] mice, implying that MC are not solely responsible for the neovascularization process *(166)*. That MC-mediated angiogenesis can be deleterious was illustrated by the presence of fewer metastases in the MC-deficient mice.

Effects of Mast Cells on the Nervous System

In tissues throughout the body, MC and nerves can be found in intimate association. The bidirectional communication between MC and nerves has been reviewed at length elsewhere *(145,167)*. MC have the potential to influence the growth and functioning of the nervous system and this has implications for neurological disorders. Indeed, MC have been implicated in the etiology of neurological diseases such as multiple sclerosis and Alzheimer's disease *(145,168)*. Mediators derived from MC, including histamine and ROI, can also alter the integrity of the blood-brain barrier, allowing the passage of leukocytes into central nervous tissue in inflammatory conditions *(168)*.

The bidirectional nature of interactions between MC and cells of the nervous system is exemplified by their production of mutually trophic factors. The MC growth factors NGF and SCF are produced by Schwann cells. MC, for their part, can secrete a number of neurotrophic factors, including NGF, LIF (a cholinergic neuronal differentiation factor), IL-6, and GM-CSF *(169)*. NGF is a shared growth factor for neurons and MC and may, therefore, play an important role in coordinating MC hyperplasia and nerve remodeling in chronic inflammation. Circumstantial evidence of such a link is the correlation between changes in MMC numbers and new nerve growth in jejunal mucosa following *N. brasiliensis* infection in the rat *(170)*.

There is an apparent association between MC accumulation and activation (degranulated appearance and increased histamine concentration in CNS tissue fluid) and inflammatory demyelination in both clinical multiple sclerosis and its major animal model, experimental allergic encephalomyelitis (EAE) *(168)*. The fact that normal MC distribution in the CNS mirrors the regions of early lesion formation in EAE *(168)* and that supernatants of compound-48/80-activated rat PMC can generate EAE-inducing peptides from intact myelin *(171)* also supports a role for the MC, at least in experimental inflammatory demyelination. MC may also be implicated in the pathogenesis of Alzheimer's disease in which an inflammation-like event may lead to the deposition of the characteristic β-protein plaques in the brain. A candidate β-protein-generating proteinase has been identified in rat brain that appears to be identical to RMCP-1 and co-localizes to areas of high density of MC in the rat brain *(172)*. The stimuli that may induce MC activation in multiple sclerosis or Alzheimer's disease are, as yet, unclear.

Mast Cells and Epithelial Function

Epithelial surfaces serve both as a barrier limiting the uptake of immunogens and to control the transport of ions, solutes, and water between the luminal space and the underlying tissues. MC, particularly MMC, have been postulated to play an important role in the pathogenesis of food allergies and inflammatory bowel disease where diarrhea is a prominent feature *(150,151)*. The evidence for this in human disease is circumstantial; however, there is experimental evidence that supports the view that MC can function as important regulators of intestinal epithelial secretion and permeability *(173,174)*.

Using isolated gut preparations, both rat jejunum *(173)* and human colon *(175)* responded to IgE-mediated stimulation with a net epithelial secretion of chloride ions, which is a central pathophysiological disturbance in most types of acute diarrhea *(176)*. As illustrated in Mast Cell Activation and Functional Regulation, MC can release many mediators, and some of these (including histamine and prostaglandins) are capable of provoking intestinal chloride ion secretion *(177)*.

Disruption of the barrier function of the epithelium, leading to increased permeability, may also result from MC activation. When NO synthesis was inhibited, rat intestinal permeability was markedly increased and this was accompanied by increased concentrations of the rat MMC-associated chymase, RMCP-2 *(178)*. The increased mucosal permeability was apparently MC-mediated since the NO synthesis inhibitor had no direct effect on permeability through monolayers of rat epithelial cells in vitro and the increased mucosal permeability was almost completely inhibited by MC stabilizers (178). The effect was mediated by prostaglandins, histamine, PAF, and the superoxide radical.

The intestinal epithelial shedding seen in rodent models of anaphylaxis and intestinal nematode expulsion has been postulated to be, at least partly, mediated by the presumed effect of RMCP-2 on epithelial basement membrane collagen *(179)*. However, a recent study has shown that no significant epithelial shedding occurred despite massive release of RMCP-2 following worm antigen challenge of ex vivo-perfused jejunum from *N. brasiliensis*-immune rats *(180)*. The authors suggest that other factors such as hypoxia following microvasular congestion in the villi may be more important in causing the loss of epithelium in intestinal anaphylaxis.

There can be little doubt that activation of MMC can effect changes in epithelial electrolyte transport and increased permeability. The significance of this for homeostasis of epithelial function is not yet clear, but the resulting intraluminal accumulation of fluid, electrolytes, and plasma proteins may have evolved as a protective response to enteric-dwelling parasites.

CONCLUSIONS

The ability of MC to secrete a vast array of cytokines and growth factors and their sensitivity to many non-IgE-mediated activators implicate these cells in a much broader range of activities than acute allergic inflammation and responses to helminth infection. It is increasingly apparent that MC, in addition to their long association with wheezes, sneezes, and parasitic diseases, play a vital role in homeostatic mechanisms such as tissue repair. It is possible that T-cell-dependent MMC hyperplasia is an adaptive response to helminth infection, whereas CTMC are concerned more with homeostasis. When these responses are inappropriately elicited or regulated, this may result in the pathology associated with asthma, Crohn's disease, tumor metastasis, and neurological disorders. As the precise role of MC in health and disease and the factors that lead to inappropriate activation of these cells become clearer, it should be possible to target therapies that reduce MC-mediated pathology while preserving their homeostatic functions.

REFERENCES

1. Galli SJ (1990) New insights into "the riddle of the mast cells": microenvironmental regulation of mast cell development and phenotypic heterogeneity. Lab Invest 62:5–33.
2. Befus AD (1994) Inflammation: mast cells. In: Ogra PL, Mestecky J, Lamm M, Strober W, McGhee J, Bienenstock J, eds. Handbook of Mucosal Immunology. Academic, San Diego, pp. 307–314.
3. Holgate ST (1991) The mast cell and its function in allergic disease. Clin Exp Allergy 21(suppl 3):1–16.
4. Schwartz L, Huff T (1993) Biology of mast cells and basophils. In: Middleton E Jr, Reed CE, Ellis EF, Adkinson NF Jr, Yunginger JW, Busse WW, eds. Allergy Principles and Practice, 4th ed. Mosby, St. Louis, pp. 135–168.
5. Echtenacher B, Männel DN, Hültner L. (1996) Critical protective role of mast cells in a model of acute septic peritonitis. Nature 381:75–77.
6. Malaviya R, Ikeda T, Ross E, Abraham SN (1996) Mast cell modulation of neutrophil influx and bacterial clearance at sites of infection through TNF-α. Nature 381:77–80.
7. Kitamura Y, Shimada M, Hatanaka K, Miyano Y (1977) Development of mast cells from grafted bone marrow cells in irradiated mice. Nature 268:442–443.
8. Rodewald H-R, Dessing M, Dvorak AM, Galli SJ (1996) Identification of a committed precursor for the mast cell lineage. Science 271:818–822.
9. Huff TF, Lantz CS, Ryan JJ, Leftwich, JA (1995) Mast cell committed progenitors. In: Kitamura Y, Yamamota S, Galli SJ, Greaves MW, eds. Biological and Molecular Aspects of Mast Cell and Basophil Differentiation and Function. Raven, New York, pp. 105–117.
10. Rottem M, Metcalfe DD (1995) Development and maturation of mast cells and basophils. In: Busse WW, Holgate ST, eds. Asthma and Rhinitis. Blackwell, Boston, pp. 167–181.
11. Lantz CS, Huff TF (1995) Differential responsiveness of purified mouse c-*kit*⁺ mast cells and their progenitors to IL-3 and stem cell factor. J Immunol 155:4024–4029.
12. Tsai M, Takeishi T, Thompson H, Langley KE, Zsebo KM, Metcalfe DD, Geissler EN, Galli SJ (1991) Induction of mast cell proliferation, maturation and heparin synthesis by the rat c-*kit* ligand, stem cell factor. Proc Natl Acad Sci USA 88:6382–6386.
13. Rennick D, Hunte B, Holland G, Thompson-Snipes L (1995) Cofactors are essential for stem cell factor-dependent growth and maturation of mast cell progenitors: comparative effects of interleukin-3 (IL-3), IL-4, IL-10, and fibroblasts. Blood 85:57–65.
14. Tsuji, K, Nakahata T, Takagi M, Kobayashi T, Ishiguro A, Kikuchi K, Naganuma K, Koike K, Miyajima A, Arai K, Akabane T (1990) Effects of interleukin-3 and interleukin-4 on the development of connective tissue-type mast cells: interleukin-3 supports their survival and interleukin-4 triggers and supports their proliferation synergistically with interleukin-3. Blood 75:421–427.
15. Haig DM, Huntley JF, Mackellar A, Newlands GFJ, Inglis L, Sangha R, Cohen D, Hapel A, Galli SJ, Miller HRP (1994) Effects of stem cell factor (*kit*-ligand) and interleukin-3 on the growth and serine proteinase expression of rat bone marrow-derived or serosal mast cells. Blood 83:72.
16. Galli SJ, Zsebo M, Geissler EN (1994) The kit ligand, stem cell factor. Adv Immunol 55:1–96.
17. Kitamura Y, Kasugai T, Nomura S, Matsuda H (1993) Development of mast cells and basophils. In: Foreman JC, ed. Immunopharmacology of Mast Cells and Basophils. Academic, London, pp. 5–27.
18. Hamaguchi Y, Kanakura Y, Fujita J, Takeda S, Nakano T, Tarui S, Horijo T, Kitamura Y (1987) Interleukin 4 as an essential factor for in vitro clonal growth of murine connective tissue-type mast cells. J Exp Med 165:268–273.
19. Takagi M, Nakahata T, Koike K, Kobayashi T, Tsuji K, Kojima S, Hirano T, Miyajima A, Arai K, Akabane T (1989) Stimulation of connective tissue-type mast cell proliferation by crosslinking of cell-bound IgE. J Exp Med 170:233–244.

20. Renauld J-C, Kermouni A, Vink A, Louahed J, Van Snick J (1995) Interleukin-9 and its receptor: involvement in mast cell differentiation and T cell oncogenesis. J Leukoc Biol 57:353–360.

21. Valent P, Besemer J, Sillaber C, Butterfield JH, Eher R, Majdic O, Kishi K, Klepetko W, Eckersberger R, Lechner K, Bettelheim P (1990) Failure to detect IL-3-binding sites on human mast cells. J Immunol 145:3432–3437.

22. Agis H, Valent P (1995) Molecules involved in the development of human basophils and mast cells. In: Kitamura Y, Yamamoto S, Galli SJ, Greaves MW, eds. Biological and Molecular Aspects of Mast Cell and Basophil Differentiation and Function Raven, New York, pp. 119–130.

23. Nilsson G, Miettinen U, Ishizaka T, Ashman LK, Irani A-M, Schwartz LB (1994) Interleukin-4 inhibits the expression of kit and tryptase during stem cell factor-dependent development of human mast cells from fetal liver cells. Blood 84:1519–1527.

24. Horigome K, Bullock ED, Johnson EM Jr (1994) Effects of nerve growth factor on rat peritoneal mast cells. Survival promotion and immediate-early gene induction. J Biol Chem 269:2695–2702.

25. Matsuda H, Yukiko K, Hiroko U, Kiso Y, Kanemoto T, Suzuki H, Kitamura Y (1991) Nerve growth factor induces development of connective tissue-type mast cells *in vitro* from murine bone marrow cells. J Exp Med 174:7–14.

26. Broide DH, SI Wasserman, J Alvaro-Garcia, NJ Zvaifler, GS Firestein (1989) Transforming growth factor-β1 selectively inhibits IL-3 dependent mast cell proliferation without affecting mast cell function or differentiation. J Immunol 143:1591–1597.

27. Bissonnette EY, Enciso JA, Befus AD (1997) TGFβ1 inhibits histamine and TNFα release by rat peritoneal mast cells. Am J Respir Cell Mol Biol 16:275–282.

28. Nafziger J, Arock M, Guillosson J-J, Wietzerbin J (1990) Specific high-affinity receptors for interferon-γ on mouse bone marrow-derived mast cells: inhibitory effect of interferon-γ on mast cell precursors. Eur J Immunol 20:113–117.

29. Hu Z-Q, Zenda N, Shimamura T (1996) Down-regulation by IL-4 and up-regulation by IFN-γ of mast cell induction from mouse spleen cells. J Immunol 156:3925–3931.

30. Ra C, Yasuda M, Kim Z, Saito H, Nakahata T, Yagita H, Okumura K (1995) Fibronectin receptor (FNR) integrins on mast cells are involved in cellular activation. In: Kitamura Y, Yamamoto S, Galli SJ, Greaves MW, eds. Biological and Molecular Aspects of Mast Cell and Basophil Differentiation and Function. Raven, New York, pp. 239–247.

31. Hamawy MM, Mergenhagen SE, Siraganian RP (1994) Adhesion molecules as regulators of mast-cell and basophil function. Immunol. Today 15:62–66.

32. Bianchine PJ, Metcalfe DD (1995) Adhesion molecules and their relevance in understanding the biology of the mast cell. In: Y Kitamura, S Yamamoto, SJ Galli, MW Greaves, eds. Biological and Molecular Aspects of Mast Cell and Basophil Differentiation and Function. Raven, New York, pp. 139–147.

33. Cohen JJ (1993) Apoptosis. Immunol Today 14:126–130.

34. Mekori YA, Oh CK, Metcalfe DD (1993) IL-3-dependent murine mast cells undergo apoptosis on removal of IL-3: prevention of apoptosis by c-kit ligand. J Immunol 151:3775–3784.

35. Iemura A, Tsai M, Ando A, Wershil BK, Galli SJ (1994) The c-kit ligand, stem cell factor, promotes mast cell survival by suppressing apoptosis. Am J Pathol 144:321–328.

36. Mekori YA, Metcalfe DD (1994) Transforming growth factor-β prevents stem cell factor-mediated rescue of mast cells from apoptosis after IL-3 deprivation. J Immunol 153:2194–2203.

37. King SJ, Miller HRP, Newlands GFJ, Woodbury RG (1985) Depletion of mucosal mast cell protease by corticosteroid: effect on intestinal anaphylaxis in the rat. Proc Nat Acad Sci USA 82:1214–1218.

38. Soda K, Kawabori S, Perdue MH, Bienenstock J (1991) Macrophage engulfment of mucosal mast cells in rats treated with dexamethasone. Gastroenterology 100:929–937.

39. Schleimer RP, Schulman ES, MacGlashan DW Jr, Peters SP, Hayes EC, Adams K III, Lichtenstein LM, Adkinson NF Jr. (1983) Effects of dexamethasone on mediator release from human lung fragments and purified human lung mast cells. J Clin Invest 71:1830–1835.

40. Berenstein EH, Garcia-Gil M, Siraganian RP (1987) Dexamethasone inhibits receptor-activated phosphoinositide breakdown in rat basophilic leukemia (RBL-2H3) cells. J Immunol 138:1914–1918.

41. Newlands GFJ, MacKellar A, Miller HRP (1990) Intestinal mucosal mast cells in *Nippostrongylus*-infected mice: lack of sensitivity to corticosteroids. Int J Parasitol 20:669–672.

42. Gibson S, Miller HRP (1986) Mast cell subsets in the rat distinguished immunohistochemically by their content of serine proteinases. Immunology 58:101–104.

43. Befus AD (1989) Mast cells are that polymorphic! Regional Immunol 2:176–187.

44. Bissonnette EY, Befus AD (1993) Modulation of mast cell function in the gastrointestinal tract. In: Wallace JL, ed. Immunopharmacology of the Gastrointestinal System. Academic, London, pp. 95–103.

45. Newlands GFJ, Lammas DA, Huntley JF, Mackellar A, Wakelin D, Miller HRP (1991) Heterogeneity of murine bone marrow-derived mast cells: analysis of their proteinase content. Immunology 72:434–439.

46. Levi-Scháffer F, Rubinchik E (1994) Mast cell/fibroblast interactions. Clin Exp Allergy 24:1016–1021.

47. Gurish MF, Ghildyal N, McNeil HP, Austen KF, Gillis S, Stevens RL (1992) Differential expression of secretory granule proteases in mouse mast cells exposed to interleukin 3 and c-kit ligand. J Exp Med 175:1003–1012.

48. Kanakura Y, Thompson H, Nakano T, Yamamura T, Asai H, Kitamura Y, Metcalfe DD, Galli SJ (1988) Multiple bidirectional alterations of phenotype and changes in proliferative potential during *in vitro* and in vivo passage of clonal mast cell populations derived from mouse peritoneal mast cells. Blood 72:877–885.

49. MacDonald AJ, Thornton EM, Newlands GFJ, Galli SJ, Moqbel R, Miller HRP (1996) Rat bone marrow-derived mast cells co-cultured with 3T3 fibroblasts in the absence of T cell-derived cytokines require stem cell factor for their survival and maintain their mucosal mast cell-like phenotype. Immunology 88:375–383.

50. McMenamin CC, Gault EA, Haig DM (1987) The effect of dexamethasone on growth and differentiation of bone marrow-derived mucosal mast cells *in vitro*. Immunology 62:29–34.

51. Benyon RC, Lowman MA, Rees PH, Holgate ST, Church MK (1989) Mast cell heterogeneity. In: Morley J, ed. Asthma Reviews Vol. 2. Academic, London, pp. 151–189.

52. Beaven MA, Metzger H (1993) Signal transduction by Fc receptors: the FcεRI case. Immunol. Today 14, 222–226.

53. Pearce FL, Befus AD, Gauldie J, Bienenstock J (1982) Mucosal mast cells. II. effects of anti-allergic compounds on histamine secretion by isolated intestinal mast cells. J Immunol 128:2481–2486.

54. Horigome K, Pryor JC, Bullock ED, Johnson EM JR (1993) Mediator release from mast cells by nerve growth factor. Neurotrophin specificity and receptor mediation. J Biol Chem 268:14881–14887.

55. Shanahan F, Denburg JA, Fox JET, Bienenstock J, Befus AD (1985) Mast cell heterogeneity: effects of neuroenteric peptides on histamine release. J Immunol 135:1331–1337.

56. Befus AD, Dyck N, Goodacre R, Bienenstock J (1987) Mast cells from the human intestinal lamina propria. Isolation, histochemical subtypes, and functional characterization. J Immunol 138:2604–2610.

57. Holgate ST, Robinson C, Church MK (1993) Mediators of immediate hypersensitivity. In: Middleton E Jr, Reed CE, Ellis EF, Adkinson NF, Yuninger JW, Busse WW, eds. Allergy, Principles and Practice. Mosby, St. Louis, pp. 267–301.

58. Befus AD, Pearce FL, Gauldie J, Horsewood P, Bienenstock J (1982) Mucosal mast cells. I. Isolation and functional characteristics of rat intestinal mast cells. J Immunol 128:2475–2480.

59. Schulman ES, Kagey-Sobotka A, MacGlashan DW, Adkinson NF, Peters SP, Schleimer RP, Lichtenstein LM (1983) Heterogeneity of human mast cells. J Immunol 131:1936–1941.

60. Kapeller-Adler R (1965) Histamine catabolism in vitro and in vivo. Fed Proc 24:757–765.

61. Moran NC, Uvnas B, Westesholm B (1962) Release of 5-hydroxytryptamine and histamine from rat mast cells. Acta Physiol Scand 56:26–41.

62. Wingren U, Enerback L, Ahlman H, Allenmark S, Dahlstrom A (1983) Amines of the mucosal mast cell of the gut in normal and nematode infected rats. Histochemistry 77:145–158.

63. Schwartz LB, Riedel C, Caulfield JP, Wasserman SI, Austen KF (1981) Cell association of complexes of chymase, heparin proteoglycan, and protein after degranulation by rat mast cells. J Immunol 126:2071–2078.

64. Befus AD, Chin B, Pick J, Evans S, Osborn S, Forstrom J (1995) Proteinases of rat mast cells: peritoneal but not intestinal mucosal mast cells express mast cell proteinase 5 and carboxypeptidase A. J Immunol 155:4406–4411.

65. Schwartz LB, Riedel C, Schratz JJ, Austen KF (1982) Localization of carboxypeptidase A to the macromolecular heparin proteoglycan-protein complex in secretory granules of rat serosal mast cells. J Immunol 128:1128–1133.

66. Haig DM, McKee TA, Jarrett EE, Woodbury R, Miller HRP (1982) Generation of mucosal mast cells in stimulated *in vitro* by factors derived from T cells of helminth-infected rats. Nature 300:188–190.

67. Lee TDG, Shanahan F, Miller HRP, Bienenstock J, Befus AD (1985) Intestinal mucosal mast cells: isolation from rat lamina propria and purification using unit gravity velocity sedimentation. Immunology 55:721–728.

68. Matsumoto R, Sali A, Ghildyal N, Karplus M, Stevens R (1995) Packaging of proteases and proteoglycans in the granules of mast cells and other hematopoietic cells, a cluster of histidines on mouse mast cell protease 7 regulates its binding to heparin serglycin proteoglycans. J Biol Chem 270:19,524–19,531.

69. Schwartz LB, Irani AA, Roller K, Castells MC, Schechter NM (1987) Quantitation of histamine, tryptase and chymase in dispersed human T and TC mast cells. J Immunol 138:2611–2615.

70. Clark JM, Abraham WM, Fishman CF, Forteza R, Ahmed A, Cortes A, Warne RL, Moore WR, Tanaka RD (1995) Tryptase inhibitors block allergen-induced airway and inflammatory responses in allergic sheep. Am J Respir Crit Care Med 152:2076–2083.

71. Molinari JF, Moore WR, Clark J, Tanaka R, Butterfield JH, Abraham WM (1995) Role of tryptase in immediate cutaneous responses in allergic sheep. J Appl Physiol 79:1966–1970.

72. Craig SS, Irani A-MA, Metcalfe DD, Schwartz LB (1993) Ultrastructural localization of heparin to human mast cells of the MC_{TC} and MC_T types by labeling with antithrombin III-gold. Lab Invest 69:552–561.

73. Stevens, RL., Lee, T.D.G., Seldin, D.C., Austen, K.F., Befus, A.D., and Bienenstock, J. (1986) Intestinal mucosal mast cells from rats infected with *Nippostrongylus brasiliensis* contain protease resistant chondroitin sulfate di-B proteoglycans. *J. Immunol.* 137:291–295.

74. Kusche M, Lindahl U, Enerback L, Roden L (1988) Identification of oversulphated galactosaminoglycans in intestinal-mucosal mast cells of rats infected with the nematode worm *Nippostrongylus brasiliensis*. Biochem J 253:885–893.

75. Henderson WR, Kaliner M (1978) Immunologic and non-immunologic generation of superoxide from mast cells and basophils. J Clin Invest 61:187–196.

76. Henderson WR, Kaliner M (1979) Mast cell granule peroxidase: location, secretion and SRS-A inactivation. J Immunol 122:1322–1328.

77. Berger RJ, Zuccarello M, Keller JT (1994) Nitric oxide synthase immunoreactivity in the rat dura mater. Neuroreport 5:519–21.

78. Bacci S, Arbi-Ricardi R, Mayer B, Rumio C, Borghi-Cirri MB (1994) Localization of nitric oxide synthase immunoreactivity in mast cells of human nasal mucosa. Histochemistry 102:89–92.

79. Bandaletova T, Brouet I, Bartsch H, Sugimura T, Esumi H, Ohshima H (1993) Immunohistochemical localization of an inducible form of nitric oxide synthase in various organs of rats treated with *Propionibacterium acnes* and lipopolysaccharide. Acta Pathol Microbiol Immunol Scand 101:330–336.

80. Hogaboam CM, Befus AD, Wallace JL (1993) Modulation of rat mast cell reactivity by IL-1β, divergent effects on nitric oxide and platelet-activating factor release. J Immunol 151:3767–3774.

81. Ambrosio G, Oriente A, Napoli C, Palumbo G, Chiariello P, Marone G, Condorelli M, Chiariello M, Triggiani M (1994) Oxygen radicals inhibit human plasma acetylhydrolase, the enzyme that catabolizes platelet-activating factor. J Clin Invest 93:2408–2416.

82. Bissonnette EY, Hogaboam CM, Wallace JL, Befus AD (1991) Potentiation of tumor necrosis factor-α-mediated cytotoxicity of mast cells by their production of nitric oxide. J Immunol 147:3060–3065.

83. Salvemini D, Masini E, Pistelli A, Mannaioni PF, Vane JR (1991) Nitric oxide: a regulatory mediator of mast cell reactivity. J Cardiovasc Pharmacol 17:S258–S264.

84. Mannaioni PF, Masini E (1988) The release of histamine by free radicals. Free Radic Biol Med 5:177–197.

85. Lin T-J, Enciso JA, Bissonnette EY, Szczepek A, Befus AD (1996) Cytokine and drug modulation of TNFα in mast cells, in *Proceedings International Symposium on Molecular Biology of Allergens and the Atopic Immune Response* (Sehon A, HayGlass KT, Kraft D, eds.), Plenum, New York, pp. 279–285.

86. Lin T-J, Befus AD (1997) Differential regulation of mast cell function by IL-10 and stem cell factor. J Immunol 159:4015–4023.

87. Selvan RS, Butterfield JH, Krangel MS (1994) Expression of multiple chemokine genes by human mast cell leukemia. J Biol Chem 269:13,893–13,898.

88. Bradding P, Okayama Y, Howarth PH, Church MK, Holgate ST (1995) Heterogeneity of human mast cells based on cytokine content. J Immunol 155:297–307.

89. Zhang Y, Ramos BF, Jakschik BA (1992) Neutrophil recruitment by tumor necrosis factor from mast cells in immune complex peritonitis. Science 258:1957–1959.

90. Gordon JR, Galli SJ (1994) Promotion of mouse fibroblast collagen gene expression by mast cells stimulated via the FcεRI. Role for mast cell-derived transforming growth factor β and tumor necrosis factor α. J Exp Med 180:2027–2037.

91. Bissonnette EY, Chin B, Befus AD (1995) Interferons differentially regulate histamine and TNF-α in rat intestinal mucosal mast cells. Immunology 86:12–17.

92. Hill PB, MacDonald AJ, Thornton EM, Newlands GFJ, Galli SJ, Miller HRP (1996) Stem cell factor enhances immunoglobulin E-dependent mediator release from cultured rat bone marrow-derived mast cells: activation of previously unresponsive cells demonstrated by a novel ELISPOT assay. Immunology 87:326–333.

93. Lin T-J, Bissonnette EY, Hirsh A, Befus AD (1996) Stem cell factor potentiates histamine secretion by multiple mechanisms, but does not affect TNFα release from rat mast cells. Immunology 89:301–307.

94. Murakami M, Austen KF, Arm JP (1995) The immediate phase of c-kit ligand stimulation of mouse bone marrow-derived mast cells elicits rapid leukotriene C_4 generation through posttranslational activation of cytosolic phospholipase A_2 and 5-lipoxygenase. J Exp Med 182:197–206.

95. Nilsson G, Butterfield JH, Nilsson K, Siegbahn A (1994) Stem cell factor is a chemotactic factor for human mast cells. J Immunol 153:3717–3723.

96. Johnston HB, Atterwill CK (1992) Nerve growth factor (NGF) receptors on mast cells: effects of the cholinergic neurotoxin ethylcholine mustard aziridinium ion (ECMA). Neurotoxicology 13:155–159.

97. Gruber BL, Marchese MJ, Kew RR (1994) Transforming growth factor-β_1 mediates mast cell chemotaxis. J Immunol 152:5860–5867.

98. Meade R, Askenase PW, Geba GP, Neddermann K, Jacoby RO, Pasternak RD (1992) Transforming growth factor-β_1 inhibits murine immediate and delayed type hypersensitivity. J Immunol 149:521–528.

99. Thompson HL, Burbelo PD, Metcalfe DD (1990) Regulation of adhesion of mouse bone marrow-derived mast cells to laminin. J Immunol 145:3425–3431.

100. Frandji P, Tkaczyk C, Oskeritzian C, Lapeyre J, Peronet R, David B, Guillet JG, Mecheri S (1995) Presentation of soluble antigens by mast cells: upregulation by interleukin-4 and granulocyte/macrophage colony-stimulating factor and downregulation by interferon γ. Cell Immunol 163:37–46.

101. Gold MR, Duronio V, Saxena SP, Schrader JW, Aebersold R (1994) Multiple cytokines activate phosphatidylinositol 3-kinase in hemopoietic cells. Association of the enzyme with various tyrosine-phosphorylated proteins. J Biol Chem 269:5403–5412.

102. Holliday MR, Banks EM, Dearman RJ, Kimber I, Coleman JW (1994) Interaction of IFNγ with IL-3 and IL-4 in the regulation of serotonin and arachidonate release from mouse peritoneal mast cells. Immunology 82:70–74.

103. Coleman JW, Buckley MG, Holliday MR, Morris AG (1991) Interferon-γ inhibits serotonin release from mouse peritoneal mast cells. Eur J Immunol 21:2559–2564.

104. Enciso JA, Bissonnette EY, Befus AD (1996) Regulation of mRNA levels of TNF-alpha and the alpha chain of the high-affinity receptor for IgE in mast cells by IFN-gamma and alpha/beta. Int Arch Allergy Immunol 110:114–123.

105. Swieter M, Ghali WA, Rimmer C, Befus AD (1989) Interferon-α/β inhibits IgE-dependent histamine release from rat mast cells. Immunology 66:606–610.

106. Mattoli S, Ackerman V, Vittori E, Marini M (1995) Mast cell chemotactic activity of RANTES. Biochem Biophys Res Commun 209:316–321.

107. Taub D, Dastych J, Inamura N, Upton J, Kelvin D, Metcalfe D, Oppenheim J (1995) Bone marrow-derived murine mast cells migrate, but do not degranulate, in response to chemokines. J Immunol 154:2393–2402.

108. Alam R, Kumar D, Anderson-Walters D, Forsythe PA (1994) Macrophage inflammatory protein-1α and monocyte chemoattractant peptide-1 elicit immediate and late cutaneous reactions and activate murine mast cells in vivo. J Immunol 152:1298–1303.

109. Yamamura H, Nabe T, Kohno S, Ohata K (1994) Endothelin-1, one of the most potent histamine releasers in mouse peritoneal mast cells. Eur J Pharmacol 265:9–15.

110. Yamamura H, Nabe T, Kohno S, Ohata K (1995) Mechanism of histamine release by endothelin-1 distinct from that by antigen in mouse bone marrow-derived mast cells. Eur J Pharmacol 288:269–275.

111. Yamamura H, Nabe T, Kohno S, Ohata K (1995) Endothelin-1 induces release of histamine and leukotriene C_4 from mouse bone marrow-derived mast cells. Eur J Pharmacol 257:235–242.

112. Uchida Y, Ninomiya H, Sakamoto T, Lee JY, Endo T, Nomura A, Hasegawa S, Hirata F (1992) ET-1 released histamine from guinea pig pulmonary but not peritoneal mast cells. Biochem Biophys Res Commun 189:1196–1201.

113. Gruber BL, Marchese MJ, Kew R (1995) Angiogenic factors stimulate mast cell migration. Blood 86:2488–2493.

114. Masini E, Bani D, Bigazzi M, Mannaioni PF, Bani-Sacchi T (1994) Effects of relaxin on mast cells. In vitro and in vivo studies in rats and guinea pigs. J Clin Invest 94:1974–1980.

115. Subramanian N, Bray MA (1987) Interleukin 1 releases histamine from human basophils and mast cells in vitro. J Immunol 138:271–275.

116. Salari H, Chan-Yeung M (1989) Interleukin-1 potentiates antigen-mediated arachidonic acid metabolite formation in mast cells. Clin Exp Allergy 19:637–641.

117. Tasaka K, Hamada M, Mio M (1994) Inhibitory effect of interleukin-2 on histamine release from rat mast cells. Agents Actions 41:C26–C27.

118. Takaishi T, Morita Y, Hirai K, Yamaguchi M, Yokota T, Arai K, Ito K, Miyamoto T (1992) Mouse IL-3 induces histamine release from mouse peritoneal mast cells. Int Arch Allergy Immunol 98:205–210.

119. Matsuura N, Zetter BR (1989) Stimulation of mast cell chemotaxis by interleukin 3. J Exp Med 170:1421–1426.

120. Murakami M, Austen KF, Bingham CO III, Friend DS, Penrose JF, Arm JP (1995) Interleukin-3 regulates development of the 5-lipoxygenase/leukotriene C_4 synthase pathway in mouse mast cells. J Biol Chem 270:22,653–22,656.

121. Ghildyal N, McNeil HP, Gurish MF, Austen KF, Stevens RL (1992) Transcriptional regulation of the mucosal mast cell-specific protease gene, MMCP-2, by interleukin 10 and interleukin 3. J Biol Chem 267:8473–8477.

122. Dvorak AM, Tepper RI, Weller PF, Morgan ES, Estrella P, Monahan-Earley RA, Galli SJ (1994) Piecemeal degranulation of mast cells in the inflammatory eyelid lesions of interleukin-4 transgenic mice. Evidence of mast cell histamine release in vivo by diamine oxidase-gold enzyme-affinity ultrastructural cytochemistry. Blood 83:3600–3612.

123. Egger D, Geuenich S, Denzlinger C, Schmitt E, Mailhammer R, Ehrenreich H, Dormer P, Hultner L (1995) IL-4 renders mast cells functionally responsive to endothelin-1. J Immunol 154:1830–1837.

124. Buckley MG, Williams CM, Thompson J, Pryor P, Ray K, Butterfield JH, Coleman JW (1995) IL-4 enhances IL-3 and IL-8 gene expression in a human leukemic mast cell line. Immunology 84:410–415.

125. Coleman JW, Buckley MG, Taylor AM, Banks EM, Williams CM, Holliday MR, Thompson J (1995) Effects of interleukin-4 or stem cell factor on mast cell mediator release and cytokine gene expression. Int Arch Allergy Immunol 107:154–155.

126. Sillaber C, Strobl H, Bevec D, Ashman LK, Butterfield JH, Lechner K, Maurer D, Bettelheim P, Valent P (1991) IL-4 regulates c-kit proto-oncogene product expression in human mast and myeloid progenitor cells. J Immunol 147:4224–4228.

127. Eklund KK, Ghildyal N, Austen KF, Stevens RL (1993) Induction by IL-9 and suppression by IL-3 and IL-4 of the levels of chromosome 14-derived transcripts that encode late-expressed mouse mast cell proteases. J Immunol 151:4266–4273.

128. Welham MJ, Duronio V, Sanghera JS, Pelech SL, Schrader JW (1992) Multiple hemopoietic growth factors stimulate activation of mitogen-activated protein kinase family members. J Immunol 149:1683–1693.

129. Louahed J, Kermouni A, Van Snick J, Renauld JC (1995) IL-9 induces expression of granzymes and high-affinity IgE receptor in murine T helper clones. J Immunol 154:5061–5070.

130. Hultner L, Moeller J (1990) Mast cell growth-enhancing activity (MEA) stimulates interleukin 6 production in a mouse bone marrow-derived mast cell line and a malignant subline. Exp Hematol 18:873–877.

131. Ghildyal N, McNeil HP, Stechschulte S, Austen KF, Silberstein D, Gurish MF, Somerville LL, Stevens RL (1992) IL-10 induces transcription of the gene for mouse mast cell protease-1, a serine protease preferentially expressed in mucosal mast cells of *Trichinella spiralis*-infected mice. J Immunol 149:2123–2129.

132. Ghildyal N, Friend DS, Nicodemus CF, Austen KF, Stevens RL (1993) Reversible expression of mouse mast cell protease 2 mRNA and protein in cultured mast cells exposed to IL-10. J Immunol 151:3206–3214.

133. Murakami M, Austen KF, Arm JP (1995) The immediate phase of c-*kit* ligand stimulation of mouse bone marrow-derived mast cells elicits rapid leukotriene C_4 generation through posttranslational activation of cytosolic phospholipase A_2 and 5-lipoxygenase. J Exp Med 182:197–206.

134. Arock M, Zuany-Amorim C, Singer M, Benhamou M, Pretolani M (1996) Interleukin-10 inhibits cytokine generation from mast cells. Eur J Immunol 26:166–170.

135. Marshall JS, Leal-Berumen I, Nielsen L, Glibetic M, Jordana M (1996) Interleukin (IL)-10 inhibits long-term IL-6 production but not preformed mediator release from rat peritoneal mast cells. J Clin Invest 97:1122–1128.

136. Bissonnette EY, Enciso JA, Befus AD (1996) Inhibitory effects of sulfasalazine and its metabolites on histamine release and TNFα production by mast cells. J Immunol 156:218–223.

137. Wershil BK, Furuta GT, Lavigne JA, Choudhury AR, Wang ZS, Galli SJ (1995) Dexamethasone or cyclosporin A suppress mast cell-leukocyte cytokine cascades, multiple mechanisms of inhibition of IgE- and mast cell-dependent cutaneous inflammation in the mouse. J Immunol 154:1391–1398.

138. Williams CMM, Coleman JW (1995) Induced expression of mRNA for IL-5, IL-6, TNFα, MIP-2 and IFNγ in immunologically activated rat peritoneal mast cells: inhibition by dexamethasone and cyclosporin A. Immunology 86:244–249.

139. Emadi-Khiav B, Mousli M, Bronner C, Landry Y (1995) Human and rat cutaneous mast cells: involvement of a G-protein in the response to peptidergic stimuli. Eur J Pharmacol 272:97–102.

140. Bissonnette EY, Mathison R, Carter L, Davison JS, Befus AD (1993) Decentralization of the superior cervical ganglia inhibits mast cell mediated TNFα-dependent cytotoxicity. 1. Potential role of salivary glands. Brain Behav Immun 7:293–300.

141. White SR, Stimler-Gerard NP, Munoz NM, Popovich KJ, Murphy TM, Blake JS, Mack MM, Leff AR (1989) Effect of beta-adrenergic blockade and sympathetic stimulation on canine bronchial mast cell response to immune degranulation in vivo. Am Rev Respir Dis 139:73–79.

142. Levi-Schaffer F, Rubinchik E (1995) Mast cell role in fibrotic diseases. Israel J Med Sci 31:450–453.

143. Meininger C (1995) Mast cells and tumor-associated angiogenesis, in Human Basophils and Mast Cells: Clinical Aspects. (Marone, G., ed.). Chem Immunol, Vol. 62. Karger, Basel, pp. 239–257.

144. Kovanen PT (1995) Role of mast cells in atherosclerosis, in Human Basophils and Mast Cells: Clinical Aspects. (Marone, G., ed.). Chem Immunol, Vol. 62. Karger, Basel, pp. 132–170.

145. Marshall JS, Waserman S (1995) Mast cells and the nerves—potential interactions in the context of chronic disease. Clin Exp Allergy 25:102–110.

146. Árnason JA, Malone DG (1995) Role of mast cells in arthritis, in Human Basophils and Mast Cells: Clincal Aspects. (Marone, G., ed.). Chem Immunol, Vol. 62. Karger, Basel, pp. 204–238.

147. Leal-Berumen I, Conlon P, Marshall JS (1994) Interleukin-6 production by rat peritoneal mast cells is not necessarily preceded by histamine release and can be induced by bacterial lipopolysaccharide. J Immunol 152:5468–5476.

148. Galli SJ, Tsai M, Gordon JR, Geissler EN, Wershil BK (1992) Analyzing mast cell development and function using mice carrying mutations at W/c-kit or Sl/MGF (SCF) loci. Ann NY Acad Sci 664:69–88.

149. Roche WR, Beasley R, Williams JH, Holgate ST (1989) Subepithelial fibrosis in the bronchi of asthmatics. Lancet 1(8637):520–524.

150. Wershil BK (1995) Role of mast cells and basophils in gastrointestinal inflammation, in Human Basophils and Mast Cells: Clinical Aspects. (Marone, G., ed.). Chem Immunol, Vol. 62. Karger, Basel, pp. 187–203.

151. Crowe SE, Perdue MH (1993) Anti-immunoglobulin E-stimulated ion transport in human large and small intestine. Gastroenterology 105:764–772.

152. Li Q-Y, Raza-Ahmad A, MacAulay MA, Lalonde LD, Rowden G, Trethewey E, Dean S (1992) The relationship of mast cells and their secreted products to the volume of fibrosis in posttransplant hearts. Transplantation 53:1047–1051.

153. Levi-Schaffer F, Rubinchik E (1995) Activated mast cells are fibrogenic for 3T3 fibroblasts. J Invest Dermatol 104:999–1003.

154. Everett ET, Pablos JL, Harley RA, LeRoy EC, Norris JS (1995) The role of mast cells in the development of skin fibrosis in skin-tight mutant mice. Comp Biochem Physiol 110:159–165.

155. Mori H, Kawada K, Zhang P, Uesugi Y, Sakamoto O, Koda A (1991) Bleomycin-induced pulmonary fibrosis in genetically mast cell-deficient WBB6F1-W/Wᵛ mice and mechanism of the suppressive effect of tranilast, an antiallergic drug inhibiting mediator release from mast cells. Int Arch Allergy Appl Immunol 95:195–201.

156. Friedman BS, Metcalfe DD (1989) Mastocytosis. In: Biochemistry of the Acute Allergic Reactions. Fifth International Symposium. (Tauber AI, Wintroub BU, Simon AS, eds.) Liss, New York. pp. 163–173.

157. Reed JA, Albino AP, McNutt NS (1995) Human cutaneous mast cells express basic fibroblast growth factor. Lab Invest 72:215–222.

158. Thompson HL, Burbelo PD, Gabriel G, Yamada Y, Metcalfe DD (1991) Murine mast cells synthesize basement membrane components—a potential role in early fibrosis. J Clin Invest 87:619–623.

159. Gruber BL, Marchese MJ, Carsons SE, Schechter NM (1990) Human mast cell chymase degrades basement membrane components laminin, fibronectin and type IV collagen. Clin Res 38, 578A (abstract).

160. Lohi J, Harvima I, Keski-Oja J (1992) Pericellular substrates of human mast cell tryptase: 72,000 dalton gelatinase and fibronectin. J Cell Biochem 50:337–349.

161. Tetlow LC, Wooley DE (1995) Distribution, activation and tryptase/chymase phenotype of mast cells in the rheumatoid lesion. Ann Rheum Disease 54:549–555.

162. Gruber BL, Schwartz LB (1990) The mast cell as an effector of connective tissue degradation: a study of matrix susceptibility to human mast cells. Biochem Biophys Res Commun 171:1272–1278.

163. Marks RM, Roche WR, Czerniecki M, Penny R, Nelson DS (1986) Mast cell granules cause proliferation of human microvascular endothelial cells. Lab Invest 55:289–294.

164. Bashkin P, Doctrow S, Klagsbrun M, Svahn CM, Folkman J, Vlodavsky I (1989) Basic fibroblast growth factor binds to subendothelial matrix and is released by heparinase and heparin-like molecules. Biochem 28:1737–1743.

165. Rüger B, Dunbar PR, Hasan Q, Sawada H, Kittelberger R, Greenhill N, Neale TJ (1994) Human mast cells produce type VIII collagen in vivo. Int J Exp Path 75:397–404.

166. Starkey JR, Crowle PK, Taubenberger S (1988) Mast cell-deficient *W/W^v* mice exhibit a decreased rate of tumor angiogenesis. Int J Cancer 42:48–52.

167. Williams RM, Bienenstock J, Stead RH (1995) Mast cells: the neuroimmune connection, in Human Basophils and Mast Cells: Clinical Aspects. (Marone, G., ed.), Chem Immunol, Vol. 61. Karger, Basel, pp. 208–235.

168. Purcell WM, Atterwill CK (1995) Mast cells in neuroimmune function: neurotoxicological and neuropharmacological perspectives. Neurochem Res 20:521–532.

169. Marshall JS, Bienenstock J (1994) The role of mast cells in inflammatory reactions of the airways, skin and intestine. Curr Opin Immunol 6:853–859.

170. Stead RH, Kosecka-Janiszewska U, Beate Oestreicher A, Dixon MF, Bienenstock J (1991) Remodelling of B-50 (GAP-43)- and NSE-immunoreactive mucosal nerves in the intestines of rats infected with *Nippostrongylus brasiliensis*. J Neurosci 11:3809–3821.

171. Dietsch GN, Hinrichs DJ (1991) Mast cell proteases liberate stable encephalitogenic fragments from intact myelin. Cell Immunol 135:541–548.

172. Nelson RB, Siman R, Iqbal MA, Potter H (1993) Identification of a chymotrypsin-like mast cell protease in rat brain capable of generating the N-terminus of the Alzheimer amyloid β-protein. J Neurochem 61:567–577.

173. Perdue MH, Kosecka U, Crowe SE (1992) Antigen-mediated effects on epithelial function. Ann NY Acad Sci 664:325–334.

174. Perdue MH, Masson S, Wershil BK, Galli SJ (1991) Role of mast cells in the ion transport abnormalities associated with intestinal anaphylaxis. Correction of the diminished secretory response in genetically mast cell-deficient *W/W^v* mice by bone marrow transplantation. J Clin Invest 87:687–693.

175. Stack WA, Keely SJ, O'Donoghue DP, Baird AW (1995) Immune regulation of human colonic electrolyte transport in vitro. Gut 36:395–400.

176. Powell DW (1991) Immunophysiology of intestinal electrolyte transport, in Handbook of Physiology. The Gastrointestinal System IV. (Schultz, S.G., ed.). American Physiologic Society, Rockville, MD, pp. 591–641.

177. Barrett KE (1992) Mechanisms of inflammatory diarrhoea. Gastroenterology 103:710–711.

178. Kanwar S, Wallace JL, Befus D, Kubes P (1994) Nitric oxide synthesis inhibition increases epithelial permeability via mast cells. Am J Physiol 266:G222–G229.

179. Miller HRP, King SJ, Gibson S, Huntley JF, Newlands GFJ, Woodbury RG (1986) Intestinal mucosal mast cells in normal and parasitised rats, in Mast cell differentiation and heterogeneity. (Befus, A.D., Bienenstock, J., and Denburg, J.A., eds.). Raven, New York, pp. 239–255.

180. Scudamore CL, Pennington AM, Thornton E, McMillan L, Newlands GFJ, Miller HRP (1995) Basal secretion and anaphylactic release of rat mast cell protease-II (RMCP-II) from ex vivo perfused rat jejunum: translocation of RMCP-II into the gut lumen and its relation to mucosal histology. Gut 37:235–241.

7

Human Langerhans Cells

Thomas Bieber, MD, PHD

Contents

INTRODUCTION

Similar to gut-associated lymphoid tissue (GALT) *(1)*, the skin has been provided, by evolutionary pressure, with a proper immune system. The so-called skin-associated lymphoid tissue (SALT) *(2)* or skin immune system (SIS) *(3)* contains all elements required for recognition and efficient immune response against foreign structures invading this interface epithelium, which is in close contact with the environment. In this first line of immunosurveillance in the epidermis, as in other interface epithelia, professional antigen-presenting cells, i.e., dendritic cells (DC), play a key role that has been best established by studying the immunobiology of Langerhans cells (LC). In this review, we will summarize the most important aspects of these cells and discuss their physiological and pathophysiological role in IgE-mediated immune reactions. (Although the vast majority of the data has been collected in animal models, e.g., in the murine system, one should be aware that there are some important discrepancies between the human and murine LC and SIS. These will be mentioned appropriately whenever necessary.)

SHORT HISTORY OF THE LANGERHANS CELLS

In 1868, in search of sensory nerve endings in the epidermis, using a gold chloride technique, the young pathologist Paul Langerhans first described these cells in the human epidermis, which carry his name *(4)*. No particular interest was focused on these cells until, about one century later, Birbeck *(5)* described the presence of a characteristic and highly specific pentalaminar organelle in the cytoplasm of LC: the so-called Birbeck granule. Concerning the

From: *Allergy and Allergic Diseases: The New Mechanisms and Therapeutics*
Edited by: J. A. Denburg © Humana Press Inc., Totowa, NJ

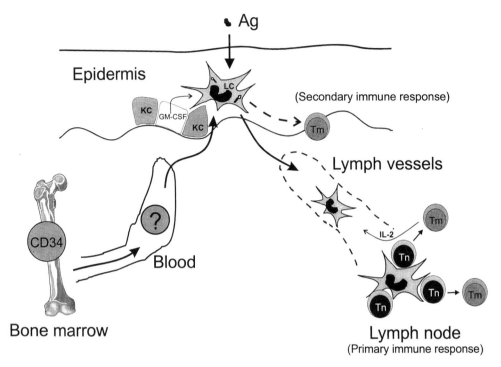

Fig. 1. Birth, life, and death of Langerhans cells. LC are derived from CD34⁺ stem cells and leave the bone marrow for the peripheral blood, in which they probably represent a minute, not-yet-identified subpopulation of monocytoid cells. The circulating LC-precursor cells migrate into the skin organ, most probably driven by epidermal-derived chemokines and supported by specific skin homing adhesion molecules. In the epidermal compartment, they apparently can stay for a relatively long period of time (almost 1 yr) and can encounter a large range of various foreign or self proteins. Such proteins (or other dangerous events) can be captured and either induce their emigration out of the skin to the regional lymph nodes, in which they are the most efficient stimulators for naive T-cells (primary immune response), or are presented directly to memory T-cells already present in the skin (secondary immune response). Finally, once they have fulfilled their duties, it is assumed that they die by apoptosis triggered by the responding T-cells, thereby avoiding chronic stimulation.

biology of LC, Stingl et al. was first reported on their functional capacity as antigen presenting cells *(6)*. The development of monoclonal antibodies in the early 1980s, and especially the description of the strong reactivity of LC with anti-CD1a antibodies *(7)*, was the starting point of a new era in the immunohistological, immunomorphological, and functional studies of these cells.

ONTOGENESIS OF LANGERHANS CELLS

Since the pioneering experiments of Katz et al. *(8)*, using a model of bone marrow transplantation in mice, it became clear that LC are of marrow origin (Fig. 1). However, the question of their circulating precursors is not definitively solved. Indeed, although several CD1a⁺ circulating cells have been reported in distinct conditions, as, for example in burn patients during epidermal recovery *(9)*, the identity of the exact precursor is not clear.

Recently, the question of the ontogeny of LC and DC arose again as new methods for the generation of DC from CD34⁺ stem cells and circulating myelo-monocytic cells were described *(10–14)*. Briefly, two nonmutually exclusive concepts have been proposed.

Some authors favor the idea that DC and LC are derived from circulating monocytes that further differentiate into DC under the influence of granulocyte macrophage-colony-stimulating factor (GM-CSF) alone or combined with interleukin-4 (IL-4) *(15)*. Because these cells lose CD14 while acquiring CD1a, they would also represent the putative precursors of LC. Thus, monocytes would represent a pluripotent cell type that, depending on the inflammatory environment, is able to either mature into macrophages or undergo another pathway of differentiation to highly potent stimulatory DC. Whether these pathways are irreversible or, alternatively, whether DC may convert into macrophages and vice versa is still not known.

On the other hand, Steinman *(16)* proposed that DC represent a separate lineage directly derived from CD34$^+$ stem cells *(16)*. This theory is supported by the recent generation of murine DC directly from bone marrow cells *(17)*. Furthermore, osteomalagic mice deficient in monocytes display epidermal LC. In the human system, Caux et al. and others have generated CD1a$^+$ DC that display all characteristics of LC, including Birbeck granules, using purified cord blood derived CD34$^+$ stem cells *(10–14)*. GM-CSF and tumor necrosis factor (TNF)-α, but not IL-4, were required for this differentiation.

FUNCTIONAL PROPERTIES OF LANGERHANS CELLS

During the last few years, a number of in vivo and in vitro studies have provided arguments supporting the concept of Schuler and Steinmann, according to which resident murine LC are functionally immature DC that need a further step of differentiation in order to acquire the full stimulatory capacity of classical DC *(18)*. Although there have been some difficulties to reproduce this functional maturation with human LC, it is assumed that this concept is valid for the human system *(19)*. It may also apply to other DC in their localization in peripheral tissue and includes three major issues: antigen uptake in the tissue, a lymph node-directed migratory function, and finally a stimulatory function in the lymph node.

Antigen Uptake

In their epidermal localization, LC provide a tight network with their dendrites that is aimed to capture or/and to detect invading proteins, allergens, haptens, bacteria, viruses, parasites, and even tumor cells (Fig. 2). It is well accepted that, as for other professional antigen-presenting cells, LC/DC may capture these structures by several pathways, including either nonspecific fluid-phase macro- or micropinocytosis or specific receptor-mediated endocytosis (RME) by either membrane immunoglobulin (mIg), Fc receptors, or mannose receptors *(20,21)*. Interestingly, pinocytosis enables LC/DC to filter large volumes of their environment. However, as for B-cells, the efficiency of processing will be dictated by the pathway used for antigen capture. In contrast to micropinocytosis, RME most probably directs the route to major histocompatibility complex (MHC) class II-rich compartments, which results in a very efficient loading into the MHC groove and, ultimately, in antigen focusing. Unlike pinocytosis, RME may also activate the cells in a specific way, depending on the type of receptor involved. This particular way of antigen capture putatively leads to the synthesis and release of mediators and/or the expression of surface molecules involved in the functional duties of LC/DC.

Functional Maturation and Migration to Regional Lymph Nodes

Once the antigen has been captured, LC will leave the epidermal compartment to reach the regional lymph node. The signals leading to the mobilization of LC are not yet identified. However, considering the presence of calcium-dependent intercellular adhesion sites

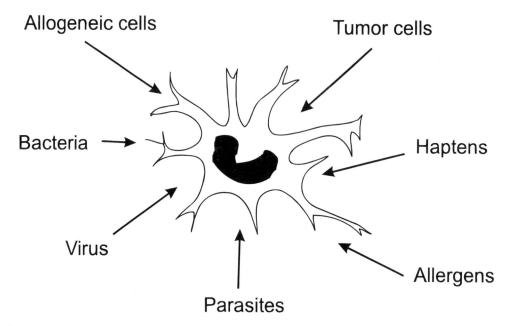

Fig. 2. Langerhans cells are the outpost of the immune system in the skin. They are able to capture a large variety of structures and to initiate a primary as well as secondary immune response.

(E-cadherins) between LC and their surrounding keratinocytes *(22,23)*, it is assumed that these signals probably induce the rupture of these LC-keratinocyte connections. Although studies in mice have suggested that TNF-α may be relevant for the emigration of LC out of the epidermis *(24)*, more recent studies with human LC have provided evidence for a role of GM-CSF as a chemokinetic factor supporting the migratory capability of LC *(25)*; other yet-to-be-defined chemotactic factors would then lead LC to migrate into lymph vessels. This migration is accompanied by profound morphologic, phenotypic *(see* Table 1), and functional alterations.

These modifications can be reproduced in vitro once LC are isolated from their epithelial environment. They irreversibly mature into lymphoid dendritic cells under the influence of GM-CSF or IL-1, either added exogenously or produced endogenously by keratinocytes in bulk epidermal cell cultures *(26)*. At the other end of this migration route, LC have to find their way to the T-cell-rich paracortical areas in the lymph node. For this purpose, they seem to use T-cell-derived IL-2 as a chemoattractant, since this cytokine exerts strong attractive activity on mature, but not on freshly isolated, LC *(27)*. Thus, migration/maturation is an obligatory step LC have to undergo before being able to fulfill their stimulatory activity toward naive T-cells in the lymph node.

Antigen Presentation

As members of the family of DC, LC are unique in their capacity not only to trigger a secondary immune response (effector phase) but, most importantly, also to stimulate naive T-cells and thereby to initiate a primary immune response (sensitization phase). However, freshly isolated LC (equivalent to resident LC) are good stimulators of memory T-cells, but poor in stimulating naive T-cells. In contrast, in vitro differentiated LC (equivalent to LC that have migrated to the regional lymph nodes) are known to be the most efficient stimulators of naive T-cells. This ability seems to be related to the expression of distinct surface molecules,

Table 1
Comparative Phenotype of Resident (Immature)
and Cultured (Mature) LC

	Resident LC	Cultured LC
Birbeck Granules	++	−
ATPase	++	±
Esterase	++	−
MHC		
Class Ia	+	+++
Class Ib		
CD1a	++++	++
CD1b	−	−
CD1c	+	−
Class II	++	++++
CD4	+	−
CD9	++	++
CD11a	±	+
CD11b	±	+
CD11c	±	+
CD18	+	+
CD24	−	+
CD25	−	++
CD32	++	±
CD40	−	++
CD45	+++ (RO)	+++ (RO/RB)
CD50	+	++
CD54	±	++
CD69	++	−
CD80/B7.1	−	++
CD86/B7.2	−	++
CD83	+	++
E-Cadherin	++	±
Stimulation of		
Naive T-cells	−	++
Memory T-cells	++	++

which enables them to easily form rosettes with naïve T-cells, a capacity obviously restricted to DC *(28)*. Once LC have fulfilled their duties, it is assumed that they die by apoptosis, most probably induced by surface receptor signals emerging from activated T-cells.

PHENOTYPE OF HUMAN LANGERHANS CELLS

LC express a wide variety of surface antigens (Table 1). Apart from CD1a, which, in normal skin, is expressed only on LC, none of these structures is specific for LC or even for cells of the DC lineage. Furthermore, this phenotype of resident LC is dramatically modulated during the maturation of LC into lymphoid dendritic cells *(29)*. Finally, resident LC are subjected to the influence of the environmental micromilieu in the skin depending on the inflammatory conditions. Thus, investigators should always be aware of these alterations when studying LC under pathological conditions, especially in allergic reactions in which infiltrating helper T-cells (TH) may secrete distinct repertoires of cytokines, depending on their subtype (TH0, TH1, TH2, or TH3).

MODULATION OF LANGERHANS CELLS BY THE SIS AND UV LIGHT

As a part of the SIS, resident LC not only are active players in the mechanisms of immune defense occurring in the skin, but also are continuously subjected to modulatory signals emerging from other cellular compartments such as keratinocytes, T-cells, fibroblasts, endothelial cells, and those cells invading the skin in the context of inflammatory reactions *(30)*. Based on this concept, we have recently proposed that the phenotype and the functions of resident LC may reflect the actual inflammatory microenvironment, specific for each disease and expressed clinically by different morphological types of skin lesions *(31)*. For example, the phenotypic profile of LC in lesional skin of atopic dermatitis is quite unique, with a strong expression of the high-affinity receptor for IgE, FcεRI *(32)*. Thus, it may be possible to characterize the type of inflammation from the phenotype of LC isolated from skin lesions.

Almost all the data collected in the field of UV light are the result of either experiments in the murine model or observations made in humans exposed to UV light for therapeutic purposes. This subject has been discussed extensively in other reviews *(33)* and is beyond the scope of the present chapter, mainly dealing with mechanisms of allergic reactions. Briefly, it has beeen shown in mice that UVB light (290–320 nm) is able to thoroughly suppress the immune response, locally as well as systemically. Furthermore, UVB light not only suppresses the function of LC, but also induces a state of tolerance that is transferable by CD8 cells, pointing to the putative role of other antigen-presenting cells with suppressive activities *(34)*. Recently, it has become evident that a major part of the biological effects of UV light observed in mice, especially in terms of immunosuppression, is a result of the UV-induced secretion of suppressive cytokines, e.g., IL-10, by keratinocytes *(35,36)*. However, the capacity of human keratinocytes to secrete IL-10 after exposure to UV light or other stimulants (including PMA) remains a matter of debate *(37,38)*. This may be, as for IL-3, an example of a cytokine mainly secreted by murine keratinocytes, but not at all (or in very limited amounts) by their human counterparts. Nonetheless, the utility of UV radiation in therapeutic regimens, especially in allergic reactions like chronic eczema or atopic dermatitis, may be related to an effect not only on the function of LC directly but also on other epidermal cells, inducing production of immunomodulatory mediators that can alter the LC function.

CYTOKINE PRODUCTION BY LANGERHANS CELLS

Our current knowledge of the cytokine repertoire of LC is limited. This area becomes even more complicated in light of the fact that the aforementioned different maturational stages of LC most probably confer distinct abilities to secrete such mediators. Whereas it has been shown that murine LC are able to synthesize and release IL-1β, IL-6, TNF-α, MIP1α, and IL-12 *(39,40)*, data in the human system suggest that LC can produce at least the pro-inflammatory cytokines IL-1, TNF-α, and IL-8 *(41–43)*. This strongly suggests that LC are involved in the initiation of inflammation, especially in the context of allergic reactions. Furthermore, mediators released either spontaneously or secondary to receptor ligation by LC most probably dictate the route of differentiation that stimulated T-cells will undergo in the context of antigen presentation. Thereby, LC contribute to direct T-cells into the TH0, TH1, TH2, or TH3 pathways, respectively.

FcεRI-EXPRESSING LANGERHANS CELLS: NEW PLAYERS IN THE ATOPIC GAME

We and others have reported that, in contrast to murine LC (Hanau et al., unpublished results), human LC express the high-affinity receptor for IgE, FcεRI *(44,45)*. The structure of the receptor differs from the classical FcεRI and its expression and the function may be highly variable, depending on the microenvironment *(46)*. Thus, one has to envisage the role of FcεRI-expressing LC in the network of IgE-mediated immunity and allergic reactions. Since LC are not equipped with any granule or preformed mediator able either to induce an immediate allergic reaction or to kill parasitic invaders, new functional duties for IgE *(47)* and for FcεRI have to be considered for these cells.

FcεRI in Antigen Processing and Presentation

Antigen uptake, processing, and presentation are the main functional characteristics of LC. As mentioned above, the FcεRI seems to enable specific antigen uptake via RME in LC. Furthermore, the high density of FcεRI on LC of patients with atopic dermatitis implies several important features (Fig. 3):

1. LC extend their ability to react with allergens by binding large amounts of IgE molecules with various specificities. This significantly enhances the probability of FcεRI-cross-link by a defined allergen at the cell surface.
2. IgE/FcεRI complexes allow the capture of rather large allergens that, under normal circumstances, are not engulfed via the usual pathway, i.e., by pinocytosis.
3. Aggregation of FcεRI on LC is followed by its internalization via receptor-mediated endocytosis into coated pits, coated vesicles and endosomes *(48)*. However, by analogy to B-cell receptors (BCR) in which Igα and Igβ are targeted to different endosomal compartments *(49)*, the route used for antigen uptake by LC, i.e., specifically via IgE and FcεRI, may dictate whether the foreign structure will be efficiently processed and targeted to MHC class II-rich compartments, ultimately leading to a higher density of specific peptides in the grooves of surface MHC class II molecules.
4. Finally, as mentioned above, LC expressing high receptor densities will display full cell activation upon FcεRI ligation, most probably inducing the synthesis and release of yet-to-be-defined mediators. Such mediators may have proinflammatory capacities and/or enhance/influence subsequent antigen presentation, or recruit inflammatory cells to sites of allergen penetration.

This scenario allows for efficient antigen presentation of even minute amounts of allergens. Indeed, whereas it has been reported that LC isolated from atopic skin use IgE for antigen uptake, followed by presentation to autologous T-cells *(50)*, formal proof that FcεRI enables antigen-presenting cells to provide IgE-mediated antigen focusing has been provided only recently for monocytes *(51,52)*, circulating DC *(53)*, as well as for LC *(54)*.

FcεRI and Immune Responses

One may speculate that FcεRI-expressing LC armed with specific IgE are able to boost the secondary immune response and to further trigger IgE synthesis by recruiting and activating more antigen-specific TH2 or TH1 cells. As mentioned above, LC are the most potent stimulators of naive T-cells, i.e., they are committed to initiate a primary immune response. At first glance, FcεRI-mediated antigen uptake and subsequent presentation would appear unlikely in the primary reaction, since specific IgE would have to be present at the very beginning.

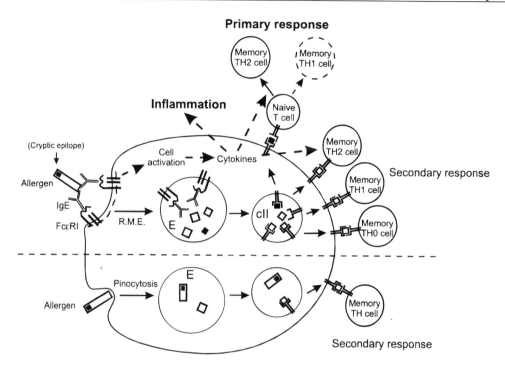

Fig. 3. Consequences of IgE/FcεRI-mediated allergen uptake by LC. Allergen uptake via pinocytosis (lower part of the diagram) leads to a limited processing in endosomes (E) and loading onto MHC class II molecules. In contrast, receptor-mediated endocytosis (R.M.E.) (upper part of the diagram) via FcεRI may result in a more efficient processing of the allergen and to the access to MHC class II-rich compartments. Furthermore, cryptic epitopes not directly recognized by allergen-specific IgE on FcεRI may be unmasked and loaded onto MHC class II molecules. This would result in a primary immune response and ultimately extend the repertoire of the IgE response. Finally, as a consequence of concomitant cell activation initiated by FcεRI-crosslinking, APC may be triggered to synthezise and release pro-inflammatory mediators that initiate inflammatory reactions and influence the efficiency/outcome (TH0, TH1, TH2, or TH3) of antigen presentation.

However, it cannot be excluded that complex allergenic structures, efficiently captured via FcεRI on LC or other DC, are processed by these cells in a way that leads to the unmasking and presentation, among others, of cryptic peptides/epitopes never encountered by T-cells. This would then initiate a primary reaction against these antigens, thereby contributing to an increase in the variety of IgE specificities. The concept of simultaneous antigen uptake and FcεRI aggregation on LC leading to the *de novo* synthesis and release of mediators capable of directing T-cells toward a defined phenotype and/or function, i.e., TH1 or TH2 cells, is a very acceptable working hypothesis, which remains to be verified especially in the light of recent findings suggesting the role of LC-derived IL-12 and PGE2 in driving TH cells into either TH1 or TH2, respectively.

FcεRI Expressing Langerhans Cells as Trigger for IgE-Mediated Delayed Type Hypersensitivity Reactions

One may speculate that FcεRI-ligation on LC putatively triggers the synthesis and release of mediators that may initiate a local inflammatory reaction, as has been demonstrated for mast cells *(55)*. From a physiopathological standpoint, FcεRI-expressing LC and related DC in the epidermis have been suspected of playing a crucial role in atopic dermatitis, since they may represent a pivotal link between transepidermis-penetrating aeroallergens and antigen-specific T-cells infiltrating the skin lesions *(56,57)*. The observation that the presence of FcεRI-expressing LC, bearing IgE molecules, is a prerequisite to provoking eczematous lesions, observed after application of aeroallergens to the skin of atopic patients, strongly supports this concept. Consequently, atopic dermatitis may represent a paradigm of IgE/FcεRI-mediated, delayed-type hypersensitivity reaction. A similar role could be attributed to other FcεRI-expressing DC in the lung.

FUTURE PERSPECTIVES: LANGERHANS CELLS AS VECTORS OR TARGETS FOR NEW IMMUNOTHERAPEUTIC STRATEGIES

Since the skin and the lung are easily accessible organs, FcεRI on LC/DC of these tissues may provide a putative target for new topical therapeutic approaches for atopic diseases. On the other hand, systemic approaches similar to those focusing on classical IgE-mediated allergic reactions, e.g., preventing the binding of IgE to its receptor with soluble recombinant receptor, recombinant human anti-IgE antibodies, or even high-affinity oligonucleotides, could also represent valuable alternatives in the management of atopic conditions. Once the mechanisms of LC/DC involvement in tolerance are more fully understood, in vitro-generated LC/DC expressing FcεRI could be used to induce allergen-specific tolerance/anergy in patients exhibiting exaggerated skin immune responses toward environmental allergens.

REFERENCES

1. McWilliams M, Philips-Quagliata JM, Lamm ME (1975) Characteristics of mesenteric lymph node cells homing to gut-associated lymphoid tissue in syngeneic mice. J Immunol 115:54–58.
2. Streilein, JW (1978) Lymphocyte traffic, T cell malignancies and the skin. J Invest Dermatol 71:167–171.
3. Bos JD, Kapsenberg ML (1993) The skin immune system: progress in cutaneous biology. Immunol Today 14:75–78.
4. Langerhans P (1868) Uber die Nerven der menschlichen Haut. *Virchows Arch.* (Pathol Anat Physiol) 44:325–337.
5. Birbeck MS, Breathnach AS, Everall JD (1961) An electronmicroscopic study of basal melanocytes and high-level clear cells (Langerhans cells) in vitiligo. J Invest Dermatol 37:51–63.
6. Stingl G, Katz SI, Clement L, Green I, Shevach EM (1978) Immunologic functions of Ia-bearing epidermal Langerhans cells. J Immunol 121:2005–2013.
7. Fithian E, Kung P, Goldstein G, Rubenfeld M, Fenoglio C, Edelson, R (1981) Reactivity of Langerhans cells with hybridoma antibody. Proc Natl Acad Sci USA 78:2541–2544.
8. Katz SI, Tamaki K, Sachs DH (1979) Epidermal Langerhans cells are derived from cells originating in bone marrow. Nature 282:324–326.
9. Gothelf Y, Hanau D, Tsur H, Sharon N, Sahar E, Cazenave JP, Gazit E (1988) T6 positive cells in the peripheral blood of burn patients: are they Langerhans cells precursors? J Invest Dermatol 90:142–148.
10. Caux C, Dezutter-Dambuyant C, Schmitt D, Banchereau J (1992) GM-CSF and TNF-alpha cooperate in the generation of dendritic Langerhans cells. Nature 360:258–261.
11. Romani N, Gruner S, Brang D, Kämpgen E, Lenz A, Trockenbacher B, Konwalika G, Fritsch P, Steinman RM, Schuler G (1994) Proliferating dendritic cell progenitors in human blood. J Exp Med 180:83–93.
12. Kulmburg P, Schaefer HE, Mertelsmann R, Lindemann A (1995) Delineation of the dendritic cell lineage by generating large numbers of Birbeck granule-positive Langerhans cells from human peripheral blood progenitor cells in vitro. Blood 86:2699–2707.
13. Strunk D, Rappersberger K, Egger C, Strobl H, Kromer E, Elbe A, Maurer D, Stingl G (1996) Generation of human dendritic cells Langerhans cells from circulating CD34[(+)] hematopoietic progenitor cells. Blood 87:1292–1302.
14. Caux C, Vanbervliet B, Massacrier C, Durand I, Banchereau J (1996) Interleukin-3 cooperates with tumor necrosis factor alpha for the development of human dendritic Langerhans cells from cord blood CD34[(+)] hematopoietic progenitor cells. Blood 87:2376–2385.

15. Sallusto F Lanzavecchia A (1994) Efficient presentation of soluble antigen by cultured human dendritic cells is maintained by granulocyte/macrophage colony-stimulating factor plus interleukin-4 and down-regulated by tumor necrosis factor-alpha. J Exp Med 179:1109–1118.

16. Steinman RM (1991) The dendritic cell system and its role in immunogenicity. Annu Rev Immunol 9:271–296.

17. Inaba K, Inaba M, Deguchi M, Hagi K, Yasumizu R, Ikehara S, Muramatsu S, Steinman RM (1993) Granulocytes, macrophages, and dendritic cells arise from a common major histocompatibility complex II-negative progenitor in mouse bone marrow. Proc Natl Acad Sci USA 90:3038–3042.

18. Schuler G, Steinman RM (1985) Murine epidermal Langerhans cells mature into potent immunostimulatory dendritic cells in vitro. J Exp Med 161:526–546.

19. Teunissen MB, Wormmeester J, Krieg SR, Peters PJ, Vogels IM, Kapsenberg ML, Bos JD (1990) Human epidermal Langerhans cells undergo profound morphologic and phenotypical changes during in vitro culture. J Invest Dermatol 94:166–173.

20. Steinman RM and Swanson J (1995) The endocytic activity of dendritic cells. J Exp Med 182:283–288.

21. Sallusto F, Cella M, Danieli C, Lanzavecchia A (1995) Dendritic cells use macropinocytosis and the mannose receptor to concentrate macromolecules in the major histocompatibility complex class II compartment: Downregulation by cytokines and bacterial products. J Exp Med 182:389–400.

22. Tang A, Amagai M, Granger LG, Stanley JR, Udey MC (1993) Adhesion of epidermal Langerhans cells to keratinocytes mediated by E-cadherin. Nature 361:82–85.

23. Blauvelt A, Katz SI, Udey MC (1995) Human Langerhans cells express E-cadherin. J Invest Dermatol 104:293–296.

24. Cumberbatch M, Kimber I (1995) Tumour necrosis factor-alpha is required for accumulation of dendritic cells in draining lymph nodes and for optimal contact sensitization. Immunology 84:31–35.

25. Rupec R, Magerstaedt R, Sander E, Bieber T (1996) Granulocyte/macrophage-colony stimulating factor induces the migration of human epidermal Langerhans cells. Exp Dermatol 5:115–119.

26. Heufler C, Koch F, Schuler G (1988) Granulocyte/macrophage colony-stimulating factor and interleukin 1 mediate the maturation of murine epidermal Langerhans cells into potent immunostimulatory dendritic cells. J Exp Med 167:700–705.

27. Strobel I, Rupec R, Wollenberg A, Bieber T (1993) IL-2 receptor on human Langerhans cells lacks the β-chain but mediates IL-2 dependent migration: evidence for a putative γ-chain. Arch Dermatol Res 285 :108

28. Inaba K, Steinman RM (1986) Accessory cell-T lymphocyte interactions. Antigen-dependent and -independent clustering. J Exp Med 163:247–261.

29. Romani N, Lenz A, Glassel H, Stossel H, Stanzl U, Majdic O, Fritsch P, Schuler G (1989) Cultured human Langerhans cells ressemble lymphoid dendritic cells in phenotype and function. J Invest Dermatol 93:600–609.

30. Luger TA, Schwarz T (1993) Epidermal growth factors and cytokines. Marcel Dekker, New York, 1993.

31. Wollenberg A, Wen SP, Bieber T (1995) Langerhans cells phenotyping: A new tool for the differential diagnosis of eczematous skin diseases. Lancet 346:1626–1627.

32. Wollenberg A, Kraft S, Hanau D, Bieber T (1996) Immunomorphological and ultrastructural characterization of Langerhans cells and a novel, inflammatory dendritic epidermal cell (IDEC) population in lesional skin of atopic eczema. J Invest Dermatol 106:446–453.

33. Kripke ML (1991) Immunological effects of ultraviolet radiation. J Dermatol 18:429–433.

34. Saijo S, Bucana CD, Ramirez KM, Cox PA, Kripke ML, Strickland FM (1995) Deficient antigen presentation and Ts induction are separate effects of ultraviolet irradiation. Cell Immunol 164:189–202.

35. Enk AH, Katz SI (1992) Identification and induction of keratinocyte-derived IL-10. J Immunol 149:92–95.

36. Enk CD, Sredni D, Blauvelt A, Katz SI (1995) Induction of IL-10 gene expression in human keratinocytes by UVB exposure in vivo and in vitro. J Immunol 154:4851–4856.

37. Grewe M, Gyufko K, Krutman J (1995) Interleukin-10 production by cultured human keratinocytes and their modulation by ultraviolet B and ultraviolet A1. J Invest Dermatol 104:3–6.

38. Jackson M, Thomson KE, Laker R, Norval M, Hunter J, Mc Kenzie RC (1996) Lack of induction of IL-10 expression in human keratinocytes. J Invest Dermatol 106:1329–1330.

39. Schreiber S, Kilgus O, Payer E, Kutil R, Elbe A, Mueller C, Stingl G (1992) Cytokine pattern of Langerhans cells isolated from murine epidermal cell cultures. J Immunol 149:3524–3534.

40. Romani N, Kampgen E, Koch F, Heufler C, Schuler G (1990) Dendritic cell production of cytokines and responses to cytokines. Int Rev Immunol 6:151–161.

41. Sauder DN, Dinarello CA, Morhenn VB (1984) Langerhans cell production of interleukin-1. J Invest Dermatol 82:605–607.

42. Larrick JW, Morhenn V, Chiang YL, Shi T (1989) Activated Langerhans cells release tumor necrosis factor. J Leukoc Biol 45:429–433.

43. Bieber T, Sticherling M, Rupec R, Schroeder JM (1991) Human epidermal Langerhans cells release the neutrophil activating peptide IL-8. J Invest Dermatol 96:1013.

44. Bieber T, de la Salle H, Wollenberg A, Hakimi J, Chizzonite R, Ring J, Hanau D, de la Salle C (1992) Human epidermal Langerhans cells express the high affinity receptor for immunoglobulin E (FcεRI). J Exp Med 175:1285–1290.

45. Wang B, Rieger A, Kilgus O, Ochiai K, Maurer D, Fodinger D, Kinet JP, Stingl G (1992) Epidermal Langerhans cells from normal human skin bind monomeric IgE via Fc epsilon RI. J Exp Med 175:1353–1365.

46. Bieber T (1996) Fc epsilon R1 on human antigen presenting cells. Curr Opin Immunol 18:773–777.

47. Mudde GC, Hansel TT, V.Reijsen FC, Osterhoff BF, Bruijnzeel-Koomen CAFM (1990) IgE: an immunoglobulin specialized in antigen capture. Immunol Today 11:440–443.

48. Jurgens M, Wollenberg A, Hanau D, De la Salle H, Bieber T (1995) Activation of human epidermal Langerhans cells by engagement of the high affinity receptor for IgE, FcεRI. J Immunol 155:5184–5189.

49. Bonnerot C, Lamkar D, Hanau D, Spehne D, Davoust J, Salamero J, Fridman WH (1995) Role of B-cell receptor Ig alpha and Ig beta subunits in MHC class II restricted antigen presentation. Immunity 3:335–347.

50. Mudde GC, van-Reijsen FC, Boland GJ, de-Gast GC, Bruijnzeel PL, Bruijnzeel-Koomen CA (1990) Allergen presentation by epidermal Langerhans cells from patients with atopic dermatitis is mediated by IgE. Immunology 69:335–341.

51. Maurer D, Fiebiger E, Reininger B, Wolffwiniski B, Jouvin MH, Kilgus O, Kinet JP, Stingl G (1994) Expression of functional high affinity immunoglobulin E receptors (FcεRI) on monocytes of atopic individuals. J Exp Med 179:745–750.

52. Maurer D, Ebner C, Reininger B, Fiebiger E, Kraft D, Kinet JP, Stingl G (1995) The high affinity IgE receptor (FcεRI) mediates IgE-dependent allergen presentation. J Immunol 154:6285–6290.

53. Maurer D, Fiebiger E, Ebner C, Reininger B, Fischer GF, Wichlas S, Jouvin M-H, Schmitt-Egenolf M, Kraft D, Kinet J-P, Stingl G (1996) Peripheral blood dendritic cells express FcεRI as a complex composed of FcεRIα- and FcεRIγ-chains and can use this receptor for IgE-mediated allergen presentation. J Immunol 157:607–616.

54. Bieber T (1997) FcεRI on human epidermal Langerhans cells: an old receptor with new structure and functions. Int Arch All Clin Immunol 113:30–34.

55. Galli SJ, Costa JJ (1995) Mast-cell-leukocyte cytokine cascades in allergic inflammation. Allergy 50:851–862.

56. Bruijnzeel-Koomen C, van Reysen F, Mudde GC (1991) IgE and atopic dermatitis. Clin Exp Allergy 21-(Suppl) 1:294–301.

57. Bieber T (1995) Role of Langerhans cells in the pathophysiology of atopic dermatitis. Pathol Biol 43:871–875.

8

Eosinophils

Redwan Moqbel, PhD, FRCPath
and Paige Lacy, PhD

CONTENTS

INTRODUCTION

When Paul Ehrlich first described the eosinophil in 1879, having detected blood white cells that bound eosin-like dyes with great affinity, he was unaware of the magnitude of subsequent interest in this cell, from both a clinical and biological point of view. Since his description, and particularly over the last two decades, a remarkable expansion in eosinophil literature has occurred. A significant association was established between the eosinophil and a number of disease conditions, including helminthiasis, allergy, asthma, drug hypersensitivity, certain neoplasia, and graft rejection *(1,2)*. It now seems that the eosinophil may have a wide spectrum of biological activities, especially in inflammation. These range from ameliorating local inflammatory reactions by either antagonizing allergic mediators or releasing repair-associated cytokines to exerting deleterious cytotoxic effects on metazoan parasitic targets and airway mucosal tissue cells. The effector function is thought to be related to the release of highly cytotoxic, granule-associated cationic proteins following stimulation of eosinophils. In spite of strong arguments in favor of either end of this spectrum, the evidence remains circumstantial; the precise role of this cell in health and disease is still in need of further elucidation. The current perspective on the role of the eosinophil in disease supports the view that it may be a key proinflammatory cell with the capacity to cause tissue damage in asthma and other related allergic diseases *(1,2)*. The recent description of the capacity of this cell to synthesize and release a battery of inflammatory cytokines, chemokines, and growth factors *(3)* has introduced a new and important regulatory dimension to the eosinophil in asthma, allergy, and inflammatory disorders. Interest in the eosinophil remains focused on providing a better understanding of its role and determining the mechanisms that regulate its differentiation, recruitment, and activation, with a view to devising novel and effective therapeutic strategies in diseases with which this cell is associated.

From: *Allergy and Allergic Diseases: The New Mechanisms and Therapeutics*
Edited by: J. A. Denburg © Humana Press Inc., Totowa, NJ

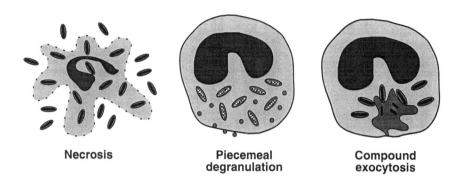

Necrosis   Piecemeal   Compound
                  degranulation   exocytosis

Fig. 1. Potential mechanisms for eosinophil degranulation.

GENERAL STRUCTURE AND MORPHOLOGY OF EOSINOPHILS

Mature eosinophils are nondividing (approx 10–15 μm in diameter) and possess bilobed or trilobed nuclei as well as primary and secondary granules acquired during growth and differentiation in the bone marrow *(4)*. The primary granules are the sole location for storage of the Charcot-Leyden crystal (CLC) protein *(5)*. The secondary granules are spherical or ovoid-shaped membrane-bound organelles (~200/cell) and contain an electron-dense crystalline core surrounded by a less dense matrix *(6)*. Eosinophils also contain non-membrane-bound lipid bodies, which contain lipids that have been esterified into glycerophospholipids, and appear to be the cell's principal store for arachidonic acid *(7)*.

The morphology of activated eosinophils varies from that of primed cells (stimulated without undergoing active secretion with only subtle differences in organelle structures) to that of fully activated, degranulating cells. Morphological markers of eosinophil activation include increased size and numbers of lipid bodies and increased numbers of primary granules, small granules, and vesiculo-tubular structures. Smooth endoplasmic reticulum and crystals of CLC protein, the latter of which are not membrane-bound, may appear in the cytoplasm. In addition, there is often a marked reduction in the number of crystalloid secretory granules, which may also appear translucent as if emptied of their contents, particularly in tissue eosinophils. Morphological differences between normal peripheral blood eosinophils and activated eosinophils have been studied in inflammatory bowel disease *(8)*, skin samples from patients with hypereosinophilic syndrome (HES) *(9,10)*, cytokine-activated peripheral blood eosinophils *(11)*, and mature cord blood-derived eosinophils *(12)*. Degranulation is a crucial event in the activation of the eosinophil. In its proinflammatory role, the eosinophil acts by releasing its granule proteins onto the surface of an invasive organism. Eosinophils can release their secretory granule contents by three possible mechanisms: necrosis, piecemeal degranulation, and compound exocytosis (Fig. 1). In necrosis, many eosinophils at sites of inflammation appear disorganized, with cells displaying nuclear lysis, centralization of granules, and loss of integrity of granules and plasma membrane. Release of intact or disrupted granules into the interstitium is likely to have toxic effects on the surrounding cells. Necrotic release of granules has been observed in the skin of patients with HES and bullous pemphigoid *(13)*.

The most commonly observed form of eosinophil degranulation *in situ* closely resembles a process known as piecemeal degranulation. In piecemeal degranulation, numerous small vesicles bud off from the larger secondary granules and move to the plasma membrane for fusion, thereby causing gradual emptying of the secondary granules to the outside of the cell. A spectrum of morphologies has been identified for piecemeal degranulation, including the apparent loss of protein from the core of the secondary granule (creating a "mottled" appearance by

Table 1
Mediators Released from Eosinophils

Cationic granule proteins
    Major basic protein
    Eosinophil cationic protein
    Eosinophil-derived neurotoxin
    Eosinophil peroxidase

Lipid mediators
    Eicosanoids
        Prostaglandins D_2, E_2, F_2
        Leukotrienes A_4, B_4, C_4, D_4, E_4
        15-HPETE
        15-HETE
    Platelet-activating factor

Cytokines, Growth Factors, and Chemokines
    Interleukins-1α, 2, 3, 4, 5, 6, 8, 10, 16
    GM-CSF, TGFα, β, TNFα (IFNγ?)
    RANTES, MIP-1α, PDGF-B

Reactive oxygen species
    O_2^-
    H_2O_2

Others
    CLC protein
    Hexosaminidase
    Arylsulfatase B
    Collagenase
    Histaminase
    Catalase

transmission electron microscopy), partial or complete loss from the matrix compartment, and total emptying of the granule contents *(14)*.

In regulated exocytosis, the crystalloid granules fuse directly with the plasma membrane prior to releasing their contents to the outside of the cell. This phenomenon is regarded as the classic form of regulated secretion, which is well characterized in anaphylactic degranulation of mast cells and basophils *(15)*. Compound exocytosis may also occur where secondary granules fuse with each other prior to release from the cell through a single fusion pore. Although these processes have been shown to occur in eosinophils from patients with inflammatory bowel disease and tissue invasive infections *(16)* as well as calcium ionophore-stimulated peripheral blood eosinophils *(17)*, it is unusual to see morphological evidence of classical or compound exocytosis in eosinophilic inflammation.

EOSINOPHIL-DERIVED MEDIATORS

Eosinophils have the capacity to secrete a number of potent mediators (Table 1). These include preformed basic proteins, which are stored in the secondary granules, de novo synthesized phospholipids, cytokines, proteases, and products of oxidative metabolism, including superoxide anions and hydrogen peroxide.

Eosinophil Granule Cationic Proteins

The remarkable and unique crystalloid granules present in eosinophils contain four basic proteins. Major basic protein (MBP) makes up fully 50% of the granule protein and is stored inclusively in the electron-dense crystal found at the core of the granule, in which it accounts for virtually all of the core protein *(18)*. Eosinophil peroxidase (EPO), eosinophil cationic protein (ECP), and eosinophil-derived neurotoxin (EDN), on the other hand, are found in the granule matrix surrounding the core *(19,20)*. The biology of these proteins has been reviewed elsewhere *(21,22)*.

MAJOR BASIC PROTEIN

MBP is a single polypeptide chain of 117 amino acids, a molecular weight of 13.8 kDa, and an alkaline pI of 10.9. Its basic nature relates to its 17 arginine residues, accounting for its basicity, and 9 cysteine residues explain its tendency to form disulfide bonds. A monoclonal antibody (MAb; BMK-13) that binds to MBP specifically has been used to quantitate total number of eosinophils, regardless of their activation status (i.e., paneosinophilic) *(23)*. MBP can be detected in biological fluids by immunoassay only after it has been reduced and alkylated. The reduced form is toxic for parasites, as is the native form, but is considerably less potent. In addition to its in vitro potent cytotoxic effects against both tissue and cells and parasite metazoan targets, MBP can act as a secretagogue for many inflammatory cells and has been shown to specifically induce noncytotoxic release of histamine from basophils (in contrast to other eosinophil granule proteins) and rat peritoneal mast cells *(24,25)*. This discovery has modified the previously held view that eosinophils can act to ameliorate the anaphylactic response in mast cells. MBP can cause neutrophil and macrophage activation *(26)*, and together with EPO is a strong agonist for platelet mediator release *(27)*. In addition, MBP is capable of stimulating eosinophil degranulation and IL-8 release *(28)*. Whereas many actions of MBP can be mimicked in some cases by other highly basic proteins, not all properties are shared, suggesting that the intrinsic positive charge of the protein is not the only factor responsible for its physiological effects.

EOSINOPHIL CATIONIC PROTEIN

ECP is a single-chain polypeptide with a similarly alkaline pI of 10.8. It displays marked heterogeneity in molecular sizing, ranging between 16 and 21.4 kDa, probably as a result of differential glycosylation. There are approx 25 pg of ECP per eosinophil, which corresponds to an order of magnitude less than MBP. Two isoforms have been identified, ECP-1 and ECP-2, using heparin Sepharose *(29)*. The amino acid sequence of ECP is 66% homologous to another eosinophil granule protein, namely, EDN, and 31% homologous to human pancreatic ribonuclease. However, the ribonuclease activity of ECP is 100 times less potent than that of EDN *(30)*.

MAbs have been used to distinguish between a form of ECP that may be found in resting eosinophils (MAb EG1) and a secreted cleaved form of ECP that is thought to correspond to the activated form of this cell (MAb EG2) *(31)*. The latter antibody, which has recently been used to identify activated eosinophils in tissue, also cross-reacts with EDN, probably through its active site (also *see* below).

At least one isoform of ECP is toxic for schistosomulae of *Schistosoma mansoni* and other helminthic parasites; it is more potent than MBP on a molar basis *(32)* and its toxicity appears to be mediated through its ability to form membrane pores *(33)*. It also exhibits toxic effects on guinea pig tracheal epithelial cells at concentrations 10 times higher than those of MBP *(34)*, and like EDN can cause a neurological syndrome called the Gordon phenomenon when injected into the cerebrospinal fluid of rabbits and rats *(35)*.

EOSINOPHIL-DERIVED NEUROTOXIN

This protein is a single-chain polypeptide with an apparent molecular weight of 18.6 kDa. EDN is also called EPX *(36)*, and like ECP possesses marked ribonuclease activity *(37)*. EDN is a member of a ribonuclease multigene family, with a sequence identical to human urinary ribonuclease *(38)*. EDN activity is not restricted to eosinophils; it is also found in mononuclear cells and possibly neutrophils, although it is not clear whether neutrophils phagocytose this protein from degranulating eosinophils. It is only weakly toxic for parasites or mammalian cells, and its only known function, other than ribonuclease activity, is its neurotoxicity exhibited by the Gordon phemonenon *(39)*.

EOSINOPHIL PEROXIDASE

EPO is a heme-containing protein composed of two subunits, a light 14-kDa and a heavy 58-kDa subunit derived from a single protein that has been subsequently cleaved. It shares a 68% homology with human neutrophil myeloperoxidase and other peroxidase enzymes, and is antigenically similar. There is approx 15 pg of EPO per eosinophil *(40)*.

In the presence of H_2O_2, EPO is able to oxidize halides to form reactive hypohalous acids with bromide as the preferred substrate. EPO is toxic for microorganisms and parasites as well as respiratory epithelium and pneumocytes, and its potency is increased 10,000-fold when it is combined with H_2O_2 and a halide *(41,42)*. However, it appears that thiocyanate, a pseudo-halide, is able to compete for EPO in physiological conditions and inhibit the effects of bromide and iodide even when the halides are present in excess *(43)*. Thus, studies demonstrating cytotoxic effects of EPO trough the H_2O_2/halide system may be in need of some revision.

EICOSANOIDS

Eicosanoids are signaling molecules produced by oxidation of arachadonic acid cleaved from phospholipids. Cleavage of a membrane or lipid body-associated phospholipid containing arachidonic acid by phospholipase A_2 results in the release of free fatty acid. Lipid bodies are the principal store for $[^3H]$-arachidonic acid after labeling in eosinophils *(44)*, and arachidonic acid is mainly incorporated into phosphatidylcholine, phosphatidylinositol, and phosphatidylethanolamine *(7)*. The main pathways of arachidonic acid metabolism in eosinophils are the cyclooxygenase-dependent pathway, producing prostaglandins and thromboxanes, and the lipoxygenase-dependent pathway, generating leukotrienes, hydroperoxyeicosatetranoic acids (HPETEs), HETEs, and diHETEs.

Eosinophils are able to generate picogram quantities of prostaglandin (PG) E_2, PGD_2, and PGF_2 *(45,46)*, although the predominant cyclooxygenase product is thromboxane B_2 (TXB_2); after stimulation with calcium ionophore, human peripheral blood eosinophils can produce over 2 ng of $TXB_2/10^6$ cells *(47)*.

Leukotriene (LT) A_4 is generated by the action of 5-lipoxygenase on arachidonic acid, and is further converted to LTC_4 after linkage of a glutathione molecule by glutathione-S-transferase in eosinophils *(48)*, which in turn may be converted to LTD_4 and LTE_4 by the actions of γ-glutamyl-transpeptidase and a dipeptidase, respectively. Eosinophils generate relatively large amounts of LTC_4 after calcium ionophore stimulation (up to 70 ng/10^6 cells), but negligible concentrations of LTB_4 *(49,50)*. LTC_4 can also be released in response to a number of physiological stimuli, including immunoglobulin (Ig) G-coated Sepharose beads *(51)*, opsonized zymosan *(52)*, and IgG-antigen complexes *(53)*. The ability of the eosinophil to release LTB_4 is apparently species-specific whereby guinea pig eosinophils are able to synthesize LTB_4, in contrast to human eosinophils *(54)*. LTC_4, D_4, and E_4 (sulfidopeptide leukotrienes) exhibit a number of biological properties that may be relevant to asthma, including smooth muscle contraction, mucus hypersecretion, and increased vascular permeability.

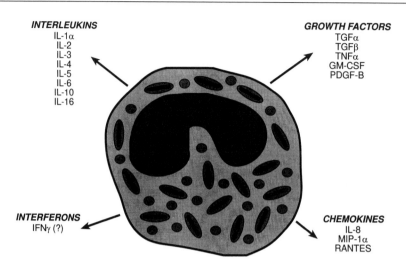

Fig. 2. Eosinophil-derived cytokines, chemokines and growth factors.

Eosinophils also contain large quantities of 15-lipoxygenase, a 70-kDa enzyme homologous to 5-lipoxygenase that can convert arachidonic acid to 15-hydroperoxyeicosatetranoic acid (15-HPETE) and subsequently to 15-HETE *(55,56)*; the latter may be of importance in asthma due to its potential to induce mucus production by cultured human airway cells *(57)*. Eosinophils from asthmatic subjects appear to generate more LTC_4 than those from normal donors *(58,59,60)*. Sulfidpeptide leukotrienes have been measured in asthmatic bronchoalveolar lavage (BAL) fluid *(61)*, at sites of allergic inflammation *(62)*, and in urine *(63)*.

Sulfidopeptide leukotriene receptor antagonists and 5-lipoxygenase inhibitors in early clinical trials are showing promising potential in reducing the severity of asthmatic symptoms *(64)*. Whether these antagonists are able to block release of eosinophil-derived mediators is yet to be determined.

PLATELET-ACTIVATING FACTOR (PAF)

PAF (1-O-alkyl-2-acetyl-sn-glycero-3-phosphocholine) is a phospholipid derived from its inactive precursor, lyso-PAF, following acetylation by a specific acetyltransferase. Rapid biodegradation of PAF via an acetyl hydrolase activity hydrolyses an acetyl group to regenerate lyso-PAF *(65)*. PAF is strongly proinflammatory and exhibits potent eosinophil chemoattraction and stimulating activity *(66)*. Eosinophils generate substantial quantities of PAF after stimulation with calcium ionophore, opsonized zymosan, and IgG-coated Sepharose beads *(67,68)*. Detecting any increased amounts of PAF in eosinophil-associated diseases is very difficult, possibly due to its rapid metabolism locally. PAF antagonists have so far been disappointing in clinical trials for the treatment of asthma.

Cytokines, Growth Factors, and Chemokines

Although eosinophils are predominantly "end-stage cells" with a presumed limited capacity to transcribe and translate new proteins, it is now clear that they can synthesize and secrete many important inflammatory and regulatory cytokines in response to physiological stimuli (Fig. 2). Cytokine expression by non-T-cells was discovered when *in situ* hybridization was applied to tissue biopsies to detect cytokine transcripts in T-cells. It is most likely that the recruitment and activation of eosinophils in inflammatory foci is dependent on T-cell-derived cytokines and chemokines, including interleukin (IL)-5, IL-3, granulocyte/macrophage-colony-stimulating factor (GM-CSF), regulated on activation, normal T expressed, and secreted (RANTES), and macrophage inflammatory protein (MIP)-1α. Whether eosinophil-derived cytokines (*see* below) contribute significantly to ongoing inflammatory reactions in allergy and/or asthma remains to be determined.

IL-1α

IL-1α is a proinflammatory cytokine product of monocytic cells and macrophages. It is involved in antigen presentation to T cells and has multipotential effects on immune and inflammatory cells. IL-1α messenger ribonucleic acid (mRNA) was first detected in murine eosinophils by the use of *in situ* hybridization *(69)* and later confirmed in human eosinophils obtained from hypereosinophilic patients *(70)*. The latter study also showed that IL-1α release was associated with cytokine-induced human leukocyte antigen-DR (HLA-DR) expression in eosinophils, suggesting a potential role for eosinophils as antigen-presenting cells.

IL-2

IL-2 is known to be an essential growth factor required for proliferation of cells in response to T-cell receptor stimulation. Human eosinophils respond to IL-2 by undergoing chemotaxis, and a subpopulation of eosinophils express IL-2 receptors (CD25) *(71)*. An average of 10% of freshly isolated, unstimulated blood eosinophils from asthmatics were shown to exhibit granular staining for IL-2 *(72)*. The amount of stored IL-2 measured in 10^6 lysed eosinophils was approx 26 pg, and only a small proportion of this was released following stimulation. Using a cell fractionation method and immunogold staining, the majority of IL-2 was shown to be associated with eosinophil granules *(72)*. Detection of IL-2 mRNA in human peripheral blood eosinophils by a combination of *in situ* reverse transcriptase polymerase chain reaction (RT-PCR) and *in situ* hybridization *(73)* suggest that these cells may participate in immune regulation through their ability to synthesize this cytokine.

IL-3

IL-3 is a pluripotential growth factor for a wide range of myelocytic cells and granulocytes. Ionomycin-stimulated eosinophils elaborate IL-3 at concentrations equivalent to 50% of the capacity of mononuclear cells *(74)*. Eosinophil-derived IL-3 appears to have autocrine effect on prolonging eosinophil survival and activation, in vitro. Treatment of eosinophils with the immunosuppressants, FK-506, and rapamycin was shown to inhibit ionophore-induced production of IL-3 and GM-CSF from eosinophils *(75)*.

IL-4

IL-4 is a critical cytokine in the initiation and maintenance of atopy, conversion of T-helper (Th) cell to Th2 phenotype and isotype switching in B-cells to IgE. IL-4 also exhibits chemotactic activity for eosinophils from atopic patients *(76)*. By RT-PCR, IL-4 message can be detected in highly purified asthmatic blood eosinophils, and approx 30% of these eosinophils showed immunoreactivity for IL-4, which appears to be localized to eosinophil granules *(77)*. Lysed eosinophils contain an average of 108 pg of IL-4/10^6 cells, 30% of which is released following physiological stimulation. The majority of eosinophils infiltrating allergen-induced cutaneous late-phase reactions are immunoreactive for IL-4 and express mRNA for this cytokine, in contrast to eosinophils recovered from the airways of asthmatic subjects *(77)*. In addition, eosinophils in bronchial mucosa and nasal polyps from atopic individuals have also been shown to express IL-4 *(78)*. These findings have important implications for the role of eosinophils in the maintenance and progress of atopy.

IL-5

Transcripts encoding IL-5, a crucial cytokine required for terminal differentiation of eosinophils from $CD34^+$ progenitors, were identified in eosinophils infiltrating mucosa of patients with active coeliac disease *(79)*. By *in situ* hybridization, eosinophils from patients with hypereosinophilic syndrome, eosinophilic cystitis, or eosinophilic heart disease also expressed IL-5 mRNA *(79,80)*. This expression was also confirmed in BAL eosinophils obtained from asthmatic subjects *(81)*. IL-5 was colocalized to eosinophilic granules by immunogold staining, suggesting that it resides intracellularly in association with eosinophil granules *(80)*. Whether it is present in the core or matrix of the granule is not clear, as two separate studies have shown distinct locations for IL-5 immunoreactivity in the granule *(82,83)*.

IL-6

IL-6 is a pleiotropic lymphokine involved in the regulation of the immune response by modulating T- and B-lymphocyte functions as well as priming granulocytes and endothelial cells. Message encoding IL-6 was detected in peripheral blood eosinophils by *in situ* hybridization and confirmed by Northern blot analysis *(84)*. The translated protein was also shown to be released following stimulation with interferon-γ (IFNγ). These results have been confirmed by using RT-PCR and *in situ* hybridization in blood eosinophils obtained from both normal and hypereosinophilic donors *(85)*. Whether IL-6 from eosinophils associated with allergic or helminth-induced inflammation contributes to the regulation or modulation of cells at local foci remains unclear.

IL-8

IL-8 is important in neutrophil chemotaxis and is a cofactor required for granulocytic differentiation. Highly purified eosinophils stimulated by calcium ionophore have been shown to release IL-8 into the supernatant *(86)*. Ionophore-induced release of IL-8 was inhibited by cyclosporin A and cycloheximide. Immunoreactivity for IL-8 was again granular in appearance, suggesting storage of preformed IL-8. Stimulation of eosinophils with C5a and fMLP induced synthesis and release of IL-8, while PAF or C-C chemokines had no effect *(87)*. Asthmatic BAL eosinophils released higher concentrations of IL-8 when compared with normal controls *(88)*.

IL-10

The known actions of IL-10 include inhibition of cytokine synthesis from Th1-subtype T-cells and enhancement of major histocompatibility complex (MHC) II expression on B-cells. By RT-PCR, mRNA expression of IL-10 was shown in eosinophils from normal donors, which was upregulated following stimulation with IL-5 *(89)*. These cells were also shown to constitutively express large quantities of stored IL-10, which appeared to diminish following in vitro culture of the cells *(89)*.

IL-16

IL-16, formerly known as lymphocyte chemoattractant factor, is a homotetrameric cytokine that binds to CD4 *(90)*. IL-16 was recently found to be produced by normal peripheral blood eosinophils after overnight stimulation with GM-CSF *(91)*. These results suggest that eosinophils have the potential to express IL-16 after physiological stimulation and thus may be involved in the events leading to infiltration and accumulation of lymphocytes at sites of allergic inflammatory reactions.

INTERFERON-γ (IFNγ)

A Th1 cytokine with an important role in regulating immune responses against tumors, viruses, and protozoan parasites, IFNγ exerts a wide range of biological activities on many immune and inflammatory cell types, including the eosinophil. Nakajima et al. *(89)* failed to detect mRNA encoding IFNγ in eosinophils from normal healthy donors in the presence or absence of stimulation. However, a subpopulation of eosinophils has been suggested to express mRNA for this cytokine, prompting the proposal that a cytokine profile-dependent dichotomy (type 1 and type 2) may exist in eosinophils akin to that recognized in T-helper cells (M. Capron, personal communication).

GRANULOCYTE MACROPHAGE-COLONY STIMULATING FACTOR

Like immune cells, a number of tissue cell types are capable of synthesizing and elaborating GM-CSF, an important cofactor in granulocyte proliferation, survival, activation, and differentiation. GM-CSF stimulates upregulation of adhesion molecules on eosinophils and therefore contributes to their activation and mobility across endothelial cells.

Peripheral blood eosinophils were shown to transcribe and translate GM-CSF mRNA after stimulation with calcium ionophore or IFNγ *(92)*. GM-CSF was released from eosinophils in response to ionomycin, and this release was blocked by cyclosporin-A treatment *(74)*. Elegant evidence was presented in this study for an autocrine effect of eosinophil-derived GM-CSF on prolongation of eosinophil survival. GM-CSF mRNA has been detected in eosinophils, in vivo, in association with nasal polyposis *(93)*, and immunoreactive GM-CSF can be identified in a 24-h culture supernatant of nasal polyp tissue. The presence of GM-CSF mRNA was confirmed in human BAL eosinophils obtained from asthmatic subjects after endobronchial allergen challenge *(81)*. GM-CSF has recently been shown to be stored in association with crystalloid granules of eosinophils obtained from asthmatic subjects *(94)*. The expression and release of GM-CSF by eosinophils at inflammatory foci may provide an autocrine pathway to maintain the viability and effector function of these cells.

TRANSFORMING GROWTH FACTOR-α AND -β (TGFα/β)

TGFα and TGFβ are released by numerous cell types during incidents of tissue trauma and are important in tissue remodeling in response to injury. TGFβ is required as a cofactor for B-cell switching to IgA-secreting phenotype. TGFα mRNA and its translated product have been colocalized in tissue eosinophils found in close proximity to the site of oral squamous carcinoma *(95)*, which is known to be associated with elevated tissue eosinophil levels. This was confirmed by findings on peripheral blood eosinophils from hypereosinophilic patients. In a rabbit wound healing model, eosinophils were shown to constitutively express mRNA for TGFα in skin tissue *(96)*. Epithelial wound healing coincided with TGFα mRNA disappearance and dispersal of eosinophils from the site. The ability of eosinophils to express TGFα was also observed in the Syrian hamster cheek pouch mucosa, while hamster bone marrow eosinophils were shown to express TGFα mRNA and its product *(97)*.

TGFβ1 is also a product of eosinophils from patients with blood eosinophilia, as demonstrated by Northern blot analysis, *in situ* hybridization, and immunocytochemistry *(98)*. Mucosal tissue from nasal polyps displayed TGFβ1 mRNA expression, and 50% of the eosinophils (as determined by Carbol chromotrope 2R staining) that accumulated in this tissue were mRNA[+] for TGFβ1 *(99)*. TGFβ1 has also been localized to eosinophils in nodular sclerosis-associated Hodgkin's disease *(100)*. Eosinophil-derived TGFβ1, with its recognized role in chronic inflammation and fibrosis, may well exert its effect in tissue repair by promoting fibroblast growth and activation.

TUMOR NECROSIS FACTOR-α (TNFα)

TNFα is a potent proinflammatory factor that can be released by a number of immune cells, particularly during viral or bacterial infection, and is itself capable of activating eosinophil cytotoxicity. Expression of TNFα mRNA was observed by *in situ* hybridization in 44–100% of eosinophils obtained from peripheral blood of normal subjects or hypereosinophilic patients *(101)*, and the stored protein could be detected by immunocytochemical staining. Purified eosinophils from atopic individuals spontaneously released TNFα, in vitro, which was inhibited by cycloheximide. In necrotizing enterocolitis, infiltrating eosinophils were shown to be TNFα[+] by immunogold labelling *(102)*, and immunogold particles were localized to the matrix compartment of the specific secondary granules of eosinophils from patients with idiopathic hypereosinophilic syndrome *(103)*. Thus, eosinophils have the potential to contribute to local effects of TNFα during invasive infections.

MACROPHAGE INFLAMMATORY PROTEIN-1α (MIP-1α)

The effects of MIP-1α include chemotactic and activating roles for monocytes and macrophages. A high percentage of blood eosinophils (39–91%) obtained from hypereosinophilic patients showed positive mRNA expression for MIP-1α *(101)*, while no MIP-1α[+] eosinophils could be detected in blood from normal donors. In vivo, the majority of eosinophils infiltrating nasal polyp tissue had strong expression for MIP-1α mRNA, which was confirmed by Northern blot analysis. However, the physiological relevance of MIP-1α expression in eosinophils has yet to be found.

RANTES

RANTES is a C-C chemokine with potent chemotactic and activating properties for eosinophils. Highly purified blood eosinophils have been shown to express mRNA for RANTES as detected by RT-PCR *(104)*. This was confirmed by *in situ* hybridization, in which 7–10% of blood eosinophils express RANTES mRNA in the absence of stimulus. Following in vitro incubation with IFN-γ, but not ionomycin, this increased to 25%. By ELISA, blood eosinophils were shown to contain a median of 7.3 ng of RANTES per 10^6 cells. Eosinophils secreted 24% of this total into culture supernatants following stimulation with serum-coated particles. The capacity of human eosinophils to synthesize and translate mRNA for RANTES in association with allergic inflammation in vivo was also demonstrated in allergen-induced late-phase cutaneous reactions in atopic volunteers *(104)*. RANTES mRNA was also detected in stimulated human blood eosinophils from atopic individuals by RT-PCR, and its translated product identified *(90)*. This was also found in eosinophils from normal individuals following 3-h stimulation with immobilized Ig, TNFα, and/or IL-5 *(91)*, suggesting that eosinophil-derived RANTES may be an important regulator of local inflammatory responses.

PLATELET-DERIVED GROWTH FACTOR-B (PDGF-B)

PDGF-B, thought to be involved in tissue remodeling, was shown to be synthesized by and co-localized to eosinophils using *in situ* hybridization in nasal polyp tissue and bronchial biopsies from severe asthmatic subjects *(105)*. However, the presence of PDGF-B protein in tissue eosinophils was not demonstrated. Ionophore-stimulated peripheral blood eosinophils, on the other hand, expressed both mRNA and immunoreactivity for PDGF-B *(105)*.

Other Eosinophil-Derived Mediators

CHARCOT-LEYDEN CRYSTAL PROTEIN (CLC PROTEIN)

A major constituent of the human eosinophil is the CLC protein. It is a 17.4-kDa hydrophobic protein that subsequently was shown to be lysophospholipase *(106)*. Approximately 10% of the total cellular protein of eosinophils consists of CLC protein *(107,108)*. The protein forms characteristic bipyramidal crystals both intracellularly and in surrounding tissues infiltrated by activated eosinophils *(109)*.

GRANULE-ASSOCIATED ENZYMES

The eosinophil also contains a number of other granule-stored enzymes whose roles have been postulated but not yet defined *(110)*. These include acid phosphatase (large amounts of which have been isolated from eosinophils), collagenase, arylsulfatase B, histaminase, phospholipase D, catalase, nonspecific esterases, vitamin B12-binding proteins, and glycosaminoglycans.

RESPIRATORY BURST PRODUCTS

Eosinophils can undergo a respiratory burst with release of superoxide ions and H_2O_2 in response to particulate stimuli (such as opsonized zymosan) and soluble mediators (such as LTB_4 and phorbol myristate acetate). Eosinophils can generate twice as much chemiluminescence as neutrophils and the capacity of eosinophils to generate reactive oxygen species is increased in cells from patients with allergic rhinitis *(111)*.

EOSINOPHIL RECEPTORS

Eosinophils possess a number of receptors to immobilized immunoglobulins, cytokines, complement proteins, and lipid mediators. It is not known which of these receptors is required for in vivo activation of eosinophils during asthma or allergic inflammation. This section contains a description of some of the most important receptors so far identified on eosinophils. Eosinophil adhesion receptors are reviewed in Chapter 18.

Receptors for Immunoglobulins

Eosinophils express receptors for IgG, IgA, IgD, and IgE. The precise molecular structures of these receptors has not yet been fully determined, and with the IgE receptor in particular there exists controversy concerning the exact nature of the IgE–eosinophil interaction.

IgG RECEPTOR (FcγR)

Eosinophils express FcγRII (CD32) but to a limited extent, but do not appear to express any FcγRI (CD64) *(112)*. Their relative lack of FcγRIII (CD16) has been exploited to allow purification of eosinophils from granulocyte preparations, as neutrophils express abundant quantities of this receptor *(113)*. FcγRII is a low-affinity receptor of 40 kDa that is widely expressed on many immune cells, including monocytes, neutrophils, eosinophils, platelets, and B-cells. Eosinophils will bind all four subclasses of IgG *(114)*. FcγRII receptor stimulation is able to induce degranulation and respiratory burst in eosinophils, although not as strongly as IgA receptor stimulation *(115)*. Stimulation of FcγRII molecules is likely to occur as part of the host response to helminthic infections, as parasitic larvae coated with IgG antibodies provide a potent stimulus for eosinophil cytotoxicity *(116)*.

IgA RECEPTOR (FcαR)

A number of studies have shown that eosinophils possess functional surface IgA receptors *(115,117,118)*. IgA, and particularly secretory IgA, is effective in stimulating substantial eosinophil degranulation and release of EDN. This effect is enhanced by preincubation of eosinophils with the cytokines GM-CSF and IL-3. This may be of physiological importance as eosinophils are often found at mucosal surfaces in the lungs.

FcαR molecules have been detected on eosinophils from normal individuals after in vitro activation as well as on unstimulated eosinophils from allergic individuals *(119)*, suggesting that in the allergic phenotype, eosinophils upregulate their expression of FcαR. The FcαR expressed by eosinophils differs from those of neutrophils and macrophages in that eosinophil FcαR has a higher content of N-linked carbohydrate moieties.

IgE Receptor (FcεR)

Many studies have shown that eosinophils express low-affinity IgE receptors (FcεRII; CD23) (120–124). It was later demonstrated that eosinophils also possess the high-affinity IgE receptor (FcεRI) in cells purified from hypereosinophilic patients (125). This finding has been difficult to reconcile with earlier studies in which no evidence of significant high-affinity IgE receptor activity was detected in these cells. In addition, all subjects in the later study had eosinophils in association with idiopathic hypereosinophilic syndrome, various skin diseases, and lymphomas. It is possible that eosinophil heterogeneity accounts for these discrepancies.

A further development has added to the complexity of this area by the description of the IgE-binding molecule Mac-2/epsilon BP on human eosinophils. This S-lectin-type molecule on eosinophils was shown to bind IgE and participate in IgE-dependent effector functions (126).

Stimulation of FcεRII on eosinophils by IgE-coated particles does not lead to a detectable degranulation response, in vitro (117). However, there is evidence to suggest that IgE may be a cofactor for other eosinophil responses (127). It is likely from these findings that the IgE-dependent component of eosinophil function has an important role within the context of allergic-type hypersensitivity disorders in which such responses are damaging.

Receptors for Complement

Eosinophils strongly express complement receptor 3 (CR3) (CD11b/CD18/Mac-1), a member of the β2 integrin family of adhesion molecules that has at least two binding sites that recognize a number of ligands, such as C3bi, ICAM-1, fibrinogen, and polysaccharides. Peripheral blood eosinophils express significantly fewer CR3 molecules than neutrophils (112). However, this receptor is integral to a number of important eosinophil functions, such as adhesion to endothelial cells (128) and IgE- and IgG-dependent schistosomula killing (129). Binding of complement-coated particles via this receptor is a potent stimulus for eosinophils to undergo respiratory burst (130) and degranulation (131).

Eosinophils also express low levels of CR1 (CD35), a glycoprotein that binds the complement fragment C3b (132). It may also be involved in killing of parasitic larvae, but possibly to a lesser degree than CR3 (133).

Receptors for Cytokines

In addition to synthesizing and releasing cytokines of their own, eosinophils respond to picomolar concentrations of GM-CSF, IL-3, and IL-5 (134–138), via high affinity cytokine receptors that have been fully characterized (139–144). Eosinophils and basophils, but not neutrophils, express IL-5 receptors, whereas GM-CSF receptors are present on both eosinophils and neutrophils. These receptors are heterodimers that share common β, but have distinct α chains (145,146). The homologous α chains (60–80 kDa) form a low-affinity association with their respective cytokines, whereas the common β chains (120–140 kDa) combine with α chains to form high-affinity binding sites (147). Cross-competition between these three receptors has been observed, which is probably explained by limiting numbers of β chains, which may in turn regulate the extent of eosinophil activation (140,144). Stimulation of cytokine receptors induces phosphorylation of a common set of proteins (148–150), which suggests that the β chain (or another common component) is responsible for directing signal transduction along similar pathways for GM-CSF, IL-3, and IL-5. (This is reviewed in Chapter 17.)

Variations in the effects of each cytokine on eosinophils may be owing to additional components associated with the α and β chains. Increased expression of mRNA for IL-5 receptor has
recently been observed in bronchial biopsies from asthmatics *(151)*. Since this expression was
almost exclusively associated with eosinophils, it is plausible to assume that these cells are the
major target for IL-5 signaling in asthmatic airways.

Purified eosinophils from hypereosinophilic syndrome patients were shown to possess
high-affinity receptors for IL-2 (CD25), which may be associated with their activation *(71)*.
This receptor has been suggested to stimulate eosinophil chemotaxis upon ligand binding by
IL-2, which was shown to be approximately fourfold more potent than PAF in eosinophil
chemotaxis. Recent studies also described the expression of an eosinophil-specific receptor for
the chemokine eotaxin *(152,153)*, described as a highly potent and specific chemotactic activity for eosinophils *(154)*.

Miscellaneous Receptors

RECEPTORS FOR ALLERGIC MEDIATORS AND SECRETAGOGUES

Specific receptors for LTB_4, PAF, C5a, and C3a are expressed on eosinophils. LTB_4 receptors on guinea pig, but not human, alveolar and peritoneal eosinophils have been shown to be
of both high and low affinity *(155)*. Human eosinophils have been reported to express receptors
of two affinities for PAF *(156,157)*. The presence of a receptor for fMLP on eosinophils has not
been demonstrated directly, but there is sufficient evidence to indicate that a low-affinity
binding site may exist that is associated with a functional response to high levels of this peptide
(158). Receptors for LTB_4, PAF, C5a, and fMLP have been recognized as belonging to a
family of seven transmembrane-spanning receptors possessing in common a binding site for
guanosine 5'-triphosphate (GTP)-binding proteins *(159,160)*. C5a receptors may also activate
phospholipase D and stimulate chemotaxis and mediator release from human eosinophils *(161)*.
Eosinophil C3a receptors induce chemotaxis, mediator release and reactive oxygen species
release as well as intracellular Ca^{2+} transport in human eosinophils following activation *(162)*.

OTHER RECEPTORS

Eosinophils also express the CD4 receptor *(163)*, which is elevated in cells from hypereosinophilic syndrome patients *(164,165)*. The association between CD4 expression on the
eosinophil surface and human immunodeficiency virus (HIV) infection is likely because
$CD4^+$ eosinophil precursors in human bone marrow cultured with IL-5 can be infected with
this virus *(166)*.

HLA-DR expression has also been reported in eosinophils *(167)* following their culture
with 3T3 fibroblasts in the presence of GM-CSF. Collateral with this, eosinophils have been
shown to act as relatively weak antigen-presenting cells *(70,168)*.

CD69 molecules have been detected in vivo on lung eosinophils from patients with
eosinophilic pneumonia *(169)*. Expression of CD69 could be induced on human peripheral
blood eosinophils by GM-CSF stimulation as early as 1h after incubation, whereas in vivo
expression of CD69 was detected in eosinophils from BAL fluid of mild asthmatic subjects
(170). These studies suggest that CD69 may be a marker of eosinophil activation by cytokines,
as it is for lymphocytes *(171)*.

Recent studies have shown expression of CD40 receptors on eosinophils from peripheral
blood and nasal polyposis. The ligation of this receptor led to the release of GM-CSF, suggesting that eosinophils may serve a hitherto unrecognized role for binding to cells expressing
the CD40 ligand *(172)*. The Fas antigen, CD95, has also been identified in human peripheral
blood eosinophils. Anti-Fas antibody treatment diminished IL-5-induced eosinophil viability
and activated apoptosis *(173)*. Other receptors expressed on eosinophils whose functions

remain ill-defined include CD31 *(174)* and CD9 *(175)*. CD9 is a 24-kDa protein found on eosinophils, platelets, and pre-B-cells, but not neutrophils, and is a potentially useful marker for separation of eosinophils from neutrophils in a mixed cell population. Its precise function in eosinophils is unknown.

RECEPTORS FOR GLUCOCORTICOIDS

Glucocorticosteroids are among the most potent drugs for suppressing the numbers of circulating eosinophils in humans, as well as for inhibiting their cytokine-induced prolonged survival *(176)*. A high-affinity but low-capacity receptor for steroids has been defined in eosinophils that, when bound, is able to mediate anti-inflammatory effects on eosinophil function *(177)*. Interestingly, eosinophils from idiopathic hypereosinophilic syndrome patients fail to respond to steroid treatment, probably because they lack receptors for these agents *(178)*.

ROLE OF EOSINOPHILS IN DISEASE

The precise role of eosinophils in health and disease remains an enigma. The range of observed in vitro and in vivo activities of this cell suggests that the eosinophil may assume different roles under different conditions and is subject to a number of factors related to the inflammatory microenvironment. These factors may include degree of inflammation, cytokine profile, cell age, and site and type of the pathological milieu. This diversity of biological activities seen in this cell involves the eosinophil in a range of reactions from homeostatic control to regulation of immune and inflammatory reactions to redundancy. Elevation in eosinophil counts, in both the peripheral blood and relevant tissue foci associated with asthma, allergic and drug reactions, helminthic parasitic infections, eosinophilic leukemia, and the hypereosinophilic syndrome have been well documented. Eosinophilia has also been associated with a number of clinical features, including endomyocardial fibrosis and vasculitis. It is very likely that these symptoms relate to the presence of eosinophils and the toxic properties of their granule contents *(179)*. Much of the work undertaken in recent years on eosinophils has concentrated on their association with helminthic infection and allergic disease, which are prevalent in the general population throughout the world. Since the emphasis of this volume is on allergic conditions, we will only briefly review the controversies regarding the role of this cell in parasitic disease.

Role of Eosinophils in Helminthic Parasite Infections

The precise role of eosinophils in the immunopathological changes associated with helminthic infections unfortunately remains incompletely understood and rather controversial. Elevated eosinophil numbers in tissue in blood, together with mastocytosis and increases in the levels of total and parasite-specific IgE, are considered the hallmarks of infection with parasitic worms, especially in their tissue migratory phases. However, it is still unclear whether the presence of eosinophils represents an event in the pathology of the disease or is part of a protective immune response mounted specifically against the relevant parasitic worm infection *(180,181)*.

EVIDENCE FOR HELMINTHIC PARASITE KILLING

The original experiments using in vitro assays demonstrated that isolated human peripheral blood eosinophils from patients infected with *Schistosoma mansoni* were able to rapidly adhere to and kill larvae of this trematode *(116,182,183)*. Similar antibody-dependent, eosinophil-mediated in vitro cytotoxicity was reported for a number of other helminthic parasites. Eosinophils act by firmly adhering to opsonized worms or larvae and discharging their granule contents onto the outside surface of the organism. The granule contents can be detected by electron microscopy following labeling of eosinophil peroxidase, for instance, as thick layers of electron-dense deposits on the organism *(184)*. This deposition results in lysis and death of the organism by the formation of pores in its outer coat. The damaging effects are mediated by the eosinophil granule cationic proteins (MBP, ECP, and EPO) at very low molar concentrations. MBP is considered to be toxic toward a number of parasitic larvae of various helminths, although ECP is 10 times more potent on a molar basis than MBP, and EPO and EDN are relatively inactive on their own. MBP is present in the granule in much larger amounts than ECP, and this may account for a higher proportion of the toxicity observed *(185)*.

Evidence of a direct in vivo killing role for eosinophils toward helminthic parasites in humans has so far proved elusive. Available in vivo data on the role of human eosinophils is largely limited to measurements of blood and tissue eosinophilia during the migration of helminth(s) to various tissue sites *(186)*. These include evidence of direct contact between eosinophils and fragments of dead skin-invading larvae of *Strongyloides ratti* hyperimmune rats after challenge with infective larvae *(187)*. Eosinophils have also been found in close contact with schistosomula of *Schistosoma haematobium* in the cutaneous tissue of immune monkeys *(188)*. Furthermore, in vivo release of allergic mediators (including LTC$_4$ and PAF) from eosinophil-rich sites during systemic parasite-induced anaphylaxis or rapid expulsion of a secondary helminthic insult has provided further supportive evidence for a possible eosinophil effector function against helminthic parasites *(189–191)*. In man, evidence suggests that eosinophils may not directly kill parasitic worms. For example, the presence of an eosinophilic infiltrate in association with human onchocerciasis has been shown to be correlated with microfilarial production from pregnant female adult *Onchocerca volvulus* worms rather than the host's immune status *(192)*. On the other hand, the rate of reinfection in African children with *S. haematobium* indicates that both IgE and eosinophils appear to contribute to resistance/ protection in that age group *(193,194)*. In a mouse animal model of helminthic infection, subsequent treatment with a neutralizing anti-IL-5 antibody abolished eosinophilia without influencing the host's protective responses against infection *(195)*. These observations have raised considerable doubts regarding the putative anti-parasitic properties of this cell. It should, however, be emphasized that the development of the mammalian host's protective response against helminths involves a complex cascade of events with the eosinophil being one among many other participants. Furthermore, eosinophils and their cytotoxic products may directly or indirectly cause parasite damage through the creation of an unfavorable local environment, which may in turn eliminate worm burden. Parasites possess ingenious adaptive mechanisms to prolong their survival within the host's tissue and help evade or manipulate the immune and inflammatory responses.

Eosinophils in Asthma and Allergic Inflammation

The association between eosinophils, asthma, and allergic disease has been documented for many years with the conclusion that large numbers of eosinophils (together with mononuclear cells) are frequently found in and around the bronchi in patients who have died of asthma *(196–198)*. Immunostaining of postmortem bronchial tissue has revealed the presence of substantial deposition of MBP in the airways *(199)*. However, this finding is not universal, since a number of case reports showed no evidence of airway eosinophilia in association with childhood asthma deaths *(200)*.

In both atopic and nonatopic chronic asthma, the presence of increased peripheral blood eosinophil numbers is well established, although this elevation is not as great as that seen in other eosinophil-associated diseases, and often the eosinophil count is within normal values. Eosinophil counts correlated with several measurements of airflow obstruction *(201)* as well as the degree of bronchial hyperreactivity in patients with a late-phase response after antigen challenge *(202)*. A similar correlation was observed in a cross sectional study of asthmatics seen at a routine chest clinic *(203)*. The concentration of ECP in the serum of asthmatics has also been found to correlate with the severity of clinical disease, and monitoring of ECP has been suggested as a useful adjunct to clinical assessment *(204)*.

STUDIES USING INVASIVE CLINICAL TECHNIQUES

The technique of fiberoptic bronchoscopy has been used to obtain BAL fluid from the airways of patients with mild to moderate asthma. This approach has helped shed new light on our appreciation of the extent of eosinophil involvement in asthma. A number of studies to measure and compare changes from baseline values in the cellular content of BAL with those obtained after allergen challenge have been conducted on asthmatics. This approach has proven to be a safe method to explore the airways providing it is conducted by experienced personnel on an appropriate patient population with adequate precautions *(205)*. This method has been successfully employed both experimentally (i.e., after exposure of atopic subjects to the relevant specific allergen) or in patients with ongoing clinical asthma during and outside the allergen season.

Challenge of some sensitized asthmatic subjects with aerosolized allergen results in a dual response. The first is an early phase of bronchoconstriction, with an immediate onset that may last up to 1 h before returning to baseline, and the second is a late-phase airway obstruction and hyperresponsiveness increasing for up to 6 h after challenge and lasting 24 h or even longer in some instances. The early phase is thought to be due to the immediate release of mast cell-derived bronchoconstricting mediators, and the late phase is thought to correspond with the influx of immune and inflammatory cells, which may closely mimic the pathology of clinical asthma *(206,207)*.

Following the segmental challenge technique, whereby allergen is directly instilled into the airways, up to 50% of the lavage cells were eosinophils 24 h after challenge *(208)*. Challenge with agents causing occupational asthma, such as plicatic acid in red cedar wood asthma and toluene diisocyanate, also generate BAL eosinophilia *(209,210)*. Despite the almost invariable finding of eosinophilia after allergen challenge, a causal relationship to the development of airway signs and symptoms remains circumstantial.

CLINICAL ASTHMA

In patients with ongoing clinical asthma, BAL fluids and endobronchial biopsies invariably reveal elevated (but modest) eosinophil numbers when compared with normal controls, and often in association with increased numbers of mast cells and epithelial cells *(211)*. However, it is now clear that even in very mild asthmatics (requiring only occasional use of bronchodilators), eosinophilic airway inflammation is evident in both BAL and biopsy material. As a consequence, anti-inflammatory drugs, particularly inhaled corticosteroids, have assumed a critical and prominent position in management and treatment strategies in asthma.

It now appears that airway eosinophils in asthma are activated (as determined by EG2 MAb immunoreactivity *(212)* and expression of the activation marker CD69 *(170)*). In addition, measurement of MBP concentrations in BAL fluid appears to give a better indication for disease activity than the number of eosinophils in BAL *(213,214)*. Indeed, a marked reduction in the levels of ECP (a marker of eosinophil activity) in asthmatic BAL was associated with clinical improvement induced by corticosteroid treatment in the absence of any effect of the drug on the number of BAL eosinophils *(215)*.

Present evidence in human studies suggests that IL-5 plays a critical role in eosinophil recruitment and eosinophil-mediated tissue damage. IL-5 mRNA$^+$ cells have been identified in bronchial biopsies *(216)* and BAL fluid *(217)* from ongoing steady-state asthmatics, as well as from asthmatics provoked by aerosolized allergen challenge *(218,219)*. Chronic severe asthmatics have elevated serum concentrations of IL-5 compared with controls, and levels were found to decrease following treatment with corticosteroids *(220,221)*. In support of these findings, a recent study using IL-5 knockout mice demonstrated lowered airway hyperresponsiveness to β-methacholine and reduced lung damage in response to aeroallergen challenge, along with markedly reduced eosinophil numbers *(222)*.

As in asthma, eosinophils are prominent in other forms of allergic inflammation, including allergic rhinitis and atopic dermatitis. Essentially, the findings in rhinitis have been similar to those in asthma, with increased numbers of activated eosinophils and their granule proteins in association with increased numbers of nasal epithelial mast cells *(219,223,224)*. However, in rhinitis, the nasal epithelium generally appears intact. Nasal polyps contain large numbers of activated eosinophils, and the syndrome of aspirin sensitivity, eosinophilia, and nasal polyposis is well recognized *(225)*. In atopic dermatitis, peripheral blood eosinophilia is a common feature, and skin lesions are characterized by marked deposition of eosinophil granule proteins, often in the absence of intact eosinophils *(226,227)*. The different morphologies of eosinophils and their surrounding tissues in these atopic diseases suggest that slightly different phenotypes of eosinophils are expressed in each tissue.

CONCLUSION

Eosinophils are almost invariably present in increased numbers at sites of allergic inflammation. They actively secrete mediators that could cause many of the pathological features of the disease process. The levels of eosinophils and their released mediators correlate broadly with disease activity, and effective treatment for asthma, particularly glucocorticoids, reduces the activity of tissue and blood eosinophils. Therefore, although there is good evidence for a proinflammatory role for eosinophils in asthma and related diseases, much of this remains circumstantial, and in some cases controversial. The discovery of pharmaceutical antagonists that specifically inhibit eosinophil accumulation or activation in tissues continues to be keenly awaited.

REFERENCES

1. Gleich GJ, Adolphson CR (1986) The eosinophilic leukocyte: structure and function. Adv Immunol 39:177–253.
2. Wardlaw AJ, Moqbel R, Kay AB (1995) Eosinophils: biology and role in disease. Adv Immunol 60:151–266.
3. Moqbel R, Levi-Schaffer F, Kay AB (1994) Cytokine generation by eosinophils. J Allergy Clin Immunol 94(Suppl):1183.
4. Dvorak AM, Ackerman SJ, Weller PF (1991) Subcellular morphology and biochemistry of eosinophils. In: Harris JR, ed. Blood Cell Biochemistry, Vol. 2, Megakaryocytes, Platelets, Macrophages and Eosinophils. Plenum, London, pp. 237–344.
5. Dvorak AM, Letourneau L, Login GR, Weller PF, Ackerman SJ (1988) Ultrastructural localization of the Charcot-Leyden crystal protein (lysophospholipase) to a distinct crystalloid-free granule population in mature human eosinophils. Blood 72:150–158.
6. Sokol RJ, Hudson G, Wales J, James NT (1991) Ultrastructural morphometry of human leucocytes in health and disease. Electron Microsc Rev 4:179–195.
7. Weller PF, Monahan-Earley RA, Dvorak HF, Dvorak AM (1991) Cytoplasmic lipid bodies of human eosinophils. Subcellular isolation and analysis of arachidonate incorporation. Am J Pathol 138:141–148.
8. Dvorak AM, Monahan RA, Osage JE, Dickersin GR (1980) Crohn's disease: transmission electron microscopic studies. II. Immunologic inflammatory response. Alterations of mast cells, basophils, eosinophils and the microvasculature. Hum Pathol 11:606–619.
9. Henderson WR, Harley JB, Fauci AS, Chi EY (1988) Hypereosinophilic syndrome human eosinophil degranulation induced by soluble and particulate stimuli. Br J Haematol 69:13–21.

10. Peters MS, Gleich GJ, Dunnette SL, Fukuda T (1988) Ultrastructural study of eosinophils from patients with the hypereosinophilic syndrome: a morphological basis of hypodense eosinophils. Blood 71:780–785.

11. Caulfield JP, Hein A, Rothenberg ME, Owen WF, Soberman RJ, Stevens RL, Austen KF (1990) A morphometric study of normodense and hypodense human eosinophils that are derived in vivo and in vitro. Am J Pathol 137:27–41.

12. Dvorak AM, Saito H, Estrella P, Kissell S, Arai N, Ishizaka T (1989) Ultrastructure of eosinophils and basophils stimulated to develop in human cord blood mononuclear cell cultures containing recombinant human interleukin-5 or interleukin-3. Lab Invest 61:116–132.

13. Dvorak AM, Mihm MC Jr, Osage JE, Kwan TH, Austen KF, Wintroub BU (1982) Bullous pemphigoid, an ultrastructural study of the inflammatory response: eosinophil, basophil and mast cell granule changes in multiple biopsies from one patient. J Invest Dermatol 78:91–101.

14. Tai P-C, Spry CJF (1981) The mechanisms which produce vacuolated and degranulated eosinophils. Br J Haematol 49:219–226.

15. Dvorak AM (1991) Degranulation of basophils and mast cells. In: Dvorak AM, ed. Blood Cell Biochemistry, Vol. 4, Basophil and Mast Cell Degranulation and Recovery. Plenum, London, pp. 101–275.

16. Dvorak AM, Onderdonk AB, McCleod RS, Monahan-Earley RA, Antonioli DA, Cullen J, Blair JE, Cisneros R, Letourneau L, Morgan E, et al. (1993) Ultrastructural identification of exocytosis of granules from human gut eosinophils in vivo. Int Arch Allergy Immunol 102:33–45.

17. Henderson WR, Chi EY (1985) Ultrastructural characterization and morphometric analysis of human eosinophil degranulation. J Cell Sci 73:33–48.

18. Lewis DM, Lewis JC, Loegering DA, Gleich GJ (1978) Localization of the guinea pig eosinophil major basic protein to the core of the granule. J Cell Biol 77:702–713.

19. Egesten A, Alumets J, von Mecklenburg C, Palmegren M, Olssen I (1986) Localization of eosinophil cationic protein, major basic protein, and eosinophil peroxidase in human eosinophils by immunoelectron microscopic technique. J Histochem Cytochem 34:1399–1403.

20. Peters MS, Rodriguez M, Gleich GJ (1986) Localization of human eosinophil granule major basic protein, eosinophil cationic protein, and eosinophil-derived neurotoxin by immunoelectron microscopy. Lab Invest 54:656–662.

21. Ackerman SJ, Corrette SE, Rosenberg HF, Bennett JC, Mastrianni DM, Nicholson-Weller A, Weller PF, Chin DT, Tenen DG (1993) Molecular cloning and characterization of human eosinophil Charcot-Leyden crystal protein (lysophospholipase). Similarities to IgE binding proteins and the S-type animal lectin superfamily. J Immunol 150:456–468.

22. Gleich GJ, Kay AB, eds. (1994) Eosinophils in Allergy and Inflammation. Marcel Dekker, New York.

23. Moqbel R, Barkans J, Bradley BL, Durham SR, Kay AB (1992) Application of monoclonal antibodies against major basic protein (BMK-13) and eosinophil cationic protein (EG1 and EG2) for quantifying eosinophils in bronchial biopsies from atopic asthma. Clin Exp Allergy 22:265–273.

24. O'Donnell MC, Ackerman SJ, Gleich GJ, Thomas LL (1983) Activation of basophil and mast cell histamine release by eosinophil granule major basic protein. J Exp Med 157:1981–1991.

25. Zheutlin LM, Ackerman SJ, Gleich GJ, Thomas LL (1984) Stimulation of basophil and rat mast cell histamine release by eosinophil granule-derived cationic proteins. J Immunol 133:2180–2185.

26. Moy JN, Gleich GJ, Thomas LL (1990) Noncytotoxic activation of neutrophils by eosinophil granule major basic protein. Effect on superoxide anion generation and lysosomal enzyme release. J Immunol 145:2626–2632.

27. Rohrbach MS, Wheatley CL, Slifman NR, Gleich GJ (1990) Activation of platelets by eosinophil granule proteins. J Exp Med 172:1271–1274.

28. Kita H, Abu-Ghazaleh RI, Sur S, Gleich GJ (1995) Eosinophil major basic protein induces degranulation and Il-8 production by human eosinophils. J Immunol 154:4749–4758.

29. Gleich GJ, Loegering DA, Bell MP, Checkel JL, Ackerman SJ, McKean DJ (1986) Biochemical and functional similarities between human eosinophil-derived neurotoxin and eosinophil cationic protein: homology with ribonuclease. Proc Natl Acad Sci USA 83:3146–3150.

30. Slifman NR, Loegering DA, McKean DJ, Gleich GJ (1986) Ribonuclease activity associated with human eosinophil-derived neurotoxin and eosinophil cationic protein. J Immunol 137:2913–2917.

31. Tai P-C, Spry CJ, Peterson C, Venge P, Olsson I (1984) Monoclonal antibodies distinguish between storage and secreted forms of eosinophil cationic protein. Nature 309:182–184.

32. McLaren DJ, McKean JR, Olsson I, Venge P, Kay AB (1981) Morphological studies on the killing of schistosomula of *Schistosoma mansoni* by human eosinophil and neutrophil cationic proteins in vitro. Parasite Immunol 3:359–373.

33. Young JDE, Peterson CGB, Venge P, Cohn ZA (1986) Mechanism of membrane damage mediated by human eosinophil cationic protein. Nature 321:613–616.

34. Motojima S, Frigas E, Loegering DA, Gleich GJ (1989) Toxicity of eosinophil cationic proteins for guinea pig tracheal epithelium in vitro. Am Rev Respir Dis 139:801–805.

35. Fredens K, Dahl R, Venge P (1982) The Gordon phenomenon induced by the eosinophil cationic protein and eosinophil protein X. J Allergy Clin Immunol 70:361–366.

36. Slifman NR, Venge P, Peterson CGB, McKean DJ, Gleich GJ (1989) Human eosinophil-derived neurotoxin and eosinophil protein X are likely the same protein. J Immunol 143:2317–2322.

37. Rosenberg HF, Tenen DG, Ackerman SJ (1989) Molecular cloning of the human eosinophil-derived neurotoxin: a member of the ribonuclease gene family. Proc Natl Acad Sci USA 86:4460–4464.

38. Beintema JJ, Hofsteenge J, Iwama M, Morita T, Ohgi K, Irie M, Sugiyama RH, Schieven GL, Dekker CA, Glitz DG (1988) Amino acid sequence of the non-secretory ribonuclease of human urine. Biochemistry 27:4530–4538.

39. Sorrentino S, Glitz DG, Hamann KJ, Loegering DA, Checkel JL, Gleich GJ (1992) Eosinophil-derived neurotoxin and human liver ribonuclease: identity of structure and linkage of neurotoxicity to nuclease activity. J Biol Chem 267:14,859–14,865.

40. Carlson MG, Peterson CGB, Venge P (1985) Human eosinophil peroxidase: purification and characterization. J Immunol 134:1875–1879.

41. Weiss SJ, Test ST, Eckman CM, Roos D, Regiani S (1986) Brominating oxidants generated by human eosinophils. Science 234:200–203.

42. Mayeno AN, Curran AJ, Roberts RL, Foote CS (1989) Eosinophils preferentially use bromide to generate halogenating agents. J Biol Chem 264:5660–5668.

43. Slungaard A, Mahoney JR Jr (1991) Thiocyanate is the major substrate for eosinophil peroxidase in physiological fluids. Implications for cytotoxicity. J Biol Chem 266:4903–4910.

44. Weller PF, Dvorak AM (1985) Arachidonic acid incorporation by cytoplasmic lipid bodies of human eosinophils. Blood 65:1269–1274.

45. Hubscher T (1975) Role of the eosinophil in allergic reactions. II. Release of prostaglandins from human eosinophilic leukocytes. J Immunol 114:1389–1393.

46. Parsons WG, Roberts LJ (1988) Transformation of prostaglandin D2 to isomeric prostaglandin F2 compounds by human eosinophils. A potential mast cell-eosinophil interaction. J Immunol 141:2413–2419.

47. Foegh ML, Maddox YT, Ramwell PW (1986) Human peritoneal eosinophils and formation of arachidonate cyclo oxygenase products. Scand J Immunol 23:599–603.

48. Samuelsson B (1983) Leukotrienes: mediators of hypersensitivity reactions and inflammation. Science 220:568–575.

49. Jorg A, Henderson WR, Murphy RC, Klebanoff SJ (1982) Leukotriene generation by eosinophils. J Exp Med 155:390–402.

50. Weller PF (1993) Eicosanoids, cytokines and other mediators elaborated by eosinophils. In: Makino S, Fukuda T, eds. Eosinophils, Biological and Clinical Aspects. CRC, Boca Raton, FL, pp. 125–154.

51. Shaw RJ, Walsh GM, Cromwell O, Moqbel R, Spry CJF, Kay AB (1985) Activated human eosinophils generate SRS-A leukotrienes following IgG-dependent stimulation. Nature 316: 150–152.

52. Bruijnzeel PL, Kok PT, Hamelink ML, Kijne AM, Verhagen J (1985) Exclusive leukotriene C_4 synthesis by purified human eosinophils induced by opsonized zymosan. FEBS Lett 189:350–354.

53. Cromwell O, Moqbel R, Fitzharris P, Kurlak L, Harvey C, Walsh GM, Shaw RJ, Kay AB (1988) Leukotriene C_4 generation from human eosinophils stimulated with IgG-*Aspergillus fumigatus* antigen immune complexes. J Allergy Clin Immunol 82:535–543.

54. Sun FF, Czuk CI, Taylor BM (1989) Arachidonic acid metabolism in guinea pig eosinophils: synthesis of thromboxane B2 and leukotriene B4 in response to soluble or particulate activators. J Leuk Biol 46:152–160.

55. Sigal E, Grunberger D, Cashman JR, Craik CS, Caughey GH, Nadel JA (1988) Arachidonate 15-lipoxygenase from human eosinophil-enriched leukocytes: partial purification and properties. Biochem Biophys Res Commun 150:376–383.

56. Weller PF (1991) Immunobiology of eosinophils. N Engl J Med 324:1110–1118.

57. Marom Z, Shelhamer JH, Sun F, Kaliner M (1983) Human airway monohydroxyeicosatetraenoic acid generation and mucus release. J Clin Invest 72:122–127.

58. Taniguchi N, Mita H, Saito H, Yui Y, Kajita T, Shida T (1985) Increased generation of leukotriene C_4 from eosinophils in asthmatic patients. Allergy 40:571–573.

59. Aizawa T, Tamura G, Ohtsu H, Takishima T (1990) Eosinophil and neutrophil production of leukotriene C_4 and B_4: comparison of cells from asthmatic subjects and healthy donors. Ann Allergy 64:287–292.

60. Kohi F, Miyagawa H, Agrawal DK, Bewtra AK, Townley RG (1990) Generation of leukotriene B_4 and C_4 from granulocytes of normal controls, allergic rhinitis and healthy donors. Ann Allergy 65:228–232.

61. Wardlaw AJ, Hay H, Cromwell O, Collins JV, Kay AB (1989) Leukotrienes, LTC_4 and LTB_4 in bronchoalveolar lavage fluid in bronchial asthma and other respiratory diseases. J Allergy Clin Immunol 84:19–26.

62. Wenzel SE, Larsen GL, Johnston K, Voelkel NF, Westcott JY (1990) Elevated levels of leukotriene C4 in bronchoalveolar lavage fluid from atopic asthmatics after endobronchial allergen challenge. Am Rev Respir Dis 142:112–119.

63. Christie PE, Tagari P, Ford-Hutchinson AW, Charlesson P, Chee P, Arm JP, Lee TH (1991) Urinary leukotriene E_4 concentrations increase after aspirin challenge in aspirin-sensitive asthmatic subjects. Am Rev Respir Dis 143:1025–1029.

64. Spector SL, Smith LJ, Glass M (1994) Effects of 6 weeks of therapy with oral doses of ICI 204,219, a leukotriene D_4 receptor antagonist, in subjects with bronchial asthma. Am J Respir Crit Care Med 150:618–623.

65. Snyder F (1985) Chemical and biochemical aspects of platelet activating factor: a novel class of acetylated ether-linked choline-phospholipids. Med Res Rev 5:107–140.

66. Wardlaw AJ, Moqbel R, Cromwell O, Kay AB (1986) Platelet activating factor: a potent chemotactic and chemokinetic factor for human eosinophils. J Clin Invest 78:1701–1706.

67. Cromwell O, Wardlaw AJ, Champion A, Moqbel R, Osei D, Kay AB (1990) IgG-dependent generation of platelet-activating factor by normal and low density human eosinophils. J Immunol 145:3862–3868.

68. Burke LA, Crea AEG, Wilkinson JRW, Arm JP, Spur BW, Lee TH (1990) Comparison of the generation of platelet-activating factor and leukotriene C4 in human eosinophils stimulated by unopsonized zymosan and the calcium ionophore A23187: the effects of nedocromil sodium. J Allergy Clin Immunol 85:26–35.

69. Del Pozo V, de Andres B, Martin E, Maruri N, Zubeldia JM, Palomino P, Lahoz C (1990) Murine eosinophils and IL-1: alpha IL-1 mRNA detection by in situ hybridization. Production and release of IL-1 from peritoneal eosinophils. J Immunol 144:3117–3122.

70. Weller PF, Rand TH, Barrett T, Elovic A, Wong DT, Finberg RW (1993) Accessory cell function of human eosinophils: HLA-DR-dependent, MHC-restricted antigen presentation and IL-1α expression. J Immunol 150:2554–2562.

71. Rand TH, Silberstein DS, Kornfield H, Weller PF (1991) Human eosinophils express functional interleukin-2 receptors. J Clin Invest 88:825–832.

72. Levi-Schaffer F, Barkans J, Newman TM, Ying S, Wakelin M, Hohenstein R, Barak V, Lacy P, Kay AB, Moqbel R (1996) Identification of interleukin-2 in human peripheral blood eosinophils. Immunology 87:155–161.

73. Bossé M, Audette M, Ferland C, Pelletier G, Chu HW, Dakhama A, Lavigne S, Boulet L-P, Laviolette M (1996) Gene expression of interleukin-2 in purified human peripheral blood eosinophils. Immunology 87:149–154.

74. Kita H, Ohnishi T, Okubo Y, Weiler D, Abrams JS, Gleich GJ (1991) Granulocyte/macrophage colony-stimulating factor and interleukin 3 release from human peripheral blood eosinophils and neutrophils. J Exp Med 174:745–748.

75. Hom JT, Estridge T (1993) FK506 and rapamycin modulate the functional activities of human peripheral blood eosinophils. Clin Immunol Immunopathol 68:293–300.

76. Dubois GR, Bruijnzeel-Koomen CA, Bruijnzeel PL (1994) IL-4 induces chemotaxis of blood eosinophils from atopic dermatitis patients, but not from normal individuals. J Invest Dermatol 102:843–846.

77. Moqbel R, Ying S, Barkans J, Newman TM, Kimmitt P, Wakelin M, Taborda-Barata L, Meng Q, Corrigan CJ, Durham SR, Kay AB (1995) Identification of messenger RNA for IL-4 in human eosinophils with granule localization and release of the translated product. J Immunol. 155:4939–4947.

78. Nonaka M, Nonaka R, Woolley K, Adelroth E, Miura K, Ohkawara Y, Glibetic M, Nakano K, O'Byrne P, Dolovich J, Jordana M (1995) Distinct immunohistological localization of IL-4 in human inflamed airway tissue. IL-4 is localized to eosinophils in vivo and is released by peripheral blood eosinophils. J Immunol 155:3234–3244.

79. Desreumaux P, Janin A, Colombel JF, Prin L, Plumas J, Emilie D, Torpier G, Capron A, Capron M (1992) Interleukin 5 messenger RNA expression by eosinophils in the intestinal mucosa of patients with coeliac disease. J Exp Med 175:293–296.

80. Dubucquoi S, Desreumaux P, Janin A, Klein O, Goldman M, Tavernier J, Capron A, Capron M (1994) Interleukin 5 synthesis by eosinophils: association with granules and immunoglobulin-dependent secretion. J Exp Med 179:703–708.

81. Broide DH, Paine MM, Firestein GS (1992) Eosinophils express interleukin 5 and granulocyte macrophage-colony-stimulating factor mRNA at sites of allergic inflammation in asthmatics. J Clin Invest 90:1414–1424.

82. Beil WJ, Weller PF, Tzizik DM, Galli SJ, Dvorak AM (1993) Ultrastructural immunogold localization of tumor necrosis factor-alpha to the matrix compartment of eosinophil secondary granules in patients with idiopathic hypereosinophilic syndrome. J Histochem Cytochem 41:1611–1615.

83. Moller GM, de Jong TA, Overbeek SE, van der Kwast TH, Postma DM, Hoogsteden HC (1996) Ultrastructural immunogold localization of interleukin 5 to the crystalloid core compartment of eosinophil secondary granules in patients with atopic asthma. J Histochem Cytochem 44:67–69.

84. Hamid Q, Barkans J, Meng Q, Ying S, Abrams JS, Kay AB, Moqbel R (1992) Human eosinophils synthesize and secrete interleukin-6, in vitro. Blood 80:1496–1501.

85. Melani C, Mattia GF, Silvani A, Care A, Rivoltini L, Parmiani G, Colombo MP (1993) Interleukin-6 expression in human neutrophil and eosinophil peripheral blood granulocytes. Blood 81:2744–2749.

86. Braun RK, Franchini M, Erard F, Rihs S, de Vries IJM, Blaser K, Hansel TT, Walker C (1993) Human peripheral blood eosinophils produce and release IL-8 on stimulation with calcium ionophore. Eur J Immunol 23:956–960.

87. Miyamasu M, Hirai K, Takahashi Y, Iida M, Yamaguchi M, Koshino T, Takaishi T, Morita Y, Ohta K, Kasahara T (1995) Chemotactic agonists induce cytokine generation in eosinophils. J Immunol 154:1339–1349.

88. Yousefi S, Hemmann S, Weber M, Holzer C, Hartung, K, Blaser K, Simon HU (1995) IL-8 is expressed by human peripheral blood eosinophils: evidence for increased secretion in asthma. J Immunol 154:5481–5490.

89. Nakajima H, Gleich GJ, Kita H (1996) Constitutive production of IL-4 and IL-10 and stimulated production of IL-8 by normal peripheral blood eosinophils. J Immunol 156:4859–4866.

90. Cruikshank WW, Center DM, Nisar N, Wu M, Natke B, Theodore AC, Kornfeld H (1994) Molecular and functional analysis of a lymphocyte chemoattractant factor: association of biological function with CD4 expression. Proc Natl Acad Sci USA 91:5109–5113.

91. Lim KG, Wan H-C, Bozza PT, Resnick MB, Wong DT, Cruikshank WW, Kornfeld H, Center DM, Weller PF (1996) Human eosinophils elaborate the lymphocyte chemoattractants. IL-16 (lymphocyte chemoattractant factor) and RANTES. J Immunol 156:2566–2570.

92. Moqbel R, Hamid Q, Ying S, Barkans J, Hartnell A, Tsicopoulos A, Wardlaw AJ, Kay AB (1991) Expression of mRNA and immunoreactivity for the granulocyte/macrophage-colony stimulating factor in activated human eosinophils. J Exp Med 174:749–752.

93. Ohno I, Lea RG, Finotto S, Marshall J, Denburg J, Dolovich J, Gauldie J, Jordana M (1991) Granulocyte/macrophage-colony stimulating factor (GM-CSF) gene expression by eosinophils in nasal polyposis. Am J Resp Cell Mol Biol 5:505–510.

94. Levi-Schaffer F, Lacy P, Severs NJ, Newman TM, North J, Gomperts B, Kay AB, Moqbel R (1995) Association of granulocyte-macrophage colony-stimulating factor with the crystalloid granules of human eosinophils. Blood 85:2579–2586.

95. Wong DT, Weller PF, Galli SJ, Elovic A, Rand TH, Gallagher GT, Chiang T, Chou MY, Matossian K, McBride J, Todd R (1990) Human eosinophils express transforming growth factor-α. J Exp Med 172:673–681.

96. Todd R, Donoff BR, Chiang T, Chou MY, Elovic A, Gallagher GT, Wong DT (1991) The eosinophil as a cellular source of transforming growth factor-α in healing cutaneous wounds. Am J Pathol 138:1307–1313.

97. Wong DT, Donoff RB, Yang J, Song BZ, Matossian K, Nagura N, Elovic A, McBride J, Gallagher G, Todd R, et al. (1993) Sequential expression of transforming growth factors-α and β1 by eosinophils during cutaneous wound healing in the hamster. Am J Pathol 143:130–142.

98. Wong DT, Elovic A, Matossian K, Nagura N, McBride J, Chou M, Gordon JR, Rand TH, Galli SJ, Weller PF (1991) Eosinophils from patients with blood eosinophilia express transforming growth factor β1. Blood 78:2702–2707.

99. Ohno I, Lea RG, Flanders KC, Clark DA, Banwatt D, Dolovich J, Denburg J, Harley CB, Gauldie J, Jordana M (1992) Eosinophils in chronically inflamed human upper airway tissues express transforming growth factor-β1 gene. J Clin Invest 89:1662–1668.

100. Kadin M, Butmarc J, Elovic A, Wong DT (1993) Eosinophils are the major source of transforming growth factor-β1 in nodular sclerosing Hodgkin's disease. Am J Path 142:11–16.

101. Costa JJ, Matossian K, Resnick MB, Beil WJ, Wong DT, Gordon JR, Dvorak AM, Weller PF, Galli SJ (1993) Human eosinophils can express the cytokines tumor necrosis factor-α and macrophage inflammatory protein-1α. J Clin Invest 91:2673–84.

102. Tan X, Hsueh W, Gonzalez-Crussi F (1993) Cellular localization of tumor necrosis factor (TNF)-α transcripts in normal bowel and in necrotizing enterocolitis. TNF gene expression by Paneth cells, intestinal eosinophils, and macrophages. Am J Path 142:1858–1865.

103. Schall TJ (1991) Biology of the RANTES/SIS cytokine family. Cytokine 3:165–183.

104. Ying S, Meng Q, Taborda-Barata L, Corrigan CJ, Barkans J, Assoufi B, Moqbel R, Durham SR, Kay AB (1996) Human eosinophils express mRNA encoding RANTES and store and release biologically active RANTES protein. Eur J Immunol 26:70–76.

105. Ohno I, Nitta Y, Yamauchi K, Hoshi H, Honma M, Woolley K, O'Byrne P, Dolovich J, Jordana M, Tamura G, Tanno Y, Shirato K (1995) Eosinophils as a potential source of platelet-derived growth factor B-chain (PDGF-B) in nasal polyposis and bronchial asthma. Am J Respir Cell Mol Biol 13:639–647.

106. Weller PF, Goetzl EJ, Austen KF (1980) Identification of human eosinophil lysophospholipase as the constituent of Charcot-Leyden crystals. Proc Natl Acad Sci USA 77:7440–7443.

107. Ackerman SJ, Weil GJ, Gleich GJ (1982) Formation of Charcot-Leyden crystals by human basophils. J Exp Med 155:1597–1609.

108. Weller PF, Bach DS, and Austen KF (1984) Biochemical characterization of human eosinophils Charcot-Leyden crystal protein (lysophospholipase). J Biol Chem 259:15,100–15,105.

109. Dvorak AM, Weller PF, Monahan-Earley RA, Letourneau L, and Ackerman SJ (1990) Ultrastructural localization of Charcot-Leyden crystal protein (lysophospholipase) and peroxidase in macrophages, eosinophils and extracellular matrix of the skin in the hypereosinophilic syndrome. Lab Invest 62:590–607.

110. Spry CJF (1988) Eosinophils. A Comprehensive Review and Guide to the Medical Literature. Oxford University Press, Oxford and London.

111. Shult PA, Graziano FM, Busse WW (1985) Enhanced eosinophil luminol-dependent chemoluminescence in allergic rhinitis. J Allergy Clin Immunol 77:702–708.

112. Hartnell A, Moqbel R, Walsh GM, Bradley B, Kay AB (1990) Fcγ and CD11/CD18 receptor expression on normal density and low density human eosinophils. Immunology 69:264–270.

113. Hansel TT, DeVries IJ, Iff T, Rihs S, Wandzilak M, Betz S, Blaser K, Walker C (1991) An improved immunomagnetic procedure for the isolation of highly purified human blood eosinophils. J Immunol Meth 145:105–110.

114. Walsh GM, Kay AB (1986) Binding of immunoglobulin classes and subclasses to human neutrophils and eosinophils. Clin Exp Immunol 63:466–472.

115. Abu-Ghazaleh RI, Fujisawa T, Mestecky J, Kyle RA, Gleich GJ (1989) IgA-induced eosinophil degranulation. J Immunol 142:2393–2400.

116. Butterworth AE, Sturrock RF, Houba V, Mahmoud AA, Sher A, Rees PH (1975) Eosinophils as mediators of antibody-dependent damage to schistosomula. Nature 256:727–729.

117. Capron M, Tomassini M, Ven der Vorst E, Kusnierz JP, Papin JP, Capron A (1988) Existence et fonctions d'un recepteur pour l'immunoglobline A sur les eosinophiles humaines. CR Acad Sci/Immunol 307:397–402.

118. Kita H, Abu-Ghazaleh R, Sanderson CJ, Gleich GJ (1991) Effect of steroids on immunoglobulin-induced eosinophil degranulation. J Allergy Clin Immunol 87:70–77.

119. Monteiro RC, Hostoffer RW, Cooper MD, Bonner JR, Gartland GL, Kubagawa H (1993) Definition of immunoglobulin A receptors on eosinophils and their enhanced expression in allergic individuals. J Clin Invest 92:1681–85.

120. Capron M, Jouault T, Prin L, Joseph M, Ameisen J-C, Butterworth AE, Papin J-P, Kusnierz J-P, Capron A (1986) Functional study of a monoclonal antibody to IgE Fc receptor (FcεRII) of eosinophils, platelets, and macrophages. J Exp Med 164:72–89.

121. Capron A, Dessaint JP, Capron M, Joseph M, Ameisen J-C, Tonnel AB (1986) From parasites to allergy: a second receptor for IgE. Immunol Today 7:15–18.

122. Capron M, Capron A (1987) The IgE receptor of human eosinophils. In: Kay AB, ed. Allergy and Inflammation. Academic Press, London, pp. 151–159.

123. Jouault T, Capron M, Balloul J-M, Ameisen J-C, Capron A (1988) Quantitative and qualitative analysis of the Fc receptor for IgE (FcεRII) on human eosinophils. Eur J Immunol 18:237–241.

124 Capron M, Truong M-J, Aldebert D, Gruart V, Suemera M, Delespesse G, Tourvieille B, Capron A (1991) Heterogeneous expression of CD23 epitopes by eosinophils from patients: relationships with IgE-mediated functions. Eur J Immunol 21:2423–2429.

125. Gounni AS, Lamkhioued B, Ochiai K, Tanaka Y, Delaporte E, Capron A, Kinet J-P, Capron M (1994) High-affinity IgE receptor on eosinophils is involved in defence against parasites. Nature 367:183–186.

126. Truong MJ, Gruart V, Kusnierz JP, Papin JP, Loiseau S, Capron A, Capron M (1993) Human neutrophils express immunoglobulin E (IgE)-binding proteins (Mac-2/epsilon BP) of the S-type lectin family: role in IgE-dependent activation. J Exp Med 177:243–248.

127. Moqbel R, Walsh GM, Nagakura T, MacDonald AJ, Wardlaw AJ, Iikura Y, Kay AB (1990) The effect of platelet-activating factor on IgE binding to, and IgE-dependent biological properties of, human eosinophils. Immunology 70:251–257.

128. Walsh GM, Hartnell A, Wardlaw AJ, Kurihara K, Sanderson CJ, Kay AB (1990) IL-5 enhances the in vitro adhesion of human eosinophils, but not neutrophils, in a leucocyte integrin (CD11/18)-dependent manner. Immunology 71:258–265.

129. Capron M, Kazatchkine MD, Fischer E, Joseph M, Butterworth AE, Kusnierz J-P, Prin L, Papin J-P, Capron A (1987) Functional role of the alpha-chain of complement receptor type 3 in human eosinophil-dependent antibody-mediated cytotoxicity against schistosomes. J Immunol 139:2059–2065.

130. Koenderman, L, Tool ATJ, Roos D, Verhoeven AJ (1990) Priming of the respiratory burst in human eosinophils is accompanied by changes in signal transduction. J Immunol 145:3883–3888.

131. Zeiger RS, Colten HR (1977) Histaminase release from human eosinophils. J Immunol 118:540–543.

132. Hartnell A, Kay AB, Wardlaw AJ (1992) Interleukin-3-induced up-regulation of CR3 expression on human eosinophils is inhibited by dexamethasone. Immunology 77:488–493.

133. Anwar ARE, Smithers SR, Kay AB (1979) Killing of schistosomula of *Schistosoma mansoni* coated with antibody and/or complement by human leucocytes in vitro: requirement for complement in preferential killing by eosinophils. J Immunol 122:628–637.

134. Silberstein DS, Owen WF, Gasson JC, DiPersio JF, Golde DW, Bina JC, Soberman R, Austen KF, David JR (1986) Enhancement of human eosinophil cytotoxicity and leukotriene synthesis by biosynthetic (recombinant) granulocyte-macrophage colony-stimulating factor. J Immunol 137:3290–3294.

135. Owen WF, Rothenberg ME, Silberstein DS, Gasson JC, Stevens RL, Austen KF, Soberman RJ (1987) Regulation of human eosinophil viability, density and function by granulocyte/macrophage colony-stimulating factor in the presence of 3T3 fibroblasts. J Exp Med 166:129–141.

136. Rothenberg ME, Owen WF, Silberstein DS, Woods J, Soberman RJ, Austen KF, Stevens RL (1988) Human eosinophils have prolonged survival, enhanced functional properties, and become hypodense when exposed to human interleukin-3. J Clin Invest 81:1986–1992.

137. Rothenberg ME, Petersen J, Stevens RL, Silberstein DS, McKenzie DT, Austen KF, Owen WF (1989) IL-5-dependent conversion of normodense human eosinophils to the hypodense phenotype uses 3T3 fibroblasts for enhanced viability, accelerated hypodensity and sustained antibody-dependent cytotoxicity. J Immunol 143:2311–2316.

138. Her E, Frazer J, Austen KF, Owen WF (1991) Eosinophil hematopoietins antagonize the programmed cell death of eosinophils. Cytokine and glucocorticoid effects on eosinophils maintained by endothelial cell-conditioned medium. J Clin Invest 88:1982–1987.

139. DiPersio J, Billing P, Kaufman S, Eghtesady P, Williams RE, Gasson JC (1988) Characterization of human granulocyte-macrophage colony-stimulating factor receptor. J Biol Chem 263:1834–1841.

140. Lopez AF, Eglinton JM, Gillis D, Park LS, Clark S, Vadas MA (1989) Reciprocal inhibition of binding between interleukin 3 and granulocyte-macrophage colony-stimulating factor to human eosinophils. Proc Natl Acad Sci USA 86:7022–7026.

141. Chihara, J, Plumas J, Gruart V, Tavernier J, Prin L, Capron A, Capron M (1990) Characterization of a receptor for interleukin 5 on human eosinophils: variable expression and induction by granulocyte/macrophage colony-stimulating factor. J Exp Med 172:1347–1351.

142. Migita M, Yamaguchi N, Mita S, Higuchi S, Hitoshi Y, Yoshida Y, Tomonaga M, Matsuda I, Tominaga A, Takatsu K (1991) Characterization of the human IL-5 receptors on eosinophils. Cell Immunol 133:484–497.

143. Ingley E, Young IG (1991) Characterization of a receptor for interleukin-5 on human eosinophils and the myeloid leukemia line HL-60. Blood 78:339–344.

144. Lopez AF, Vadas MA, Woodcock JM, Milton SE, Lewis A, Elliott MJ, Gillis D, Ireland R, Olwell E, Park LS (1991) Interleukin-5, interleukin-3, and granulocyte-macrophage colony-stimulating factor cross-compete for binding to cell surface receptors on human eosinophils. J Biol Chem 266:24,741–24,747.

145. Tavernier J, Devos R, Cornelis S, Tuypens T, Van der Heyden J, Fiers W, Plaetinck G (1991) A human high affinity interleukin-5 receptor (IL-5R) is composed of an IL-5-specific alpha chain and a beta chain shared with the receptor for GM-CSF. Cell 66:1175–1184.

146. Lopez AF, Elliott MJ, Woodcock J, Vadas MA (1992) GM-CSF, IL-3 and IL-5: cross-competition on human haemopoietic cells. Immunol Today 13:495–500.

147. Miyajima A, Kitamura T, Harada N, Yokota T, Arai K (1992) Cytokine receptors and signal transduction. Annu Rev Immunol 10:295–331.

148. Kanakura, Y, Druker B, Cannistra SA, Furukawa Y, Torimoto Y, Griffin JD (1990) Signal transduction of the human granulocyte-macrophage colony-stimulating factor and interleukin-3 receptors involves tyrosine phosphorylation of a common set of cytoplasmic proteins. Blood 76:706–715.

149. Linnekin D, Farrar WL (1990) Signal transduction of human interleukin 3 and granulocyte-macrophage colony-stimulating factor through serine and tyrosine phosphorylation. Biochem J 271:317–324.

150. Murata, Y, Takaki S, Migita M, Kikuchi Y, Tominaga A, Takatsu K (1992) Molecular cloning and expression of the human interleukin-5 receptor. J Exp Med 175:341–351.

151. Ploysongsang Y, Humbert M, Ying S, Yasruel Z, Durham S, Kay AB, Hamid Q (1995) Increased expression of interleukin-5 receptor gene in asthma. J Allergy Clin Immunol 95:279 (abstract 555).

152. Daugherty BL, Siciliano SJ, DeMartino JA, Malkowitz L, Sirotina A, Springer MS (1996) Cloning, expression, and characterization of the human eosinophil eotaxin receptor. J Exp Med 183:2349–2354.

153. Ponath PD, Qin S, Post TW, Wang J, Wu L, Gerard NP, Newman W, Gerard C, Mackay CR (1996) Molecular cloning and characterization of a human eotaxin receptor expressed selectively on eosinophils. J Exp Med 183:2437–2448.

154. Jose PJ, Griffiths-Johnson DA, Collins PD, Walsh DT, Moqbel R, Totty NF, Truong O, Hsuan JJ, Williams TJ (1994) Eotaxin: a potent eosinophil chemoattractant cytokine detected in a guinea pig model of allergic airways inflammation. J Exp Med 179:881–887.

155. Sehmi R, Rossi AG, Kay AB, Cromwell O (1992) Identification of receptors for leukotriene B_4 expressed on guinea pig peritoneal eosinophils. Immunology 77:129–135.

156. Kroegel C, Yukawa T, Dent G, Venge P, Chung KF, Barnes PJ (1989) Stimulation of degranulation from human eosinophils by platelet-activating factor. J Immunol 142:3518–3526.

157. Kurihara K, Wardlaw AJ, Moqbel R, Kay AB (1989) Inhibition of platelet-activating factor (PAF)-indued chemotaxis and PAF binding to human eosinophils and neutrophils by the specific ginkgolide-derived PAF antagonist, BN52021. J Allergy Clin Immunol 83:83–90.

158. Yazdanbakhsh M, Eckmann CM, Koenderman L, Verhoeven AJ, Roos D (1987) Eosinophils do respond to fMLP. Blood 70:379–383.

159. Gerard NP, Gerard C (1991) The chemotactic receptor for human C5a anaphylatoxin. Nature 349:614–617.

160. Honda Z, Nakamura M, Miki I, Minami M, Watanabe T, Seyama Y, Okado H, Toh H, Ito K, Miyamoto T, Shimizu T (1991) Cloning by functional expression of platelet-activating receptor from guinea pig lung. Nature 349:342–346.

161. Minnicozzi M, Anthes JC, Siegel MI, Billah MM, Egan RW (1990) Activation of phospholipase D in normodense human eosinophils. Biochem Biophys Res Commun 170:540–547.

162. Elsner J, Oppermann M, Czech W, Dobos G, Schopf E, Norgauer J, Kapp A (1994) C3a activates reactive oxygen radical species production and intracellular calcium transients in human eosinophils. Eur J Immunol 24:518–522.

163. Riedel D, Lindemann A, Brach M, Mertelsmann R, Herrmann F (1990) Granulocyte-macrophage colony-stimulating factor and interleukin-3 induce surface expression of interleukin-2 receptor p55-chain and CD4 by eosinophils. Immunology 70:258–261.

164. Lucey DR, Dorsky DI, Nicholson-Weller A, Weller PF (1989) Human eosinophils express CD4 protein and bind human immunodeficiency virus 1 gp120. J Exp Med 169:327–332.

165. Rand TH, Cruikshank WW, Center DM, Weller PF (1991) CD4-mediated stimulation of human eosinophils: lymphocyte chemoattractant factor and other CD4-binding ligands elicit eosinophil migration. J Exp Med 173:1521–1528.

166. Freedman AR, Gibson FM, Fleming SC, Spry CJF, Griffin GE (1991) Human immunodeficiency virus infection of eosinophils in human bone marrow cultures. J Exp Med 174:1661–1664.

167. Lucey DR, Nicholson-Weller A, Weller PF (1989) Mature human eosinophils have the capacity to express HLA-DR. Proc Natl Acad Sci USA 86:1348–1351.

168. Weller PF, Rand TH, Finberg RW (1991) Human eosinophils function as HLA-DR dependent, MHC-restricted antigen-presenting cells. FASEB J 5:A640.

169. Nishikawa K, Morii T, Ako H, Hamada K, Saito S, Narita N (1992) In vivo expression of CD69 on lung eosinophils in eosinophilic pneumonia: CD69 as a possible activation marker for eosinophils. J Allergy Clin Immunol 90:169–174.

170. Hartnell A, Robinson DS, Kay AB, Wardlaw AJ (1993) CD69 is expressed by human eosinophils activated in vivo in asthma and in vitro by cytokines. Immunology 80:281–286.

171. Corte G, Moretta L, Damiani G, Mingari MC, Bargellesi A (1981) Surface antigens specifically expressed by activated T cells in humans. Eur J Immunol 11:162–164.

172. Ohkawara Y, Lim KG, Xing Z, Glibetic M, Nakano K, Dolovich J, Croitoru K, Weller PF, Jordana M (1996) CD40 expression by human peripheral blood eosinophils. J Clin Invest 97:1761–1766.

173. Matsumoto K, Schleimer RP, Saito H, Iikura Y, Bochner BS (1995) Induction of apoptosis in human eosinophils by anti-Fas antibody treatment in vitro. Blood 86:1437–1443.

174. Tanaka Y, Albelda SM, Horgan KJ, van Seventer GA, Shimizu Y, Newman W, Hallam J, Newman PJ, Buck CA, Shaw S (1992) CD31 expressed on distinctive T cell subsets is a preferential amplifier of β1 integrin-mediated adhesion. J Exp Med 176:245–253.

175. Kim JT, Gleich GJ, Kita H (1997) Roles of CD9 molecules in survival and activation of human eosinophils. J Immunol 159:926–933.

176. Schleimer RP (1993) An overview of gluocorticosteroid anti-inflammatory actions. Eur J Clin Pharm 45:3–7.

177. Peterson AP, Altman LC, Hill JS, Gosney K, Kadin ME (1981) Glucocorticoid receptors on normal human eosinophils: comparisons with neutrophils. J Allergy Clin Immunol 68:212–217.

178. Prin L, Lefebvre P, Gruart V, Capron M, Storme L, Formstecher P, Loiseau S, Capron A (1989) Heterogeneity of human eosinophil glucocorticoid receptor expression in hypereosinophilic patients: absence of detectable receptor correlates with resistance to corticotherapy. Clin Exp Immunol 78:383–389.

179. Spry CJF (1993) The idiopathic hypereosinophilic syndrome. In: Makino S, Fukuda T, eds. Eosinophils: Biological and Clinical Aspects. CRC, Boca Raton, pp. 403–420.

180. Kay AB, Moqbel R, Durham SR, MacDonald AJ, Walsh GM, Shaw RJ, Cromwell O, Mackay J (1985) Leucocyte activation initiated by IgE-dependent mechanisms in relation to helminthic parasitic disease and clinical models of asthma. Int Archs Allergy Appl Immunol 77:69–72.

181. Finkelman FD, Pearce EJ, Urban JF, Sher A (1991) Regulation and biological function of helminth-induced cytokine responses. In: Ash C, Gallagher RB, eds. Immunoparasitology Today. Elsevier, Cambridge, pp. A62–A66.

182. Butterworth AE, Richardson BA (1985) Factors affecting the levels of antibody- and complement-dependent eosinophil-mediated damage to schistosomula of *Schistosoma mansoni* in vitro. Parasite Immunol 7:119–131.

183. Butterworth AE, Thorne KJI (1993) Eosinophils and parasitic diseases. In: Smith H, Cook RM, eds. Immunopharmacology of Eosinophils. Academic, London, pp. 119–150.

184. McLaren DJ, MacKenzie CD, Ramalho-Pinto FJ (1977) Ultrastructural observations on the in vitro interaction between rat eosinophils and some parasitic helminths (*Schistosoma mansoni, Trichinella spiralis* and *Nippostrongylus brasiliensis*). Clin Exp Immunol 30:105–118.

185. Ackerman SJ, Gleich GJ, Loegering DA, Richardson BA, Butterworth AE (1985) Comparative toxicity of purified human eosinophil granule cationic proteins for schistosomula of *Schistosoma mansoni*. Am J Trop Med Hyg 34:735–745.

186. Wardlaw AJ, Moqbel R (1992) The eosinophil in allergic and helminth-related inflammatory responses. In: Moqbel R, ed. Allergy and Immunity to Helminths. Common Mechanisms or Divergent Pathways? Taylor and Francis, London, pp. 154–186.

187. Moqbel R (1980) Histopathological changes following primary, secondary and repeated infections of rats with *Strongyloides ratti*, with special reference to tissue eosinophils. Parasite Immunol 2:11–27.

188. Hsu SY, Hsu HF, Mitros FA, Helms CM, Solomon RI (1980) Eosinophils as effector cells in the destruction of *Schistosoma mansoni* eggs in granulomas. Ann Trop Med Parasitol 74:179–183.

189. Moqbel R, King SJ, MacDonald AJ, Miller HRP, Cromwell O, Shaw RJ, Kay AB (1986) Enteral and systemic release of leukotrienes during anaphylaxis of *Nippostongylus brasiliensis*-primed rats. J Immunol 137:296–301.

190. Moqbel R, Wakelin D, MacDonald AJ, King SJ, Grencis RK, Kay AB (1987) Release of leukotrienes during rapid expulsion of *Trichinella spiralis* from immune rats. Immunology 60:425–430.

191. Moqbel R, MacDonald AJ, Kay AB (1989) Platelet activating factor (PAF) release during intestinal anaphylaxis in rats. FASEB J 3, A1337 (abstract 6454).

192. Wildenburg G, Krömer M, Büttner, DW (1996) Dependence of eosinophil granulocyte infiltration into nodules on the presence of microfilariae producing *Onchocerca volvulus*. Parasitol Res 82:117–124.

193. Hagan P, Blumenthal UJ, Dunn D, Simpson AJ, Wilkins HA (1991) Human IgE, IgG4 and resistance to reinfection with *Schistosoma haematobium*. Nature 349:243–245.

194. Woolhouse MEJ, Taylor P, Matanhire D, Chandiwana SK (1991) Acquired immunity and epidemiology of *Schistosoma haematobium*. Nature 351:757–759.

195. Sher A, Coffman RL, Hieny S, Cheever AW (1990) Ablation of eosinophil and IgE responses with anti-IL-5 or anti-IL-4 antibodies fails to affect immunity against *Schistosoma mansoni* larvae in the mouse. J Immunol 145:3911–3916.

196. Ellis AG (1908) The pathologic anatomy of bronchial asthma. Am J Med Sci 136:407.

197. Dunnill MS (1978) The pathology of asthma. In: Middleton E Jr, Reed CE, Ellis EF, eds. Allergy: Principles and Practice. Mosby, St Louis, p. 678–686.

198. Huber HL, Koessler KK (1922) The pathology of bronchial asthma. Arch Int Med 30:689–760.

199. Filley WV, Holley KE, Kephart GM, Gleich GJ (1982) Identification by immunofluorescence of eosinophil granule major basic protein in lung tissue of patients with bronchial asthma. Lancet 2:11–16.

200. Sur S, Crotty TB, Kephart GM, Hyrna BA, Colby TV, Reed CE, Hunt LW, Gleich GJ (1993) Sudden-onset fatal asthma. A distinct entity with few eosinophils and relatively more neutrophils in the airway submucosa? Am Rev Respir Dis 148:713–719.

201. Horn BR, Robin ED, Theodore J, Van Kessel A (1975) Total eosinophil counts in the management of bronchial asthma. N Engl J Med 292:1152–1155.

202. Durham SR, Kay AB (1985) Eosinophils, bronchial hyperreactivity and late-phase asthmatic reactions. Clin Allergy 15:411–418.

203. Taylor KJ, Luksza AR (1987) Peripheral blood eosinophil counts and bronchial hyperresponsiveness. Thorax 42:452–456.

204. Venge P (1993) Human eosinophil granule proteins: structure, function and release. In: Smith H, Cook RM, eds. Immunopharmacology of Eosinophils. Academic, London, pp. 43–55.

205. NHLBI Workshop Summaries (1985) Summary and recommendations of a workshop on the investigative use of fibreoptic bronchoscopy and bronchoalveolar lavage in asthmatics. Am Rev Respir Dis 132:180–182.

206. Dolovich J, Hargreave FE, Jordana M, Denburg J. (1989) Late-phase airway reaction and inflammation. J Allergy Clin Immunol 83:521–524.

207. Durham SR (1991) The significance of late responses in asthma. Clin Exp Allergy 21:3–7.

208. Metzger WJ, Zavala D, Richerson HB, Moseley P, Iwamota P, Monick M, Sjoerdsma K, Hunninghake GW (1987) Local allergen challenge and bronchoalveolar lavage of allergic asthmatic lungs. Description of the model and local airway inflammation. Am Rev Respir Dis 135:433–440.

209. Fabbri LM, Boschetto P, Zocca E, Milani G, Pivirotto F, Plebani M, Burlina A, Licata B, Mapp CE (1987) Bronchoalveolar neutrophilia during late asthmatic reactions induced by toluene diisocyanate. Am Rev Respir Dis 136:36–42.

210. Lam S, LeRiche J, Phillips D, Chan-Yeung M, et al. (1987) Cellular and protein changes in bronchial lavage fluid after late asthmatic reaction in patients with red cedar asthma. J Allergy Clin Immunol 80:44–50.

211. Djukanovic R, Roche WR, Wilson JW, Beasley CRW, Twentyman OP, Howarth PH and Holgate, ST (1990) Mucosal inflammation in asthma. Am Rev Respir Dis 142:434–457.

212. Azzawi M, Bradley B, Jeffery PK, Frew AJ, Wardlaw AJ, Knowles G, Assoufi B, Collins JV, Durham S, Kay AB (1990) Identification of activated T lymphocytes and eosinophils in bronchial biopsies in stable atopic asthma. Am Rev Respir Dis 142:1407–1413.

213. Wardlaw AJ, Dunnette S, Gleich GJ, Collins JV, Kay AB (1988) Eosinophils and mast cells in bronchoalveolar lavage in subjects with mild asthma. Relationship to bronchial hyperreactivity. Am Rev Respir Dis 137:62–69.

214. De Monchy JGR, Kauffman HF, Venge P, Koeter GH, Jansen HM, Sluiter HJ, de Vries K (1985) Bronchoalveolar eosinophilia during allergen-induced late asthmatic reactions. Am Rev Respir Dis 131:373–376.

215. Adelroth E, Rosenhall L, Johansson S, Linden M, Venge P (1990) Inflammatory cells and eosinophilic activity in asthma investigated by bronchoalveolar lavage. The effects of antiasthmatic treatment with budesonide or terbutaline. Am Rev Respir Dis 142:91–99.

216. Hamid Q, Azzawi M, Ying S, Moqbel R, Wardlaw AJ, Corrigan CJ, Bradley B, Durham SR, Collins JV, Jeffery PK, Quint DJ, Kay AB (1991) Expression of mRNA for interleukin-5 in mucosal bronchial biopsies from asthma. J Clin Invest 87:1541–1546.

217. Robinson DS, Hamid Q, Ying S, Tsicopoulos A, Barkans J, Bentley AM, Corrigan CJ, Durham SR, Kay AB (1992) Predominant T_{H2}-type bronchoalveolar lavage T-lymphocyte population in atopic asthma. N Engl J Med 326:298–304.

218. Bentley AM, Maestrelli P, Saetta M, Fabbri LM, Robinson DS, Bradley BL, Jeffery PK, Durham SR, Kay AB (1992) Activated T-lymphocytes and eosinophils in the bronchial mucosa in isocyanate-induced asthma. J Allergy Clin Immunol 89:821–829.

219. Bentley AM, Menz G, Storz C, Robinson DS, Bradley B, Jeffery PK, Durham SR, Kay AB (1992) Identification of T lymphocytes, macrophages, and activated eosinophils in the bronchial mucosa in intrinsic asthma. Relationship to symptoms and bronchial responsiveness. Am Rev Respir Dis 146:500–506.

220. Corrigan CJ, Haczku A, Gemou-Engesaeth V, Doi S, Kikuchi Y, Takatsu K, Durham SR, Kay AB (1993) CD4 T-lymphocyte activation in asthma is accompanied by increased serum concentrations of interleukin-5. Effect of glucocorticoid therapy. Am Rev Respir Dis 147:540–547.

221. Robinson D, Hamid Q, Ying S, Bentley A, Assoufi B, Durham SR, Kay AB (1993) Prednisolone treatment in asthma is associated with modulation of bronchoalveolar lavage cell interleukin-4, interleukin-5 and interferon-gamma cytokine gene expression. Am Rev Respir Dis 148:401–406.

222. Foster PS, Hogan SP, Ramsay AJ, Matthaei KI, Young IG (1996) Interleukin 5 deficiency abolishes eosinophilia, airways hyperreactivity, and lung damage in a mouse asthma model. J Exp Med 183:195–201.

223. Viegas M, Gomez E, Brooks J, Gatland D, Davies RJ (1987) Effect of the pollen season on nasal mast cells. Br Med J 294:414

224. Pipkorn U, Karlsson G, Enerback L (1988) The cellular response of the human allergic mucosa to natural allergen exposure. J Allergy Clin Immunol 82:1046–1054.

225. Slavin RG (1993) Upper respiratory tract. In: Weiss EB, Stein M, eds. Bronchial Asthma. Mechanisms and Therapeutics. Boston, Little Brown, pp. 533–544.

226. Leiferman KM, Ackerman SJ, Sampson HA, Haugen HS, Venencie PY, Gleich GJ (1985) Dermal deposition of eosinophil-granule major basic protein in atopic dermatitis. Comparison with onchocerciasis. N Engl J Med 313:282–285.

227. Bruyjnzeel-Koomen CAF, Van Wichen DF, Spry CJF, Venge P, Bruyjnzeel PLB (1988) Active participation of eosinophils in patch test reactions to inhalant allergens in patients with atopic dermatitis. Br J Dermatol 118:229–238.

9

Role of Basophils in Allergic Reactions

Peter Valent, MD

CONTENTS

INTRODUCTION

A number of previous and more recent studies have shown that basophil granulocytes are effector cells of allergic reactions *(1–3)*. These cells store histamine in their granules and express high-affinity immunoglobulin E (IgE) binding sites *(3,4)*. In addition, blood basophils can release their mediators in response to an allergen or other stimuli. In patients with allergic asthma, rhinitis, or contact dermatitis, basophils can be detected at the sites of disease and frequently show signs of anaphylactoid degranulation *(5–7)*. Basophils may also accumulate in affected tissues during the late phase of an allergic reaction following antigen challenge *(5,8)*. During the past few years, major advances in basophil research have been made and novel concepts have emerged. In contrast to mast cell research most of these data stem from research on human cells. This article gives a short overview of the role of blood basophils in allergic reactions.

ORIGIN OF BASOPHILS

A well-established concept is that blood basophils originate from multipotent hemopoietic progenitor cells *(2,9)*. Under normal physiologic conditions, the multilineage progenitors (colony-forming unit [CFU]-MIX) and the basophil-committed progenitor cells (CFU-ba) undergo differentiation in the bone marrow *(2)* (Fig. 1). However, progenitor cells giving rise to basophils can also be detected in the peripheral blood *(10)*. Interleukin-3 (IL-3) is the most potent growth factor for bone marrow derived basophils *(11)* (Fig. 1). Other cytokines that may be involved in the development of human basophils are IL-5, granulocyte-macrophage colony-stimulating factor (GM-CSF), nerve growth factor (NGF), stem cell factor (SCF), and transforming growth factor (TGF)-β *(12–16)*.

From: *Allergy and Allergic Diseases: The New Mechanisms and Therapeutics*
Edited by: J. A. Denburg © Humana Press Inc., Totowa, NJ

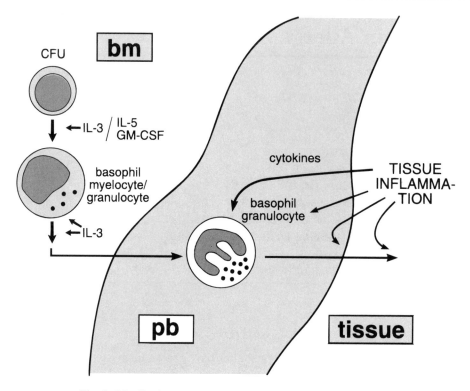

Fig. 1. Distribution and fate of basophils and their progenitors.

Interestingly, the basophil differentiation factor IL-3, as well as GM-CSF and IL-5, can be detected at the sites of ongoing inflammation or allergy *(17,18)*. These factors are considered to trigger survival and activation of local cells *(19)*. Whether these factors also induce basophil differentiation from progenitor cells in inflamed tissues remains unknown.

The number of circulating blood basophils in allergic patients may be normal or may be increased. During glucocorticoid treatment, the numbers of basophils and eosinophils usually decline. There is no evidence that a moderate increase in blood basophils *per se* would cause or contribute to the course of an allergic disease. However, in the case of a massive increase of basophils, as seen in chronic myeloid leukemia, a life-threatening mediator syndrome may occur during allergic reactions *(20)*.

HOW DO BASOPHILS ENTER THE TISSUES?

A number of studies have shown that basophils can leave the blood stream during an allergic reaction. These basophils can enter the affected tissues and appear at the sites of ongoing disease, for example on the epithelial surface of the airways during allergen challenge *(21,22)*.

The infiltration of blood cells into tissues during an inflammatory response is regulated by various molecules and preceded by distinct functional alterations of blood cells and endothelial cells (EC) *(23)*. Both types of cells (the endothelial cells and the leukocytes) must undergo activation before transmigration and extravasation occur. Also, these cells must express recognition molecules that can facilitate rolling, cell–cell attachment, and transmigration *(23)*. The endothelial-cell-agonists that can induce activation and cause binding of leukocytes are well-known mediators of inflammation and allergy. For example, histamine causes expression of

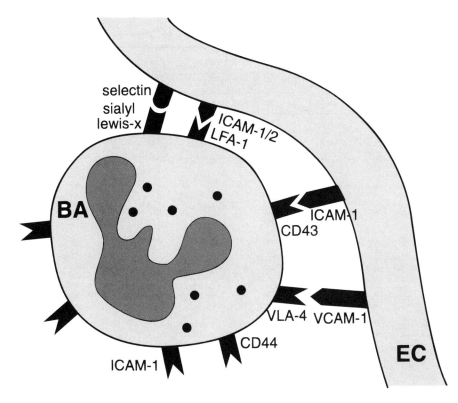

Fig. 2. Adhesion molecules expressed on basophils.

selections in EC, and tumor necrosis factor (TNF), interferons (IFNs), and several interleukins upregulate intercellular adhesion molecule (ICAM)-1 and vascular cell adhesion molecule (VCAM)-1 expression in EC.

In common with other blood leukocytes, human basophils constitutively express a number of adhesion molecules that can interact with EC-antigens. In particular, human basophils express the β2 integrin LFA-1 (leukocyte function antigen-1, CD11b/CD18), the counter receptor of ICAM-1 (CD54) expressed on vascular endothelial cells *(24,25)* (Fig. 2). Basophils also express VLA-4 (very late antigen-4, CD49d/CD29, the counter-receptor of VCAM-1), sialyl-lewis-X, CD54, CD43, CD44, and several other adhesion molecules *(26–28)*. The current concept is that basophils, like all other leukocytes, undergo a stepwise process: first, they start to roll on an EC selectin (E-selectin) via sialyl-lewis-X (margination); then, they attach to activated endothelium via LFA-1-ICAM-1 and/or VLA-4-VCAM-1 interaction(s) (Fig. 2). Ultimately, the basophils leave the blood stream and transmigrate through the endothelial cell layer. Then, chemotactic factors may be present that guide the basophils into the center of an inflammatory (allergic) reaction. Many other agonists may also be around and promote survival, attachment, degranulation, or mediator production in the recruited basophil (*see* below). A detailed review of the roles of adhesion molecules in allergic reactions is presented in Chapter 18.

BASOPHIL AGONISTS

A number of basophil agonists have been identified. The IgE-dependent activation of basophils through a specific allergen is a well-defined process *(4)*. A second class of basophil

Table 1
Response of Human Basophils to Various Agonists

	Agonist-effects (time after which an effect is measured)			
Agonists	*Effect on differentiation[a]*	*Histamine release*	*Release priming*	*Effect on migration*
IL-2	–	–	–	nk[b]
IL-3	+ (14 d)	–/+[c]	+ (15 min)	+
IL-4	–	–	–	nk
IL-5	+/– (14 d)	–	+ (15 min)	+
GM-CSF	+/– (14 d)	–/+[c]	+ (15 min)	+
NGF	–/+ (14 d)	–	+ (15 min)	nk
IGF	nk	–	+ (15 min)	nk
IFNs	– (inhibits)	–	+ (12 h)	nk
C5a	–	+ (15 min)	–/+[d]	+
IL-8	–	+/–	–/+[d]	+
MCAF	–	+ (15 min)	– (+)[d]	+
MIP-1α	–	–	– (+)[d]	+
RANTES	–	–	– (+)[d]	+
GROα/β/γ	–	–	–	+

[a]In vitro differentiation from bone marrow progenitor cells.
[b]nk, not known.
[c]IL-3 did not induce a significant histamine release in normal basophils.
[d]Priming with IL-3 makes cells responsive to this (incomplete) agonist.

agonists are the complement (C) cleavage products C5a and C3a (anaphylatoxins). The cytokines IL-3, IL-5, GM-CSF, and NGF, as well as the IGFs (insulin-like growth factors) and the IFNs, can augment the IgE-dependent release of histamine in human basophils *(29–36)*. In the case of allergic donors, some of these cytokines (IL-3) may act as complete agonists and induce mediator secretion *per se (31,37)*. Many basophil-active cytokines not only trigger mediator secretion in basophils but also survival, chemotaxis, adherence to endothelium, and leukotriene formation.

The chemokine family of proinflammatory mediators can also trigger basophil functions. These substances can act as complete or incomplete agonists on basophils and promote mediator release and chemotaxis *(38–45)*. For example, IL-8 can induce histamine release in IL-3 primed basophils, but not in unstimulated cells *(38,39)*. In contrast, the chemokine MCAF directly induces mediator release from human basophils *(40–42)*. Table 1 gives an overview of basophil agonists. Many of the basophil agonists may be coproduced during an inflammatory or allergic response. Therefore, the situation in vivo is complicated by the fact that many agonists act on basophils. Moreover, most of these molecules trigger not only basophil functions, but also those of a number of other cells (lymphocytes, eosinophils, macrophages). Therefore, the contribution of basophils and their response to a certain agonist in a given allergic reaction is difficult to estimate *(21,22)*.

The effects of the cytokines on human basophils are mediated via specific cell surface membrane receptors. Human basophils express receptors for IL-2, IL-3, IL-4, IL-5, and IL-8 (Table 2) *(39,47–50)*. They do not express receptors for G-CSF or M-CSF. There is no absolute correlation between expression of cytokine binding sites on human basophils and the response of the cells to the respective ligands. Thus, under the same experimental conditions,

Table 2
Expression of Some Cytokine Receptors (R) on Human Blood Basophils

Cytokine R	CD	Expression on basophils	Assessed by
IL-2Rα/TAC	25	+	MAb, Northern
IL-2Rβ	122	–	MAb
IL-4Rα	124	+/–	MAb, radio-R
IL-7Rα	127	–	MAb
IL-3Rα	123	+	MAb, radio-R
IL-5Rα	125	+	Radio-R
GM-CSFRα	116	+/–	MAb, radio-R
IL-3-5/GM-CSFRβ	131	+	MAb
IL-6Rα	126	–	MAb
IL-6/-11Rβ/pg130	130	–	MAb
IL-8R	128	+/–	MAb, radio-R
M-CSFR	115	–	MAb
G-CSFR	114	–	MAb
SCFR/c-*kit*	117	–/+*	MAb

MAb, monoclonal antibodies; radio-R, radioreceptor assay.
*Low c-*kit* expression on basophils has been described by Columbo et al. *(46)*.

IL-3 is a basophil agonist, whereas IL-2 and IL-4 do not induce or augment mediator release in human basophils *(37,38)*.

BASOPHIL-DERIVED MEDIATORS

A number of mediators are produced in human blood basophils. A subset of them (histamine) are synthesized during cell maturation and are stored in the granules of the mature cells. Other mediators (lipid mediators) are produced and released during an allergic response. Basophil mediators are important regulators of the immediate-type response to an allergen, or the late phase of an allergic response (*see* Chapter 26).

A novel important issue is that basophils can produce significant amounts of interleukin-4 (IL-4) *(51–53)*. This molecule is produced in the basophils in response to IgE-dependent *(51,52)* or IL-3/C5a-dependent *(53)* cell activation and can be detected in the supernatants of isolated basophils after challenge with a specific antigen. The production and release of IL-4 by human basophils has several pathophysiologic implications. In particular, IL-4 is a multifunctional regulator of the immune response and plays an essential role in the pathophysiology of allergic reactions. Specifically, IL-4 is an important regulator of B-cells and is involved in the regulation of IgE synthesis *(54)*. Thus, IL-4 release from basophils may represent an important step in the generation of an allergic response.

BASOPHIL DEACTIVATING DRUGS

A number of anti-inflammatory drugs and signal transduction inhibitors appear to inhibit mediator release from human basophils and other basophil cell functions. For example, glucocorticoids can suppress the IgE-induced mediator release in basophils *(55)* as well as basophil migration into tissue and accumulation of basophils *(56,57)*. Interestingly, the anti-inflammatory drugs cyclosporin A and FK-506 can also interfere with basophil activation and mediator release *(58–60)*. A detailed analysis of signaling in basophils is found in Chapter 21.

CONCLUDING REMARKS

Accumulating evidence exists that basophils play an important role in allergic reactions and that basophil-derived molecules can trigger both the immediate response to an allergen and a specific secondary response of the immune system via release of specific cytokines, such as IL-4. The knowledge of novel basophil-dependent pathways in allergy should enable scientists to screen for specific inhibitors that can interfere with basophil activation in allergic diseases.

REFERENCES

1. Lichtenstein LM, Bochner BS (1991) The role of basophils in asthma. Ann NY Acad Sci 629:48–61.
2. Valent P, Bettelheim P (1990) The human basophil. Crit Rev Oncol Hematol 10:327–352.
3. Serafin WE, Austen KF (1987) Mediators of immediate hypersensitivity reactions. N Engl J Med 317:30–34.
4. Ishizaka T, Ishizaka K (1984) Activation of mast cells for mediator release through IgE receptors. Prog Allergy 34:188–235.
5. Dvorak HF, Simpson BA, Bast RC, Leskowitz S (1971) Cutaneous basophil hypersensitivity. III. Participation of the basophil in hypersensitivity to antigen-antibody complexes, delayed hypersensitivity and contact allergy. J Immunol 107:138–148.
6. Dvorak HF, Mihm MC (1972) Basophilic leukocytes in allergic contact dermatitis. J Exp Med 135:235–254.
7. Mitchell EB, Askenase PW (1983) Basophils in human disease. Clin Rev Allergy 1:427–448.
8. Charlesworth EN, Hood AF, Soter NA, Kagey-Sobotka, Norman PS, Lichtenstein LM (1989) Cutaneous late-phase response to allergen: mediator release and inflammatory cell infiltration. J Clin Invest 83:1519–1526.
9. Denburg JA (1992) Basophil and mast cell lineages in vitro and in vivo. Blood 79:846–860.
10. Denburg JA, Richardson M, Telizyn S, Bienenstock J (1983) Basophil/mast cell precursors in human peripheral blood. Blood 61:775–780.
11. Valent P, Schmidt G, Besemer J, Mayer P, Zenke G, Liehl E, Hinterberger W, Lechner K, Maurer D, Bettelheim P (1989) Interleukin-3 is a differentiation factor for human basophils. Blood 73: 1763–1769.
12. Denburg JA, Silver JE, Abrams JS (1991) Interleukin-5 is a human basophilopoietin: induction of histamine content and basophilic differentiation of HL-60 cells and of peripheral blood basophil-eosinophil progenitors. Blood 77:1462–1468.
13. Mayer P, Valent P, Schmidt G, Liehl E, Bettelheim P (1989) The in vivo effects of recombinant human interleukin-3: demonstration of basophil differentiation factor, histamine-producing activity, and priming of GM-CSF-responsive progenitors in nonhuman primates. Blood 74:613–621.
14. Matsuda H, Coughlin MD, Bienenstock J, Denburg, JA (1988) Nerve growth factor promotes human hemopoietic colony growth and differentiation. Proc Natl Acad Sci USA 85:6508–6512.
15. Tsuda T, Wong D, Dolovich J, Bienenstock J, Marshall J, Denburg JA (1991) Synergistic effects of nerve growth factor and granulocyte-macrophage colony-stimulating factor on human basophilic cell differentiation. Blood 77:971–979.
16. Sillaber C, Geissler K, Scherrer R, Kaltenbrunner R, Bettelheim P, Lechner K, Valent P (1992) Type β transforming growth factors promote interleukin-3 (IL-3)-dependent differentiation of human basophils but inhibit IL-3 dependent differentiation of human eosinophils. Blood 80:634–641.
17. Bradding P, Roberts JA, Britten KM, Montefort S, Djukanovic R, Mueller R, Heusser CH, Howarth PH, Holgate ST (1994) Interleukin-4, -5, -6 and tumor necrosis factor-alpha in normal and asthmatic airways: evidence for the human mast cell as a source of these cytokines. Am J Respir Cell Mol Biol 10:471–480.
18. Kay AB, Ying S, Varney V, Gaga M, Durham SR, Moqbel R, Wardlaw AJ, Hamid Q (1991) Messenger RNA expression of the cytokine gene cluster, interleukin-3 (IL-3), IL-4, IL-5, and granulocyte/

macrophage colony-stimulating factor, in allergen-induced late-phase cutaneous reactions in atopic subjects. J Exp Med 173:775–778.

19. Denburg JA, Woolley M, Leber B, Linden M, O'Byrne P (1994) Basophil and eosinophil differentiation in allergic disease. J Allergy Clin Immunol 94:1135–1141.

20. Rosenthal S, Schwartz JH, Canellos GP (1977) Basophilic chronic granulocytic leukemia with hyperhistaminaemia. Br J Haematol 36:367–372.

21. Iliopoulos O, Baroody FM, Naclerio RM, Bochner BS, Kagey-Sobotka A, Lichtenstein LM (1992) Histamine-containing cells obtained from the nose hours after antigen challenge have functional and phenotypic characteristics of basophils. J Immunol 148:2223–2228.

22. Guo CB, Liu MC, Galli SJ, Bochner BS, Kagey-Sobotka A, Lichtenstein LM (1994) Identification of IgE-bearing cells in the late-phase response to antigen in the lung as basophils. Am. J Respir Cell Mol Biol 10:384–390.

23. Springer TA (1990) Adhesion receptors of the immune system. Nature 346:425–434.

24. Stain C, Stockinger H, Scharf M, Jäger U, Gössinger H, Lechner K, Bettelheim P (1987) Human blood basophils display a unique phenotype including activation linked membrane structures. Blood 70:1872–1879.

25. Bochner BS, McKelvey AA, Sterbinsky SA, Hildreth JEK, Derse CP, Klunk DA, Lichtenstein LM, Schleimer RP (1990) Il-3 augments adhesiveness for endothelium and CD11b expression in human basophils but not neutrophils. J Immunol 145:1832–1837.

26. Bochner BS, Sterbinsky SA, Knol EF, Katz BJ, Lichtenstein LM, MacGlashan DW, Schleimer RP (1994) Function and expression of adhesion molecules on human basophils. J Allergy Clin Immunol 94:1157–1162.

27. Valent P, Bettelheim P (1992) Cell surface structures on human basophils and mast cells: biochemical and functional characterization. Adv Immunol 52:333–423.

28. Valent P, Majdic O, Maurer D, Bodger M, Muhm M, Bettelheim P (1990) Further characterization of surface membrane structures expressed on human basophils and mast cells. Int Arch Allergy Appl Immunol 91:198–203.

29. Hirai K, Morita Y, Misaki Y, Ohta K, Takaishi T, Suzuki S, Motoyoshi K, Miyamoto T (1988) Modulation of human basophil histamine release by hemopoietic growth factors. J Immunol 14:3958–3964.

30. Valent P, Besemer J, Muhm M, Majdic O, Lechner K, Bettelheim P (1989) Interleukin 3 activates human blood basophils via high affinity binding sites. Proc Natl Acad Sci USA 86:5542–5546.

31. Schleimer RP, Derse CP, Friedman B, Gillis S, Plaut M, Lichtenstein LM, MacGlashan DW (1989) Regulation of human basophil mediator release by cytokines. J Immunol 143:1310–1317.

32. Kurimoto A, De Weck AL, Dahinden CA (1989) Interleukin 3-dependent mediator release in basophils triggered by C5a. J Exp Med 170:467–479.

33. Bischoff SC, Dahinden CA (1992) Effect of nerve growth factor on the release of inflammatory mediators by mature human basophils. Blood 79:2662–2669.

34. Hirai K, Miyamasu M, Yamaguchi M, Nakajima K, Ohtoshi T, Koshino T, Takaishi T, Morita Y, Ito K (1993) Modulation of human basophil histamine release by insuline-like growth factors. J Immunol 150:1503–1508.

35. Ida S, Hooks JJ, Siraganian RP, Notkins AL (1977) Enhancement of IgE-mediated histamine release from human basophils by viruses: role of interferon. J Exp Med 145:892–906.

36. Hernandez-Asensio M, Hooks JJ, Ida S, Siraganian RP, Notkins AL (1979) Interferon induced enhancement of IgE-mediated histamine release from human basophils requires RNA synthesis. J Immunol 122:1601–1603.

37. Haak-Frendscho M, Arai N, Arai K, Baeza ML, Finn A, Kaplan AP (1988) Human recombinant granulocyte-macrophage colony stimulating factor and interleukin 3 cause basophil histamine release. J Clin Invest 82:17–20.

38. Dahinden CA, Kurimoto Y, de Weck AL, Lindley I, Dewald B, Baggiolini M (1989) The neutrophil-activating peptide NAF/NAP-1 induces histamine and leukotriene release by interleukin 3-primed basophils. J Exp Med 170:1787–1792.

39. Krieger M, Brunner T, Bischoff SC, Tscharner V, Walz A, Moser B, Baggiolini M, Dahinden CA (1992) Activation of human basophils through the IL-8 receptor. J Immunol 149:2662–2667.

40. Kuna P, Reddigari SR, Schall TJ, Rucinski D, Sadick M, Kaplan AP (1993) Characterization of the human basophil response to cytokines, growth factors, and histamine releasing factors of the intercrine/chemokine family. J Immunol 150:1932–1943.

41. Bischoff SC, Krieger M, Brunner T, Dahinden CA (1992) Monocyte chemotactic protein 1 is a potent activator of human basophils. J Exp Med 175:1271–1275.

42. Alam R, Lett-Brown MA, Forsythe PA, Anderson-Walters DJ, Kenamore C, Kormos C, Grant JA (1992) Monocyte chemotactic and activating factor is a potent histamine-releasing factor for basophils. J Clin Invest 89:723–728.

43. Alam R, Forsythe PA, Stafford S, Lett-Brown MA, Grant JA (1992) Macrophage inflammatory protein-1α activates basophils and mast cells. J Exp Med 176:781–786.

44. Bischoff SC, Krieger M, Brunner T, Rot A, vonTscharner V, Baggiolini M, Dahinden CA (1993) RANTES and related chemokines activate human basophil granulocytes through different G protein-coupled receptors. Eur J Immunol 23:761–767.

45. Geiser T, Dewald B, Ehrengruber MU, Clark-Lewis I, Baggiolini M (1993) The interleukin-8-related chemotactic cytokines GROα, GROβ, and GROγ activate human neutrophil and basophil leukocytes. J Biol Chem 268:15,419–15,424.

46. Columbo M, Horowitz EM, Botana LM, MacGlashan DW, Bochner BS, Gillis S, Zsebo KM, Galli SJ, Lichtenstein LM (1992) The human recombinant c-kit receptor ligand, rhSCF, induces mediator release from human cutaneous mast cells and enhances IgE-dependent mediator release from both skin mast cells and peripheral blood basophils. J Immunol 149:599–608.

47. Stockinger H, Valent P, Majdic O, Bettelheim P, Knapp W (1990) Human blood basophils synthesize interleukin-2 binding sites. Blood 75:1820–1826.

48. Valent P, Besemer J, Kishi K, diPadova F, Geissler K, Bettelheim P (1990) Human basophils express interleukin-4 receptors. Blood 76:1734–1738.

49. Lopez AF, Lyons AB, Eglinton JM, Park LS, To LB, Clark SC, Vadas MA (1990) Specific binding of human interleukin-3 and granulocyte-macrophage colony-stimulating factor to human basophils. J Allergy Clin Immunol 85:99–102.

50. Lopez AF, Eglinton, JM, Lyons AB, Tapley PM, To LB, Park LS, Clark SC, Vadas MA (1990) Human interleukin-3 inhibits the binding of granulocyte-macrophage colony-stimulating factor and interleukin-5 to basophils and strongly enhances their functional activity. J Cell Physiol 145:69–77.

51. MacGlashan DW, White JM, Huang SK, Ono SJ, Schroeder JT, Lichtenstein LM (1994) Secretion of IL-4 from human basophils. J Immunol 152:3006–3016.

52. Brunner T, Heusser CH, Dahinden CA (1993) Human peripheral blood basophils primed by interleukin 3 (IL-3) produce IL-4 in response to immunoglobulin E receptor stimulation. J Exp Med 177:605–611.

53. Ochensberger B, Rihs S, Brunner T, Dahinden C (1995) IgE-independent interleukin-4 expression and induction of a late phase of leukotriene C4 formation in human blood basophils. Blood 86:4039–4049.

54. Paul WE (1991) Interleukin-4 A prototypic immunoregulatory lymphokine. Blood 77:1859–1870.

55. Schleimer RP, Lichtenstein LM, Gillespie E (1981) Inhibition of basophil histamine release by anti-inflammatory steroids. Nature 292:454–455.

56. Yamaguchi M, Hirai K, Nakajima K, Ohtoshi T, Takaishi T, Ohta K, Morita Y, Ito K (1994) Dexamethasone inhibits basophil migration. Allergy 49:371–375.

57. Charlesworth EN, Kagey-Sobotka A, Schleimer RP, Norman PS, Lichtenstein LM (1991) Prednisone inhibits the appearance of inflammatory mediators and the influx of eosinophils and basophils associated with the cutaneous late-phase response to allergen. J Immunol 146:671–676.

58. de Paulis A, Cirillo R, Ciccarelli A, Condorelli M, Marone G (1991) FK-506, a potent novel inhibitor of the release of proinflammatory mediators from human FcεRI⁺ cells. J Immunol 146:2374–2381.

59. Cirillo R, Triggiani M, Siri L, Ciccarelli A, Pettit GR, Condorelli M, Marone G (1990) Cyclosporin A rapidly inhibits mediator release from human basophils presumably by interacting with cyclophilin. J Immunol 144:3891–3897.

60. Casolaro V, Spadaro G, Patella V, Marone G (1993) In vivo characterization of the anti-inflammatory effect of cyclosporin A on human basophils. J Immunol 151:5563–5573.

10

Neurogenic Inflammation in Allergic Disease

Peter J. Barnes, DM, DSc, FRCP

INTRODUCTION

There is a close association between the allergic inflammatory response and neural control mechanisms. Inflammatory products may activate sensory nerves to cause symptoms, such as cough and chest tightness, sneezing, and itching, which are among the most troublesome aspects of allergic diseases. Sensory nerves themselves may also release neurotransmitters that increase inflammation, and this is termed neurogenic inflammation. The phenomenon of neurogenic inflammation is well established in the skin and in the respiratory tract of rodents, although there is less certainty about its role in human airway diseases. The peptides substance P (SP), neurokinin A (NKA), and calcitonin gene-related peptide (CGRP) are localized to a population of sensory neurons in the respiratory tract and the skin *(1–4)*. These peptides have potent effects on the circulation, secretions, airway smooth muscle tone, and inflammatory and immune cells. Although some clues to the physiological and pathophysiological role of sensory neuropeptides are provided by their localization and functional effects, their role in allergic diseases will only become apparent when specific inhibitors are used in clinical studies. Depletion studies using capsaicin have proved to be very helpful in elucidating the role of sensory neuropeptides in animal models, but the recent development of specific receptor antagonists and other inhibitors is proving to be critical in understanding the role of neurogenic inflammation in the respiratory tract and skin. Most studies have concentrated on the lower airways and asthma *(5)*, but there is increasing information about the nose and skin *(4,6)*.

NONADRENERGIC NONCHOLINERGIC NERVES

The role of cholinergic (parasympathetic) and adrenergic (sympathetic) nerves in the respiratory tract has been well documented, but there are neural mechanisms that are not blocked

From: *Allergy and Allergic Diseases: The New Mechanisms and Therapeutics*
Edited by: J. A. Denburg © Humana Press Inc., Totowa, NJ

by adrenergic or cholinergic blockers, the so called nonadrenergic noncholinergic (NANC) nerves. It was once believed that this was a third type of nervous system with specific nerves releasing neurotransmitters, but it is now apparent that NANC neural mechanisms are mediated by the release of cotransmitters from classical autonomic nerves. Thus parasympathetic nerves release acetylcholine but also vasoactive intestinal peptide (VIP), sympathetic nerves release norepinephrine but also neuropeptide Y, and sensory nerves release glutamate but also SP, NKA, and CGRP. In human airways, there is a prominent bronchodilator NANC neural pathway, and the neurotransmitter is nitric oxide (NO), probably released from parasympathetic nerves *(7,8)*. In rodents there is a bronchoconstrictor NANC neural pathway (e-NANC) that is mediated via the release of tachykinins from sensory nerves *(9)*.

TACHYKININS

Localization

SP and NKA, but not neurokinin B, are localized to sensory nerves in the airways of several species. SP-immunoreactive nerves are abundant in rodent airways, but are very sparse in human airways *(10–12)*. Rapid enzymatic degradation of SP in airways, and the fact that SP concentrations may decrease with age and possibly after cigarette smoking, could explain the difficulty in demonstrating this peptide in some studies. SP-immunoreactive nerves in the airway are found beneath and within the airway epithelium, around blood vessels, and, to a lesser extent, within airway smooth muscle. SP-immunoreactive nerves fibers also innervate parasympathetic ganglia, suggesting a sensory input that may modulate ganglionic transmission and so result in ganglionic reflexes. In the nose, SP-immunoreactive nerves innervate blood vessels and mucus glands *(13)*.

SP in the airways is localized predominantly to capsaicin-sensitive unmyelinated nerves in the airways, but chronic administration of capsaicin only partially depletes the lung of tachykinins, indicating the presence of a population of capsaicin-resistant SP-immunoreactive nerves, as in the gastrointestinal tract *(14,15)*. Similar capsaicin denervation studies are not possible in human airways, but after extrinsic denervation by heart-lung transplantation there appears to be a loss of SP-immunoreactive nerves in the submucosa *(16)*.

Effects

Tachykinins have many different effects on the respiratory tract that may be relevant to asthma and rhinitis. These effects are mediated via NK_1-receptors (preferentially activated by SP) and NK_2-receptors (preferentially activated by NKA), whereas there is little evidence of NK_3-receptors.

Airway Smooth Muscle

Tachykinins constrict smooth muscle of human airways in vitro via NK_2-receptors *(17,18)*. The contractile response to NKA is significantly greater in smaller human bronchi than in more proximal airways, indicating that tachykinins may have a more important constrictor effect in peripheral airways *(19)*, whereas cholinergic constriction tends to be more pronounced in proximal airways. This is consistent with the autoradiographic distribution of tachykinin receptors, which are distributed to small and large airways. In vivo SP does not cause bronchoconstriction or cough, either by intravenous infusion *(20,21)* or by inhalation *(20,22)*, whereas NKA causes bronchoconstriction both after intravenous administration *(21)* and after inhalation in asthmatic subjects *(22)*. Inhalation of SP increased airway responsiveness to methacholine in asthmatic subjects, an effect that has been ascribed to airway edema *(23)*. Mechanical removal of airway epithelium potentiates the bronchoconstrictor response to tachykinins *(24,25)*, largely because the ectoenzyme neutral endopeptidase 24.11 (NEP), which is a key enzyme in the degradation of tachykinins in airways, is strongly expressed on epithelial cells.

SECRETIONS

SP stimulates mucus secretion from submucosal glands in ferret and human airways in vitro *(26,27)* and is a potent stimulant to goblet cell secretion in guinea pig airways *(28)*. Indeed SP is likely to mediate the increase in goblet cell discharge after vagus nerve stimulation and exposure to cigarette smoke *(29,30)*. SP induces serous and mucus gland secretion from human nasal explants in vitro *(13)* and nasal secretions in allergic rhinitis patients *(31)*.

Stimulation of the vagus nerve in rodents causes microvascular leakage, which is prevented by prior treatment with capsaicin or by a tachykinin antagonist, indicating that release of tachykinins from sensory nerves mediates this effect. Among the tachykinins, SP is most potent at causing leakage in guinea-pig airways *(32)* and NK_1-receptors have been localized to postcapillary venules in the airway submucosa *(33)*. Inhaled SP also causes microvascular leakage in guinea pigs, and its effect on the microvasculature is more marked than its effect on airway smooth muscle *(34)*. It is difficult to measure airway microvascular leakage in human airways, but SP causes a weal in human skin when injected intradermally, indicating the capacity to cause microvascular leak in human postcapillary venules; NKA is less potent, indicating that an NK_1-receptor mediates this effect *(35)*. SP administration to the nose has little effect in normal individuals, but increases the secretion of albumin and causes nasal obstruction in patients with allergic rhinitis, presumably owing to an effect on the microvasculature *(31)*.

VASCULAR EFFECTS

Tachykinins have potent effects on airway blood flow. Indeed the effect of tachykinins on airway blood flow may be the most important physiological and pathophysiological role of tachykinins in airways. In canine and porcine trachea both SP and NKA cause a marked increase in blood flow *(36,37)*. Tachykinins also dilate canine bronchial vessels in vitro, probably via an endothelium-dependent mechanism *(38)*. Tachykinins also regulate bronchial blood flow in pig; stimulation of the vagus nerve causes a vasodilation mediated by the release of sensory neuropeptides, and it is likely that CGRP as well as tachykinins are involved *(37)*.

EFFECTS ON NERVES

In guinea-pig trachea, tachykinins also potentiate cholinergic neurotransmission at postganglionic nerve terminals, and an NK_2-receptor appears to be involved *(39)*. There is also potentiation at ganglionic level *(40,41)*, which appears to be mediated via an NK_1-receptor *(41)*. There is also evidence that NK_3-receptors are involved *(42)*. Endogenous tachykinins may also facilitate cholinergic neurotransmission since capsaicin pretreatment results in a significant reduction in cholinergic neural responses both in vitro and in vivo *(43,44)*. However in human airways there is no evidence for a facilitatory effect on cholinergic neurotransmission *(45)*, although such an effect has been reported in the presence of potassium channel blockers *(46)*.

In conscious guinea pigs, very low concentrations of inhaled SP are reported to cause cough and this effect is potentiated by NEP inhibition *(47)*. Citric acid-induced cough is blocked by a nonpeptide NK_2-receptor antagonist (SR 48968), suggesting the involvement of NK_2-receptor although these may be centrally located *(48)*.

IMMUNOLOGICAL EFFECTS

Tachykinins may also interact with inflammatory and immune cells *(49,50)*, although whether this is of pathophysiological significance remains to be determined. There is likely to be increasing research in the area of neuroimmune interaction and in some species there is already evidence for neuropeptide innervation of bronchus-associated lymphoid tissue *(51)*. SP degranulates certain types of mast cell, such as those in human skin, although this is not mediated via a tachykinin receptor *(52)*. There is no evidence that tachykinins degranulate lung mast cells *(53)*. SP has a degranulating effect on eosinophils *(54)*; again the degranulation is related to high concentrations of peptide and, as for mast cells, is not mediated via a tachykinin receptor. At lower concentrations tachykinins have been reported to enhance eosinophil chemotaxis *(55)*. Tachykinins may activate alveolar macrophages *(56)* and monocytes to release inflammatory cytokines, such as IL-6 *(57)*. Topical application of SP to human nasal mucosa results in increased expression of several cytokines, suggesting that SP may have important chronic immune effects *(58)*, and these deserve further study. Tachykinins and vagus nerve stimulation also cause transient vascular adhesion of neutrophils in the airway circulation *(59)* and in human skin *(60)*.

STRUCTURAL EFFECTS

SP stimulates proliferation of blood vessels (angiogenesis) *(61)* and may therefore be involved in the new vessel formation that is found in asthmatic airways *(62)*. SP and NKA also stimulate the proliferation and chemotaxis of human lung fibroblasts, suggesting that tachykinins may contribute to the fibrotic process in chronic asthma *(63)*. These effects appear to be mediated by both NK_1- and NK_2-receptors.

Metabolism

Tachykinins are subject to degradation by at least two enzymes, angiotensin-converting enzyme (ACE) and NEP *(64)*. ACE is predominantly localized to vascular endothelial cells and therefore breaks down intravascular peptides. ACE inhibitors, such as captopril, enhance bronchoconstriction owing to intravenous SP *(65,66)*, but not inhaled SP *(67)*. NKA is not a good substrate for ACE; however. NEP appears to be the most important enzyme for the breakdown of tachykinins in tissues. NEP is expressed in human airways and nose and is localized to many cell types, including epithelial cells, glands, and airway smooth muscle *(68,69)*.

Inhibition of NEP by phosphoramidon or thiorphan markedly potentiates bronchoconstriction in vitro in animal *(70)* and human airways *(71)* and, after inhalation, in vivo *(67)*. NEP inhibition also potentiates mucus secretion in response to tachykinins in human airways in vitro *(26)*. NEP inhibition enhances e-NANC and capsaicin-induced bronchoconstriction, owing to the release of tachykinins from airways sensory nerves *(24,72)*.

The activity of NEP in the airways appears to be an important factor in determining the effects of tachykinins; any factors that inhibit the enzyme or its expression may be associated with increased effects of exogenous or endogenously released tachykinins. Several of the stimuli known to induce bronchoconstrictor responses in asthmatic patients have been found to reduce the activity of airway NEP *(64)* (Fig. 1).

CALCITONIN GENE-RELATED PEPTIDE

Localization

CGRP-immunoreactive nerves are abundant in the respiratory tract of several species. CGRP is costored and colocalized with SP in afferent nerves *(73)*. CGRP has been extracted from and is localized to human airways *(12,74)*. CGRP-immunoreactive nerve fibers appear to be more abundant than SP fibers, possibly because CGRP has greater stability, and is also present in some nerves that do not contain SP. CGRP is found in trigeminal, nodose-jugular, and dorsal root ganglia *(75)* and has also been detected in neuroendocrine cells of the lower airways.

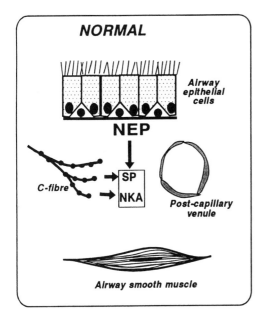
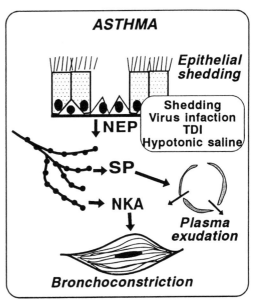

Fig. 1. Interaction of tachykinins with airway epithelium. When epithelium is intact, neutral endopeptidase (NEP) degrades substance P (SP) and neurokinin A (NKA) released from sensory nerves (**left panel**). In asthmatic airways, when epithelium is shed or NEP downregulated, any tachykinins released will have an exaggerated effect (**right panel**).

Effects

CGRP is a potent vasodilator that has long-lasting effects. CGRP is an effective dilator of human pulmonary vessels in vitro and acts directly on receptors on vascular smooth muscle *(76)*. It also potently dilates bronchial vessels in vitro *(76)* and produces a marked and long-lasting increase in airway blood flow in anesthetized dogs *(77)* and conscious sheep in vivo *(78)*. Receptor mapping studies have demonstrated that CGRP receptors are localized predominantly to bronchial vessels rather than to smooth muscle or epithelium in human airways *(79)*. It is possible that CGRP may be the predominant mediator of arterial vasodilatation and increased blood flow in response to sensory nerve stimulation in the bronchi *(37)*. CGRP may be an important mediator of airway hyperemia in asthma.

By contrast, CGRP has no direct effect of airway microvascular leak *(32)*. In the skin, CGRP potentiates the leakage produced by SP, presumably by increasing the blood delivery to the sites of plasma extravasation in the postcapillary venules *(80)* (Fig. 2). This does not occur in guinea-pig airways when CGRP and SP are coadministered, possibly because blood flow in the airways is already high *(32)*, although an increased leakage response has been reported in rat airways *(81)*. It is possible that potentiation of leak may occur when the two peptides are released together from sensory nerves.

CGRP causes constriction of human bronchi in vitro *(74)*. This is surprising, since CGRP normally activates adenylyl cyclase, an event that is usually associated with bronchodilatation. Receptor mapping studies suggest few, if any, CGRP receptors over airway smooth muscle in human or guinea pig airways and this suggests that the paradoxical bronchoconstrictor response reported in human airways may be mediated indirectly. In guinea pig airways, CGRP has no consistent effect on tone *(82)*. The variable effects of CGRP on airways may be explained by the fact that it may release other mediators that have effects on tone. Thus CGRP may release both NO and endothelin in airways *(83)*.

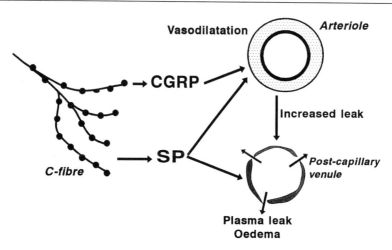

Fig. 2. Effect of sensory neuropeptides in vessels. Substance P causes vasodilatation and plasma exudation, whereas calcitonin gene-related peptide causes vasodilatation of arterioles, which may theoretically increase plasma extravasation by increasing blood delivery to leaky postcapillary venules.

CGRP has a weak inhibitory effect on cholinergically stimulated mucus secretion in ferret trachea *(84)* and on goblet cell discharge in guinea pig airways *(28)*. This is probably related to the low density of CGRP receptors on mucus secretory cells, but does not preclude the possibility that CGRP might increase mucus secretion in vivo by increasing blood flow to submucosal glands.

CGRP injection into human skin causes a persistent flare, but biopsies have revealed an infiltration of eosinophils *(85)*. CGRP itself does not appear to be chemotactic for eosinophils, but proteolytic fragments of the peptide are active *(86)*, suggesting that CGRP released into the tissues may lead to eosinophilic infiltration.

CGRP inhibits the proliferative response of T-lymphocytes to mitogens, and specific receptors have been demonstrated on these cells *(87)*. CGRP also inhibits macrophage secretion and the capacity of macrophages to activate T-lymphocytes *(88)*. This suggests that CGRP has potential anti-inflammatory actions in the airways. CGRP also induces proliferation of guinea-pig airway epithelial cells and may therefore be involved in healing the airway after epithelial shedding in asthma *(89)*.

NEUROGENIC INFLAMMATION

The weal and flare response in human skin is an example of neurogenic inflammation. In rodents there is now considerable evidence for neurogenic inflammation in the respiratory tract owing to the antidromic release of neuropeptides from nociceptive nerves or C-fibers via an axon reflex *(9,90,91)* (Fig. 3) and it is possible that it may contribute to the inflammatory response in asthma *(92,93)* (Fig. 4).

Neurogenic Airway Inflammation in Animal Models

There are several lines of evidence that neurogenic inflammation may be important in animal models that may have relevance to asthma. These models have usually been in rodents, in which tachykinin effects are pronounced, and may not be predictive of the role of tachykinins in human airways, however. There are four main experimental approaches that have been used to assess the role of sensory neuropeptides in animal models of asthma; these include studies

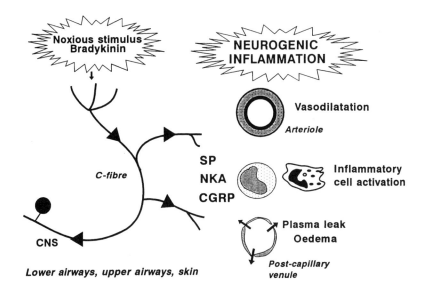

Fig. 3. Neurogenic inflammation.

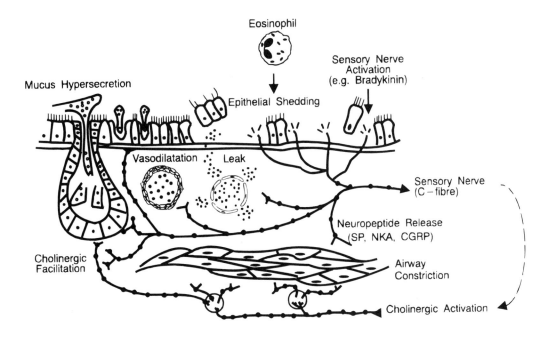

Fig. 4. Possible neurogenic inflammation in asthmatic airways via retrograde release of peptides from sensory nerves via an axon reflex. Substance P (SP) causes vasodilatation, plasma exudation, and mucus secretion, whereas neurokinin A (NKA) causes bronchoconstriction and enhanced cholinergic reflexes, and calcitonin gene-related peptide (CGRP) vasodilatation.

of depletion with capsaicin depletion, enhancement with inhibitors of NEP, tachykinin receptor antagonists, and inhibitors of sensory neuropeptide release.

Capsaicin Depletion Studies

Capsaicin pretreatment is used to deplete neuropeptides from C-fibers, either in neonatal animals (which results in degeneration of C-fibers) or in acute treatment in adult animals (resulting in depletion of sensory neuropeptides). In rat trachea capsaicin pretreatment inhibits the microvascular leakage induced by irritant gases, such as cigaret smoke (94), and inhibits goblet cell discharge and microvascular leak induced by cigaret smoke in guinea pigs (30). Capsaicin-sensitive nerves may also contribute to the bronchoconstriction and microvascular leak induced by isocapnic hyperventilation (95), hypocapnia (96), inhaled sodium metabisulfite (97), and nebulized hypertonic saline (98) and toluene diisocyanate (99) in rodents. In guinea pigs capsaicin pretreatment has little or no effect on the acute bronchoconstrictor or plasma exudation response to allergen inhalation in sensitized animals (100). Administration of capsaicin increases airway responsiveness in guinea pigs to cholinergic agonists, and this effect is prevented by prior treatment with capsaicin, suggesting that capsaicin-sensitive nerves release products that increase airway responsiveness (101). Similarly, in a virus model of airway hyperresponsiveness in guinea pigs capsaicin pretreatment completely blocks the virus-induced hyperesponsiveness (102). In pigs capsaicin pretreatment inhibits the vasodilator response to allergen (which may be mediated by the release of CGRP) (103). In allergic sheep capsaicin pretreatment prevents the airway hyperresponsiveness to both allergen and cholinergic agonists (104). In a model of chronic allergen exposure in guinea pigs capsaicin pretreatment results in complete inhibition of airway hyperresponsiveness, without any change in the eosinophil inflammatory response (105) and also prevents the increased responsiveness to ovalbumin in vitro (106). In rabbits neonatal capsaicin treatment inhibits the airway hyperresponsiveness associated with neonatal allergen sensitization, although this does not appear to be associated with any change in content of sensory neuropeptides in lung tissue (107). This suggests that capsaicin-sensitive nerves may play a role in chronic inflammatory responses to allergen.

There has been speculation that mast cells in the airways might be influenced by capsaicin-sensitive nerves. Histological studies have demonstrated a close proximity between mast cells and sensory nerves in airways (108). There is also evidence that antidromic stimulation of the vagus nerve leads to mast cell mediator release in canine airways (109). Furthermore allergen exposure has effects on ion transport in guinea pig airways that are dependent on capsaicin-sensitive nerves (110).

Inhibition of Neuropeptide Metabolism

The activity of NEP may be an important determinant of the extent of neurogenic inflammation in airways, and inhibition of NEP in rodent by thiorphan or phosphoramidon has been shown to enhance neurogenic inflammation in various rodent models. NEP is not specific to tachykinins and is also involved in the metabolism of other bronchoactive peptides, including kinins and endothelins. Certain virus infections enhance eNANC responses in guinea pigs (111), and mycoplasma infection enhances neurogenic microvascular leakage in rats (91), an effect that is mediated by inhibition of NEP activity. Influenza virus infection of ferret trachea in vitro and guinea pigs in vivo inhibits the activity of epithelial NEP and markedly enhances the bronchoconstrictor responses to tachykinins (112). Similarly Sendai virus infection potentiates neurogenic inflammation in rat trachea (113). This may explain why respiratory tract virus infections are so deleterious to patients with asthma. Hypertonic saline also impairs epithelial NEP function, leading to exaggerated tachykinin responses (98), and cigaret smoke

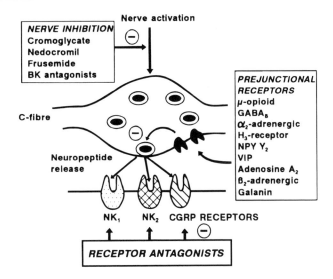

Fig. 5. Modulation of neurogenic inflammation in airway sensory nerves.

exposure has a similar effect, which can be explained by an oxidizing effect on the enzyme *(114)*. Toluene diisocyanate, albeit at rather high doses, also reduces NEP activity, and this may be a mechanism contributing to the airway hyperresponsiveness that may follow exposure to this chemical *(115)*. Inhalation of IL-1β is associated with increased responsiveness to bradykinin, and this may be owing to inhibition of NEP expression *(116)*. Ozone also induces airway hyperresponsiveness and this is mediated in part by impaired function of NEP *(117)*. Thus, many of the agents that lead to exacerbations of asthma appear to reduce the activity of NEP at the airway surface, thus leading to exaggerated responses to tachykinins (and other peptides) and thus to increased airway inflammation.

Antagonists

Specific antagonists of tachykinin receptors have now been developed and provide a more specific tool to investigate the role of tachykinins in animal models. Several highly potent and stable peptide and nonpeptide tachykinin antagonists have recently been developed that are highly selective for either NK_1- or NK_2-receptors *(118)*. The NK_1-receptor antagonist CP 96,345 is able to block the plasma exudation response to vagus nerve stimulation and to cigaret smoke in guinea pig airways *(119,120)*, without affecting the bronchoconstrictor response, which is blocked by the NK_2-antagonist SR 48,968 *(18)*. Similar results have been obtained with the very potent NK_1-selective antagonist FK-888 *(121)*. CP 96,345 also blocks hyperpnea- and bradykinin-induced plasma exudation in guinea pigs *(122,123)*, but has no effect on the acute plasma exudation induced by allergen in sensitized animals *(123)*. These specific antagonists are very useful new tools in probing the involvement of tachykinins in disease and will be invaluable in clinical studies in the future.

Inhibition of Sensory Neuropeptide Release

Several agonists act on prejunctional receptors on airway sensory nerves to inhibit the release of neuropeptides and neurogenic inflammation *(124)* (Fig. 5). Opioids are the most effective inhibitory agonists, acting via prejunctional μ-receptors, and have been shown to inhibit cigaret smoke-induced discharge from goblet cells in guinea-pig airways in vivo *(125)* and to inhibit ozone-induced hyperreactivity in guinea pigs, which appears to be mediated via sensory nerves *(126)*. Several other agonists are also effective and may act by opening a common calcium-activated large-conductance potassium channel in sensory nerves *(127)*. Openers of other potassium channels that achieve the same hyperpolarization of the sensory nerve are also effective in blocking neurogenic inflammation in rodents *(128)* and have been shown to block cigaret smoke-induced goblet cell secretion in guinea pigs *(129)*.

NEUROGENIC INFLAMMATION IN ALLERGIC DISEASES

Although it was proposed several years ago that neurogenic inflammation and peptides released from sensory nerves might be important as an amplifying inflammation in asthma and rhinitis *(92)*, there is little direct evidence to date to support this idea, despite the extensive work in rodent models *(130,131)*. This is partly because it has proved difficult to apply the same approaches that have been used in animals to human volunteers.

Sensory Nerves in Human Respiratory Tract

In comparison with rodent airways, SP- and CGRP-immunoreactive nerves are very sparse in the human respiratory tract. Quantitative studies indicate that SP-immunoreactive fibers constitute only 1% of the total number of intraepithelial fibers, whereas in guinea pig they make up 60% of the fibers *(132)*. This raises the possibility that sensory nerves in humans may contain some unidentified transmitter that may be involved in neurogenic inflammation. Chronic inflammation may lead to changes in the pattern of innervation, through the release of neurotrophic factors from inflammatory cells. Thus in chronic arthritis and inflammatory bowel disease there is an increase in the density of SP-immunoreactive nerves *(133,134)*. A striking increase in SP-like immunoreactive nerves has been reported in the airway of patients with fatal asthma *(135)*. This increased density of nerves is particularly noticeable in the submucosa. Whether this apparent increase results from proliferation of sensory nerves or from increased synthesis of tachykinins has not yet been established. However, other studies have failed to confirm an increased in SP in lungs from patients with asthma *(136)*. After nasal challenge with allergen an increase in SP in nasal lavage fluid has been reported *(137)*. Recently, elevated concentrations of SP in bronchoalveolar lavage of patients with asthma have been reported, with a further rise after allergen challenge *(138)*, suggesting that there may be an increase in SP in the airways of asthmatic patients. Similarly, SP has been detected in the sputum of asthmatic patients after hypertonic saline inhalation *(139)*. SP also increases in the bronchoalveolar lavage of normal volunteers exposed to ozone, possible because of a reduction in NEP activity *(140)*. Both SP and CGRP increase in nasal secretions after allergen challenge *(137)*.

Cultured sensory neurons are stimulated by nerve growth factor (NGF), which markedly increases the transcription of preprotachykinin A gene, the major precursor peptide for tachykinins *(141)*. Similarly, adjuvant-induced inflammation in rat spinal cord increases the gene expression of PPT-A *(142)*. Preliminary studies suggest that allergen challenge is associated with a doubling in PPT-A messenger ribonucleic acid (mRNA) positive neurons in nodose ganglia of guinea pigs and an increase in SP-immunoreactivity in the lungs *(143)*. However, bronchial biopsies of mild asthmatic patients have not revealed any evidence of increased SP-immunoreactive nerves *(144)*. This may indicate that the increased innervation *(135)* may be a feature of either prolonged or severe asthma and indicates the need for more studies.

Sensory Nerve Activation

Sensory nerves may be activated in asthma and rhinitis and may be responsible for the symptoms of coughing and sneezing. In asthmatic airways the epithelium is often shed, thereby exposing sensory nerve endings. Sensory nerves in asthmatic airways may be "hyperalgesic" as a result of exposure to inflammatory mediators such as prostaglandins and certain cytokines (such as IL-1β and TNF-α) *(145)*. Hyperalgesic nerves may then be activated more readily by other mediators, such as kinins.

Capsaicin induces bronchoconstriction and plasma exudation in guinea pigs *(14)* and increases airway blood flow in pigs *(103)*. In humans capsaicin inhalation causes cough and a *transient* bronchoconstriction that is inhibited by cholinergic blockade and probably results from a laryngeal reflex *(146,147)*. This suggests that neuropeptide release does not occur in human airways, although it is possible that insufficient capsaicin reaches the lower respiratory tract because the dose is limited by coughing. In patients with asthma, there is no evidence that capsaicin induces a greater degree of bronchoconstriction than in normal individuals *(146)*.

Bradykinin is a potent bronchoconstrictor in asthmatic patients and also induces coughing and a sensation of chest tightness that closely mimics a naturally occurring asthma attack. Yet it is a weak constrictor of human airways in vitro, suggesting that its potent constrictor effect is mediated indirectly. Bradykinin is a potent activator of bronchial C-fibers in dogs *(148)*, and releases sensory neuropeptides from perfused rodent lungs *(149)*. In guinea pigs bradykinin instilled into the airways causes bronchoconstriction that is reduced significantly by a cholinergic antagonist (as in asthmatic patients *(150)*), and also by capsaicin pretreatment *(151)*. The plasma leakage induced by inhaled bradykinin is inhibited by an NK_1-antagonist, and bronchoconstriction by an NK_2-antagonist *(123,152)*. This indicates that bradykinin activates sensory nerves in the airways and that part of the airway response is mediated by release of constrictor peptides from capsaicin-sensitive nerves. In asthmatic patients the inhaled nonselective tachykinin antagonist FK-224 has recently been shown to reduce the bronchoconstrictor response to inhaled bradykinin and also to block the cough response in those subjects that coughed in response to bradykinin *(153)*.

Studies with NEP Inhibitors

In rodents, inhibition of NEP with thiorphan or phosphoramidon results in striking potentiation of tachykinin and sensory nerve-induced effects, and has been used as an approach to explore the potential for neurogenic inflammation in disease *(64)*. Intravenous acetorphan, which is hydrolyzed to thiorphan, was administered to asthmatic subjects, and although there was potentiation of the weal and flare response to intradermal SP, there was no effect on baseline airway caliber or on bronchoconstriction induced by the "neurogenic" trigger sodium metabisulfite *(154)*. The lack of effect could be due to inadequate inhibition of NEP in the airways, and particularly at the level of the epithelium. Nebulized thiorphan has been shown to potentiate the bronchoconstrictor response to inhaled NKA in normal and asthmatic subjects *(155,156)*, but there was no effect on baseline lung function in asthmatic patients *(156)*, indicating that there is unlikely to be any basal release of tachykinins. Similarly, acetorphan potentiates the nasal secretory response to SP in normal and rhinitic subjects to a similar extent and has no baseline effect *(157)*. NEP is strongly expressed in the human airway *(68,69)*, but there is no evidence based on immunocytochemical staining or *in situ* hybridization that it is defective in asthmatic or rhinitic airways (Baraniuk J and Barnes PJ: unpublished observations), and the fact that after inhaled thiorphan the bronchoconstrictor response to inhaled NKA is further enhanced in asthmatic subjects provides supportive functional data that NEP function may not be impaired, at least in mild asthma *(156)*. Of course, it is possible that NEP may become dysfunctional after viral infections or exposure to oxidants and thus contribute to asthma exacerbations.

Tachykinin Responsiveness

In inflammatory bowel disease there is evidence for a marked upregulation of tachykinin receptors, particularly in the vasculature, suggesting that chronic inflammation may lead to changes in tachykinin receptor expression *(158,159)*. In patients with allergic rhinitis an increased vascular response to nasally applied SP is observed *(31,160)*. There is evidence that NK_1-receptor gene expression may be increased in the lungs of asthmatic patients *(161)*. This might be owing to increased transcription in response to activation of transcription factors, such as AP-1, which are activated by cytokines such as tumor necrosis factor-α. A consensus sequence for AP-1 binding has been identified upstream of the NK_1-receptor gene *(162)*. Corticosteroids conversely reduce NK_1-receptor gene expression *(163)* presumably via an inhibitory effect on AP-1 activation.

MODULATION OF NEUROGENIC INFLAMMATION

Apart from tachykinin receptor antagonists neurogenic inflammation may be modulated by either preventing activation of sensory nerves or preventing the release of neuropeptides. Both approaches may be tried in asthmatic patients, using currently available drugs, although these approaches are not as specific as tachykinin antagonists, since the drugs used have additional effects.

Activation of sensory nerves may be inhibited by local anesthetics, but it has proved to be very difficult to achieve adequate local anesthesia of the respiratory tract. Inhalation of local anesthetics, such as lidocaine, have not been found to have consistent inhibitory effects on various airway challenges, and indeed may even promote bronchoconstriction in some patients with asthma *(164)*. This paradoxical bronchoconstriction may be due to the greater anesthesia of laryngeal afferents that are linked to a tonic NANC bronchodilator reflex *(165,168)*. Other drugs may inhibit the activation of airway sensory nerves. Cromolyn sodium and nedocromil sodium may have direct effects on airway C-fibers *(167,168)* and this might contribute to their antiasthma effect. Nedocromil sodium is highly effective against bradykinin-induced and sulfur dioxide-induced bronchoconstriction in asthmatic patients *(167,169)* which are believed to be mediated by activation of sensory nerves in the airways. In addition, nedocromil sodium, and to a much lesser extent cromolyn sodium, inhibit the eNANC neural bronchoconstriction due to tachykinin release form sensory nerves in guinea pig bronchi in vitro, indicating an effect on release of sensory neuropeptides as well as on activation *(170)*. The loop diuretic furosemide (frusemide) given by nebulization behaves in a fashion similar to nedocromil sodium and inhibits metabisulfite-induced bronchoconstriction in asthmatic patients *(171)* and also eNANC and cholinergic bronchoconstriction in guinea pig airways in vitro *(172)*. In addition, nebulized furosemide also inhibits certain types of cough *(173)*, providing further evidence for an effect on sensory nerves.

Many drugs act on prejunctional receptors to inhibit the release of neuropeptides, as discussed above. Opioids are the most effective inhibitors, but an inhaled μ-opioid agonist, the pentapeptide BW443C, was found to be ineffective in inhibiting metabisulfite-induced bronchoconstriction, which is believed to act via neural mechanisms *(174)*. One problem with BW443C is that is may be degraded by NEP in the airway epithelium and therefore may not reach a high enough concentration in the vicinity of the airway sensory nerves. Another agent that has a prejunctional modulatory effect in guinea pigs is the H_3-receptor agonist α-methyl histamine *(175)*. However, inhalation of α-methyl histamine had no effect on either resting tone or metabisulfite-induced bronchoconstriction in asthmatic patients *(176)*.

CONCLUSIONS

Neurogenic inflammation may contribute to the inflammatory responses in allergic disease of the respiratory tract and skin. Tachykinins and CGRP released from C-fibers result in vasodilatation, plasma exudation, mucus secretion, and bronchoconstriction. Although the role of neurogenic inflammation is well established in rodents, there is less evidence in humans. There is evidence for release of tachykinins in allergic rhinitis and asthma, and topical application of tachykinins has inflammatory effects. However it is unclear whether endogenous tachykinins and CGRP are important in comparison with the myriad of other mediators produced in allergic inflammation. The role of neurogenic inflammation in allergic disease will only be revealed by the use of specific inhibitors. Several drugs, including tachykinin antagonists and opioids, are already in clinical trial. It is possible that neurogenic inflammation is restricted to certain patients and may not be relevant in mild disease, on which novel drugs are usually tested, however.

REFERENCES

1. Uddman R, Hakanson R, Luts A, Sundler F (1997) Distribution of neuropeptides in airways. In: Bames PJ, ed. Autonomic Control of the Respiratory System. Harvard Academic, London, pp. 21–37.
2. Barnes PJ, Baraniuk J, Belvisi MG (1991) Neuropeptides in the respiratory tract. Am Rev Respir Dis 144:1187–1198, 1391–1399.
3. Kaliner M, Barnes PJ, Kunkel GHH, Baraniuk JN (1994) Neuropeptides in Respiratory Medicine. Marcel Dekker, New York, p. 693.
4. Pincelli C, Fantini F, Giannetti A (1993) Neuropeptides and skin inflammation. Dermatology 187: 153–158.
5. Barnes PJ (1991) Neuropeptides and asthma. Am Rev Respir Dis 143:S28–32.
6. Baraniuk JN (1990) Neural control of human nasal secretion. Pulmon Pharmacol 4:20–31.
7. Belvisi MG, Stretton CD, Barnes PJ (1992) Nitric oxide is the endogenous neurotransmitter of bronchodilator nerves in human airways. Eur J Pharmacol 210:221–222.
8. Ward JK, Belvisi MG, Fox AJ, et al. (1993) Modulation of cholinergic neural bronchoconstriction by endogenous nitric oxide and vasoactive intestinal peptide in human airways in vitro. J Clin Invest 92:736–743.
9. Solway J, Leff AR (1991) Sensory neuropeptides and airway function. J Appl Physiol 71:2077–2087.
10. Martling CR, Theodorsson-Norheim E, Lundberg JM (1987) Occurrence and effects of multiple tachykinins: substance P, neurokinin A, and neuropeptide K in human lower airways. Life Sci 40: 1633–1643.
11. Laitinen LA, Laitinen A, Panula PA, Partanen M, Tervo K, Tervo T (1983) Immunohistochemical demonstration of substance P in the lower respiratory tract of the rabbit and not of man. Thorax 38:531–536.
12. Komatsu T, Yamamoto M, Shimokata K, Nagura H (1991) Distribution of substance-P-immunoreactive and calcitonin gene-related peptide-immunoreactive nerves in normal human lungs. Int Arch Allergy Appl Immunol 95:23–28.
13. Baraniuk JN, Lundgren JD, Mullol J, Okayama M, Merida M, Kaliner M (1991) Substance P and neurokinin A (NKA) in human nasal mucosa. Am J Respir Cell Mol Biol 4:228–236.
14. Lundberg JM, Saria A, Lundblad L, et al. (1987) Bioactive peptides in capsaicin-sensitive C-fiber afferents of the airways: functional and pathophysiological implications. In: Neural Control of Airways. Kaliner M, Barnes PJ, eds. New York: Marcel Decker, pp. 417–445.
15. Dey RD, Altemus JB, Michalkiewicz M (1991) Distribution of vasoactive intestinal peptide- and substance P-containing nerves originating from neurons of airway ganglia in cat bronchi. J Comp Neurol 304:330–340.
16. Springall DR, Polak JM, Howard L, et al. (1990) Persistence of intrinsic neurones and possible phenotypic changes after extrinsic denervation of human respiratory tract by heart-lung transplantation. Am Rev Respir Dis 141:1538–1546.
17. Naline E, Devillier P, Drapeau G, et al. (1989) Characterization of neurokinin effects on receptor selectivity in human isolated bronchi. Am Rev Respir Dis 140:679–686.
18. Advenier C, Naline E, Toty L, et al. (1992) Effects on the isolated human bronchus of SR 48968, a potent and selective non-peptide antagonist of the neurokinin A (NK$_2$) receptors. Am Rev Respir Dis 146:1177–1181.
19. Frossard N, Barnes PJ (1988) Effects of tachykinins on small human airways and the influence of thiorphan. Am Rev Respir Dis 137:195A.
20. Fuller RW, Maxwell DL, Dixon CMS, et al. (1987) The effects of substance P on cardiovascular and respiratory function in human subjects. J Appl Physiol 62:14731–1479.

21. Evans TW, Dixon CM, Clarke B, Conradson TB, Barnes PJ (1988) Comparison of neurokinin A and substance P on cardiovascular and airway function in man. Br J Pharmacol 25:273–275.

22. Joos G, Pauwels R, van der Straeten ME (1987) Effect of inhaled substance P and neurokinin A in the airways of normal and asthmatic subjects. Thorax 42:779–783.

23. Cheung D, van der Veen H, den Hartig J, Dijkman JH, Sterk PJ (1995) Effects of inhaled substance P on airway responsiveness to methacholine in asthmatic subjects. J Appl Physiol 77:1325–1332.

24. Frossard N, Rhoden KJ, Barnes PJ (1989) Influence of epithelium on guinea pig airway responses to tachykinins: role of endopeptidase and cyclooxygenase. J Pharmacol Exp Ther 248:292–298.

25. Devillier P, Advenier C, Drapeau G, Marsac J, Regoli D (1988) Comparison of the effects of epithelium removal and of an enkephalinase inhibitor on the neurokinin-induced contractions of guinea pig isolated trachea. Br J Pharmacol 94:675–684.

26. Rogers DF, Aursudkij B, Barnes PJ (1989) Effects of tachykinins on mucus secretion on human bronchi in vitro. Eur J Pharmacol 174:283–286.

27. Ramnarine SI, Hirayama Y, Barnes PJ, Rogers DF (1994) "Sensory-efferent" neural control of mucus secretion: characterization using tachykinin receptor antagonists in ferret trachea in vitro. Br J Pharmacol 113:1183–1190.

28. Kuo H, Rhode JAL, Tokuyama K, Barnes PJ, Rogers DF (1990) Capsaicin and sensory neuropeptide stimulation of goblet cell secretion in guinea pig trachea. J Physiol 431:629–641.

29. Tokuyama K, Kuo H, Rohde JAL, Barnes PJ, Rogers DF (1990) Neural control of goblet cell secretion in guinea pig airways. Am J Physiol 259:L108–L115.

30. Kuo H, Barnes PJ, Rogers DF (1992) Cigarette smoke-induced airway goblet cell secretion: dose dependent differential nerve activation. Am J Physiol 7:L161–L167.

31. Braunstein G, Pajac I, Lacronique J, Frossard N (1991) Clinical and inflammatory responses to exogenous tachykinins in allergic rhinitis. Am Rev Respir Dis 144:630–636.

32. Rogers DF, Belvisi MG, Aursudkij B, Evans TW, Barnes PJ (1988) Effects and interactions of sensory neuropeptides on airway microvascular leakage in guinea pigs. Br J Pharmacol 95:1109–1116.

33. Sertl K, Wiedermann CJ, Kowalski ML, et al. (1988) Substance P: the relationship between receptor distribution in rat lung and the capacity of substance P to stimulate vascular permeability. Am Rev Respir Dis 133:151–159.

34. Lövall JO, Lemen RJ, Hui KP, Barnes PJ, Chung KF (1990) Airflow obstruction after substance P aerosol: contribution of airway and pulmonary edema. J Appl Physiol 69:1473–1478.

35. Fuller RW, Conradson T, Dixon CMS, Crossman DC, Barnes PJ (1987) Sensory neuropeptide effects in human skin. Br J Pharmacol 92:781–788.

36. Salonen RO, Webber SE, Widdicombe JG (1988) Effects of neuropeptides and capsaicin on the canine tracheal vasculature in vivo. Br J Pharmacol 95:1262–1270.

37. Matran R, Alving K, Martling CR, Lacroix JS, Lundberg JM (1989) Effects of neuropeptides and capsaicin on tracheobronchial blood flow in the pig. Acta Physiol Scand 135:335–342.

38. McCormack DG, Salonen RO, Barnes PJ (1989) Effect of sensory neuropeptides on canine bronchial and pulmonary vessels in vitro. Life Sci 45:2405–2412.

39. Hall AK, Barnes PJ, Meldrum LA, Maclagan J (1989) Facilitation by tachykinins of neurotransmission in guinea-pig pulmonary parasympathetic nerves. Br J Pharmacol 97:274–280.

40. Undem BJ, Myers AC, Barthlow H, Weinreich D (1991) Vagal innervation of guinea pig bronchial smooth muscle. J Appl Physiol 69:1336–1346.

41. Watson N, Maclagan J, Barnes PJ (1993) Endogenous tachykinins facilitate transmission through parasympathetic ganglia in guinea-pig trachea. Br J Pharmacol 109:751–759.

42. Myers AC, Undem BJ (1993) Electrophysiological effects of tachykinins and capsaicin on guinea-pig parasympathetic ganglia. J Physiol 470:66–679.

43. Martling C, Saria A, Andersson P, Lundberg JM (1984) Capsaicin pretreatment inhibits vagal cholinergic and noncholinergic control of pulmonary mechanisms in guinea pig. Naunyn Schmiedeberg Arch Pharm 325:343–348.

44. Stretton CD, Belvisi MG, Barnes PJ (1992) The effect of sensory nerve depletion on cholinergic neurotransmission in guinea pig airways. J Pharmacol Exp Ther 260:1073–1080.

45. Belvisi MG, Patacchini R, Barnes PJ, Maggi CA (1994) Facilitatory effects of selective agonists for tachykinin receptors on cholinergic neurotransmission: evidence for species differences. Br J Pharmacol 111:103–110.

46. Black JL, Johnson PR, Alouvan L, Armour CL (1990) Neurokinin A with K^+ channel blockade potentiates contraction to electrical stimulation in human bronchus. Eur J Pharmacol 180:311–317.

47. Kohrogi H, Graf PPD, Sekizawa K, Borson DB, Nadel JA (1988) Neutral endopeptidase inhibitors potentiate substance P and capsaicin-induced cough in awake guinea pigs. J Clin Invest 82:2063–2070.
48. Advenier C, Girard V, Naline E, Vilain P, Emons-Alt X (1992) Antitussive effect of SR 48968, a non-peptide tachykinin NK_2 receptor antagonist. Eur J Pharmacol 250:169–171.
49. McGillis JP, Organist ML, Payan DG (1987) Substance P and immunoregulation. Fed Proc 14:120–123.
50. Daniele RP, Barnes PJ, Goetzl EJ, et al. (1992) Neuroimmune interactions in the lung. Am Rev Respir Dis 145:1230–1235.
51. Nohr D, Weihe E (1991) The neuroimmune link in the bronchus-associated lymphoid tissue (BALT) of cat and rat: peptides and neural markers. Brain Behav Immun 5:84–101.
52. Lowman MA, Benyon RC, Church MK (1988) Characterization of neuropeptide-induced histamine release from human dispersed skin mast cells. Br J Pharmacol 95:121–130.
53. Ali H, Leung KBI, Pearce FL, Hayes NA, Foremean JC (1986) Comparison of histamine releasing activity of substance P on mast cells and basophils from different species and tissues. Int Arch Allergy 79:121–124.
54. Kroegel C, Giembycz MA, Barnes PJ (1990) Characterization of eosinophil activation by peptides. Differential effects of substance P, mellitin, and f-met-leu-phe. J Immunol 145:2581–2587.
55. Numao T, Agrawal DK (1992) Neuropeptides modulate human eosinophil chemotaxis. J Immunol 149:3309–3315.
56. Brunelleschi S, Vanni L, Ledda F, Giotti A, Maggi CA, Fantozzi R (1990) Tachykinins activate guinea pig alveolar macrophages: involvement of NK_2 and NK_1 receptors. Br J Pharmacol 100:417–420.
57. Lotz M, Vaughn JH, Carson DM (1988) Effect of neuropeptides on production of inflammatory cytokines by human monocytes. Science 241:1218–1221.
58. Okamoto Y, Shirotori K, Kudo K, Ishikawa K, Ito E, Togawa K (1995) Cytokine expression after the topical administration of substance P to human nasal mucosa. J Immunol 151:4391–4398.
59. Umeno E, Nadel JA, Huang HT, McDonald DM (1989) Inhibition of neutral endopeptidase potentiates neurogenic inflammation in the rat trachea. J Appl Physiol 66:2647–2652.
60. Smith CH, Barker JNWH, Morris RW, McDonald DM, Lee TH (1993) Neuropetides induce rapid expression of endothelial cell adhesion molecules and elicit granulocytic infiltration in human skin. J Immunol 151:3274–3282.
61. Fan T, Hu DE, Guard S, Gresham GA, Watling KJ (1993) Stimulation of angiogenesis by substance P and Interleukin-1 in the rat and its inhibition by NK_1 or interleukin-1 receptor antagonists. Br Pharmacol 110:43–49.
62. Kuwano K, Boskev CH, Paré PD, Bai TR, Wiggs BR, Hogg JC (1993) Small airways dimensions in asthma and chronic obstructive pulmonary disease. Am Rev Respir Dis 148:1220–1225.
63. Harrison NK, Dawes KE, Kwon OJ, Barnes PJ, Laurent GJ, Chung KF (1995) Effects of neuropeptides in human lung fibroblast proliferation and chemotaxis. Am J Physiol 12:L278–283.
64. Nadel JA (1991) Neutral endopeptidase modulates neurogenic inflammation. Eur Resp J 4:745–754.
65. Shore SA, Stimler-Gerard NP, Coats SR, Drazen JM (1988) Substance P induced bronchoconstriction in guinea pig. Enhancement by inhibitors of neutral metalloendopeptidase and angiotensin converting enzyme. Am Rev Respir Dis 137:331–336.
66. Martins MA, Shore SA, Gerard NP, Gerald C, Drazen JM (1990) Peptidase modulation of the pulmonary effects of tachykinins in tracheal superfused guinea pig lungs. J Clin Invest 85:170–176.
67. Lötvall JO, Skoogh B, Barnes PJ, Chung KF (1990) Effects of aerosolized substance P on lung resistance in guinea pigs: a comparison between inhibition of neutral endopeptidase and angiotensin-converting enzyme. Br J Pharmacol 100:69–72.
68. Baraniuk JN, Ohkubo K, Kwon OJ, et al. (1993) Localization of neutral endopeptidase mRNA in human nasal mucosa. J Appl Physiol 74:272–279.
69. Baraniuk JN, Ohkubo O, Kwon OJ, et al. (1995) Localization of neutral endopeptidase (NEP) mRNA in human bronchi. Eur Respir J 8:1458–1464.
70. Sekizawa K, Tamaoki J, Graf PD, Basbaum CB, Borson DB, Nadel JA (1987) Enkephalinase inhibitors potentiate mammalian tachykinin-induced contraction in ferret trachea. J Pharmacol Exp Ther 243:1211–1217.
71. Black JL, Johnson PRA, Armour CL (1988) Potentiation of the contractile effects of neuropeptides in human bronchus by an enkephalinase inhibitor. Pulmon Pharmacol 1:21–23.
72. Djokic TD, Nadel JA, Dusser DJ, Sekizawa K, Graf PD, Borson DB (1989) Inhibitors of neutral endopeptidase potentiate electrically and capsaicin-induced non-cholinergic contraction in guinea pig bronchi. J Pharmacol Exp Ther 248:7–11.

73. Martling CR (1987) Sensory nerves containing tachykinins and CGRP in the lower airways: functional implications for bronchoconstriction, vasodilation, and protein extavasation. Acta Physiol Scand Suppl 563:1–57.

74. Palmer JBD, Cuss FMC, Mulderry PK, et al. (1987) Calcitonin gene-related peptide is localized to human airway nerves and potently constricts human airway smooth muscle. Br J Pharmacol 91:95–101.

75. Uddman R, Luts A, Sundler F (1985) Occurrence and distribution of calcitonin gene related peptide in the mammalian respiratory tract and middle ear. Cell Tissue Res 214:551–555.

76. McCormack DG, Mak JCW, Coupe MO, Barnes PJ (1989) Calcitonin gene-related peptide vasodilation of human pulmonary vessels: receptor mapping and functional studies. J Appl Physiol 67:1265–1270.

77. Salonen RO, Webber SE, Widdicombe JG (1988) Effects of neuropeptides and capsaicin on the canine tracheal vasculature in vivo. Br J Pharmacol 95:1262–1270.

78. Parsons GH, Nichol GM, Barnes PJ, Chung KF (1992) Peptide mediator effects on bronchial blood velocity and lung resistance in conscious sheep. J Appl Physiol 72:1118–1122.

79. Mak JCW, Barnes PJ (1988) Autoradiographic localization of calcitonin gene-related peptide binding sites in human and guinea pig lung. Peptides 9:957–964.

80. Khalil Z, Andrews PV, Helme RD (1988) VIP modulates substance P induced plasma extravasation in vivo. Eur J Pharmacol 151:281–287.

81. Brockaw JJ, White GW (1992) Calcitonin gene-related peptide potentiates substance P-induced plasma extravasation in the rat trachea. Lung 170:89–93.

82. Martling CR, Saria A, Fischer JA, Hokfelt T, Lundberg JM (1988) Calcitonin gene related peptide and the lung: neuronal coexistence and vasodilatory effect. Regulatory Peptides 20:125–139.

83. Ninomiya H, Uchida Y, Endo T, et al. (1995) Calcitonin gene-related peptide is a bronchoconstrictor or a bronchodilator? Am J Respir Crit Care Med 151:A108.

84. Webber SG, Lim JCS, Widdicombe JG (1991) The effects of calcitonin gene related peptide on submucosal gland secretion and epithelial albumin transport on ferret trachea in vitro. Br J Pharmacol 102:79–84.

85. Pietrowski W, Foreman JC (1986) Some effects of calcitonin gene related peptide in human skin and on histamine release. Br J Dermatol 114:37–46.

86. Haynes LW, Manley C (1988) Chemotactic response of guinea pig polymorphonucleocytes in vivo to rat calcitonin gene related peptide and proteolytic fragments. J Physiol 43:79P.

87. Umeda Y, Arisawa H (1989) Characterization of the calcitonin gene related peptide receptor in mouse T lymphocytes. Neuropeptides 14:237–242.

88. Nong YH, Titus RG, Riberio JM, Remold HG (1989) Peptides encoded by the calcitonin gene inhibit macrophage function. J Immunol 143:45–49.

89. White SR, Hershenson MB, Sigrist KS, Zimmerman A, Solway J (1993) Proliferation of guinea pig tracheal epithelial cells induced by calcitonin gene-related peptide. Am J Respir Cell Mol Biol 8:592–596.

90. Barnes PJ (1990) Neurogenic inflammation in airways and its modulation. Arch Int Pharmacodyn 303:67–82.

91. McDonald DM (1987) Neurogenic inflammation in the respiratory tract: actions of sensory nerve mediators on blood vessels and epithelium of the airway mucosa. Am Rev Respir Dis 136:S65–S72.

92. Barnes PJ (1986) Asthma as an axon reflex. Lancet i:242–245.

93. Barnes PJ (1991) Sensory nerves, neuropeptides and asthma. Ann NY Acad Sci 629:359–370.

94. Lundberg JM, Saria A (1983) Capsaicin-induced desensitization of the airway mucosa to cigarette smoke, mechanical and chemical irritants. Nature 302:251–253.

95. Ray DW, Hernandez C, Leff AR, Drazen JM, Solway J (1989) Tachykinins mediate bronchoconstriction elicited by isocapnic hyperpnea in guinea pigs. J Appl Physiol 66:1108–1112.

96. Reynolds AM, McEvoy RD (1989) Tachykinins mediate hypocapnia-induced bronchoconstriction in guinea pigs. J Appl Physiol 67:2454–2460.

97. Sakamoto T, Elwood W, Barnes PJ, Chung KF (1992) Pharmacological modulation of inhaled metabisulphite-induced airway microvascular leakage and bronchoconstriction in guinea pig. Br J Pharmacol 107:481–488.

98. Umeno E, McDonald DM, Nadel JA (1990) Hypertonic saline increases vascular permeability in the rat trachea by producing neurogenic inflammation. J Clin Invest 85:1905–1908.

99. Thompson JE, Scypinski LA, Gordon T, Sheppard D (1987) Tachykinins mediate the acute increase in airway responsiveness by toluene diisocyanate in guinea-pigs. Am Rev Respir Dis 136:43–49.

100. Lötvall JO, Hui KP, Löfdahl C, Barnes PJ, Chung KF (1991) Capsaicin pretreatment does not inhibit allergen-induced airway microvascular leakage in guinea pig. Allergy 46:105–108.

101. Hsiug T, Garland A, Ray DW, Hershenson MB, Leff AR, Solway J (1992) Endogenous sensory neuropeptide release enhances non specific airway responsiveness in guinea pigs. Am Rev Respir Dis 146:148–153.

102. Ladenius ARC, Folkerts G, van der Linde HJ, Nijkamp FP (1995) Potentiation by viral respiratory infection of ovalbumin-induced guinea-pig tracheal hyperresponsiveness: role for tachykinins. Br J Pharmacol 115:1048–1052.

103. Alving K, Matran R, Lacroix JS, Lundberg JM (1988) Allergen challenge induces vasodilation in pig bronchial circulation via a capsaicin sensitive mechanism. Acta Physiol Scand 134:571–572.

104. Abraham WM, Ahmed A, Cortes A, Delehunt JC (1993) C-fiber desensitization prevents hyperresponsiveness to cholinergic and antigen stimuli after antigen challenge in allergic sheep. Am Rev Respir Dis 147:A478.

105. Matsuse T, Thomson RJ, Chen X, Salari H, Schellenberg RR (1991) Capsaicin inhibits airway hyperresponsiveness, but not airway lipoxygenase activity nor eosinophilia following repeated aerosolized antigen in guinea pigs. Am Rev Respir Dis 144:368–372.

106. Ladenius ARC, Nijkamp FP (1993) Capsaicin pretreatment of guinea pigs in vivo prevents ovalbumin-induced tracheal hyperreactivity in vitro. Eur J Pharmacol 235:127–131.

107. Riccio MM, Manzini S, Page CP (1993) The effect of neonatal capsaicin in the development of bronchial hyperresponsiveness in allergic rabbits. Eur J Pharmacol 232:89–97.

108. Bienenstock J, Perdue M, Blennerhassett M, et al. (1988) Inflammatory cells and epithelium: mast cell/nerve interactions in lung in vitro and in vivo. Am Rev Respir Dis 138:S31–S34.

109. Leff AR, Stimler NP, Munoz NM, Shioya T, Tallet J, Dame C (1982) Augmentation of respiratory mast cell secretion of histamine caused by vagal nerve stimulation during antigen challenge. J Immunol 136:1066–1073.

110. Sestini P, Bienenstock J, Crowe SE, et al. (1990) Ion transport in rat tracheal ganglion in vitro. Role of capsaicin-sensitive nerves in allergic reactions. Am Rev Respir Dis 141:393–397.

111. Saban R, Dick EC, Fishlever RI, Buckner CK (1987) Enhancement of parainfluenza 3 infection of contractile responses to substance P and capsaicin in airway smooth muscle from guinea pig. Am Rev Respir Dis 136:586–591.

112. Jacoby DB, Tamaoki J, Borson DB, Nadel JA (1988) Influenza infection increases airway smooth muscle responsiveness to substance P in ferrets by decreasing enkephalinase. J Appl Physiol 64:2653–2658.

113. Piedimonte G, Nadel JA, Umeno E, McDonald DM (1990) Sendai virus infection potentiates neurogenic inflammation in the rat trachea. J Appl Physiol 68:754–760.

114. Dusser DJ, Djocic TD, Borson DB, Nadel JA (1989) Cigarette smoke induces bronchoconstrictor hyperresponsiveness to substance P and inactivates airway neutral endopeptidase in the guinea pig. J Clin Invest 84:900–906.

115. Sheppard D, Thompson JE, Scypinski L, Dusser DJ, Nadel JA, Borson DB (1988) Toluene diisocyanate increases airway responsiveness to substance P and decreases airway neutral endopeptidase. J Clin Invest 81:1111–1115.

116. Tsukagoshi H, Sun J, Kwon O, Barnes PJ, Chung KF (1995) Role of neutral endopeptidase in bronchial hyperresponsiveness to bradykinin induced by IL-1β. J Appl Physiol 78:921–927.

117. Tsugoshi H, Haddad E, Sun J, Barnes PJ, Chung KF (1995) Ozone-induced airway hyperresponsiveness: role of superoxide anions, neutral endopeptidase, and bradykinin receptors. J Appl Physiol 78:1015–1022.

118. Watling KJ (1992) Non peptide antagonists heralded a new era in tachykinin research. Trends Pharmacol Sci 13:266–269.

119. Lei Y, Barnes PJ, Rogers DF (1992) Inhibition of neurogenic plasma exudation in guinea pig airways by CP-96,345, a new non-peptide NK$_1$-receptor antagonist. Br J Pharmacol 105:261,262.

120. Delay-Goyet P, Lundberg JM (1991) Cigarette smoke-induced airway oedema is blocked by the NK$_1$-antagonist CP-96,345. Eur J Pharmacol 203:157–158.

121. Hirayama Y, Lei YH, Barnes PJ, Rogers DF (1993) Effects of two novel tachykinin antagonists FK 224 and FK 888 on neurogenic plasma exudation, bronchoconstriction and systemic hypotension in guinea pigs in vivo. Br J Pharmacol 108:844–851.

122. Solway J, Kao BM, Jordan JE, et al. (1993) Tachykinin receptor antagonists inhibit hypernea-induced bronchoconstriction in guinea pigs. J Clin Invest 92:315–323.

123. Sakamoto T, Barnes PJ, Chung KF (1993) Effect of CP-96,345, a non-peptide NK_1-receptor antagonist against substance P-, bradykinin-, and allergen-induced airway microvascular leak and bronchoconstriction in the guinea pig. Eur J Pharmcol 231:31–38.

124. Barnes PJ, Belvisi MG, Rogers DF (1990) Modulation of neurogenic inflammation: novel approaches to inflammatory diseases. Trends Pharmacol Sci 11:185–189.

125. Kuo H, Rohde J, Barnes PJ, Rogers DF (1992) Differential effects of opioids on cigarette smoke, capsaicin and electrically-induced goblet cell secretion in guinea pig trachea. Br J Pharmacol 105:361–366.

126. Yeadon M, Wilkinson D, Darley-Usmar V, O'Leary VJ, Payne AN (1992) Mechanisms contributing to ozone-induced bronchial hyperreactivity in guinea pigs. Pulmon Pharmacol 5:39–50.

127. Stretton CD, Miura M, Belvisi MG, Barnes PJ (1992) Calcium-activated potassium channels mediate prejunctional inhibition of peripheral sensory nerves. Proc Natl Acad Sci USA 89:1325–1329.

128. Ichinose M, Barnes PJ (1990) A potassium channel activator modulates both noncholinergic and cholinergic neurotransmission in guinea pig airways. J Pharmacol Exp Ther 252:1207–1212.

129. Kuo H, Rohde JAL, Barnes PJ, Rogers DF (1992) K^+ channel activator inhibition of neurogenic goblet cell secretion in guinea pig trachea. Eur J Pharmacol 221:385–388.

130. Barnes PJ (1994) Neuropeptides and asthma. In: Kaliner MA, Barnes PJ, Kunkel GHH, Baraniuk, JN, eds. Neuropeptides in Respiratory Medicine, New York: Marcel Dekker, pp. 285–311.

131. Joos GF, Germonpre PR, Pauwels RA (1995) Neurogenic inflammation in human airways: is it important? Thorax 50:217–219.

132. Bowden J, Gibbins IL (1992) Relative density of substance P-immunoreactive nerve fibres in the tracheal epithelium of a range of species. FASEB J 6:A1276.

133. Levine JD, Dardick SJ, Roizan MF, Helms C, Basbaum AI (1986) Contribution of sensory afferents and sympathetic efferents to joint injury in experimental arthritis. J Neurosci 6:3423–3429.

134. Holzer P (1988) Local effector functions of capsaicin-sensitive sensory nerve endings: involvement of tachykinins, calcitonin gene related peptide, and other neuropeptides. Neuroscience 24:739–768.

135. Ollerenshaw SL, Jarvis D, Sullivan CE, Woolcock AJ (1991) Substance P immunoreactive nerves in airways from asthmatics and non-asthmatics. Eur Resp J 4:673–682.

136. Lilly CM, Bai TR, Shore SA, Hall AE, Drazen JM (1995) Neuropeptide content of lungs from asthmatic and nonasthmatic patients. Am J Respir Crit Care Med 151:548–553.

137. Mosiman BL, White MV, Hohman RJ, Goldrich MS, Kaulbach HC, Kaliner MA (1993) Substance P, calcitonin gene-related peptide and vasoactive intestinal peptide increase in nasal secretions after allergen challenge in atopic patients. J Allergy Clin Immunol 92:95–104.

138. Nieber K, Baumgarten CR, Rathsack R, Furkert J, Oehame P, Kunkel G (1992) Substance P and b-endorphin-like immunoreactivity in lavage fluids of subjects with and without asthma. J Allergy Clin Immunol 90:646–652.

139. Tomaki M, Ichinose M, Miura M, et al. (1995) Elevated substance P content in induced sputum from patients with asthma and patients with chronic bronchitis. Am J Respir Crit Care Med 151:613–617.

140. Hazbun ME, Hamilton R, Holian A, Eschenbacher WL (1993) Ozone-induced increases in substance P and 8 epi-prostaglandin F_{2a} in the airways of human subjects. Am J Resp Cell Mol Biol 9:568–572.

141. Lindsay RM, Harmar AJ (1989) Nerve growth factor regulates expression of neuropeptide genes in sensory neurons. Nature 337:362–364.

142. Minami M, Kuraishi Y, Kawamura M, Yamaguchi T, Masu Y, Nakanishi S (1989) Enhancement of preprotachykinin A gene expression by adjuvant-induced inflammation in the rat spinal cord: possible inducement of substance P-containing spinal neurons in nociceptor. Neurosci Lett 98:105–110.

143. Fischer A, Philippin B, Saria A, McGregor G, Kummer W (1994) Neuronal plasticity in sensitized and challenged guinea pigs: neuropeptides and neuropeptide gene expression. Am J Resp Crit Care Med 149:A890.

144. Howarth PH, Djukanovic R, Wilson JW, Holgate ST, Springall DR, Polak JM (1991) Mucosal nerves in endobronchial biopsies in asthma and non-asthma. Int Arch Allergy Appl Immunol 94:330–333.

145. Cunha FQ, Poole S, Lorenzetti BB, Ferreira SH (1992) The pivotal role of tumour necrosis factor a in the development of inflammatory hyperalgesia. Br J Pharmacol 107:660–664.

146. Fuller RW, Dixon CMS, Barnes PJ (1985) The bronchoconstrictor response to inhaled capsaicin in humans. J Appl Physiol 85:1080–1084.

147. Midgren B, Hansson L, Karlsson JA, Simonsson BG, Persson CGA (1992) Capsaicin-induced cough in humans. Am Rev Respir Dis 146:347–351.

148. Kaufman MP, Coleridge HM, Coleridge JCG, Baker DG (1980) Bradykinin stimulates afferent vagal C-fibers in intrapulmonary airways of dogs. J Appl Physiol 48:511–517.

149. Saria A, Martling CR, Yan Z, Theodorsson-Norheim E, Gamse R, Lundberg JM (1988) Release of multiple tachykinins from capsaicin-sensitive nerves in the lung by bradykinin, histamine, dimethyl-phenylpiperainium, and vagal nerve stimulation. Am Rev Respir Dis 137:1330–1335.

150. Fuller RW, Dixon CMS, Cuss FMC, Barnes PJ (1987) Bradykinin-induced bronchoconstriction in man: mode of action. Am Rev Respir Dis 135:176–180.

151. Ichinose M, Belvisi MG, Barnes PJ (1990) Bradykinin-induced bronchoconstriction in guinea-pig in vivo: role of neural mechanisms. J Pharmacol Exp Ther 253:1207–1212.

152. Sakamoto T, Tsukagoshi H, Barnes PJ, Chung KF (1993) Role played by NK_2 receptors and cyclooxygenase activation in bradykinin B_2 receptor-mediated airway effects in guinea pigs. Ag Act 111:117.

153. Ichinose M, Nakajima N, Takahashi T, Yamauchi H, Inoue H, Takishima T (1992) Protection against bradykinin-induced bronchoconstriction in asthmatic patients by a neurokinin receptor antagonist. Lancet 340:1248–1251.

154. Nichol GM, O'Connor BJ, Le Compte JM, Chung KF, Barnes PJ (1992) Effect of neutral endopeptidase inhibitor on airway function and bronchial responsiveness in asthmatic subjects. Eur J Clin Pharmacol 42:495–498.

155. Cheung D, Bel EH, den Hartigh J, Dijkman JH, Sterk PJ (1992) An effect of an inhaled neutral endopep-tidase inhibitor, thiorphan, on airway responses to neurokinin A in normal humans in vivo. Am Rev Respir Dis 145:1275–1280.

156. Cheung D, Timmers MC, Bel EH, den Hartigh J, Dijuman JH, Sterk PJ (1992) An isolated neutral endopeptidase inhibitor, thiorphan, enhances airway narrowing to neurokinin A in asthmatic subjects in vivo. Am Rev Respir Dis 195:A682.

157. Lurie A, Nadel JA, Roisman G, Siney H, Dusser DJ (1994) Role of neutral endopeptidase and kininase II in substance P-induced increase in nasal obstruction in patients with allergic rhinitis. Am J Respir Crit Care Med 149:113–117.

158. Mantyh CR, Gates TS, Zimmerman RP, et al. (1988) Receptor binding sites for substance P but not sub-stance K or neuromedin K are expressed in high concentrations by arterioles, venules and lymph nodes in surgical specimens obtained from patients with ulcerative colitis and Crohns disease. Proc Natl Acad Sci USA 85:3235–3259.

159. Mantyh PW (1991) Substance P and the inflammatory and immune response. Ann NY Acad Sci 632:263–271.

160. Devillier P, Dessanges JF, Rakotashanaka F, Ghaem A, Boushey HA, Lockhart A (1988) Nasal response to substance P and methacholine with and without allergic rhinitis. Eur Respir J 1:356–361.

161. Adcock IM, Peters M, Gelder C, Shirasaki H, Brown CR, Barnes PJ (1993) Increased tachykinin recep-tor gene expression in asthmatic lung and its modulation by steroids. J Mol Endocrinol 11:1–7.

162. Nakanishi S (1991) Mammalian tachykinin receptors. Ann Rev Neurosci 14:123–136.

163. Ihara H, Nakanishi S (1990) Selective inhibition of expression of the substance P receptor mRNA in pancreatic acinar AR42J cells by glucocorticoids. J Biol Chem 36:22,441–22,445.

164. McAlpine LG, Thomson NC (1989) Lidocaine-induced bronchoconstriction in asthmatic patients. Relation to histamine airway responsiveness and effect of preservative. Chest 96:1012–1015.

165. Lammers J, Minette P, McCusker M, Chung KF, Barnes PJ (1988) Nonadrenergic bronchodilator mech-anisms in normal human subjects in vivo. J Appl Physiol 64:1817–1822.

166. Lammers J-WJ, Minette P, McCusker M, Chung KF, Barnes PJ (1989) Capsaicin-induced broncho-dilatation in mild asthmatic subjects: possible role of nonadrenergic inhibitory system. J Appl Physiol 67:856–861.

167. Dixon N, Jackson DM, Richards IM (1979) The effect of sodium cromoglycate on lung irritant recep-tors and left ventricular receptors in anaesthetized dogs. Br J Pharmacol 67:569–574.

168. Jackson DM, Norris AA, Eady RP (1989) Nedocromil sodium and sensory nerves in the dog lung. Pulmon Pharmacol 2:179–184.

169. Dixon CMS, Fuller RW, Barnes PJ (1987) The effect of nedocromil sodium on sulphur dioxide induced bronchoconstriction. Thorax 42:462–465.

170. Verleden GM, Belvisi MG, Stretton CD, Barnes PJ (1991) Nedocromil sodium modulates non-adrenergic non-cholinergic bronchoconstrictor nerves in guinea-pig airways in vitro. Am Rev Respir Dis 143:114–118.

171. Nichol GM, Alton EWFW, Nix A, Geddes DM, Chung KF, Barnes PJ (1990) Effect of inhaled furosemide on metabisulfite- and methacholine induced bronchoconstriction and nasal potential differ-ence in asthmatic subjects. Am Rev Respir Dis 142:576–580.

172. Elwood W, Lötvall JO, Barnes PJ, Chung KF (1991) Loop diuretics inhibit cholinergic and non-cholinergic nerves in guinea pig airways. Am Rev Respir Dis 143:1340–1344.

173. Ventresca GP, Nichol GM, Barnes PJ, Chung KF (1990) Inhaled furosemide inhibits cough induced by low chloride content solutions but not by capsaicin. Am Rev Respir Dis 142:143–146.

174. O'Connor BJ, Chen-Wordsell M, Barnes PJ, Chung KF (1991) Effect of an inhaled opioid peptide on airway responses to sodium metabisulphite in asthma. Thorax.

175. Ichinose M, Belvisi MG, Barnes PJ (1990) Histamine H_3-receptors inhibit neurogenic microvascular leakage in airways. J Appl Physiol 68:21–25.

176. O'Connor BJ, Lecomte JM, Barnes PJ (1993) Effect of an inhaled H_3-receptor agonist on airway responses to sodium metabisulphite in asthma. Br J Clin Pharmacol 35:55–57.

11

Inflammation
Th1/Th2 Cells

Sergio Romagnani, MD

INTRODUCTION

Atopic allergy is a genetically determined disorder characterized by an increased ability of B-lymphocytes to form immunoglobulin E (IgE) antibodies to certain groups of ubiquitous antigens that can activate the immune system after inhalation or ingestion, and perhaps after penetration through the skin (allergens). IgE antibodies are able to bind to high-affinity (type I) Fcε receptors (FcεRI) present on the surface of mast cells/basophils, and allergen-induced FcεRI cross linking triggers the release of vasoactive mediators, chemotactic factors, and cytokines that are responsible for the allergic cascade. In addition to IgE-producing B-cells and IgE-binding mast cells/basophils, eosinophils also appear to be involved in the pathogenesis of allergic reactions, since these cells usually accumulate in the sites of allergic inflammation and the toxic products they release significantly contribute to the induction of tissue damage. The mechanisms accounting for the joint involvement of IgE-producing B-cells, mast cells/basophils, and eosinophils in the pathogenesis of allergic reactions had remained unclear until the existence of two polarized forms of the cluster differentiation (CD)4+ T-helper (Th) cell-mediated specific immune response, based on their profile of cytokine production and defined as type 1 T-helper (Th1) and type 2 T-helper (Th2), was discovered *(1)*.

DEFINITION OF CD4+ Th1 AND Th2 CELLS

Th1 cells produce interferon γ (IFNγ), interleukin (IL)-2, and tumor necrosis factor (TNF) β, and promote the production of opsonizing and complement-fixing antibodies, macrophage activation, antibody-dependent cell cytotoxicity, and delayed-type hypersensitivity (DTH) *(1)*.

From: *Allergy and Allergic Diseases: The New Mechanisms and Therapeutics*
Edited by: J. A. Denburg © Humana Press Inc., Totowa, NJ

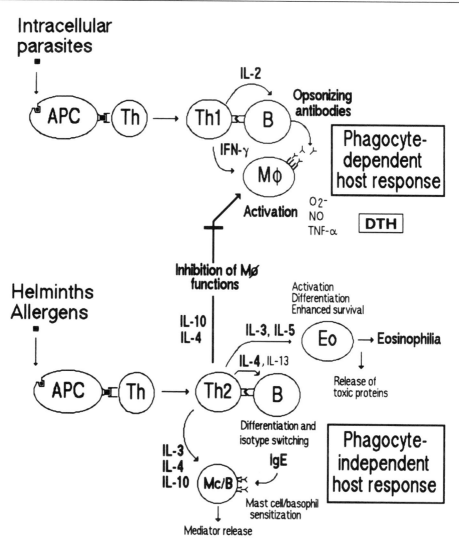

Fig. 1. Two main pathways of specific Th cell-mediated immunity based on their dependence on or independence of phagocyte recruitment in the effector response. Here and in Fig. 2: Th, CD4[+] helper T-lymphocyte; CD8[+], CD8[+] T-lymphocyte; NK, natural killer cell; B, B-lymphocyte; DTH, delayed type hypersensitivity; Eo, eosinophil; APC, antigen-presenting cell; Mc/B, cell of the mast cell/basophil lineage; CD4[+] NK1.1[+] cell, cell subset showing both T-cell and NK cell markers. (Adapted with permission from ref. *3*.)

For these reasons, Th1 cells can be considered as responsible for the phagocyte-dependent host response *(1–3)* (Fig. 1). On the other hand, Th2 cells produce IL-4, IL-5, IL-6, IL-9, IL-10, and IL-13 and provide optimal help for humoral immune responses, including IgE and IgG$_1$ isotype switching, and mucosal immunity, through production of mast cell and eosinophil growth and differentiation and facilitation to IgA synthesis. Moreover, some Th2-derived cytokines, such as IL-4, IL-10, and IL-13 inhibit several macrophage functions *(1,2)*. Therefore, it is possible to refer to Th2 cells as responsible for the phagocyte-independent host responses *(1–3)* (Fig. 1). In the absence of clear polarizing signals, CD4[+] T-cell subsets with a less differentiated lymphokine profile than Th1 or Th2 cells, designated Th0, usually arise, which mediate intermediate effects depending on the ratio of lymphokines produced and the nature of the responding cells (1,2). Th0 cells probably represent an heterogenous population of effector cells. The cytokine response of the single Th0 cell can remain mixed or further differentiate into the polarized Th1 or Th2 pathway in subjects with a particular genetic background or under the influence of strong (and/or chronic) microenvironmental signals (4). Another possibility is that cytokine profiles are largely random at the clonal level and the exogenous signals that appear to direct T-cells to differentiate into Th1 or Th2 cells act by incresing the probability of expression of certain cytokine genes at the population level, rather than by activating the expression of a cassette of transcriptionally linked genes in the individual cell (5). Finally, we often speak of CD4$^+$ T-cells that have been differentiated to produce IL-4 but not IFNγ as Th2 (or Th2-like) cells and those that produce IFNγ but not IL-4 as Th1 (or Th1-like) cells, without taking into account the other set of Th1 or Th2 cytokines. With all these points in mind, the Th1/Th2 model provides a useful paradigm for the understanding of several pathophysiologic processes and possibly for the development of novel immunotherapeutic strategies.

FUNCTIONAL AND PHENOTYPIC PROPERTIES OF Th1 AND Th2 CELLS

There is strong evidence for the existence of human CD4$^+$ Th cells with cytokine patterns and functions that are comparable to murine Th1 and Th2 cells (6–8), although in humans the expression of some cytokines, such as IL-2, IL-6, IL-10, and IL-13, may be less restricted (Table 1). Human Th1-like and Th2-like cells also differ in their cytolytic potential, mode of help for B-cell antibody synthesis, as well as the ability to activate monocytic cells (Table 1). More recently, we have shown that two activation markers, CD30 and lymphocyte activation gene-3 (LAG-3), are preferentially associated with activated Th2 and Th1 cells, respectively.

CD30, a member of the TNF receptor family (9), is consistently expressed, and its soluble form (sCD30) released, by activated Th2 and Th0 clones, whereas Th1 clones usually showed poor or no CD30 expression (10). Accordingly, costimulation of Th0 or Th2 clones with an agonistic anti-CD30 monoclonal antibody resulted in increase of antigen (Ag)-induced proliferation and cytokine production, whereas it had no significant effects on either proliferative response or cytokine production by Th1 clones (11). Finally, CD30 ligation induced activation of nuclear factor (NF)κB transcription factors in TH0 and Th2, but not in Th1, clones (12). A preferential association of CD30 expression with T-cell responses characterized by the production of Th2 cytokines has also been demonstrated in vivo. First, a few CD4$^+$CD30$^+$ T-cells were detected in the circulation of atopic grass pollen-sensitive donors during seasonal exposure to grass pollens that developed into T-cell lines able to proliferate in response to grass pollen allergens and to produce IL-4 and IL-5, but not IFNγ and TNFβ, upon polyclonal stimulation (10). More importantly, high numbers of CD30$^+$ T-cells were detected in lymph node and skin biopsies from three children with Omenn's syndrome (OS) (a rare congenital SCID, in which a polyclonal activation of Th2 cells has been suggested to play a pathogenic role) (13), as well as in the lymph node and peripheral blood (PB) of a fourth child with Omenn's-like syndrome (OLS) (14). However, no accumulation of CD30$^+$ cells was observed in bronchial biopsies from patients with allergic asthma or in conjunctival biopsies from patients with vernal conjunctivitis, which are also considered as Th2-mediated disorders. From these results, we conclude that CD30, although preferentially associated with the production of Th2 cytokines, does not represent an operational Th2 marker in vivo in all disease models. That follows also because it is unlikely that in diseases sustained by Ag-specific (oligoclonal) activation of Th2 cells remarkable numbers of CD30$^+$ cells accumulate in target organs, where they usually act as effector cells without significant proliferation.

Table 1
**Main Functional and Phenotypic Properties of Human Th1 and Th2
Cell Clones**[a]

Property	Th1	Th2
Cytokine secretion		
IFNγ	+++	−
TNFβ	+++	−
IL-2	+++	++
TNFα	+++	++
GM-CSF	++	++
IL-3	++	+++
IL-10	++	+++
IL-13	++	+++
IL-4	−	+++
IL-5	−	+++
Cytolytic potential	+++	−
B-cell help for Ig synthesis		
IgM, IgG1, IgG2, IgG3, IgA		
At low T:B-cell ratios	+++	++
At high T:B-cell ratios	−	+++
IgE, IgG4	−	+++
Monocyte activation		
Induction of PCA	+++	−
TF production	+++	−
Inhibition of TF production	−	+++
Surface expression		
CD30	+/−	+++
LAG-3	+++	+/−
Release in biological fluids		
sCD30	+/−	+++
sLAG-3	+++	+/−

[a]PCA, procoagulant activity; TF, tissue factor.

The LAG-3, a member of the immunoglobulin superfamily *(15)*, showed a different Th expression in comparison with CD30. First, LAG-3 expression correlated with IFN-γ, but not IL-4, production in Ag-stimulated T-cells. Moreover, LAG-3 expression was strongly up-regulated by IL-12, a powerful Th1-inducing agent *(see* below). Finally, most activated CD4[+] T-cell clones with established Th1 profile of cytokine secretion expressed LAG-3 (but not CD30) on their surface, whereas the great majority of Th2 clones showed neither surface LAG-3 nor LAG-3 mRNA expression. Th0 clones usually showed both CD30 and LAG-3 expression *(16)*. So far, however, the physiologic meaning of LAG-3, as well as the reason for its preferential expression in Th1-like cells, remain unclear.

PREFERENTIAL DEVELOPMENT OF ALLERGEN-SPECIFIC
Th2 CELLS IN ATOPIC SUBJECTS

Because of their ability to produce IL-3, granulocyte-macrophage colony stimulating factor (GM-CSF), IL-4, IL-5, and IL-10, Th2 cells represent an excellent candidate to explain why the mast cell/eosinophil/IgE-producing B-cell triad is involved in the pathogenesis of allergy. IL-3, IL-4, and IL-10 are growth factors for mast cells; IL-3, GM-CSF, and IL-5 favor the differentiation, activation, and *in situ* survival of eosinophils. Moreover, it has clearly been shown that IgE synthesis results from collaboration between Th2 cells and B-cells. To this end, Th2 cells provide B-cells with at least two signals: one is delivered by IL-4; the other is represented by a T–B cell-to-cell physical interaction, occurring between the CD40L expressed on the activated Th cell and the CD40 molecule constitutively expressed on the B-cell. The Th2 cell-derived IL-4 induces germ line ε expression on the B-cell, whereas CD40L/CD40 interaction is required for the expression of productive mRNA and for the synthesis of IgE protein. Recently, it has been demonstrated that another cytokine, IL-13, is also able to induce germ line ε expression, but its production does not seem to be restricted to the Th2 subset. On the other hand, Th1 cells that produce IFNγ but not IL-4, as well as Th0 cells that produce high concentrations of IFNγ in addition to IL-4 and/or IL-13, are unable to support, or rather suppress, IL-4-dependent IgE synthesis (reviewed in refs. *17,18*).

Strong evidence has been accumulated to suggest that atopic allergic reactions are initiated by a Th2-type response:

1. Allergens preferentially expand Th cells showing a Th2-like profile in atopic subjects *(19,20)*;
2. Th2-like cells accumulate in the target organs of allergic patients *(21–24)*;
3. Allergen-challenge results in local activation and recruitment of allergen-specific Th2-like cells *(25,26)*; and
4. Successful specific immunotherapy associates with changes in the cytokine profile of allergen-reactive Th cells *(27–29)*. More recently, it was found that allergen-reactive Th2 cells expressing membrane CD30, an activation marker preferentially associated with the production of Th2-type cytokines, are present in the circulation of allergic patients during seasonal allergen exposure (10). Moreover, CD30+ T-cells are present in the lesional skin of patients with atopic dermatitis, and high levels of soluble CD30 are detectable in the serum of patients with atopic dermatitis *(30)*.

The mechanisms responsible for the preferential development of allergen-reactive Th2 cells in atopic subjects have not yet been clarified. Attention has been focused on the possible role of antigen-presenting cells (APCs), the T-cell receptor (TCR) repertoire, and cytokines present in the microenvironment at the time of allergen presentation. It is highly probable that Langherans cells (LC) present in the skin, as well as dendritic cells that are localized in the respiratory mucosa, represent the primary point of contact between the immune system and allergens coming into contact with the skin and the respiratory airways, respectively. Skin LC and mucosal dendritic cells (DC) are probably involved in allergen transport to regional lymph nodes where allergen presentation to allergen-specific CD4+ T-cells occurs. Some data suggest that atopic patients with asthma may have higher numbers of intraepithelial DC than nonasthmatic subjects and that in the presence of allergen molecules these cells can induce T-cell activation and release of IL-4 and IL-5 *(31)*. However, the actual role played by APC in driving the development of allergen-reactive Th2-like cells remains to be elucidated. Although the role of the TCR repertoire in determining the development of Th1- or Th2-type responses is controversial, evidence for the pivotal role of specific Vβ-expressing T-cell subsets in the stimulation of IgE production and increased airways responsiveness induced by ragweed allergen has been reported *(32)*. Thus, it cannot be excluded that the recognition of allergen by the TCR provides a signal or sets of signals that drive the T-cells in a certain direction, e.g., to produce IL-4 or, alternatively, IFNγ. So far, however, in both mice and humans, IL-4 produced at the time of T-cell activation appears to be the most dominant factor in determining the likelihood for Th2-cell polarization *(4,33,34)*. Accordingly, IL-4-gene-targeted mice fail to generate mature Th2 cells in vivo or to produce IgE antibodies *(35)*, suggesting that early IL-4 production by a cell type distinct from the Th2 cell must be involved. Possible candidates include mast cells/basophils and eosinophils, which have been shown to release stored IL-4 in response to FcεR triggering *(36–41)*, the CD4$^+$ NK (natural killer) 1.1$^+$ T-cell subset *(42)*, or the naive Th cells themselves *(43–46)*. With regard to the role of mast cells/basophils, it is unlikely that parasites or allergens would be able to crosslink their receptors prior to a specific immune response that had produced parasite-specific IgG and IgE antibodies. On the other hand, mast cell-deficient mice develop normal Th2 responses *(47)*. Finally, in IL-4-deficient mice only those mice that are reconstituted with IL-4-producing T- (but not with IL-4-producing non-T-) cells produce antigen-specific IgE *(48)*. Thus, IL-4 production by mast cells/basophils or eosinophils triggered by antigen-IgE antibody immune complexes may play a role in amplifying secondary responses to parasites, but cannot account for the Th2 development in primary immune responses. A way out of this dilemma may be a pathway of IL-4 secretion independent of FcεR crosslinking. It has been suggested that both helminth products and some allergens may induce FcεRI$^+$ cells to release IL-4 because of their proteolytic activity *(49)*; however, obvious mechanisms of FcεR-independent IL-4 production by these cells have not been identified yet.

A second possibility is that the endogenous source of IL-4 required for the Th2 development is the CD4$^+$ NK1.1$^+$ T-cell subset. These cells appear to represent a specialized population of CD4$^+$ T-cells that are particularly effective in producing cytokines, which are positively selected by recognition of CD1, a nonpolymorphic major histocompatibility complex (MHC) class I-like molecule *(50)*. Interestingly, indeed, β$_2$-microglobulin-deficient mice (which are also deficient in CD1 expression) produce neither IL-4 nor IgE; moreover, SJL mice that are unable to produce IgE, neither possess CD4$^+$NK1.1$^+$ T cells nor express IL-4 following in vivo injection of anti-CD3 antibody *(51,52)*. Therefore, it is possible that immunogens having associated superantigens that could interact with a sufficiently large fraction of these cells may promote a pulse of IL-4 that is available at the time naive CD4$^+$ T-cells are responding to antigen for the first time. It is unlikely, however, that all antigens able to promote the differentiation of naive Th cells into the Th2 pathway should necessarily activate CD4$^+$ NK1.1$^+$, CD1-restricted, T-cells.

A final possibility is that the source of IL-4 in the primary response is the naive CD4$^+$ T-cells themselves. This possibility has recently been supported by several findings. First, low-intensity signaling of TCR, such as that mediated by low peptide doses or by mutant peptides, led to secretion of low levels of IL-4 by murine naive T-cells *(43)*. Second, human CD45RA$^+$ (naive) adult PB T-cells, as well as human neonatal T-cells, were found to develop into IL-4-producing cells in the absence of any pre-existing source of IL-4 and in spite of the presence of anti-IL-4 antibodies *(44–46)*. Finally, high proportions of T-cell clones showing a clear-cut Th2 profile of cytokine production could be generated from single CD4$^+$ T-cells isolated from the thymus of small children *(53)*. Thus, evidence is accumulating suggesting that the maturation of naive T-cells into the Th2 pathway depends mainly on the levels and kinetics of IL-4 production by naive T-cells themselves at priming. These are likely to be determined by: the genetic background of the individual and the nature and intensity of TCR signaling by the peptide ligand. Obviously, when CD1-restricted antigens are expressed on APC, CD4$^+$NK1.1$^+$ T-cells, which rapidly release high amounts of IL-4, may also contribute to the development of the Th2 pathway.

POSSIBLE GENETIC ALTERATIONS FAVORING ALLERGEN-SPECIFIC Th2 RESPONSES IN ATOPIC SUBJECTS

The demonstration that production of IgE antibodies is strictly dependent on the production of IL-4 (and/or IL-13) *(54,55)* suggests that the mechanism(s) underlying heightened IgE responsiveness seen in atopic diseases (i.e., noncognate regulation of IgE responsiveness) could primarily involve the development and/or functional capability of Th cells. Indeed, CD4$^+$ T-cell clones from atopic individuals are able to produce noticeable amounts of IL-4 and IL-5 in response to bacterial antigens, such as purified protein derivative (PPD) and streptokinase, that usually evoke responses with a restricted Th1-like cytokine profile in nonatopic individuals *(56)*. Moreover, T-cell clones generated from cord blood lymphocytes of newborns with atopic parents produced higher IL-4 concentrations than neonatal lymphocytes of newborns with nonatopic parents. More recently, large panels of *Parietaria officinalis* group 1 (Par O 1)-specific T-cell clones were generated from donors with low or high serum IgE levels and assessed for their profile of cytokine production and reactivity to two immunodominant Par O 1 peptides (p92 and p96). Interestingly, both p92- and p96-specific T-cell clones generated from "high IgE" donors produced remarkable amounts of IL-4 and low IFNγ. In contrast, T-cell clones generated from "low IgE" donors showed a different profile of cytokine production: the majority of those specific for p96 produced high amounts of both IL-4 and IFNγ, whereas most p92-specific T-cell clones showed a Th1-like profile (high IFNγ and low IL-4) *(57)*. Taken together, these data strongly suggest that allergen peptide ligand can influence the cytokine profile of Th cells; however, the mechanisms underlying noncognate regulation of IgE responsiveness are overwhelming.

The genetic alterations possibly responsible for immune disorders of atopic individuals are still unclear. Regarding a genetic link between atopy and specific IgE response, several studies have underlined the potential role of MHC class II haplotype *(58)*, but the data remain controversial. With regard to TCR repertoire, a gene (or genes) in the α/δ complex has been described that influences the development of a specific IgE response in allergic subjects *(59)*. A restricted usage of Vα13 by T-cell clones specific for *Lolium perenne* group 1 (Lol p 1) has also been reported *(60)*. More recently, we found an intra- and interindividually restricted TCR-Vβ usage in both Lol p 1- and *Poa pratensis* group 9 (Poa p 9)-specific T-cell lines *(57)*. On the other hand, the evidence for a linkage of overall IgE to markers in chromosome 5q31.1, especially to the IL-4 gene *(61)*, suggests that one or more polymorphisms exist in a coding region or, more probably, a regulatory region of the IL-4 gene. Several studies have identified potential mechanisms governing the IL-4 gene expression in human and murine T-cells. Transcription of IL-4 gene is stringently regulated by multiple promoter elements acting together *(62,63)*. Thus, the more likely possibility is that atopic subjects have an altered regulation at the level of the IL-4 gene. However, several genes map within 5q31.1, including IL-5, IL-9, and IL-13, which might influence IgE production and the other abnormalities characteristic of the atopic state. Some additional candidates are IRF1, whose gene product upregulates interferon regulatory factor (IFN)α, which in turn can downregulate IgE production and inhibit Th2 cell development *(64,65)*, and IL-12B, which encodes the β chain of IL-12, a known inducer of IFN-γ production by CD4$^+$ and CD8$^+$ T-cells and NK cells *(66)*, as well as a powerful inducer of Th1 responses *(67,68)*. In this respect, it is noteworthy that depletion of a subpopulation of IFN-γ-producing CD8$^+$ T-cells with a sublethal dose of ricin results in a massive increase in serum IgE *(69)*. More importantly, IFN-γ released by MHC class I-restricted CD8$^+$ γδ$^+$ T-cells prevents the development of Th2-like cells in response to non-replicating antigens presented at mucosal surfaces *(70,71)*. Recent experiments suggest a possible role of CD8$^+$ T-cells in controlling the allergen-specific Th2 response in humans, as

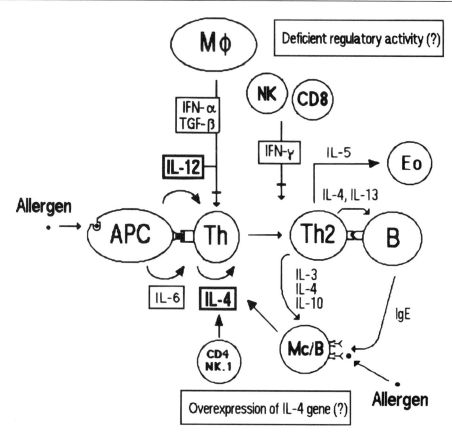

Fig. 2. Regulatory mechanisms involved in the differentiation of antigen-reactive CD4+ T-cells into the Th2 phenotype. Locally produced cytokines have a positive (arrows) or negative (flat-headed projections) regulatory influence on the development of CD4+ T-cells into Th2 cells, the early production of IL-4 by a still uncharacterized cell type (the CD4+ NK1.1+ subset?) being the most critical factor for Th2 cell development. Genetic alterations favoring the overexpression of the IL-4 gene or the deficient activity of regulatory cytokines (IL-12, IFNγ, IFNα, TGFβ), or both, might account for the preferential development of allergen-reactive CD4+ T-cells into the Th2 phenotype in atopic subjects. (Adapted with permission from ref. *17*.)

well. First, the Par O 1 peptide 92 (*see* above) expanded higher numbers of CD8+ T-cell clones in "low" than in "high" IgE producers. In addition, lactalbumin expanded higher numbers of CD8+ T-cell clones in nonatopic than in atopic milk-sensitive donors (*58*), suggesting that allergen-specific CD8+ T-cells may play an important role (via IFNγ production?) in shifting the response of CD4+ Th cells to the same allergen from Th2 to Th1.

Thus, alterations of molecular mechanisms directly involved in the regulation of IL-4 gene expression, or deficient regulatory activity of cytokines responsible for inhibition of Th2-cell development (such as IFNα/γ and IL-12), or both, may account for the preferential Th2-type response toward environmental allergens in atopic people. An overexpression of other cytokine genes (IL-3, IL-5, GM-CSF, and IL-9) located together with IL-4 and IL-13 within the same cluster of chromosome 5 may also be involved. The overexpression of the above genes can account for the preferential development of Th2 cells in response to allergens, as well as for the production by Th2 cells and even by other cell types of cytokines involved in allergic inflammation and therefore explain the persistent histological, pathophysiological, and clinical aspects of allergic disorders (Fig. 2).

ROLE OF Th2 CELLS IN THE PATHOGENESIS
OF ALLERGIC DISEASES
Vernal Conjunctivitis

The first description of the cytokine profile of T-cells from tissue in allergic disease was in vernal conjunctivitis, a condition of papillary hypertrophy of the conjunctivae with eosinophil and lymphocyte infiltration and associated high serum IgE. T-cell clones were made from tissues by initial expansion with phytohemagglutinin (PHA) followed by addition of IL-2. Clones from the conjunctival tissue of three patients were mostly CD4[+] and produced IL-4, but little IFNγ. These clones supported IgE synthesis in vitro *(21)*. Interestingly, an allergic-like blepharitis (inflammation of the eyelid) with a mononuclear cell infiltrate was observed in a cohort of IL-4 transgenic mice expressing IL-4 at the level of B- (or T-) lymphocytes *(72)*.

Allergic Rhinitis

Nasal allergen provocation followed by nasal mucosa biopsy 24 h after allergen challenge in patients with allergic rhinitis is associated with a cellular infiltrate in which CD4[+] T-cells and eosinophils are preeminent *(73)*. By use of the complementary techniques of immunohistology and *in situ* hybridization, an increase in cytokine mRNA expression for IL-3, IL-4, IL-5, and GM-CSF was found, which correlated with the degree of local eosinophilia, suggesting that the latter may occur as a consequence of the release of Th2 cytokines by allergen-specific infiltrating T-cells *(74)*. Accordingly, most CD4[+] T-cell clones generated from the nasal mucosa after allergen challenge, many of which were specific for the allergen used in the challenge test, showed a Th2 profile *(26)*. However, in another study performed on patients with perennial allergic rhinitis, a complete lack of any cytokine immunoreactivity localized to tissue lymphocytes was found. Mast cells accounted for >90% of IL-4- and IL-6- and >50% of IL-5-immunoreactive cells *(75)*. These findings leave open the question of whether allergic inflammation in the mucosa of patients with allergic rhinitis is initiated by Th2 cells that, however, do not accumulate Th2 cytokines in sufficient concentrations to be consistently detected by immunohistochemical methods, or by mast cells, which may be able to secrete Th2 cytokines rapidly and in high concentrations.

Allergic Asthma

Bronchial asthma (BA) is a complex disorder characterized by intermittent, reversible airway obstruction, and by airway hyperresponsiveness and inflammation. Although its cause(s) remains unknown, we now recognize that asthma is a syndrome whose common pathologic expression is inflammation of the airways *(76)*. Based on clinical and laboratory findings, BA may be divided into allergic (extrinsic) and nonallergic (intrinsic) forms. Allergic BA usually starts during childhood and is characterized by allergen-dependent, often seasonal symptoms with positive skin tests to allergens and elevated total and allergen-specific serum IgE. In contrast, nonallergic BA usually begins in adulthood, is perennial nd more severe, has no elevation in serum IgE, and is often associated with sinusitis and nasal polyposis. Both allergic and intrinsic BA are characterized by infiltration of the bronchial mucosa with large numbers of activated eosinophils and the presence of elevated concentrations of eosinophil-derived proteins, such as major basic protein (MBP) and eosinophil cationic protein (ECP) *(77)*.

By specific immunostaining of bronchial mucosal biopsies obtained via a fibrotic bronchoscope, a significant increase in the number of IL-2 receptor-positive (activated) T-cells in the airways of mild, steady-state asthmatics was observed *(78)*. Using an *in situ* hybridization technique, cells showing mRNA for Th2, but not Th1, lymphokines were found at the site of late phase reactions in skin biopsies from atopic patients *(79)*, and in mucosal bronchial biopsies or bronchoaveolar lavage (BAL) of patients with atopic BA *(24,25)*. By use of immunomagnetic separation the majority of IL-4 and IL-5 mRNA in BAL cells from asthmatic subjects was shown to be associated with CD2+ T-cells *(25)*. Interestingly, corticosteroid treatment in BA resulted in the downregulation of BAL cells expressing mRNA for IL-4 and IL-5, whereas the number of cells expressing mRNA for IFN-γ was increased *(80)*. Glucocorticoids and the immunosuppressants KK506 and cyclosporin A also suppress IL-5 production by peripheral blood mononuclear cells (PBMC) from mite-sensitive atopic asthmatics *(81)*. In contrast, no effect in the number of BAL cells expressing mRNA for IL-4 and IL-5 was observed either, suggesting that steroid-resistant BA may be associated with a dysregulation of the expression of the genes encoding for Th2/Th1 cytokines in airway cells *(82)*. In order to assess whether the T-cell response to inhaled allergens induced activation and recruitment of allergen-specific Th2 cells in the airway mucosa of patients with respiratory allergy, biopsy specimens were obtained from the bronchial mucosa of patients with grass pollen-induced BA or rhinitis 48 h after a positive bronchial provocation test with the relevant allergen. T-cell clones were derived from these specimens and from biopsy specimens taken from the bronchial mucosa of patients with toluene-diisothiocyanate (TDI)-induced BA 48 h after a positive bronchial provocation test with TDI and were assessed for allergen-specificity and cytokine secretion profile. Proportions ranging from 14–22% of CD4+ T-cell clones derived from stimulated mucosae of grass-allergic patients were specific for grass allergens and most of them exhibited a definite Th2 profile and induced IgE production by autologous B-cells in the presence of the specific allergen *(26)*. In contrast, none of the T-cell clones derived from the bronchial mucosa of patients with TDI-induced BA were specific for grass allergens and the majority of them were CD8+ T-cells producing IFNγ and IL-2 or IFNγ, IL-2, and IL-5, but no IL-4 *(26)*. Likewise, allergen inhalation challenge resulted in activation of CD4+ T-cells, increased Th2-type cytokine mRNA expression, and eosinophil recruitment in BAL of patients with atopic BA *(80,83)*.

Because many studies addressing abnormalities of T-lymphocyte cytokine secretion in BA have been performed on subjects who are also atopic, the question of whether disordered cytokine synthesis by T-lymphocytes in asthmatics simply reflects the existence of atopy or implies a role in BA pathogenesis is still unsolved. In a recent study, PBMC from atopic and nonatopic asthmatic children were stimulated with PHA in vitro and concentrations of both IL-4 and IFN-γ released into cell supernatants were measured. Although stimulated PBMC from the atopic asthmatics secreted significantly more IL-4 and significantly less IFN-γ than those from both the nonatopic asthmatics and the normal controls, no significant differences were observed in the secretion of both cytokines by cells from the nonatopic asthmatics and the normal controls *(84)*, suggesting that the imbalance of cytokine secretion relates to the atopic state rather than specifically to the presence of BA and that "intrinsic" BA is a distinct immunopathological entity *(85)*. Indeed, whereas increased levels of IL-4 and IL-5 were measured in the BAL of allergic asthmatics, in nonallergic asthmatics IL-2 and IL-5 predominated *(86)*. Accordingly, CD8+ T-cell clones producing IFNγ and IL-5, but not IL-4, were generated from the bronchial mucosa of nonatopic patients with TDI-induced BA *(26)*. Moreover, CD4+ and CD8+ T-cell lines generated from the BAL of asthmatics secreted significantly higher quantities of IL-5 and GM-CSF than T-cell lines from atopic and nonatopic controls *(87)*. Taken together, these data suggest that elevated IL-4 synthesis by T-lymphocytes is a feature of the atopic state and is not a prerequisite for the development of BA, whereas elevated secretion of IL-5 is a feature of asthmatic patients and may occur in asthmatic patients in the absence of elevated IL-4 secretion. Thus, the Th1/Th2 model does not appear to be sufficiently flexible to account for the behavior of T-cells in the pathogenesis of BA. The picture is further complicated by the acculumulating evidence that IL-4 and IL-5 may originate from mast cells, basophils, and eosinophils in the bronchial mucosa of asthmatics.

Atopic Dermatitis (AD)

AD is the cutaneous manifestation of atopic allergy owing to chronic exposure to foreign proteins resulting in chronic inflammation of the skin. The majority of patients with AD (>80%) have positive intracutaneous skin test reactions to one or more environmental allergens and elevated serum IgE levels, which represent antibodies specific to the allergens concerned. The histological appearance of lesional AD skin is characterized by dermal perivascular infiltrates of mononuclear cells, mainly consisting of CD4$^+$ T-cells and eosinophils *(88,89)*. However, the relationship between allergy and the pathogenesis of the skin lesions in AD is unclear. By using the polymerase chain reaction (PCR) technique, spontaneous mRNA IL-4 expression was found in PBMC from AD patients *(90)*, whereas IL-13, another IgE-switching cytokine, was not produced *(91)*. IFNγ mRNA expression was increased in PBMC from AD patients, but IFNγ production was reduced, suggesting a posttranscriptional defect of IFN-γ secretion *(92)*. IFNγ production by PBMC from AD patients was also found to be deficient in response to stimulation with toxic shock syndrome toxin-1 (TSST-1) or IL-12, whereas both IL-12 production and IL-12 receptor (IL-12R) expression in the same patients were normal *(93)*. However, neutralization of IL-4, and even more of IL-10, activity caused strong augmentation of IFNγ production. These data suggest that PBMC from these patients, despite normal levels of IL-12 production and IL-12R expression, are unable to generate normal IL-12-induced IFNγ responses, which may be related to the excess production of IL-4 and IL-10 *(93)*.

High proportions of *Dermatophagoides pteronyssinus* (Dp)-specific Th2-like CD4$^+$ T-cell clones were obtained from the skin lesions of patients with AD, indicating accumulation or expansion of these T-cells in lesional skin *(22,94)*. Interestingly, Dp-specific Th2-like clones were also derived from biopsy specimens of intact skin taken after contact challenge with Dp, suggesting that percutaneous sensitization to aeroallergens may play a role in the induction of skin lesions in patients with AD *(95,96)*. More recent data partially confirm both Dp specificity and Th2-type profile of high proportions of T-cell clones derived from Dp-induced patch test lesions of AD patients. Interestingly, most Dp-specific Th2-like T-cell clones were CD30$^+$. CD30 positivity was also found in AD skin biopsies by using immunohistochemistry, and high levels of soluble CD30 could be detected in the serum of the great majority of AD patients *(30)*. However, the majority of T-cell clones derived from the lesional skin of patients with AD have a mixed (Th0-like) phenotype and only a minority of them are specific for Dp. A proportion of T-cell clones derived from lesional skin exhibited high IFNγ production and some appeared to be specific for bacterial antigens. More importantly, the presence of both Dp-specific and Th2-like cells in the skin of AD patients did not correlate with the presence in the serum of Dp-specific IgE antibody or the serum levels of IgE protein *(97)*. Accordingly, by using the PCR technique, overexpression of IL-10, but not IL-4, was found in AD lesions in comparison with allergic contact dermatitis lesions and tuberculin reactions *(98)*. Moreover, when the kinetics of T-cell-derived cytokine production was assessed, the results showed that in the initiation phase IL-4 production was predominant over IFN-γ production, but in the late and chronic phase (lesional skin) the situation was reversed and IFNγ production predominated over

IL-4 production *(99)*. Taken together, these data suggest that Th2-like responses against Dp or other aeroallergens at skin level may be involved in the initiation of skin lesions, but there is a subsequent influx of Th1 cells, which is responsible for the aggravation of the inflammation. However, the relationship between aeroallergen sensitization and pathogenesis of AD still remains unclear.

CONCLUDING REMARKS

In the last few years, evidence has been accumulated suggesting that allergen-reactive Th2 cells play a triggering role in the activation and/or recruitment of IgE antibody-producing B-cells, mast cells, and eosinophils, the cellular triad involved in allergic inflammation. The question of how these Th2 cells are selected in atopic patients is still unclear. Both the nature of the TCR signaling provided by the allergen peptide ligand and dysregulation of IL-4 production can influence the cytokine profile of allergen-specific Th cells. However, alterations resulting in the overexpression of IL-4 gene and/or in defective regulatory control of Th2 cells in atopic subjects are probably overwhelming. These new findings might represent the basis for novel immunotherapeutic strategies in allergic disorders.

REFERENCES

1. Mosmann TR, Coffman RL (1989) TH1 and TH2 cells: different patterns of lymphokine secretion lead to different functional properties. Ann Rev Immunol 7:145–173.
2. Romagnani S (1994) Lymphokine production by human T cells in disease states. Ann Rev Immunol 12:227–257.
3. Romagnani S (1994) Th1 versus Th2 responses in AIDS. Curr Opin Immunol 6:616–622.
4. Seder RA, Paul WE (1994) Acquisition of lymphokine-producing phenotype by CD4+ T cells. Annu Rev Immunol 12:635–674.
5. Kelso A (1995) Th1 and Th2 subsets: paradigm lost? Immunol Today 16:374–379.
6. Romagnani S (1991) Human T_H1 and T_H2: doubt no more. Immunol Today 12:256–257.
7. Kapsenberg ML, Wierenga EA, Bos JD, Jansen HM (1991) Functional subsets of allergen-reactive human CD4+ T cells. Immunol Today 12:392–395.
8. Del Prete GF, De Carli M, Mastromauro C, Macchia D, Biagiotti R, Ricci M, Romagnani S (1991) Purified protein derivative of Mycobacterium tuberculosis and excretory-secretory antigen(s) of Toxocara canis expand in vitro human T cells with stable and opposite (type 1 T helper or type 2 T helper) profile of cytokine production. J Clin Invest 88:346–351.
9. Smith CA, Gruss H-J, Davis T, Anderson D, Farrah T, Baker E, Sutherland GR, Brannan CI, Copeland NG, Jenkins NA, Grabstein KH, Gliniak B, McAllister IB, Fanslow W, Alderson M, Falk B, Gimpel S, Gillis S, Din WS, Goodwin R, Armitage RJ (1993) CD30 antigen, a marker for Hodgkin's lymphoma, is a receptor whose ligand defines an emerging family of cytokines with homology to TNF. Cell 73:1349–1360.
10. Del Prete, G-F, De Carli M, Almerigogna F, Daniel KC, D'Elios MM, Zancuoghi D, Vinante E, Pizzolo G, Romagnani S (1995) Preferential expression of CD30 by human CD4+ T cells producing Th2-type cytokines. FASEB J 9:81–86.
11. Del Prete G-F, De Carli M, D'Elios MM, Daniel KC, Smith CA, Thomas E, Romagnani S (1995) CD30-mediated signalling promotes the development of human Th2-like T cells. J Exp Med 182:1–7.
12. McDonald PP, Cassatella MA, Bald A, Maggi E, Romagnani S, Gruss H-J, Pizzolo G (1995) CD30 ligation induces nuclear factor-κB activation in human T cell lines. Eur J Immunol 25:2870–2876.
13. Schandené L, Ferster A, Mascart-Lemone F, Crusiaux A, Gerard C, Marchant A, Lybin M, Velu T, Sariban E, Goldman M (1993) T helper type 2-like cells and therapeutic effects of interferon-γ in combined immunodeficiency with hypereosinophilia (Omenn's syndrome). Eur J Immunol 23:56–60.
14. Chilosi M, Facchetti F, Notarangelo LD, Romagnani S, Del Prete G-F, Almerigogna F, De Carli M, Pizzolo G (1995) CD30 cell expression and abnormal soluble CD30 serum accumulation in Omenn's syndrome. Evidence for a Th2-mediated condition. Eur J Immunol 26:329–334.
15. Triebel F, Jitsukawa S, Baixeras E, Roman-Roman S, Genevee C, Viegas-Pequignot E, Hercend T (1990) LAG-3, a novel lymphocyte activation gene closely related to CD4. J Exp Med 171:1393–1405.

16. Annunziato F, Manetti R, Tomasevic L, Giudizi M-G, Biagiotti R, Giannò V, Germano P, Mavilia C, Maggi E, Romagnani S (1996) Expression and release of LAG-3-encoded protein by human CD4+ T-cells are associated with IFN-production. FASEB J 10:769–776.

17. Romagnani S (1994) Regulation of the development of type 2 T-helper cells in allergy. Curr Opin Immunol 6:838–846.

18. Romagnani S (1995) Atopic allergy and other hypersensitivities. Editorial overview: Technological advances and new insights into pathogenesis prelude novel therapeutic strategies. Curr Opin Immunol 7:745–750.

19. Wierenga EA, Snoek M, de Groot C, Chretien I, Bos JD, Jansen HM, Kapsenberg ML (1990) Evidence for compartmentalization of functional subsets of CD4+ T-lymphocytes in atopic patients. J Immunol 144:4651–4656.

20. Parronchi P, Macchia D, Piccinni M-P, Biswas P, Simonelli C, Maggi E, Ricci M, Ansari AA, Romagnani S (1991) Allergen- and bacterial antigen-specific T-cell clones established from atopic donors show a different profile of cytokine production. Proc Natl Acad Sci USA 88:4538–4542.

21. Maggi E, Biswas P, Del Prete GF, Parronchi P, Macchia D, Simonelli C, Emmi L, De Carli M, Tiri A, Ricci M, Romagnani S (1991) Accumulation of Th2-like helper T-cells in the conjunctiva of patients with vernal conjunctivitis. J Immunol 146:1169–1174.

22. van der Heijden FL, Wierenga EA, Bos JD, Kapsenberg ML (1991) High frequency of IL-4-producing CD4+ allergen-specific T lymphocytes in atopic dermatitis lesional skin. J Invest Dermatol 97:389–394.

23. Hamid Q, Azzawi M, Ying S, Moqbel R, Wardlaw AJ, Corrigan CJ, Bradley B, Durham SR, Collins JV, Jeffrey PK, Quint DJ, Kay AB (1991) Expression of mRNA for interleukin-5 in mucosal bronchial biopsies from asthma. J Clin Invest 87:1541–1546.

24. Robinson DS, Hamid Q, Ying S, Tsicopoulos A, Barkans J, Bentley AM, Corrigan CJ, Durham SR, Kay AB (1992) Predominant Th2-like bronchoalveolar T-lymphocyte population in atopic asthma. New Engl J Med 326:295–304.

25. Del Prete GF, De Carli M, D'Elios MM, Maestrelli P, Ricci M, Fabbri L, Romagnani S (1993) Allergen exposure induces the activation of allergen-specific Th2 cells in the airway mucosa of patients with allergic respiratory disorders. Eur J Immunol 23:1445–1449.

26. Robinson D, Hamid Q, Bentley A, Ying S, Kay AB, Durham SR (1993) Activation of CD4+ T-cells, increased Th2-type cytokine mRNA expression, and eosinophil recruitment in bronchoalveolar lavage after allergen inhalation challenge in patients with atopic asthma. J Allergy Clin Immunol 92:313–324.

27. Varney VA, Hamid Q, Gaga M, Ying S, Jacobson M, Frew AJ, Kay AB, Durham SR (1993) Influence of grass pollen immunotherapy on cellular infiltration and cytokine mRNA expression during allergen-induced late-phase cutaneous responses. J Clin Invest 92:644–651.

28. Secrist H, Chelen CJ, Wen Y, Marshall JD, Umetsu DT (1993) Allergen immunotherapy decreases interleukin 4 production in CD4+ T-cells from allergic individuals. J Exp Med 178:2123–2130.

29. Jutel M, Pichler WJ, Skrbic D, Urwyler A, Dahinden C, Muller UR (1995) Bee venom immunotherapy results in decrease of IL-4 and IL-5 and increase of IFN-γ secretion in specific allergen-stimulated T-cell cultures. J Immunol 154:4187–4194.

30. Caproni M, Bianchi B, D'Elios HH, DeCarli H, Ameolei A, Fabbri, P (1997) In vivo relevance of CD30 in atopic dermatitis. Allergy 52:1063–1070.

31. Holt PG, Oliver J, McMenamin C, Bilik N, Kraal G, Thepen T (1993) The antigen presentation functions of lung dendritic cells are downmodulated in situ by soluble mediators from pulmonary alvelolar macrophages. J Exp Med 177:397–402.

32. Renz H, Saloga J, Bradley KL, Loader JE, Greenstein JL, Larsen G, Gelfand EW (1993) Specific VT cell subsets mediate the immediate hypersensitivity response to ragweed allergen. J Immunol 151:1907–1917.

33. Swain SL (1993) IL-4 dictates T-cell differentiation. Res Immunol 144:616–620.

34. Maggi E, Parronchi P, Manetti R, Simonelli C, Piccinni M-P, Santoni-Rugiu F, De Carli M, Ricci M, Romagnani S (1992) Reciprocal regulatory role of IFN-γ and IL-4 on the in vitro development of human Th1 and Th2 clones. J Immunol 148:2142–2147.

35. Kopf M, Le Gros G, Bachmann M, Lamers MC, Bluthmann H, Kohler G (1993) Disruption of the murine IL-4 gene blocks Th2 cytokine responses. Nature 362:245–248.

36. Piccinni M-P, Macchia D, Parronchi P, Giudizi M-G, Bani D, Aterini R, Grossi A, Ricci M, Maggi E, Romagnani S (1991) Human bone marrow non-B, non-T-cells produce interleukin-4 in response to cross-linkage of Fc and Fc receptors. Proc Natl Acad Sci USA 88:8656–8660.

37. Bradding P, Feather IH, Howarth PH, Mueller R, Roberts JA, Britten K, Bews JPA, Hunt TC, Okayama Y,

Heusser CH, Bullock GR, Church MK, Holgate ST (1992) Interleukin 4 is localized and released by human mast cells. J Exp Med 176:1381–1386.

38. Brunner T, Heusser CH, Dahinden CA (1993) Human peripheral blood basophils primed by interleukin 3 (IL-3) produce IL-4 in response to immunoglobulin E receptor stimulation. J Exp Med 177:605–611.

39. MacGlashan D, White JM, Huang S-K, Ono SJ, Schroeder JT, Lichtenstein LM (1994) Secretion of IL-4 from human basophils: the relationship between IL-4 mRNA and protein in resting and stimulated basophils. J Immunol 152:3006–3016.

40. Okayama Y, PettéFrère C, Kassel O, Semper A, Quint D, Tunon-de-Lara MJ, Bradding P, Holgate ST, Church MK (1995) IgE-dependent expression of mRNA for IL-4 and IL-5 in human lung mast cells. J Immunol 155:1796–1808.

41. Moqbel R, Ying S, Barkans J, Newman TM, Kimmitt P, Vakelin M, Taborda-Barata L, Meng Q, Corrigan CJ, Durham SR, Kay AB (1995) Identification of mRNA for interleukin-4 in human eosinophils with granule localization and release of the translated product. J Immunol 155:4939–4947.

42. Yashimoto T, Paul WE, (1994) CD4pos, NK1.1pos T cells promptly produce interleukin 4 in response to in vivo challenge with anti-CD3. J Exp Med 179:1285–1295.

43. Pfeiffer C, Stein J, Southwood S, Ketelaar H, Sette A, Bottomly K (1995) Altered peptide ligands can control CD4 T lymphocyte differentiation in vivo. J Exp Med 181:1569–1574.

44. Kalinski P, Hilkens CMU, Wierenga EA, van der Pouw-Kraan TCTM, van Lier RAW, Bos JD, Kapsenberg ML, Snijdewint FGM (1995) Functional maturation of human naive T helper cells in the absence of accessory cells: generation of IL-4-producing T-helper cells does not require exogenous IL-4. J Immunol 154:3753–3760.

45. Demeure CE, Yang LP, Byun DG, Ishihara H, Vezzio N, Delespesse G (1995) Human naive CD4 T-cells produce interleukin-4 at priming and acquire a Th2 phenotype upon repetitive stimulations in neutral conditions. Eur J Immunol 25:2722–2725.

46. Croft M, Swain SL (1995) Recently activated naive CD4 T cells can help resting B cells, and can produce sufficient autocrine IL-4 to drive differentiation to secretion of T-helper 2-type cytokines. J Immunol 154:4269–4282.

47. Wershil BK, Theodos CM, Galli SJ, Titus RG (1994) Mast cells augment lesion size and persistence during experimental leishmania major infection in the mouse. J Immunol 152:4563–4571.

48. Schmitz J, Thiel A, Kuhn R, Rajewsky K, Muller W, Assenmacher M, Radbruch A (1994) Induction of interleukin 4 (IL-4) expression in T helper (Th) cells is not dependent on IL-4 from non-T Cells. J Exp Med 179:1349–1353.

49. Finkelman FD, Urban JF (1992) Cytokines: making the right choice. Parasitol Today 8:311–314.

50. Bendelac A, Killeen N, Littman DR, Schwartz RH (1994) A subset of CD4⁺ thymocytes selected by MHC class I molecules. Science 263:1774–1778.

51. Yashimoto T, Bendelac A, Watson C, Hu-Li J, Paul WE (1995) CD-1-specific, NK1.1ᵖᵒˢ T-cells play a key in vivo role in a Th2 response and in IgE production. Science 270:1845–1847.

52. Yoshimoto T, Bendelac A, Hu-Li J, Paul WE (1995) Defective IgE production by SJL mice is linked to the absence of a subset of T-cells that promptly produce IL-4. Science 270:1845–1847.

53. Mingari, M-C, Maggi E, Cambiaggi A, Annunziato F, Schiavetti F, Manetti R, Moretta L, Romagnani S (1996) In vitro development of human CD4⁺ thymocytes into functionally mature Th2 cells. Exogenous IL-12 is required for priming thymocytes to the production of both Th1 cytokines and IL-10. Eur J Immunol 26:1083–1086.

54. Del Prete, G-F, Maggi E, Parronchi P, Chretien I, Tiri A, Macchia D, Ricci M, Romagnani S (1988) IL-4 is an essential factor for the IgE synthesis induced in vitro by human T-cell clones and their supernatants. J Immunol 140:4193–4198.

55. Punnonen J, Aversa G, Cocks BG, McKenzie ANJ, Menon S, Zurawski G, de Waal Malefyt R, de Vries JE (1993) Interleukin 13 induces interleukin 4-independent IgG4 and IgE synthesis and CD23 expression by human B cells. Proc Natl Acad Sci USA 90:3730–3734.

56. Parronchi P, De Carli M, Manetti R, Simonelli C, Piccinni M-P, Macchia D, Maggi E, Del Prete G-F, Ricci M, Romagnani S (1992) Aberrant interleukin (IL)-4 and IL-5 production in vitro by CD4⁺ helper T-cells from atopic subjects. Eur J Immunol 22:1615–1620.

57. Parronchi P, Sampognaro S, Annunziato F, Brugnolo F, Radbruch A, DiModugno F, Ruffilli A, Romagnani S, Maggi E (1998) Influence of both T cell receptor repertoire and severity of the atopic status on the cytokine secretion profile of Parietaria officinalis-specific T cells. Eur J Immunol (In Press).

58. Marsh DG, Lockhart A, Holgate ST (1993) The Genetics of Asthma. Blackwell Scientific Publications, Oxford.

59. Moffatt MF, Hill MR, Cornelis F, Schou C, Faux JA, Young RP, James AL, Ryan G, le Souef P, Musk AW, Hopkin JM, Cookson WOCM (1994) Genetic linkage of T-cell receptor a/d complex to specific IgE response. Lancet 343:1597–1600.

60. Mohapatra SS, Mohapatra S, Yang M, Ansari AA, Parronchi P, Maggi E, Romagnani S (1994) Molecular basis of cross-reactivity among allergen-specific human T-cells: T-cell receptor V gene usage and epitope structure. Immunology 81:15–20.

61. Marsh DG, Neely JD, Breazeale DR, Ghosh B, Freidhoff LR, Ehrlich-Kautzky E, Schou C, Krishnaswamy G, Beaty TH (1994) Linkage analysis of IL-4 and other chromosome 5q31.1 markers and total serum immunoglobulin E concentrations. Science 264:1152–1156.

62. Murphy KM, Murphy TL, Gold JS, Szabo SJ (1993) Current understanding of IL-4 gene regulation in T cells. Res Immunol 144:575–578.

63. Matsuda I, Nato Y, Arai K, Arai N (1993) The structure of IL-4 gene and regulation of its expression. Res Immunol 144:569–574.

64. Parronchi P, De Carli M, Manetti R, Simonelli C, Sampognaro, S, Piccinni M-P, Macchia D, Maggi E, Del Prete G-F, Romagnani S (1992) IL-4 and IFN(s) (alpha and gamma) exert opposite regulatory effects on the development of cytolytic potential by Th1 or Th2 human T-cell clones. J Immunol 149:2977–2982.

65. Parronchi P, Mohapatra S, Sampognaro S, Giannarini L, Wahn U, Chong P, Mohapatra SS, Maggi E, Renz H, Romagnani S (1996) Modulation by IFN-α of cytokine profile, T cell receptor repertoire and peptide reactivity of human allergen-specific T-cells. Eur J Immunol 26:697–703.

66. Chehimi J, Trinchieri G (1994) Interleukin-12: a bridge between innate resistance and adaptive immunity with a role in infection and acquired immunodeficiency. J Clin Immunol 14:149–161.

67. Manetti R, Parronchi P, Giudizi M-G, Piccinni M-P, Maggi E, Trinchieri G, Romagnani S (1993) Natural killer cell stimulatory factor (interleukin 12) induces T-helper type 1 (Th1)-specific immune responses and inhibits the development of IL-4-producing Th cells. J Exp Med 177:1199–1204.

68. Hsieh C-S, Macatonia SE, Tripp CS, Wolf SF O'Garra A, Murphy KM (1993) Development of TH1 CD4+ T-cells through IL-12 produced by *Leisteria*-induced macrophages. Science 260:547–49.

69. Kemeny M (1993) The role of CD8+ T-cells in the regulation of IgE. Clin Exper Allergy 23:466–470.

70. McMenamin C, Holt PG (1993) The natural immune response to inhaled soluble protein antigens involves major histocompatibility complex (MHC) class I-restricted CD8+ T-cell-mediated but MHC class-II-restricted CD4+ T-cell-dependent immune deviation resulting in selective suppression of immunoglobulin E production. J Exp Med 178:889–899.

71. McMenamin C, McKersey M, Kühnlein P, Hünig T, Holt PG (1997) γδ T cells down-regulate primary IgE responses in rats to inhaled soluble protein antigens. J Immunol 154:4390–4394.

72. Tepper RI, Levinson DA, Stonger BL, Campos-Torres J, Abbas AK, Leder P (1990) IL-4 induces allergic-like inflammatory disease and alters T-cell development in transgenic mice. Cell 62:457–467.

73. Varney VA, Jacobson MR, Sudderinck MR, Robinson DS, Irani A-MA, Scwartz LB, Mackay IS, Kay AB, Durham SR (1992) Immunohistology of the nasal mucosa following allergen-induced rhinitis: identification of activated T-lymphocytes, eosinophils and neutrophils. Am Rev Respir Dis 146:170–176.

74. Durham SR, Ying S, Varney VA, Jacobson MR, Sudderick RM, Mackay IS, Kay AB, Hamid QA (1992) Cytokine messenger RNA expression for IL-3, IL-4, IL-5, and granulocyte/macrophage colony-stimulating factor in the nasal mucosa after local allergen provocation: relationship to tissue eosinophilia. J Immunol 148:2390–2394.

75. Bradding P, Feather IH, Wilson S, Bardin PG, Heusser CH, Holgate ST, Howarth PH (1993) Immunolocalization of cytokines in the nasal mucosa of normal and perennial rhinitic subjects: the mast cells as a source of IL-4, IL-5, and IL-6 in human allergic mucosal inflammation. J Immunol 151:3853–3860.

76. Drazen JM, Arm JP, Austen KF (1996) Sorting out the cytokines of asthma. J Exp Med 183:1–5.

77. Wardlaw AJ, Dunnette S, Gleich GJ, Collins JV, Kay AB (1988) Eosinophils and mast cells in bronchoalveolar lavage in mild asthma. Relationship to bronchial hyperreactivity. Am Rev Respir Dis 137:62–69.

78. Azzawi M, Bradley B, Jeffery PK, Frew AJ, Wardlaw AJ, Knowles GK, Assoufi B, Collins JV, Durham SR, Kay AB (1990) Identification of activated T lymphocytes and eosinophils in bronchial biopsies in stable atopic asthma. Am Rev Respir Dis 142:1407–1413.

79. Kay AB, Ying S, Varney V, Gaga M, Durham SR, Moqbel R, Wardlaw AJ, Hamid Q (1991) Messenger RNA expression of the cytokine gene cluster interleukin-3 (IL-3), IL-4, IL-5, and granulocyte/macrophage colony-stimulating factor, in allergen-induced late-phase reactions in atopic subjects. J Exp Med 173:775–778.

80. Robinson D, Hamid Q, Ying S, Bentley A, Assoufi B, Durham SR, Kay AB (1993) Prednisolone treatment in asthma is associated with modulation of bronchoalveolar lavage cell interleukin-4, interleukin-5, and interferon-γ cytokine gene expression. Am Rev Respir Dis 148:401–406.

81. Mori A, Suko M, Nishizaki Y, Kaminuma O, Kobayashi S, Matsuzaki G, Yamamoto K, Ito K, Tsuruoka N, Okudaira H (1995) IL-5 production by CD4⁺ T cells of asthmatic patients is suppressed by gluocorti-coids and the immunosuppressants FK506 and cyclosporin A. Intern Immunol 7:449–457.

82. Leung DYM, Martin RJ, Szefler SJ, Sher ER, Kay AB, Hamid Q (1995) Dysregulation of interleukin-4, interleukin-5, and interferon-γ gene expression in steroid-resistant asthma. J Exp Med 181:33–40.

83. Ying S, Durham SR, Corrigan CJ, Hamid Q, Kay AB (1995) Phenotype of cells expressing mRNA for Th2-type (interleukin-4 and interleukin-5) and Th1-type (interleukin-2 and interferon-γ) cytokines in bronchoalveolar lavage and bronchial biopsies from atopic asthmatic and normal control subjects. Am J Respir Cell Mol Biol 12:477–487.

84. Tang MLK, Coleman J, Kemp AS (1995) Interleukin-4 and interferon-gamma production in atopic and non-atopic children with asthma. Clin Exp Allergy 25:515–521.

85. Corrigan CJ (1995) Elevated interleukin-4 secretion by T lymphocytes: a feature of atopy or asthma? Clin Exp Allergy 25:485–487.

86. Walker C, Bode E, Boer L, Hansel TT, Blaser K, Virchow J-C (1992) Allergic and nonallergic asthmat-ics have distinct patterns of T-cell activation and cytokine production in peripheral blood and bron-choalveolar lavage. Am Rev Respir Dis 146:109–115.

87. Till S, Li B, Durham SR, Humbert M, Assoufi B, Huston D, Dickinson R, Jeannin P, Kay AB, Corrigan C (1995) Secretion of the eosinophil-active cytokines interleukin-5, granulocyte/macrophage colony-stimulating factor and interleukin-3 by bronchoalveolar lavage CD4⁺ and CD8⁺ T cell lines in atopic asth-matics, and atopic and non-atopic controls. Eur J Immunol 25:2727–2731.

88. Zachary CB, MacDonald DM (1983) Quantitative analysis of T lymphocyte subsets in atopic eczema, using monoclonal antibodies and flow cytometry. Br J Dermatol 108:411–422.

89. Sillevis Smitt JH, Bos JD, Hulsebosch HJ, Krieg SR (1986) *In situ* immunophenotyping of antigen presenting cells and T cell subsets in atopic dermatitis. Clin Exper Dermatol 11:159–168.

90. Tang M, Kemp A (1994) Production and secretion of interferon-gamma in children with atopic dermatitis. Clin Exp Immunol 95:66–72.

91. Kimata H, Fujimoto M, Furusho K (1995) Involvement of interleukin (IL)-13, but not IL-4, in sponta-neous IgE and IgG4 production in nephrotic syndrome. Eur J Immunol 25:1497–1501.

92. Tang MLK, Varigos G, Kemp AS (1994) Reduced interferon-gamma (IFN-γ) secretion with increased IFN-γ mRNA expression in atopic dermatitis: evidence for a post-transcriptional defect. Clin Exp Immunol 97:483–490.

93. Lester MR, Hofer MF, Gately M, Trumble A, Leung DYM (1995) Down-regulating effects of IL-4 and IL-10 on the IFN-γ response in atopic dermatitis. J Immunol 154:6174–6181.

94. Reinhold U, Kukel S, Goeden B, Neumann C, Kreysel HW (1991) Functional characterization of skin-infiltrating lymphocytes in atopic dermatitis. Clin Exp Immunol 86:444–448.

95. Van Reijsen FC, Bruijnzeel-Koomen CAFM, Kalthoff FS, Maggi E, Romagnani S, Westland JKT, Mudde GC (1992) Skin-derived aeroallergen-specific T-cell clones of Th2 phenotype in patients with atopic dermatitis. J Allergy Clin Immunol 90:184–192.

96. Sager N, Feldmann A, Schilling G, Kreitsch P, Neumann C (1992) House dust mite-specific T cells in the skin of subjects with atopic dermatitis: frequency and lymphokine profile in the allergen patch test. J Allergy Clin Immunol 89:801–810.

97. Virtanen T, Maggi E, Manetti R, Piccinni M-P, Sampognaro S, Parronchi P, De Carli M, Zuccati G, Romagnani S (1995) No relationship between skin-infiltrating Th2-like cells and allergen-specific IgE response in atopic dermatitis. J Allergy Clin Immunol 96:411–420.

98. Ohmen JD, Hanifin JM, Nickoloff BJ, Rea TH, Wyzykowski R, Kim J, Jullien D, McHugh T, Nassif AS, Chan SC, Modlin RL (1995) Overexpression of IL-10 in atopic dermatitis. Contrasting cytokine patterns with delayed-type hypersensitivity reactions. J Immunol 154:1956–1963.

99. Thepen T, Langeveld-Wildschut EG, Bihari IC, van Wichen DF, van Reijsen FC, Mudde GC, Bruijnzeel-Koomen, CAFM (1996) Bi-phasic response against aeroallergen in atopic dermatitis showing a switch from an initial Th2 response into a Th1 response *in situ*: an immuno-cytochemical study. J Allergy Clin Immunol 97:828–837.

12

T-Cells in the Pathogenesis of Asthma and Allergic Diseases

Marc Humbert, MD
and Stephen R. Durham, MD, FRCP

Contents

INTRODUCTION

T-cells have a central role to play in an antigen-driven inflammatory process, since they are the only cells capable of recognizing antigenic material after processing by antigen presenting cells. CD4$^+$ and CD8$^+$ T lymphocytes activated in this manner elaborate a wide variety of protein mediators, including cytokines, which have the capacity to orchestrate the differentiation, recruitment, accumulation, and activation of specific granulocytes at mucosal surfaces. T-cell derived products can also influence immunoglobulin production by plasma cells. There now exists considerable support for the hypothesis that allergic diseases and asthma represent specialized forms of cell-mediated immunity, in which cytokines secreted predominantly by activated T-cells but also by other leukocytes such as mast cells and eosinophils bring about the specific accumulation and activation of eosinophils. This observation has important implications for future therapeutic procedures since it suggests that drugs modulating T-lymphocyte function may be of considerable interest in allergic conditions and asthma. This chapter summarizes the possible role of T-cells in allergic diseases and possible therapeutic manipulation of inappropriate T-cell activation in humans.

T-CELL-DERIVED CYTOKINES AND T-CELL SUBSETS

Antigenic peptides are presented to T-cell receptors as a high-affinity complex of peptide and major histocompatibility complex (MHC) molecules. As a general rule, the abilities of MHC class I and II to present peptides differ in that MHC class I bind peptides generated from endogenously synthesised molecules (including viral proteins) whereas MHC class II

From: Allergy and Allergic Diseases: The New Mechanisms and Therapeutics
Edited by: J. A. Denburg © Humana Press Inc., Totowa, NJ

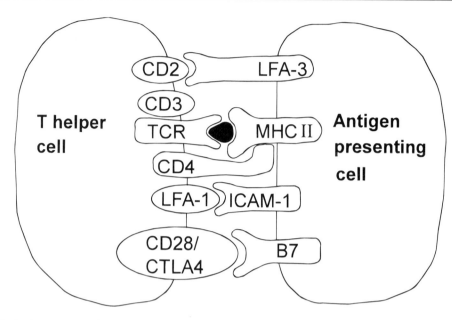

Fig. 1. Antigen presentation on the surface of MHC class II molecule to T-cell receptor and costimulatory signals involved.

molecules bind peptides generated by the proteolytic cleavage of exogenous proteins in lysosomal compartments *(1)*. Exceptions to these processing pathways have been documented but are less common. T-cells can be broadly divided into two groups based on their recognition of peptide in the context of either MHC class I gene or MHC II gene products. T-cells recognizing endogenously generated peptides, presented with class I molecules, express the CD8 molecule, which binds to class I molecules, thus increasing the avidity of the interaction. The expression of CD4 by T-cells indicates recognition of peptides in the context of class II molecules to which CD4 is able to bind (Fig. 1). From a teleogical view it is the source of antigenic peptides, i.e., endogenous vs. exogenous, that determines the nature of the T-cell response that is required. For example, expression of nonself peptides by class I molecules suggests that nonself proteins (viral, for example) are being generated within the cell and that the cell should, therefore, be eliminated. Elimination requires a cytotoxic T-cell response restricted to the peptide in question but also to class I MHC. Thus, most cytotoxic T-cells have the $CD8^+$ phenotype. In contrast, exogenous antigens are not, by definition, generated within host cells and these cells, therefore, do not require elimination. Exogenous antigens such as bacteria require neutralization with antibodies. For this reason, peptides presented in the context of class II MHC proteins generally elicit a T helper ($CD4^+$ T-lymphocyte) response.

T-helper cells can be further subdivided according to the pattern of cytokines elaborated following activation (Fig. 2) *(2–4)*. Great progress in the knowledge of phenotypic and functional activities of different T-cell subsets in mice and humans has been made recently. T-cells secreting cytokines such as interleukin (IL)-2, interferon-γ (IFNγ) and tumor necrosis factor β (TNF-β) are referred to as T-helper 1 (Th1) cells. The cytokines produced by these cells promote cytotoxic T-cell responses and inhibit allergic responses. T-cells producing IL-4, IL-5, and IL-10 but not IFN-γ are referred to as T-helper 2 (Th2) cells. These cells provide B-cell help for isotype switching to immunoglobulin E (IgE) and eosinophil maturation,

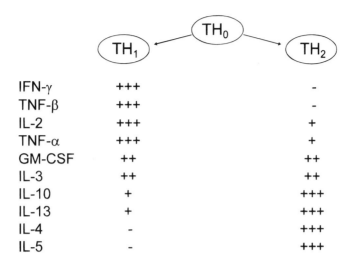

	TH$_1$	TH$_2$
IFN-γ	+++	-
TNF-β	+++	-
IL-2	+++	+
TNF-α	+++	+
GM-CSF	++	++
IL-3	++	++
IL-10	+	+++
IL-13	+	+++
IL-4	-	+++
IL-5	-	+++

Fig. 2. Profile of cytokines produced by "TH$_1$-type" and "TH$_2$-type" T lymphocytes.

survival and activation. Both T helper lymphocyte subtypes can produce eosinophil-active cytokines granulocyte-macrophage colony stimulating factor (GM-CSF) and IL-3. Th2-type lymphocytes are the predominant T-helper phenotype associated with allergic inflammation. Increasing evidence demonstrates that IL-12 (produced predominantly by macrophages and B-cells) and, to a lesser extent, IFN-γ direct CD4$^+$ T-cells to differentiate into Th1 cells (5,6). In contrast IL-4 priming is necessary to direct CD4$^+$ T-cells to differentiate into Th2 cells. Therefore the local cytokine expression is critical to direct the polarization of T-cells toward CD4$^+$ T helper subsets.

In atopic subjects allergens preferentially expand T-cell clones with a Th2 phenotype of cytokine secretion. T-cell clones established from peripheral blood of atopics can produce concordant concentrations of IL-3, IL-4, IL-5, and GM-CSF (7). Moreover, a predominant Th2-like bronchoalveolar T-lymphocyte population has been demonstrated in atopic asthma (8). A recent study using semiquantitative reverse transcriptase–polymerase chain reaction (RT-PCR) demonstrated that the number of IL-5 mRNA copies relative to β-actin in bronchial biopsies of atopic asthmatics correlated with several indicators of disease severity such as asthma (Aas) score, baseline FEV$_1$, baseline peak expiratory flow rate, and histamine PC$_{20}$ (9). In contrast elevated bronchial mucosal IL-4 mRNA expression correlated with total IgE concentrations in both atopic and nonatopic variants of asthma (10). These observations suggest that IL-4 (and possibly local IgE synthesis) is necessary but not sufficient for development of asthma, whereas IL-5 production correlated clearly with markers of asthma severity presumably via eosinophil-dependent mechanisms. Double immunohistochemistry/in situ hybridization clearly established that the majority of both IL-4 and IL-5 mRNA$^+$ cells corresponds to T-cells (mainly CD4$^+$ T lymphocytes) (11,12). Moreover, bronchoalveolar lavage CD4$^+$ T-cell lines from atopic asthmatics synthesized elevated quantities of IL-5 (13). Interestingly CD8$^+$ T-cell lines (as well as CD8$^+$ T-lymphocytes in bronchial biopsies of atopic asthmatics) were also capable of producing significant IL-5 (although fewer than CD4$^+$ cells) as compared with nonatopic nonasthmatic controls (12,13). Taken together these observations are consistent with the view that T-lymphocyte activation and expression of Th2-type cytokines may contribute to tissue eosinophilia and local IgE-dependent events during human allergic diseases.

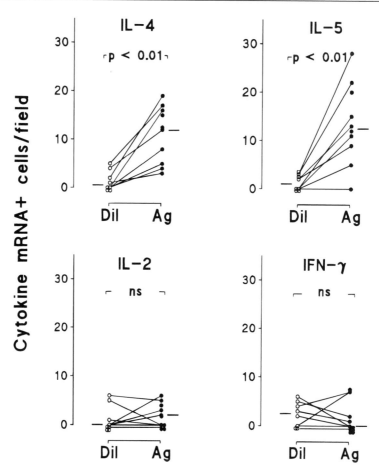

Fig. 3. Cytokine messenger RNA + cells in the nasal mucosa 24 h after nasal provocation with allergen (AG) and diluent (DIL). *In situ* hybridization was performed using antisense rhiboprobes directed against interleukin-4 (IL-4), IL-5, IL-2, and interferon-γ.

T-CELL RECRUITMENT AT SITES OF ALLERGIC INFLAMMATION

The allergen-induced cutaneous late-phase reaction is a useful model of atopic allergic inflammation. By applying the technique of immunohistochemistry to full-thickness skin biopsies, the late-phase reaction was shown to be associated with the infiltration of CD3+, CD4+, and CD8+ T-cells, CD45RO+ memory cells, EG2+ eosinophils, and CD68+ macrophages *(14,15)*. It is well established that late-phase cutaneous reactions to allergens are associated with activation of the IL-3, IL-4, IL-5, and GM-CSF chromosome 5 gene cluster *(16)*.

In the nasal epithelium and submucosa, CD4+ and CD8+ T lymphocytes are the most numerous cells in both normal and atopic subjects. Following allergen provocation, CD4+ T-lymphocyte and eosinophil numbers increase at 24 *(17,18)*. CD25+ cells also increase, although in small numbers, after allergen. Double immunostaining has shown that the majority of these CD25+ cells are indeed T-cells *(19)*. *In situ* hybridization studies have confirmed elevated numbers of cells expressing mRNA for IL-4 and IL-5 but not IL-2 or IFN-γ (Fig. 3) *(20)*. IL-4 protein-containing cells, predominantly mast cells, have also been shown in perennial allergic rhinitis *(21)*. Th2-type cytokines have also been detected in nasal lavage fluid following allergen challenge *(22)*.

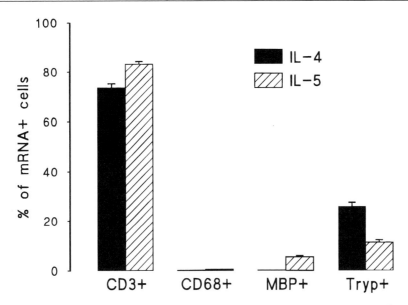

Fig. 4. Phenotype of cells expressing cytokine messenger RNA by *in situ* hybridization of nasal biopsies obtained 24 h after local allergen provocation. The majority of cells are T-lymphocytes (CD3+) with contributions from mast cells (tryptase positive) and eosinophils (major basic protein; MBP+) but not macrophages (CD68+).

Immunohistological studies of fiberoptic bronchoscopic bronchial mucosal biopsies from atopic asthmatics demonstrated elevated numbers of activated EG2+ eosinophils and CD25+ T-lymphocytes *(23–26)*. *In situ* hybridization studies demonstrated an increase in IL-4 and IL-5 mRNA+ bronchial mucosal cells *(8)*. Sequential immunohistochemistry followed by *in situ* hybridization of bronchial biopsies from asthmatics and nasal biopsies from rhinitis demonstrated that the majority of cells expressing IL-4 and IL-5 mRNA were T lymphocytes (70–80%) with lesser contributions from mast cells and eosinophils (Fig. 4) *(11)*. In patients with asthma the number of CD25+ bronchoalveolar lavage T lymphocytes correlated significantly with several markers of disease severity *(27,28)*. Studies of bronchoalveolar lavage during the late responses following allergen provocation have shown increases in BAL CD4+ T-cells up to 48 h after challenge *(29)*. T-lymphocyte recruitment activation and expression of eosinophil-modifying cytokines such as IL-5 and GM-CSF at both the mRNA and protein levels occur during human late asthmatic responses *(30–33)*. A close correlation was demonstrated between the numbers of CD25+ lymphocytes, IL-5 mRNA expression, and the numbers of activated eosinophils in bronchoalveolar lavage *(33)*.

The precise mechanisms for the recruitment of T-cells, eosinophils, and other inflammatory cells into allergen-injected sites are still unknown. However, present evidence suggests that this process involves selective cell adhesion, chemotaxis, and prolonged survival of specific inflammatory cells consequent to the local release of cytokines and other mediators from IgE-sensitized mast cells and allergen-specific T-cells *(26,34,35)*. Indeed, leukocyte trafficking comprises successive events, including rolling, firm adhesion, and extravasation, presumably in response to a chemoattractant gradient in which chemokines are thought to play a critical role *(35–39)*. Chemokines are polypeptides of relatively small molecular weight (8–14 kDa) that have been assigned to different subgroups by structural criteria: with the exception of the newly described lymphotactin, chemokines have four conserved cysteines in which the first two cysteines either are separated by one additional amino acid in one subgroup ("CXC chemokines": IL-8, …) or are adjacent to each other in the second subgroup ("CC chemokines": released from activated normal T-cells, expressed and secreted (RANTES), monocyte activated protein (MCP)-1, -2, -3, …) *(35–39)*. Interestingly, chemokines are distinguished from classical chemoattractants by a certain cell-target specificity: the CXC chemo-kines tend to act more on neutrophils, whereas the CC chemokines tend to act more on monocytes and in some cases basophils, lymphocytes, and eosinophils *(35–39)*. Owing to the effects of some CC-chemokines on basophils and eosinophils, their ability to attract and activate monocytes, and their potential role in lymphocyte recruitment, these molecules have emerged as the most potent stimulators of effector-cell accumulation and activation in allergic inflammation *(36,40–42)*.

We have tested the hypothesis that allergen-induced infiltration of T-cells, eosinophils, and macrophages in the skin of atopics is accompanied by the appearance of mRNA$^+$ cells for RANTES and MCP-3 genes *(43)*. In contrast to diluent controls, allergen provoked a significant increase in mRNA$^+$ cells for MCP-3, which peaked at 6 h and progressively declined at 24 and 48 h. This paralleled the kinetics of total and activated eosinophil infiltration. The allergen-induced expression of mRNA+ cells for RANTES was also clearly demonstrable at 6 h. However, the numbers were maximal at 24 h and declined slightly at the 48-h time point. The number of mRNA$^+$ cells for RANTES paralleled the kinetics of infiltration of CD3$^+$, CD4$^+$, and CD8$^+$ T-cells *(43)*. Although these observations give no definite information concerning the cellular source of the chemokine mRNA, they are compatible with the hypotheses that MCP-3 and RANTES are important in eosinophil and T-cell recruitment, or that these cells are a possible source of these chemokines. Interestingly, the majority of CD4$^+$ T-cells infiltrating the sites of allergen-induced cutaneous late-phase response (LPR) are of the "memory" (CD45RO$^+$) phenotype, phenotype that could be recruited by locally released RANTES *(44)*. This could also apply to asthma, a condition charaterized by combined bronchial mucosal expression of CC chemokines (RANTES and MCP-3), together with eosinophilactive cytokines (IL-5, GM-CSF, and IL-3) *(45)*.

T-CELL RECEPTOR

The antigen-specific arm of the immune response is effected by lymphocytes and in a limited fashion by natural killer cells. T- and B-lymphocytes recognize antigens by means of specific receptors generated by a process of gene rearrangement culminating in the juxtaposition of gene fragment encoding constant and variable regions of the T-cell receptor (TCR) or B-cell receptor. Identifying the antigen-specific receptors on B-cells was relatively easy because, after stimulation, B-cells secrete their receptors as soluble immunoglobulin molecules. By contrast, T-cells do not secrete their receptors. T-cells recognize small peptidic fragments of native proteins generated by antigen-presenting cells such as dendritic cells, monocytes, and B-cells. In addition, peptides are only recognized by T-cells when presented to them bound to molecules of the MHC.

T-cell receptors exist in two forms, both consisting of transmembrane heterodimers. In humans the αβ heterodimer forms 95% of the expressed peripheral repertoire, the other 5% being composed of γδ receptors *(46–50)*. Ontogenetically, the first receptor genes to rearrange are the γ and δ genes. If rearrangements at both alleles fail to generate viable receptor chains, in terms of both structure and specificity, α and β chain genes will be rearranged. T-cell receptor heterodimers are expressed on the surface of the T-cell together with a number of other molecules that act as signal transduction apparatus and are referred to as γ, δ, ε, and ζ chains (the γ and δ chains being distinct from those of the T-cell receptor). An additional chain, η, may also be present in the complex as a disulfide-linked homodimer or as a heterodimer with ζ.

Crosslinking of T-cell receptors leads to tyrosine phosphorylation of members of the CD3 complex and activation of intracellular signaling proteins such as Ras, Raf, and the mitogen-activated protein kinase system. Concomitant hydrolysis of membrane phospholipids leads to the activation of protein kinase C and an increase in intracellular calcium through release from intracellular stores and extracellular influx (51).

Although the discovery of γδ T-cells has generated wide interest, the function of these cells is still largely a mystery. Unlike αβ T-cells, γδ T-cells are CD4⁻ CD8⁻ (although a small proportion are CD4⁻ CD8⁺). γδ T-cells are relatively rare in lymphoid tissue but are conspicuous in epithelial tissue. γδ T-cells show a propensity to react to heat-shock protein and could have a "surveillance" role by destroying damaged cells through recognition of heat-shock proteins on these cells. Indirect evidence implicates γδ T-cells in the cross-regulation of CD4⁺ αβ T-cell response in mice. Adoptive transfer of small numbers of γδ T-cells from ovalbumin-tolerant mice selectively suppressed Th2-dependent IgE production without affecting IgG responses (52). Challenge of these γδ T-cells in vitro with specific antigen resulted in production of high levels of IFN-γ (52). Therefore antigen-specific γδ T-cells may have an important role in the maintenance of immunological homeostasis in the lung and airways by selective suppression of potentially pathogenic Th2-dependent responses while preserving the host's capacity to produce specific IgG antibody. It is possible that γδ T-cells may play a similar role in protection against primary allergic sensitization to environmental antigens associated with allergic rhinitis and asthma. However, exaggerated γδ T-cell responses at mucosal surfaces in normals as opposed to allergic individuals has yet to be demonstrated. In contrast elevated numbers of double negative (CD4⁻ CD8⁻) γδ T lymphocytes have been shown in the nasal mucosa of patients with allergic rhinitis (53). Moreover, a recent study has suggested increased allergen-specific, steroid-sensitive γδ T-cells in bronchoalveolar lavage fluid from patients with asthma (54). These cells could be either passive bystanders recruited by the cytokine milieu present in the lungs of asthmatic patients or T-cells responding to a particular antigenic stimulus and playing a role in atopic asthma. In light of other studies that show responses of cloned γδ T-cells to *Dermatophagoides pteronyssinus (55)*, the presence of a proliferative response of the bronchoalveolar cells to the allergen in *D. pteronyssinus*-sensitive asthmatics suggests that γδ T-cells could be immunopathologically important in asthma. However, it remains unclear whether the regulatory role of γδ T-cells in asthma is beneficial or harmful (52,54,56).

The antigen-combining region of the TCR gene is assembled by recombination of variable (V), diversity (D), and joining (J) segments (46,47). The Vα and Vβ gene segments can be clustered into families that share common genetic features and whose protein products can be identid by family-specific monoclonal antibodies. Peripheral-blood T-cell populations may not reflect the compartmentalized repertoire in diseased organs and it is assumed that analysis of the TcR repertoire at sites of inflammation may yield insight into the nature of the stimulus. Antigen-driven T-cell proliferation may result in expansion of oligoclonal T-cell populations. In contrast, nonspecific T-cell recruitment would result in a heterogeneous TCR repertoire at the inflammatory sites. Many examples of TCR repertoire selection at sites of autoimmune disease have been reported in man and in animal models (57). In atopic asthma, preliminary data show that variable patterns of T-cell receptor mRNA expression can be found in bronchoalveolar lavage from patients with mild disease (58). Although it is widely accepted that allergen exposure promotes T-cell activation in atopic asthma, the mechanisms by which T-cells (harvested by bronchoalveolar lavage or bronchial biopsy) are activated in nonatopic asthmatics is unknown (59). In this situation, studying TCR clonotypes would be of great interest to determine whether T-cells are clonally activated by putative unidentified antigen. A recent report on TcR Vβ gene expression in nonatopic asthma demonstrates that the numbers of T-cell clones expressing TcR Vβ3, Vβ6, Vβ13, Vβ14, Vβ15, and Vβ17 genes in bronchoalveolar lavage fluid specifically increased in comparison to those in peripheral-blood lymphocytes *(60)*. This is compatible with the hypothesis that infiltrating T-cells in the airway may expand after antigen-driven stimulation.

COSTIMULATORY FACTORS

It is now clearly established that ligation of TCR is not sufficient to deliver a full activation signal to the cell and further signals are required *(61,62)*. Such noncognate (nonantigen-specific) interactions are collectively referred to as costimulation, the molecules involved including CD4, CD8, lymphocyte-function associated (LFA)-1, and cytotoxic T-lymphocyte-associated molecule CD28/(CTL)A4 on the T-cell and MHC class I and II, intercellular adhesion molecule (ICAM)-1 and -2, and the B7 homologs on the antigen-presenting cell (Fig. 1).

One of the most extensively studied T-cell costimulation systems is that of CD28 and its ligands, the B7 family composed of at least two members of the immunoglobulin supergene family, B7-1 (CD80) and B7-2 (CD86) *(61–63)*. Ligation of CD28 by members of the B7 family, expressed on antigen-presenting cells, is an obligate requirement for the synthesis and secretion of the T-cell growth factor IL-2 *(64)*. Triggering through the T-cell receptor in the absence of appropriate signals from CD28 results in a nonresponsive state known as anergy, which may last for several days and may even result in cell death.

Increasing evidence suggests that CD28-mediated costimulatory signals are important at several stages of T-cell differentiation *(61–64)*. To initiate their first proliferative cycle, naive T-cells require TcR signaling and a second signal, which can be provided by CD28, resulting in secretion of IL-2 *(64)*. Following additional exposures to TcR and CD28-mediated signaling, IL-2-secreting T-cells differentiate into Th0 T-cells capable of secreting multiple cytokines *(63)*. Several murine studies demonstrate that the CD28 pathway is critical for the development of IL-4-producing T cells *(65–67)*. More precisely, a selectivity of B7-1 for promoting Th1 responses and B7-2 for promoting Th2 responses in the murine system has been suggested *(63)*. Nevertheless, the importance of the CD28-B7 costimulatory pathway in T-cell responses to allergens remains poorly defined. In human peripheral-blood mononuclear cells, production of cytokines such as IFN-γ, IL-4, IL-5, and IL-13 can be inhibited by monoclonal antibodies against B7-2 but not B7-1, suggesting that secretion of these cytokines is dependent on B7-2 costimulation in this system *(68,69)*. Further studies are needed to conclude on the in vivo relevance of this important determinant of T-cell activation.

T-cells also provide costimulation or help for B-cell activation and antibody production. Soluble mediators such as IL-4, IL-6, and IL-13 produced by T-cells act directly on B-cells, via cell surface receptors, inducing proliferation and differentiation and also modulating the antibody response *(70–72)*. Th2-type cytokine-induced B-cell activation and subsequent IgE production is believed to be a critical characteristic of patients with atopy. As indicated above, several studies have shown that atopic individuals are characterized by elevated gene expression and protein production of Th2-type cytokines as compared to nonatopic controls. An interesting situation is that of nonatopic asthma, which has been considered as a distinct pathogenic varient of asthma since these patients are skin test-negative to common aeroallergens and have normal total serum IgE *(59)*. However, the recent demonstration of elevated numbers of cells expressing the high-affinity IgE receptor in bronchial biopsies from atopic and nonatopic asthmatics *(73)* together with epidemiological evidence indicating that serum IgE concentrations relate closely to the prevalence of asthma regardless of atopic status *(74)* suggests that IgE-mediated mechanisms may be important in the pathogenesis of both atopic and nonatopic asthma. Furthermore, both variants of the disease are associated with eosinophilic inflammation *(73,75)*. We have recently compared the expression of IL-4 mRNA and protein product using semiquantitative RT-PCR amplification, *in situ* hybridization, and immuno-histochemistry in bronchial biopsies from atopic and nonatopic symptomatic asthmatics and compared our findings to atopic and nonatopic controls *(76)*. The results showed that, compared with controls, elevated numbers of IL-4 mRNA copies relative to β-actin were detected by RT-PCR in biopsies from both groups of asthmatics. Similarly, *in situ* hybridization and immunohistochemistry demonstrated increased numbers of cells expressing IL-4 mRNA and protein in asthma, irrespective of their atopic status. Therefore, elevated IL-4 production is associated with both the atopic and nonatopic variants of asthma. IgE-dependent mechanisms involving Th2-type cytokines might be a feature of intrinsic as well as extrinsic asthma. These results are in contrast to those of Walker et al. *(77)*, who found that, unlike atopic asthma, IL-4 protein was not elevated in concentrated bronchoalveolar lavage fluid in nonatopic asthma when compared to controls. The reasons for this apparent discrepancy are unclear but they may be related to methodological problems, e.g., differences in protein recovery during concentration of bronchoalveolar lavage and the possible presence of inhibitors in bronchoalveolar lavage fluid that might interfere with the protein assay. Using double *in situ* hybridization/immunohistochemistry, we have clearly demonstrated that a majority of IL-4 (and IL-5) mRNA was T-cell-derived in atopic as well as nonatopic asthma *(11,12)*. Moreover it appears that IL-13 gene expression is similar in asthmatics, irrespective of their atopic status, and elevated as compared to controls *(78)*. These results support the concept that these subtypes of asthma, despite showing some distinct clinical features, might have common immunopathological mechanisms.

Help is also provided through interaction of cell surface structures, particularly the CD40 ligand on T-cells, which interacts with CD40 on the B-cell surface *(79)*. Isotype switching of immunoglobulin is dependent on this molecular interaction, dysfunction in this pathway giving rise to X-linked hyper-IgM syndrome, an immunodeficiency that is characterized by an inability to switch immunoglobulin isotypes and a consequent lack of IgG, IgA, and IgE in affected individuals *(80)*.

ALTERING T-CELL RESPONSE
WITH ALLERGEN-SPECIFIC IMMUNOTHERAPY

Allergen-specific immunotherapy is recommended in patients with defined IgE-mediated allergies who do not respond to conventional antiallergic medications *(81,82)*. An important and hitherto unanswered question is whether immunotherapy may induce long-lived immunological changes that translate into modification of the natural history of allergic disease. The mechanism of immunotherapy is still unknown. Earlier studies demonstrated changes in serum antibody measurements with blunting of seasonal increases in IgE following pollen immunotherapy and increases in so-called "blocking" allergen-specific IgG concentrations *(83,84)*. More recently, immunotherapy has been shown to reduce the numbers of "effector" cells at mucosal sites. For example, ragweed immunotherapy inhibited allergen-induced immediate and late nasal responses and the associated production of mediators of hypersensitivity *(85)* and eosinophil accumulation *(86)*. Immunotherapy in mite-sensitive subjects reduced the numbers of mast cells in the nasal epithelium *(87)*. In birch pollen-sensitive asthmatics, immunotherapy inhibited seasonal increases in bronchial hyperresponsiveness and the associated increase in the number of bronchoalveolar eosinophils and eosinophil cationic protein concentrations *(88)*.

We hypothesized that these changes in antibodies and effector cells induced by immunotherapy may occur indirectly as a consequence of modulation of the T-cell response to allergen exposure *(89)*. Previous studies demonstrated a decrease in allergen-induced pro-

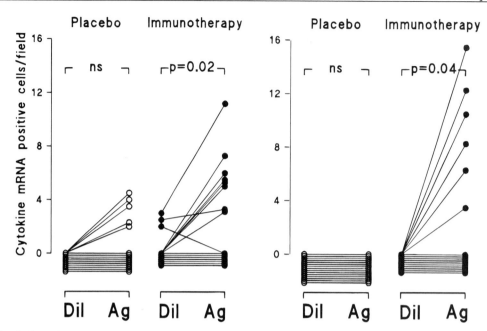

Fig. 5. Cytokine messenger RNA + cells in cutaneous biopsies obtained 24 h after intradermal challenge with allergen (AG) or control challenge diluent (DIL). The influence of 9 mo of immunotherapy with a depot grass pollen extract is compared with patients treated with placebo injections for 9 mo in a double-blind trial. Results are shown for interleukin-2 (IL2) and interferon-γ (IFN-γ).

liferation of peripheral-blood T lymphocytes following immunotherapy and an increase in the number of circulating CD8[+] T lymphocytes *(90)*. A characteristic feature of immunotherapy is its ability to inhibit allergen-induced late responses. We have used the late response in the skin and nose for assessing the effects of immunotherapy on T-lymphocyte responses *(91,92)*. We hypothesized that immunotherapy may act by reducing Th2 responses (with a decrease in local IL-4 and IL-5 expression) or increasing Th1 responses (with an increase in IFN-γ production). Studies in pollen and bee venom-sensitive patients treated with immunotherapy have shown a decrease in Th2-type cytokine secretion following allergen stimulation of cultured peripheral-blood T lymphocytes *(93,94)*. By use of immunohistochemistry and *in situ* hybridization of tissue biopsies obtained during cutaneous and nasal late-phase responses we have shown preferential increases in local allergen-induced Th1 responses *(95)*. This double-blind placebo controlled trial showed that grass pollen immunotherapy was highly effective in reducing seasonal symptoms and medication requirements. Clinical improvement was accompanied by a marked reduction in immediate allergen sensitivity in the skin and nose and inhibition of allergen-induced late cutaneous and nasal responses. At control sites following immunotherapy, a decrease in cutaneous mast cells and an increase in CD8[+] T-cells was observed. Following allergen challenge, inhibition of the late cutaneous response was associated with a decrease in CD4[+] T lymphocytes and an increase in the number of CD25[+] (IL-2 receptor-bearing) cells and Human Leukocyte Antigen-DR (HLA-DR[+]) cells (antigen-presenting cells). By *in situ* hybridization, that inhibition of the late response in the actively treated group was accompanied by an increase in allergen-induced cells expressing IL-2 and IFN-γ mRNA (Fig. 5). Immunotherapy similarly inhibited allergen-induced early and late nasal responses and resulted in a reduction in tissue recruitment of CD4[+] T lymphocytes and

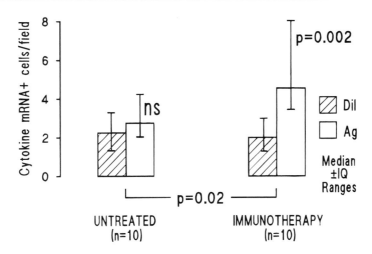

Fig. 6. Cytokine messenger RNA + cells obtained 24 h after allergen (open bars) or a control challenge (diluent, DIL; hatched bars). Interleukin-12 (IL-12) positive cells for patients who had received grass pollen immunotherapy using a depot extract for a period of 4 yr were compared with matched untreated hayfever patients. Immunotherapy was highly effective in inhibiting the late response (data not shown).

eosinophils and an increase in local IFN-γ mRNA+ cells 24 h after allergen challenge. These results suggest that inhibition of IgE-dependent mechanisms and decreased tissue eosinophilia following immunotherapy may result from modulation of T-lymphocyte responses in favor of local increases in IFN-γ.

As indicated above, IL-12 (a product of macrophages and B-cells) is known to promote Th1-type responses both in vitro and in vivo *(5,6)*. In order to test the hypothesis that IL-12 may promote and sustain long-lived Th1-type responses during immunotherapy, we repeated cutaneous biopsies 24 h after cutaneous challenge and at control sites in patients following 4 yr immunotherapy and matched control patients who had not received immunotherapy. The late cutaneous response was almost completely inhibited following immunotherapy. *In situ* hybridization of cutaneous biopsies was performed using a riboprobe directed against IL-12. Inhibition of the late response was associated with a marked increase in IL-12 mRNA+ cells in all patients tested (Fig. 6). These differences were highly significant, compared with untreated hayfever sufferers who developed late responses. Associations were sought among the number of cells expressing mRNA for IL-12, IL-4, and IFN-γ. The number of IL-12 mRNA+ cells correlated positively with that of IFN-γ mRNA+ cells and inversely with that of IL-4 mRNA+ cells. The principal source of IL-12 mRNA was determined using sequential immunostaining followed by *in situ* hybridization. Sixty to 80% of IL-12 mRNA+ cells were CD68+ tissue macrophages. We therefore suggested that changes in antibody responses and effector cells during immunotherapy may occur as a consequence of altered T-cell response (Fig. 7). Taken together, these results suggest that immunotherapy induces a switch from dominant Th2-type response to a Th1-type response following allergen exposure. These altered Th1 responses might be promoted or sustained by IL-12 produced principally from activated tissue macrophages. Moreover IFN-γ may act by inhibiting IL-4-induced IgE synthesis and/or alternatively promoting increased IgG₄ synthesis. Future treatment might include local strategies directed against IL-4, or against IgE or its high-affinity receptor in the airways mucosa. A trial of topical IFN-γ or IL-12 may also be indicated.

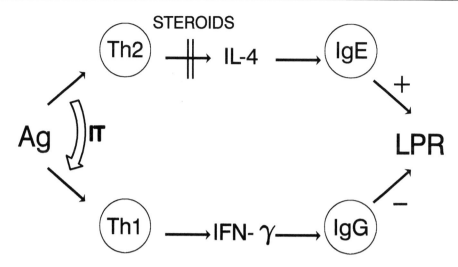

Fig. 7. Hypothesis on the mechanism of the action of topical corticosteroids compared with allergen injection immunotherapy on allergen-induced late nasal responses.

TARGETING T-CELLS IN GLUCOCORTICOID-DEPENDENT ASTHMA

Corticosteroids are the mainstay treatment for asthma, but some patients with chronic severe asthma are refractory to their effects despite oral therapy *(96,97)*. Systemic corticosteroid treatment places these patients at risk from long-term unwanted side effects such as osteoporosis, and therefore any intervention that reduces patients' requirements for corticosteroids would have important implications for future management of severe asthma. Activated $CD4^+$ T lymphocytes and their products are believed to play a pivotal role in asthma and correlate with markers of disease severity. Pharmacological targeting of T-cells could therefore form the basis of a novel approach to the treatment of asthma.

Cyclosporin A, a lipophilic undecapeptide isolated from fungal cultures, is believed to exert its immunosuppressive action primarily by inhibition of antigen-induced T-lymphocyte activation and the transcription and translation of mRNA for several cytokines, including IL-2, IL-5, and GM-CSF *(98)* In addition, cyclosporin A has effects on eosinophils, inhibiting IL-5-dependent survival and cytokine-enhanced degranulation in vitro, as well as the release of cytokines into culture supernatants by stimulated eosinophils *(98,100)*. Lastly, cyclosporin A rapidly modulates the release of preformed and *de novo* synthesized mediators from human mast cells in vitro and also from basophils ex vivo and has also been shown to suppress cytokine release from murine mast cell lines *(101–103)*.

Low doses of cyclosporin are effective in the treatment of various diseases thought to be mediated by activated T lymphocytes, including psoriasis, atopic dermatitis, and Crohn's disease *(104–106)*. In patients with chronic asthma that was clinically resistant to oral corticosteroids, dexamethasone did not inhibit mitogen-induced T-lymphocyte proliferation or lymphokine release, whereas cyclosporin significantly inhibited both processes *(107)*. A randomized, double-blind, placebo-controlled, crossover trial established that cyclosporin improves lung function in patients with corticosteroid-dependent chronic severe asthma, suggesting a role for activated lymphocytes in the pathogenesis of asthma *(108)*. The corticosteroid-sparing properties of cyclosporin A in corticosteroid-dependent asthma have been investigated recently in a double-blind, placebo-controlled study *(109)*. Compared with placebo, a 36-wk treatment with cyclosporin (initial dose 5 mg/kg/d adjusted to maintain whole-blood trough cyclosporin concentrations of 100–200 µg/L) resulted in a significant reduction in median daily prednisolone dosage and total prednisolone intake. In addition morning peak expiratory flow rate improved significantly in the active treatment group but not in the placebo group. However, these reductions were not possible in all patients and the improvements achieved were sometimes mild. Another study indicated that following cyclosporin administration a slight beneficial effect on some subjective parameters of asthma severity were observed, with no beneficial effect on pulmonary function *(110)*. Using placebo-controlled, double-blind conditions Sihra et al. *(111)* showed that cyclosporin A inhibited the late, but not the early, bronchoconstrictor response to inhaled allergen challenge of sensitized mild atopic asthmatics. This in vivo model suggests that cyclosporin A exerts its antiasthmatic effects mainly through inhibition of transcription and translation of cytokines by T-lymphocyte rather than by significantly inhibiting release of mediators from mast cells. Although the use of oral cyclosporin A in mild asthma is rarely justified because of its poor risk: benefit ratio, these observations suggest that a safe drug directed against the T-lymphocyte would be an effective therapy for asthma.

ACKNOWLEDGMENTS

The authors thank A. B. Kay and colleagues from the Department of Allergy and Clinical Immunology, National Heart and Lung Institute, London, UK.

REFERENCES

1. Germain RN (1993) Antigen processing and presentation. In: Paul WE, ed. Fundamental Immunology, 3rd ed. Raven, New York, pp. 629–676.
2. Mossmann TR, Coffman RL (1987) Two types of mouse helper T cell clone: implication for immune regulation. Immunol Today 8:223–227.
3. Mossmann TR, Sad S (1996) The expanding universe of T-cell subsets: Th1, Th2 and more. Immunol Today 17:138–146.
4. Romagnani S (1994) Lymphokine production by human T cells in disease states. Annu Rev Immunol 12:227–257.
5. Maneti R, Parronchi P, Giudzi MG, et al. (1993) Natural killer cell stimulating factor (interleukin 12) (IL-12) induces T helper type 1 (TH$_1$) specific immune responses and inhibits development of IL-4 producing TH cells. J Exp Med 177:1199–1204.
6. Trinchieri G (1994) Interleukin-12: a cytokine produced by antigen-presenting cells with immunoregulatory functions in the generation of T-helper cells type 1 and cytotoxic lymphocytes. Blood 84:4008–4024.
7. Parronchi P, Manetti R, Simonelli C, et al.(1991) Cytokine production by allergen (Der pI)-specific CD4$^+$ T cell clones derived from a patient with severe atopic disease. Int J Clin Lab Res 21:186–189.
8. Robinson DS, Hamid Q, Ying S, et al. (1992) Predominant T$_{H2}$-like bronchoalveolar T-lymphocyte population in atopic asthma. N Engl J Med 326:298–304.
9. Humbert M, Durham SR, Kimmitt P, et al. (1996) Relationship between bronchial mucosal IL-5 mRNA expression with disease severity in atopic asthma. Am J Respir Crit Care Med 153:A217 (abstract).
10. Humbert M, Corrigan CJ, Kimmitt P, Till SJ, Kay AB, Durham SR (1997) Relationship between bronchial mucosal interleukin-4 and interleukin-5 expression and disease severity in atopic asthma. Am J Resp Crit Care Med 156:704–708.
11. Ying S, Durham SR, Jacobson MR, Rak S, Masuyama K, Lowhagen O, Kay AB, Hamid Q (1994) T-lymphocytes and mast cells express messenger RNA for interleukin-4 in the nasal mucosa in allergen-induced rhinitis. Immunology 82:200–204.
12. Ying S, Durham SR, Corrigan CJ, Hamid Q, Kay AB (1995) Phenotype of cells expressing mRNA for TH2-type (interleukin-4 and interleukin-5) and TH1-type (interleukin-2 and interferon-gamma) cytokines in bronchoalveolar lavage and bronchial biopsies from atopic asthmatics and normal control subjects. Am J Respir Cell Mol Biol 12:477–487.

13. Till S, Li B, Durham S, et al. (1995) Secretion of the eosinophil-active cytokines (IL-5, GM-CSF and IL-3) by bronchoalveolar lavage CD4$^+$ and CD8$^+$ T cell lines in atopic asthmatics and atopic and non-atopic controls. Eur J Immunol 25:2727–2731.

14. Frew AJ, Kay AB (1988) The relationship between infiltrating CD4$^+$ lymphocytes, activated eosinophils, and the magnitude of the allergen-induced late-phase cutaneous reaction in man. J Immunol 141:4158–4164.

15. Ying S, Taborda-Barata L, Meng Q, Humbert M, Kay AB (1995) The kinetics of allergen-induced transcription of messenger RNA for monocyte chemotactic protein-3 and RANTES in the skin of human atopic subjects: relationship to eosinophil, T-cell, and macrophage recruitment. J Exp Med 181:2153–2159.

16. Kay AB, Ying S, Varney V, et al. (1991) Messenger RNA expression of the cytokine gene cluster, inter-leukin 3 (IL-3), IL-4, IL-5 and granulocyte/macrophage colony stimulating-factor, in allergen-induced late-phase reactions in atopic subjects. J Exp Med 173:775–778.

17. Varney VA, Jacobson MR, Sudderick RM, et al. (1992) Immunohistology of the nasal mucosa following allergen-induced rhinitis: identification of activated T lymphocytes, eosinophils and neutrophils. Am Rev Respir Dis 145:170–175.

18. Lim MC, Taylor RM, Naclerio RM (1995) The histology of allergic rhinitis and its comparison to cel-lular changes in nasal lavage. Am J Respir Crit Care Med 151:136–144.

19. Hamid Q, Barkans J, Robinson DS, Durham SR, Kay AB (1992) Co-expression of CD25 and CD3 in atopic allergy and asthma. Immunology 75:659–663.

20. Durham SR, Ying S, Varney V, et al. (1992) Cytokine messenger RNA expression for IL-3, IL-4, IL-5 and GM-CSF in the nasal mucosa after local allergen provocation: relationship to tissue eosinophilia. J Immunol 148:2390–2394.

21. Bradding PL, Feather IH, Howarth PH, et al. (1992) Interleukin 4 is localised to and released by human mast cells. J Exp Med 176:1381–1386.

22. Sim TC, Reece LM, Hilsmeier KA, Grant JA, Allam R (1995) Secretion of chemokines and other cytokines in allergen-induced nasal responses: inhibition by topical steroid treatment. Am J Respir Crit Care Med 152:927–933.

23. Bousquet J, Chanez P, Lacoste J-Y, et al. (1990) Eosinophilic inflammation in asthma. N Engl J Med 323:1033–1039.

24. Azzawi M, Bradley B, Jeffery PK et al. (1990) Identification of activated T lymphocytes and eosinophils in bronchial biopsies in stable atopic asthma. Am Rev Respir Dis 142:1407–1413.

25. Djukanovic R, Wilson JW, Britten KM (1990) Mucosal inflammation in asthma. Am Rev Respir Dis 142:434–457.

26. Corrigan CJ, Kay AB (1992) T cells and eosinophils in the pathogenesis of asthma. Immunol Today 13:501–507.

27. Walker C, Kaegi MK, Braun P, Blaser K (1991) Activated T cells and eosinophilia in bronchoalveolar lavages from subjects with asthma correlated with disease severity. J Allergy Clin Immunol 88:935–942.

28. Robinson DS, Bentley AM, Hartnell A, Kay AB, Durham SR (1993) Activated memory T helper cells in bronchoalveolar lavage fluid from patients with atopic asthma: relation to asthma symptoms, lung function, and bronchial responsiveness. Thorax 48:26–32.

29. Gonzalez MC, Diaz P, Galleguillos FR, Ancic P, Cromwell O, Kay AB (1987) Allergen-induced recruit-ment of bronchoalveolar helper (OKT4) and suppressor (OKT8) T-cells in asthma. Am Rev Respir Dis 136:600–604.

30. Broide DH, Firestein GS (1991) Endobronchial allergen challenge in asthma: demonstration of cellular source of granulocyte macrophage colony-stimulating factor by in situ hybridization. J Clin Invest 88:1048–1053.

31. Broide DH, Paine MM, Firestein GS (1992) Eosinophils express interleukin-5 and granulocyte macrophage colony-stimulating factor mRNA at sites of allergic inflammation in asthmatics. J Clin Invest 90:1414–1424.

32. Bentley AM, Meng Q, Robinson DS, Hamid Q, Kay AB, Durham SR (1993) Increases in activated T lymphocytes, eosinophils, and cytokine mRNA expression for interleukin-5 and granulocyte/macrophage colony-stimulating factor in bronchial biopsies after allergen inhalation in atopic asthmat-ics. Am J Respir Cell Mol Biol 8:35–42.

33. Robinson DS (1993) Cytokines in asthma. Thorax 48:845–853.

34. Schleimer RP, Sterbinsky SA, Kaiser J, et al. (1992) IL-4 induces adherence of human eosinophils and basophils but not neutrophils to endothelium: association with expression of VCAM-1. J Immunol 148:1086–1092.

35. Baggiolini M, Dewald B, Moser B (1994) Interleukin-8 and related chemokines: CXC and CC chemokines. Adv Immunol 55:97–179.

36. Springer TA (1994) Traffic signals for lymphocyte recirculation and leukocyte emigration: the multi-step paradigm. Cell 76:301–314.

37. Baggiolini M, Dahinden CA (1994) CC chemokines in allergic inflammation. Immunol Today 15:127–133.

38. Schall TJ, Bacon KB (1994) Chemokines, leukocyte trafficking, and inflammation. Cur Opin Immunol 6:865–873.

39. Prieschl EE, Kulmburg PA, Baumruker T (1995) The nomenclature of chemokines. Int Arcl. Allergy Immunol 107:475–483.

40. Alam R, Stafford S, Forsythe P, et al. (1993) RANTES is a chemotactic and activating factor for human eosinophils. J Immunol 150:3442–3447.

41. Ebisawa N, Yamada T, Bickel C, Klunk D, Schleimer RP (1994) Eosinophilic transendothelial migration induced by cytokines: effect of the chemokine RANTES. J Immunol 153:2153–2160.

42. Dahinden CA, Geiser T, Brunner T, et al. (1994) Monocyte chemotactic protein 3 is a most effective basophil- and eosinophil-activating cytokine. J Exp Med 179:751–756.

43. Ying S, Taborda-Barata L, Meng Q, Humbert M, Kay AB (1995) The kinetics of allergen-induced transcription of messenger RNA for monocyte chemotactic protein-3 and RANTES in the skin of human atopic subjects: relationship to eosinophil, T-cell, and macrophage recruitment. J Exp Med 181:2153–2159.

44. Schall TJ, Bacon K, Toy KJ, Goeddel TV (1990) Selective attraction of monocytes and T lymphocytes of the memory phenotype by cytokine RANTES. Nature 347:669–671.

45. Humbert M, Ying S, Corrigan C, et al. (1997) Bronchial mucosal gene expression of the CC chemokines RANTES and MCP-3 in symptomatic atopic and non-atopic asthmatics: relationship to the eosinophil-active cytokines IL-5, GM-CSF and IL-3. Am J Respir Cell Mol Biol 16:1–8.

46. Kruisbeek AM (1993) Development of alpha beta T cells. Curr Opin Immunol 5:227–234.

47. Leiden JM (1993) Transcriptional regulation of T cell receptor genes. Annu Rev Immunol 11:539–570.

48. Spits H (1994) Early stages in human and mouse T cell development. Curr Opin Immunol 6:212–221.

49. Augustin A, Kubo RT, Sim GK (1989) Resident pulmonary lymphocytes expressing the γ/δ T-cell receptor. Nature 340:239–241.

50. Fajac I, Tazi A, Hance AJ, et al. (1992) Lymphocytes infiltrating normal human lung and lung carcinomas rarely express γδ T cell antigen receptor. Clin Exp Immunol 87:127–131.

51. Chan AC, Desai DM, Weiss A (1994) The role of protein tyrosine kinases and protein tyrosine phosphatases in T cell antigen receptor signal transduction. Annu Rev Immunol 12:555–592.

52. McMenamin C, Pimm C, McKersey M, Holt PG (1994) Regulation of IgE responses to inhaled antigen in mice by antigen-specific γδ T cells. Science 265:1869–1871.

53. Okuda M, Pawankar R (1992) Flow cytometric analysis of intraepithelial lymphocytes in the human nasal mucosa. Allergy 47:255–259.

54. Spinozzi F, Agea E, Bistoni O, et al. (1996) Increased allergen-specific, steroid sensitive γδ T cells in bronchoalveolar lavage fluid from patients with asthma. Ann Int Med 124:223–227.

55. Pawankar R, Okuda M, Asuma M, et al. (1995) Characterization of nasal γδ T cells in perennial allergic rhinitis. J Allergy Clin Immunol 95:190.

56. Rossman MD, Carding SR (1996) γδ T cells in asthma. Ann Int Med 124:266–267.

57. Marguerie C, Lunardi C, So A (1992) PCR-based analysis of the TCR repertoire in human autoimmune diseases. Immunol Today 13:336–339.

58. Frew AJ, Dasmahapatra J (1995) T cell receptor genetics, autoimmunity and asthma. Thorax 10:919–922.

59. Rackeman FM (1947) A working classification of asthma. Am J Med 3:601–606.

60. Umibe T, Kita Y, Nakao A, et al. (1996) Analysis of T cell receptor clonotypes in bronchoalveolar lavage fluids of nonatopic asthmatics. J Allergy Clin Immunol 97:309 (Abstract 505).

61. June CH, Bluestone JA, Nadler LM, Thompson CB (1994) The B7 and CD28 receptor families. Immunol Today 15:321–331.

62. Thompson CB (1995) Distinct roles for the costimulatory ligands B7-1 and B7-2 in T helper cell differentiation? Cell 81:979–982.

63. Freeman GJ, Boussiotis VA, Anumanthan A, et al. (1995) B7-1 and B7-2 do not deliver identical costimulatory signals, since B7-2 but not B7-1 preferentially costimulates the initial production of IL-4. Immunity 2:523–532.

64. Ehlers S, Smith KA (1991) Differentiation of T cell lymphokine gene expression: the in vitro acquisition of T cell memory. J Exp Med 173:25–36.

65. Lu P, Zhou XD, Chen SJ, et al. (1994) CTLA-4 ligands are required to induce an in vivo interleukin 4 response to a gastrointestinal nematode parasite. J Exp Med 180:693–698.

66. Corry DB, Reiner SL, Linsley PS, Locksley RM (1994) Differential effects of blockade of CD28-B7 on the development of Th1 or Th2 effector cell in experimental Leishmaniasis. J Immunol 153:4142–4148.

67. Milich D, Linsley P, Hughes J, Jones J (1994) Soluble CTLA-4 can suppress autoantibody production and elicit long term responsiveness in a novel transgenic model. J Immunol 153:429–435.

68. Bungre J, Till S, Larché M, et al. (1996) IL-5 secretion by allergen-specific CD4$^+$ cells in short-term culture: dissociation from allergen-induced proliferation and dependence on B7-2 co-stimulation. J Allergy Clin Immunol 97:359 (Abstract 708).

69. Till SJ, Larché M, Corrigan C, Dickason R, Huston D, Kay AB, Robinson DS. Dependence of allergen-induced T cell proliferation and cytokine production on CD28/CD86 costimulation. Clin Exp Immunol (submitted).

70. Del Prete GF, Maggi E, Parronchi P, et al. (1988) IL-4 is an essential co-factor for the IgE synthesis induced in vitro by human T cell clones and their supernatants. J Immunol 140:4193–4198.

71. Hirano T, Akira S, Taga T, Kishimoto T (1990) Biological and clinical aspects of interleukin-6. Immunol Today 443–449.

72. Zurawski G, de Vries JE (1994) Interleukin 13, an interleukin 4-like cytokine that acts on monocytes and B cells, but not on T cells. Immunol Today 15:19–26.

73. Humbert M, Grant JA, Taborda-Barata L, et al. (1996) High affinity IgE receptor (FcεRI)-bearing cells in bronchial biopsies from atopic and non-atopic asthma. Am J Respir Crit Care Med 153:1931–1937.

74. Burrows B, Martinez FD, Halonen M, Barbee RA, Cline MG (1989) Association of asthma with serum IgE levels and skin-test reactivity to allergens. N Engl J Med 320:271–277.

75. Bentley AM, Menz G, Storz C, et al. (1992) Identification of T lymphocytes, macrophages, and activated eosinophils in the bronchial mucosa of intrinsic asthma: relationship to symptoms and bronchial responsiveness. Am Rev Respir Dis 146:500–506.

76. Humbert M, Durham SR, Ying S, et al. (1996) IL-4 and IL-5 mRNA and protein in bronchial biopsies from atopic and non-atopic asthmatics: evidence against "intrinsic" asthma being a distinct immunopathological entity. Am J Respir Crit Care Med 154:1497–1504.

77. Walker C, Bode E, Boer L, Hansel TT, Blaser K, Virchow Jr J-C (1992) Allergic and non-allergic asthmatics have distinct patterns of T-cell activation and cytokine production in peripheral blood and bronchoalveolar lavage. Am Rev Respir Dis 146:109–115.

78. Humbert M, Durham SR, Kimmitt P, et al. (1998) Elevated expression of mRNA encoding interleukin-13 in the bronchial mucosa of atopic and non-atopic asthmatics. J Allergy Clin Immunol (in press).

79. Jabara HH, Fu SM, Geha RS, Vercelli D (1990) CD40 and IgE: synergism between anti-CD40 MAb and IL-4 in the induction of IgE synthesis by highly purified human B cells. J Exp Med 172:1861–1864.

80. DiSanto JP, Bonnefoy JY, Gauchat JF, Fischer A, de Saint Basile G (1993) CD40 ligand mutations in X-linked immunodeficiency with hyper IgM. Nature 361:541–543.

81. EAACI (1993) Immunotherapy position paper. Allergy 48(Suppl 14):1–35.

82. BSACI Working Party (1993) Position paper on allergen immunotherapy. Clin Exp Allergy 23 (Suppl 3):1–44.

83. Lichtenstein LM, Ishizaka K, Norman PS, Sobobka AK, Hill BM (1973) IgE antibody measurements in ragweed hayfever: relationship to clinical severity and the results of immunotherapy. J Clin Invest 52:472–482.

84. Djurup R (1985) The subclass nature and clinical significance of the IgE antibody response in the patients undergoing allergen specific immunotherapy. Allergy 40:469–486.

85. Creticos P, Franklin Adkinson N Jr, Kagey-Sobobka A, et al. (1985) Nasal challenge with ragweed in hayfever patients: effects of immunotherapy. J Clin Invest 76:2247–2253.

86. Furin MJ, Norman PS, Creticos P, et al. (1991) Immunotherapy decreases antigen-induced eosinophil migration into the nasal cavity. J Allergy Clin Immunol 88:27–32.

87. Otsuka H, Mezawa A, Ohnishi M, Okubo K, Seki H, Okuda M (1991) Changes in nasal metachromatic cells during allergen immunotherapy. Clin Exp Allergy 21:115–119.

88. Rak S, Lowhagen O, Venge P (1988) The effect of immunotherapy on bronchial hyperresponsiveness and eosinophil cationic protein in pollen allergic patients. J Allergy Clin Immunol 82:470–480.

89. Durham SR, Varney V, Gaga M, Trew AS, Jacobson M, Kay AB (1991) Immunotherapy and allergic inflammation. Clin Exp Allergy 21:206–210.

90. Rocklin RE, Sheffer AL, Greineder DR, Melmon KL (1980) Generation of antigen-specific suppressor cells during allergy desensitization. N Engl J Med 302:1213–1219.

91. Varney V, Gaga M, Frew AJ, Aber VA, Kay AB, Durham SR (1991) Usefulness of immunotherapy in patients with severe hayfever uncontrolled by antiallergic drugs. Br Med J 302:265–269.

92. Varney VA, Hamid QA, Gaga M, et al. (1993) Influence of grass pollen immunotherapy on cellular infiltration and cytokine mRNA expression during allergen-induced late-phase cutaneous response. J Clin Invest 92:644–651.

93. Secrist H, Chelen CJ, Wen Y, Marshall JD, Umetsu DT (1993) Allergen immunotherapy decreases interleukin 4 production in CD4+ T cells from allergic individuals. J Exp Med 178:2123–2130.

94. Jutel M, Pichler WJ, Skrbic D, Urwyler A, Dahinden C, Mutter VR (1995) Bee venom immunotherapy results in decrease of IL-4 and IL-5 and increase of IFN-g secretion in specific allergen-stimulated T-cell cultures. J Immunol 154:4187–4194.

95. Durham SR, Varney VA, Jacobson MR, Sudderick RM, Kay AB (1993) Effect of grass pollen immunotherapy on allergen-induced early and late nasal responses. J Allergy Clin Immunol 91:290 (abstract).

96. Durham SR, Asoufi B, Corrigan C (1996) Patterns of response to corticosteroids. In: Szefler SJ, Leung DYM, eds. Severe Asthma: Pathogenesis and Clinical Management. Marcel Dekker, New York, pp. 243–253.

97. Leung DYM (1996) The glucocorticoid receptor as a target in the pathogenesis of steroid resistant asthma. In: Szefler SJ, Leung DYM, eds. Severe Asthma: Pathogenesis and Clinical Management. Marcel Dekker, New York, pp. 285–311.

98. Schreiber SL, Crabtree GR (1992) The mechanism of action of cyclosporin A and FK506. Immunol Today 13:136–142.

99. Kita H, Ohnishi T, Okubo Y, Weiler D, Abrams JS, Gleich GJ (1991) Granulocyte/macrophage colony-stimulating factor and interleukin-3 release from peripheral blood eosinophils and neutrophils. J Exp Med 174:745–8.

100. Meng Q, Ying S, Assoufi B, Moqbel R, Kay AB (1996) Effects of dexamethasone, cyclosporin A and rapamycin on eosinophil degranulation and survival. J Allergy Clin Immunol 97:277 (Abstract 379).

101. Triggiani M, Cirillo R, Lichtenstein LM, Maroni G (1989) Inhibition of histamine and prostaglandin D2 release from human lung mast cells by cyclosporin A. Int Arch Allergy Appl Immunol 88:253–255.

102. Casolaro C, Spadaro G, Patella V, Maroni G (1993) In vivo characterisation of the anti-inflammatory effect of cyclosporin A on human basophils. J Immunol 151:5563–5573.

103. Hatfield SM, Roehm NW (1992) Cyclosporin and FK506 inhibition of murine mast cell cytokine production. J Pharm Exp Therap 260:280–288.

104. Ellis CN, Fradin MS, Messana JM, et al. (1991) Cyclosporin for plaque-type psoriasis: results of a multidose, double-blind trial. N Engl J Med 324:277–284.

105. Sowden JM, Berth-Jones J, Ross JS, et al. (1991) Double-blind, controlled, cross-over study of cyclosporin in adults with severe refractory atopic dermatitis. Lancet 338:137–140.

106. Brynskov J, Freund L, Rasmussen SN, et al. (1989) A placebo-controlled, double-blind, randomised trial of cyclosporin therapy in active Crohn's disease. N Engl J Med 321:845–850.

107. Corrigan CJ, Brown PH, Barnes NC, Tsai J-J, Frew AJ, Kay AB (1991) Glucocorticoid resistance in chronic asthma: peripheral blood T lymphocyte activation and comparison of the T lymphocyte inhibitory effects of glucocorticoids and cyclosporin A. Am Rev Respir Dis 144:1026–1032.

108. Alexander AG, Barnes NC, Kay AB (1992) Trial of cyclosporin on corticosteroid-dependent asthma. Lancet 339:324–328.

109. Lock S, Kay AB, Barnes NC (1996) Double-blind, placebo-controlled study of cyclosporin A as a corticosteroid-sparing agent in corticosteroid-dependent asthma. Am J Respir Crit Care Med 153:509–514.

110. Nizankowska E, Soja J, Pinis G, et al. (1995) Treatment of steroid-dependent bronchial asthma with cyclosporin. Eur Respir J 8:1091–1099.

111. Sihra B, Walker SM, Kon OM, Barnes NC, Kay AB (1996) Inhibition of the allergen-induced late phase asthmatic reaction by oral cyclosporin A. J Allergy Clin Immunol 97:242 (Abstract 240).

13

Role of CD8+ T-Cells in the Regulation of Immunoglobulin E

Paul A. MacAry, BSC
and David M. Kemeny, BSC, PHD, MRCPATH

INTRODUCTION

Asthma and other allergic diseases have become increasingly common in the latter part of the 20th century. Allergic reactions in the airways are triggered by immunoglobulin E (IgE)-sensitized mast cells and T-helper 2 (Th2) CD4+ T-cells, whose activation leads to the infiltration of other inflammatory cells, which contribute to tissue damage. One-third of all circulating T-cells are CD8+/CD4−. These cells are found at all immune sites and are particularly prominent in mucosal tissues, where they provide a first line of defense fulfilling an immunological gatekeeper function *(1,2)*. CD8+ T-cells recognize intracellular antigens presented via major histocompatibility complex (MHC) class I and are more cytolytic than CD4+ T-cells, producing perforin and degradative enzymes such as granzyme B. CD8+ T-cells can kill MHC class-I peptide-bearing target cells via the Fas-dependent "kiss-of-death" pathway. In this chapter we will review the role of CD8+ T-cells in IgE regulation.

B-CELL SWITCHING TO IgE

B-cell immunoglobulin class switching is regulated by cytokines, two of which have been shown to selectively promote switching to IgE, IL-4 *(3,4)* and IL-13 *(5)* and have been discussed extensively in Chapters 1 and 2. Other cytokines such as interleukin (IL)-10 and transforming growth factor (TGF)-β promote switching to IgG1 and IgG3 *(6)* and IgA *(7)*, respectively. Interferon (IFN)γ and IFNα *(4)* inhibit IgE transcription. IL-4 was be shown to be essential for IgE synthesis in vivo in mice infected with the nematode *Nippostrongylus braziliensis* in that anti-IL-4 *(8)* and anti-IL-4 receptor (IL-4R) antibody inhibited IgE synthesis *(9,10)*. Ongoing IgE responses in animals sensitized with the nematode *Heligmosomoides polygyrus*, which induces a chronic IgE response, are inhibited with anti-IL-4 *(8)*, indicating that IL-4 continues to be required for IgE production. The requirement of IL-4 for IgE synthesis has been confirmed in IL-4 knockout mice *(11)*, which are unable to produce IgE.

From: *Allergy and Allergic Diseases: The New Mechanisms and Therapeutics*
Edited by: J. A. Denburg © Humana Press Inc., Totowa, NJ

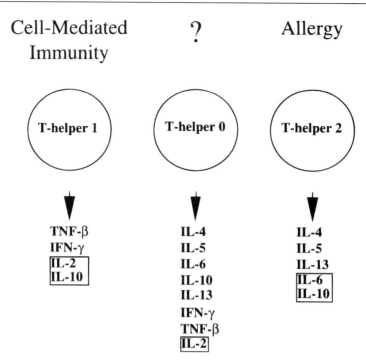

Fig. 1. Subsets of CD4[+] Th cells. Th1 cells secrete IFN-γ, TNF-β, and IL-2 and support cell-mediated immunity, and Th2 cells secrete IL-4, IL-5, IL-13, IL-6, and IL-10, support humoral immunity, and mediate allergy. Cells with an unrestricted cytokine profile, termed Th0 cells, have also been defined. The boxes represent cytokines that are defined as Th1 or Th2 in mice but are not solely associated with these subsets in rats or humans.

Th1 and Th2 CD4[+] T-Cells

T-cells are the principal source of IgE regulatory cytokines; this subject has been reviewed in detail in Chapters 11 and 12. CD4[+] T-cells can be subdivided into Th1 and Th2 *(12,13)* on the basis of the cytokines that they produce. Th1 cells make IFN-γ, IL-2, and TNF-β and effect cell-mediated immunity. Th2 cells make IL-4, IL-5, IL-6, and IL-10, support IgE responses, and cause eosinophilia. Some cytokines, including IL-3, tumor necrosis factor α (TNFα), and granulocyte-macrophage colony stimulating factor (GM-CSF), are secreted in similar amounts by both subsets (Fig. 1). In addition to Th1 and Th2 cells there are other subtypes such as Th0, which exhibit an unrestricted cytokine profile *(14)*.

The cytokine profile of human T-cell clones resembles that seen in the mouse *(15–17)*. Some human Th1 clones, however, make appreciable amounts of IL-6 *(18)*. As well as T-cells, a number of other cells make IL-4, including mast cells *(19)*, basophils *(20)*, and bone marrow and splenic non-T non-B cells *(21)*. IL-4-producing mast cells have been identified in the lung *(22)* and the nasal mucosae *(23)*, and in parasite-infested animals, there is a significant increase in IgE receptor positive non-T non-B cells in the spleen, from 0.53% to 3.8%, 8–9 wk after infection with *Schistosoma mansoni*. These cells, although present in smaller numbers than T-cells (approx 70%), secrete similar amounts of IL-4 *(24)*.

CD8[+] T-CELLS AND IgE REGULATION

The earliest report suggesting that CD8[+] T-cells were able to inhibit IgE was by Tada *(25–27)*, who showed that radiation-sensitive mouse Lyt2[+] (CD8) T-cells inhibited rat IgE responses. Subsequently Holt and colleagues *(28,29)* showed that following inhalation of antigen, T-cells that inhibited IgE were produced in the rat and that these cells were CD8$^+$. Conflicting reports and the lack of molecular evidence has made the concept of CD8$^+$ T-cell-mediated immuneregulation relatively unfashionable in recent years, especially since the discovery of clonal anergy *(30)* and the "veto" phenomenon *(31)* in in vitro systems, which might provide alternative mechanisms for immunological tolerance. However, the recent discovery of CD8$^+$ T-cell subsets *(32)*, as well as an improving understanding of the factors influencing the functional polarization of T-cell responses, combined with a growing literature demonstrating the sensitization of MHC class I restricted CD8$^+$ T-cells by exogenous antigens, has reawakened interest in the immunoregulatory potential of CD8$^+$ T-cells within the context of immune deviation and in other models of inducible tolerance.

Castor Bean Allergy

Our attention was drawn to immunoregulatory CD8$^+$ T-cells while investigating the mechanism of castor bean sensitization. Virtually all people exposed to castor bean dust, regardless of their genetic background, make IgE antibodies to castor bean proteins *(33–35)*. Rats immunized with castor bean extract became sensitized to castor bean proteins *(36)*. The substance responsible is ricin, a toxic lectin that, when injected together with a bystander antigen, potentiated the IgE, but not the IgG, antibody response to bystander antigen *(37,38)*. The IgE response thus induced can be boosted by repeated injection of ricin and antigen and is long-lived *(39)* (Fig. 2).

In these animals there was a profound (>50%) reduction in the number of CD8$^+$ T-cells in the spleen. These appear to have been targeted because they bore an increased number of ricin-binding glycoproteins on their surface 12–24 h after immunization *(40)*. When adoptively transferred to naive, syngeneic recipients, early-activated CD8$^+$ T-cells suppressed the IgE response by up to 95% *(40)*. Sedgwick and Holt *(28,29)* have shown that IgE regulatory CD8$^+$ T-cells are generated following inhalation of ovalbumin. Such cells bear the γδ form of the T-cell receptor *(41,42)*.

CD8 Cell Depletion

The effect of in vivo CD8$^+$ T-cell depletion on IgE production was therefore investigated in the rat. Following immunization of IgE hyporesponsive rats with ovalbumin complexed to the adjuvant, aluminum hydroxide (OVA-alum), CD8$^+$ T-cells were depleted in vivo by the administration of the anti-rat CD8-specific monoclonal antibody (OX-8) at different times. Depletion of CD8$^+$ T-cells 7 d after immunization failed to enhance the IgE response, but depletion of CD8$^+$ T-cells 12–18 d after immunization resulted in an increase in the magnitude and duration of the ensuing IgE response. Subsequent CD8$^+$ T-cell depletion on d 35 postimmunization extended the duration of the IgE response to over 1 yr, indicating that these cells may also play a role in the established IgE response *(43)*. The increase in IgE in CD8$^+$ T-cell depleted rats could also be correlated with decreased IFN-γ and increased IL-4 production from splenic T-cells following in vitro stimulation with antigen *(43)*.

That the effects of CD8$^+$ cell depletion were the result of CD8$^+$ T-cells was confirmed by adoptive transfer of CD8$^+$ T-cells from OVA-alum immunized rats. Following adoptive transfer, these cells effected a significant decrease in the IgE response in CD8-depleted recipients (Fig. 3). In common with data from McMenamin and Holt *(42)*, the IgE inhibitory effects of these cells could be titrated down to as few as 1000 cells *(43)*.

Discrepancies between the effects of CD8$^+$ T-cell depletion on the early and later stages of the immune response are not uncommon. In the mercuric chloride-induced model of autoimmune disease *(44)*, depletion of CD8$^+$ T-cells did not prevent disease but rendered animals more susceptible to rechallenge. Depletion of CD8$^+$ T-cells had no apparent effect on

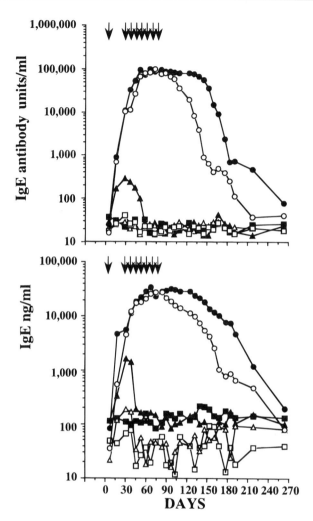

Fig. 2. The levels of IgE anti-PLA$_2$ [Phospholipase A$_2$] (top) and total IgE (bottom) in groups of 4 Wistar and Brown Norway rats immunized intraperitoneally (ip) with PLA2± ricin at the times indicated by the arrows. The standard deviation has been omitted for clarity but did not exceed 18% for total IgE or 17% for IgE anti-PLA2. The results for animals given ricin alone are not shown but were identical to those for animals given saline. Wistar: ○, ricin + antigen; △, antigen; □, ricin. Brown Norway: ●, ricin + antigen; ▲, antigen; ■, ricin.

Plasmodium chabaudi infection, although it increased recurring parasitemia (45). Furthermore, depletion of CD8$^+$ T-cells alone was insufficient to prevent reinfection with *Toxoplasma gondii* despite the finding that in vitro killing of mastocytoma cells infected with *T. gondii* was completely dependent on the presence of CD8$^+$ T-cells (46,47).

CLONING OVA-SPECIFIC CD8$^+$ T-CELLS

Ovalbumin-specific CD8$^+$ T-cell clones could be generated from the posterior mediastinal and parathymic lymph nodes, which drain the peritoneal cavity, of d 14 OVA-alum immunized PVG RT7^b rats (48,49). At this time, in vivo CD8 depletion is known to enhance the IgE response, and an activated population of CD3$^+$ T-cells could be distinguished that were

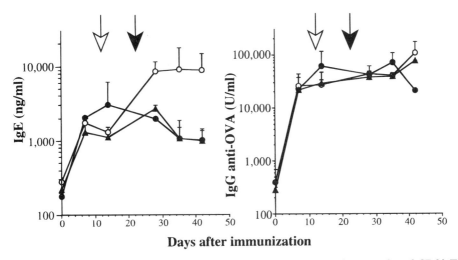

Days after immunization

Fig. 3. Enhancement of IgE by CD8-depletion and inhibition by adoptive transfer of CD8+ T-cells. Groups of four Lister Hooded rats were immunized ip with 100 μg of OVA-alum (open circles and closed triangles) or 100 μL of saline (closed circles). CD8+ T-cells were depleted by the injection of 0.5 mg of antirat CD8 (OX8) on d 12 (open arrow) in animals indicated by open circles and closed triangles. To the latter group 1 × 10^7 CD8+ T-cells from parallel immunized animals were adoptively transferred on d 22 as indicated by the closed arrow.

CD8^high and CD25^high. When purified, these cells exhibited a moderate proliferative response to trypsinated OVA pulsed antigen-presenting cells (APCs) and a strong proliferative response to OVA transfected APCs *(49)*. The OVA-specific CD8+ T-cell clones generated could be separated into two groups based on their cytokine secretion following antigen stimulation. All of the clones secreted IFNγ and IL-2. A small number also secreted IL-4. The OVA-specific CD8+ T-cell clones generated following the peritoneal introduction of OVA-alum were αβ TCR+, γδ TCR−, CD8+, CD4−, CD3+ (Table 1). This is in contrast to models based on the inhalation of antigen, which indicate that IgE immunoregulatory CD8+ T-cells produced following inhalation of soluble OVA express the T-cell receptor γδ chains *(51)*. All the clones tested by adoptive transfer effected a significant decrease in OVA-alum induced IgE in vivo without affecting the levels of OVA-specific IgG. In contrast to recent reports *(52,53)* in which cytotoxic CD8+ T-cells reduce the magnitude of the antigenic stimulus by killing APCs, the degree of IgE inhibition was not related to the cytolytic activity of the clones; nor was it correlated with the level of IFNγ production *(54)*.

MHC Class I Restriction

The responding CD8+ T-cells were MHC class-I restricted (Table 1) and bore the α/β T-cell receptor. The precursor frequency of OVA-specific CD8+ T-cell clones was much lower than that for the corresponding CD4+ T-cells purified at the same time and cultured under comparable conditions (approx 1:6 responding CD4:CD8 cells). This suggests that most of the exogenous OVA introduced into the peritoneum is directed, via the conventional MHC class II pathway, to OVA-specific CD4+ T-cells.

Antigen Processing

Inherent in our understanding of these data is the concept that the exogenous OVA introduced into the peritoneal cavity is able to stimulate CD8+ T-cells in the context of MHC class I (Fig. 4). The production of most peptides destined for the presentation by MHC class I begins

Table 1^a

Clone no.	CD8	CD4	CD3	αβ TCR	γδ TCR	IFN-γ, ng/mL	IL-4, SI	IL-2, U/mL
16	++	–	+++	+++	–	25.42	81.04	16.7
24	++	–	+++	+++	–	26.74	<2.0	18.4
32	++	–	+++	++	–	50.95	67.70	17.2
40	++	–	+++	+++	–	67.10	<2.0	22.5
45	++	–	+++	+++	–	69.05	<2.0	16.8
53	++	–	+++	+++	–	62.60	<2.0	7.6

[a]TCR denotes T-cell receptor. Cell surface marker expression and cytokine profile of IgE inhibitory OVA-specific CD8$^+$ T-cell clones determined by cytofluorometric analysis. –, negative; +, weakly positive; ++, moderately positive, and +++, strongly positive. Cytokines were measured following stimulation of 1×10^6 cloned cells with OVA by enzyme-linked immunosorbent assay (ELISA) (IFN-γ) and by bioassay (IL-4 and IL-2) *(50)*.

in the cytosol with the limited hydrolysis of antigenic proteins. Until recently, it was thought that this pathway was solely reserved for endogenously synthesized antigen. However, it is now clear from studies of murine macrophage and dendritic cells that exogenous protein antigens can gain entry to the cytosol of potential APCs, via the MHC class I pathway *(55,56)*, and that this occurs quite naturally in vivo as part of an important immunological defense against pathogens that reside in the phagosomal intracellular compartment *(57)*. There are a number of reports that indicate that CD8$^+$ CTLs can be primed by exogenous antigens *(58,59)* and that CD8$^+$ T-cells primed with soluble OVA in vivo mediate the transfer of oral and nasal tolerance *(60)*. The concept that antigen-specific CD8$^+$ T-cells may influence the functional outcome of a T-cell response is supported by Tuttosi and colleagues *(61)*, who reported antigen-specific CD8$^+$ T-cells that suppress antibody responses and induce development of delayed type hypersensitivity (DTH)-mediating cells, and by data from Renz and colleagues *(59)*, who demonstrated that mononuclear cells from recipients of antigen-primed CD8$^+$ T-cells secreted less IgE and IgG1, but more IgG2a, than controls.

CD8$^+$ T-CELL SUBSETS

The discovery by Mosmann and Coffman *(12)* that long-term CD4$^+$ T-cell clones could be segregated depending on their patterns of cytokine secretion initiated extensive investigation into the functional characteristics and generation of these subsets and their role in disease. IL-4 is required for Th2 development, and IL-12 for generation of Th1 responses, as has been described in Chapters 11 and 12. Similar investigations into CD8$^+$ T-cells revealed the existence of functionally distinct subsets within the CD8$^+$ T-cell pool, with good evidence from transgenic mouse and rat systems *(62–65)*. CD8$^+$ T-cells are reported most commonly to produce Th1 cytokines, particularly IFN-γ *(66)*. However, some instances of CD8$^+$ T-cell secretion of Th2 cytokines such as IL-4 *(67,68)* and IL-5 *(69)* have been described (Fig. 5). The strongest evidence for the existence of different subsets of CD8$^+$ T-cells in humans comes from studies of leprosy and HIV infection. Recent reports have suggested that HIV-1-specific Tc1 cytotoxic cells have a protective role against the onset of AIDS *(70)*, and the appearance of IL-4-secreting Tc2 CD8$^+$ T-cells has been associated with a downregulation in cytolytic activity and the onset of disease *(71)*.

The existence of Tc0 CD8$^+$ T-cells was first demonstrated by clones specific for *Mycobacterium leprae* that were derived from the skin biopsies of patients with leprosy, which

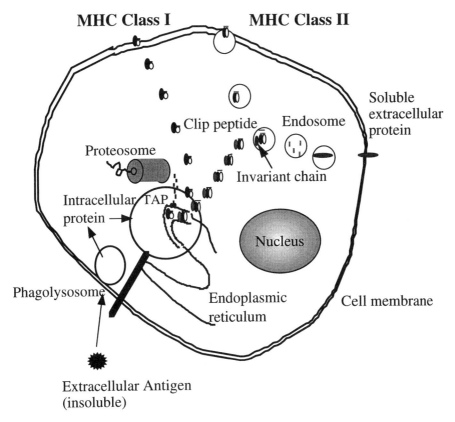

MHC Class I   **MHC Class II**

Soluble extracellular protein

Clip peptide   Endosome

Proteosome

Invariant chain

Intracellular TAP protein →

Nucleus

Phagolysosome

Endoplasmic reticulum   Cell membrane

Extracellular Antigen (insoluble)

Fig. 4. The cellular processes involved in processing of soluble and insoluble extracellular antigens are displayed below. Soluble extracellular protein antigens are taken up by endocytosis and are degraded in the intracellular endosome to constituent peptides. Newly formed MHC class II molecules leave the endoplasmic reticulum with an invariant chain and the associated clip peptide blocking the antigen binding site. On contact with antigenic peptides within the endosome, the invariant chain and the clip peptide are removed to facilitate binding of antigenic peptide to the MHC class II molecule. The MHC class II/peptide complex is then transported to the surface for display to other immune cells. Intracellular proteins are processed by the proteosome and the peptides delivered to the endoplasmic reticulum. Here they form complexes with β2 microglobulin and newly formed MHC class I α chains. The MHC class I/peptide complex is then delivered to the surface and displayed.

could be divided into two subtypes based on their cytokine secretion. Type 1 (Tc1) CD8+ T-cell clones were derived from healed lesions of patients with tuberculoid leprosy, were cytotoxic, and secreted IFNγ, but not IL-4 *(72)*. However, it should be noted that in most of the above studies, the ability to detect IL-4 production from CD8+ T-cell clones usually involved the employment of strong polyclonal stimulants, and most of the CD8+ T-cell clones described are mitogen- rather than antigen-derived. The subsets of antigen-specific CD8+ T-cells or the cytokine profiles of CD8+ T-cells at sites of immune activation have yet to be defined and their role in the immune system adequately resolved.

CD8+ T-cells are also able to influence CD4+ T-cell differentiation in vitro. Splenic T-cells were cultured for 4 d with Con A and various cytokines before isolating CD4+ T-cells by positive selection and determining their cytokine profiles following restimulation. It was observed that prior removal of CD8+ T-cells enhanced the capacity of CD4+ T-cells to produce IL-4 and

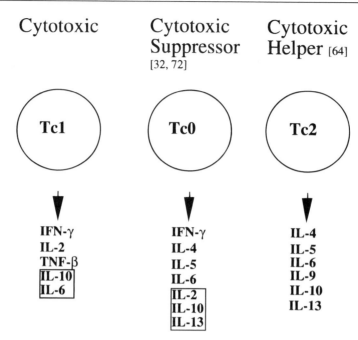

Fig. 5. Subsets of CD8[+] T-cells based on the cytokine profiles defined largely from data in rodent models and more recently from human disease systems implicating IFN-γ and IL-4 secretion as representing two polar extremes of CD8[+] T-cell differentiation, respectively. Hence Tc1 cells secrete IFN-γ, IL-2, IL-6, and IL-10. Tc2 cells secrete IL-4, IL-5, IL-10, and IL-13. A third subset defined as Tc0 has an unrestricted cytokine profile. All of these subtypes have been shown to display cytolytic activity in vitro.

IL-5 and increased the ability of these cells to proliferate in response to recombinant IL-4 *(73)*. However, removal of CD8[+] T-cells also increases the capacity of Th1 CD4[+] T-cells to produce IFN-γ, and it is not clear whether these different effects are mediated by the same or different CD8[+] T-cell subsets.

MECHANISM OF CD8[+] T-CELL-MEDIATED IgE REGULATION

There are several potential mechanisms whereby antigen-specific CD8[+] T-cells may regulate the magnitude and duration of IgE responses. Secretion of IFN-γ into the extracellular milieu during the formative stages of a CD4[+] T-cell response could inhibit the growth of Th2 cells directly, though favoring the expansion of Th1 cells, a form of immune deviation *(42,51,54)*. IFN-γ is known to stimulate macrophages to produce nitric oxides as part of a nonspecific suppressive process *(74)* that could potentially switch off or kill antigen-stimulated CD4[+] T-cells or newly activated B-cells. CD8[+] T-cell-derived IFN-γ could act directly on B-cells to inhibit immunoglobulin synthesis *(4)*. Cytolytic CD8[+] T-cells could target IgE-specific B-cells and directly limit the magnitude of antigen-specific stimulation by lysing APCs (Fig. 6). Alternatively, the suppression of IgE could be brought about by the production of antigen-specific suppressor factors. Yamaguchi and colleagues *(75)* have demonstrated the inhibition of both IgE and IgG antibody responses by antigen-specific suppressor factors; these may bind peptide or antigen in the absence of MHC molecules, but their production is MHC-restricted.

The ability of OVA-specific IgE-regulatory CD8[+] T-cell clones to inhibit IgE appeared to be unrelated to the levels of IFNγ they produced or to their in vitro cytolytic activity for OVA pulsed targets. Hence it seems likely that the mechanisms underlying the IgE-specific

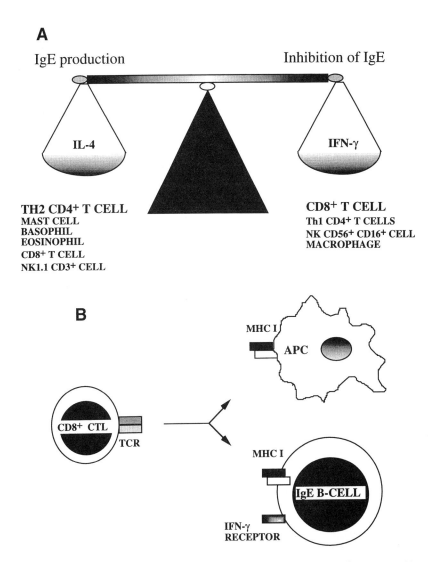

Fig. 6. The processes displayed above represent pathways by which a CD8⁺ T cell could exert a regulatory effect on an IgE immune response. The first pathway (**A**) details the potential immunoregulatory effects of IFN-γ secretion during the formative period of a Th2-like response in which localized production of IFN-γ could potentially effect a deviation of an allergen-specific immune response toward Th1 and away from the Th2 phenotype. The second mechanism (**B**) is based on the cytotoxic potential of antigen-specific CD8⁺ T-cells. By directly lysing IgE-specific B-cells, allergen-specific CD8⁺ T-cells could significantly reduce both the magnitude and duration of the ensuing response. Localized IFN-γ could potentially switch off or kill IgE-specific B-cells that express the IFN-γ receptor. Alternatively, by destroying antigen-presenting cells that drive an MHC class II-restricted Th2 CD4⁺ T-cell response, the CD8⁺ T-cell could reduce the amount of Th2 help available to below the threshold required for IgE class switching.

immunoregulatory activity of CD8[+] T-cells are complex and multifaceted and that several factors, including specific cytokines, limited cytotoxicity, cell motility, and survival, could combine to mediate the in vivo effect of these cells on IgE production.

REFERENCES

1. Hughes DP, Hayday A, Craft JE, Owen MJ, Crispe IN (1995) T-cells with gamma/delta T-cell receptors (TCR) of intestinal type are preferentially expanded in TCR-alpha-deficient lpr mice. J Exp Med 182:233–241.
2. Lundqvist C, Baranov V, Teglund S, Hammarstrom S, Hammarstrom ML (1994) Cytokine profile and ultrastructure of intraepithelial gamma delta T-cells in chronically inflamed human gingiva suggest a cytotoxic effector function. J Immunol 153:2302–2312.
3. Coffman RL, Ohara J, Bond MW, Carty J, Zlotnik A, Paul WE (1986) B cell stimulatory factor-1 enhances the IgE response of lipopolysaccharide-activated B cells. J Immunol 136:4538–4541.
4. Snapper CM, Paul WE (1987) Interferon-γ and B cell stimulatory factor-1 reciprocally regulate Ig isotype production. Science 236:944–947.
5. Punnonen J, Aversa G, Cocks BG, McKenzie ANJ, Menon S, Zurawski G, De Waal-Malefyt R, De Vries JE (1993) Interleukin 13 induces interleukin 4-independent IgG4 and IgE synthesis and CD23 expression by human B cells. Proc Natl Acad Sci USA 90:3730–3734.
6. Briere F, Servet-Delprat C, Bridon JM, Saint-Remy JM, Banchereau J (1994) Human interleukin 10 induces naive surface immunoglobulin D[+] (sIgD[+]) B cells to secrete IgG1 and IgG3. J Exp Med 179:757–762.
7. van Vlasselaer P, Punnonen J, de Vries JE (1992) Transforming growth factor-beta directs IgA switching in human B cells. J Immunol 148:2062–2067.
8. Urban J Jr, Katona IM, Paul WE, Finkelman FD (1991) Interleukin 4 is important in protective immunity to a gastrointestinal nematode infection in mice. Proc Natl Acad Sci USA 88:5513–5517.
9. Finkelman FD, Katona IM, Urban JF, Holmes J, Ohara J, Tung AS, Sample JV, Paul WE (1988) IL4 is required to generate and sustain in vivo IgE responses. J Immunol 141:2335–2341.
10. Finkelman FD, Svetic A, Gresser I, Snapper CM, Holmes J, Trotta PP, Katona IM, Gause WC (1991) Regulation by interferon alpha of immunoglobulin isotype selection and lymphokine production in mice. J Exp Med 174:1179–1188.
11. Kuhn R, Rajewsky K, Muller W (1991) Generation and analysis of interleukin-4 deficient mice. Science 254:707–710.
12. Mosmann TR, Cherwinski H, Bond MW, Giedlin MA, Coffman RL (1986) Two types of murine helper T-cell clones. 1. Definition according to profiles of lymphokine activities and secreted proteins. J Immunol 135:2348–2357.
13. Mosmann TR (1992) T lymphocyte subsets, cytokines, and effector functions. Ann NY Acad Sci 664:89–92.
14. Firestein GS, Roeder WD, Laxer JA, Townsend KS, Weaver CT, Hom JT, Linton J, Torbett BE, Glasebrook AL (1989) A new murine CD4[+] T-cell subset with an unrestricted cytokine profile. J Immunol 143:518–525.
15. Parronchi P, Macchia D, Piccinni MP, Biswas P, Simonelli C, Maggi E, Ricci M, Ansari AA, Romagnani S (1991) Allergen- and bacterial antigen-specific T-cell clones established from atopic donors show a different profile of cytokine production. Proc Natl Acad Sci USA 88:4538–4542.
16. Wierenga EA, Snoek M, De Groot C, Chretien I, Bos JD, Jansen HM, Kapsenberg ML (1990) Evidence for compartmentalization of functional subsets of CD4[+] T-lymphocytes in atopic patients. J Immunol 144:4651–4656.
17. Del Prete GF, De Carli M, Ricci M, Romagnani S (1991) Helper activity for immunoglobulin synthesis of T helper type 1 (Th1) and T helper type 1 (Th2) human T-cell clones: the help of Th1 clones is limited by their cytolytic capacity. J Exp Med 174:809–813.
18. Wierenga EA, Snoek M, Jansen HM, Bos JD, Van Lier RAW, Kapsenberg ML (1991) Human atopen-specific types 1 and 2 T helper cell clones. J Immunol 147:2942–2949.
19. Plaut M, Pierce JH, Watson CJ, Hanley-Hyde J, Nordan R, Paul WE (1989) Mast cell lines produce lymphokines in response to cross-linkage of Fc epsilon RI or to calcium ionophores. Nature 339:64–67.
20. Brunner T, Heusser CH, Dahinden CA (1993) Human peripheral blood basophils primed by interleukin-3 (IL-3) produce IL-4 in response to immunoglobulin E receptor stimulation. J Exp Med 177:605–611.

21. Ledermann F, Heusser C, Schlienger C, Le Gros G (1992) Interleukin-3-treated non-B, non-T-cells switch activated B cells to IgG1/IgE synthesis. Eur J Immunol 22:2783–2787.

22. Bradding P, Feather IH, Howarth PH, Mueller R, Roberts JA, Britten K, Bews JPA, Hunt TC, Okayama Y, Heusser CH, Bullock GR, Church MK, Holgate ST (1992) Interleukin 4 is localized to and released by human mast cells. J Exp Med 176:1381–1386.

23. Bradding P, Feather IH, Wilson S, Bardin PG, Heusser CH, Holgate ST, Howarth PH (1993) Immunolocalization of cytokines in the nasal mucosa of normal and perennial rhinitic subjects. The mast cell as a source of IL-4, IL-5, and IL-6 in human allergic mucosal inflammation. J Immunol 151:3853–3865.

24. Williams ME, Kullberg MC, Barbieri S, Caspar P, Berzofsky JA, Seder RA, Sher A (1993) Fc epsilon receptor-positive cells are a major source of antigen-induced interleukin-4 in spleens of mice infected with Schistosoma mansoni. Eur J Immunol 23:1910–1916.

25. Tada T, Taniguchi M, Okumura K (1971) Regulation of homocytotropic antibody formation in the rat. II. Effect of X-irradiation. J Immunol 106:1012–1018.

26. Taniguchi M, Tada T (1971) Regulation of homocytotropic antibody formation in the rat. IV. Effects of various immunosuppressive drugs. J Immunol 107:579–585.

27. Okumura KO, Tada T (1971) Regulation of homocytotrophic antibody formation in the rat. IV. Inhibitory effect of thymocytes on the homocytotrophic antibody response. J Immunol 107:1682–1689.

28. Sedgwick JD, Holt PG (1984) Suppression of IgE responses in inbred rats by repeated respiratory tract exposure to antigen: responder phenotype influences isotype specificity of induced tolerance. Eur J Immunol 14:893–897.

29. Sedgwick JD, Holt PG (1985) Induction of IgE-secreting cells and IgE isotype-specific suppressor T-cells in the respiratory lymph nodes of rats in response to antigen inhalation. Cell Immunol 94:182–194.

30. Schwartz RH (1990) A cell culture model for T lymphocyte clonal anergy. Science 248:1349–1356.

31. Jameson SC, Carbone FR, Bevan MJ (1993) Clone-specific T-cell receptor antagonists of major histocompatibility complex class I-restricted cytotoxic T-cells. J Exp Med 177:1541–1550.

32. Salgame P, Abrams JS, Clayberger C, Goldstein H, Convit J, Modlin RL, Bloom BR (1991) Differing lymphokine profiles of functional subsets of human CD4 and CD8 T-cell clones. Science 254:279–282.

33. Thorpe SC, Kemeny DM, Panzani R, Lessof MH (1987) The relationship between total serum IgE and castor bean-specific IgE antibodies in castor bean-sensitive patients from Marseilles. Int Arch Allergy Appl Immunol 82:3,4.

34. Thorpe SC, Kemeny DM, Panzani R, Lessof MH (1988) Allergy to castor bean. I. Its relationship to sensitization to common inhalant allergens (atopy). J Allergy Clin Immunol 82:62–66.

35. Thorpe SC, Kemeny DM, Panzani RC, McGurl B, Lord M (1988) Allergy to castor bean. II. Identification of the major allergens in castor bean seeds. J Allergy Clin Immunol 82:67–72.

36. Thorpe SC, Murdoch RD, Kemeny DM (1989) The effect of the castor bean toxin, ricin, on rat IgE and IgG responses. Immunology 68:307–311.

37. Diaz-Sanchez D, Kemeny DM (1990) The sensitivity of rat CD8⁺ and CD4⁺ T-cells to ricin in vivo and *in vitro* and their relationship to IgE regulation. Immunology 69:71–77.

38. Hellman L (1994) Profound reduction in allergen sensitivity following treatment with a novel allergy vaccine. Eur J Immunol 24:415–420.

39. Diaz-Sanchez D, Kemeny DM (1991) Generation of a long-lived IgE response in high and low responder strains of rat by co-administration of ricin and antigen. Immunology 72:297–303.

40. Diaz-Sanchez D, Lee TH, Kemeny DM (1993) Ricin enhances IgE responses by inhibiting a subpopulation of early-activated CD8⁺ T-cells. Immunology 78:226–236.

41. McMenamin C, Oliver J, Girn B, Holt BJ, Kees UR, Thomas WR, Holt PG (1991) Regulation of T-cell sensitization at epithelial surfaces in the respiratory tract: suppression of IgE responses to inhaled antigens by CD3⁺ Tcr alpha-/beta-lymphocytes (putative gamma/delta T-cells). Immunology 74:234–239.

42. McMenamin C, Pimm C, McKersey M, Holt PG (1994) Regulation of IgE responses to inhaled antigen in mice by antigen-specific gamma delta T-cells. Science 265:1869–1871.

43. Holmes BJ, MacAry PA, Kemeny DM (1997) In vivo depletion of CD8⁺ T-cells following the primary immune response results in a high and persistent IgE response in IgE hyporesponsive rats. Eur J Immunol 27:2657–2665.

44. Mathieson PW, Stapleton KJ, Oliveira DB, Lockwood CM (1991) Immunoregulation of mercuric chloride-induced autoimmunity in Brown Norway rats: a role for CD8⁺ T-cells revealed by in vivo depletion studies. Eur J Immunol 21:2105–2109.

45. Podoba JE, Stevenson MM (1991) CD4⁺ and CD8⁺ T lymphocytes both contribute to acquired immunity to blood-stage Plasmodium chabaudi AS. Infect Immun 59:51–58.

46. Subauste CS, Koniaris AH, Remington JS (1991) Murine CD8+ cytotoxic T lymphocytes lyse Toxoplasma gondii-infected cells. J Immunol 147:3955–3959.

47. Gazzinelli R, Xu Y, Hieny S, Cheever A, Sher A (1992) Simultaneous depletion of CD4+ and CD8+ T-lymphocytes is required to reactivate chronic infection with Toxoplasma gondii. J Immunol 149:175–180.

48. MacAry PA, Holmes BJ, Kemeny DM (1997) Generation of rat MHC class-I restricted ovalbumin-specific IgE inhibitory CD8+ T-cell clones. Int Archs All Appl Immunol 113:279,280.

49. MacAry PA, Holmes BJ, Kemeny DM (1998) IgE inhibitory ovalbumin-specific MHC class I-restricted, α/β TcR positive rat Tc1 and Tc0 CD8+ T-cell clones generated using lipid solubilised ovalbumin peptides. J Immunol 113:279,280.

50. Noble A, Kemeny DM (1995) IL-4 and IFN-γ regulate differentiation of CD8+ T-cells into populations with divergent cytokine profiles. Int Archs All Appl Immunol 107:186–188.

51. McMenamin C, McKersey M, Kuhnlein P, Hunig T, Holt PG (1995) Gamma delta T-cells down-regulate primary IgE responses in rats to inhaled soluble protein antigens. J Immunol 154:4390–4394.

52. Simpson E (1988) Suppression of the immune response by cytotoxic T-cells. Nature 336:426.

53. McCormack JM, Sun D, Walker WS (1991) A subset of mouse splenic macrophages can constitutively present alloantigen directly to CD8+ T-cells. J Immunol 147:421–427.

54. McMenamin C, Holt PG (1993) The natural immune response to inhaled soluble protein antigens involves major histocompatibility complex (MHC) class-I-restricted CD8+ T-cell mediated, but MHC class II-restricted CD4+ T-cell-dependent immune deviation resulting in selective suppression of immunoglobulin E production. J Exp Med 178:889–899.

55. Kovacsovics-Bankowski M, Rock KL (1995) A phagosome-to-cytosol pathway for exogenous antigens presented on MHC class I molecules. Science 267:243–246.

56. Brown ML, Fields PE, Kurlander RJ (1992) Metabolic requirements for macrophage presentation of Listeria monocytogenes to immune CD8 cells. J Immunol 148:555–61.

57. Staerz UD, Karasuyama H, Garner AM (1987) Cytotoxic T lymphocytes against a soluble protein. Nature 329:449–451.

58. Yefenof E, Zehavi-Feferman R, Guy R (1990) Control of primary and secondary antibody responses by cytotoxic T lymphocytes specific for a soluble antigen. Eur J Immunol 20:1849–1853.

59. Renz H, Lack G, Saloga J, Schwinzer R, Bradley K, Loader J, Kupfer A, Larsen GL, Gelfand EW (1994) Inhibition of IgE production and normalization of airways responsiveness by sensitized CD8 T-cells in a mouse model of allergen-induced sensitization. J Immunol 152:351–360.

60. Miller A, Lider O, Roberts AB, Sporn MB, Weiner HL (1992) Suppressor T-cells generated by oral tolerization to myelin basic protein suppress both in vitro and in vivo immune responses by the release of transforming growth factor beta after antigen-specific triggering. Proc Natl Acad Sci USA 89:421–425.

61. Tuttosi S, Bretscher PA (1992) Antigen-specific CD8+ T-cells switch the immune response induced by antigen from an IgG to a cell-mediated mode. J Immunol 148:397–403.

62. Noble A, MacAry PA, Kemeny DM (1995) IFN-γ and IL-4 regulate the differentiation of CD8+ T-cells into subpopulations with distinct cytokine profiles. J Immunol 155:2928–2937.

63. Sad S, Marcotte R, Mosmann TR (1995) Cytokine-induced differentiation of precursor mouse CD8+ T-cells into cytotoxic CD8+ T-cells secreting Th1 or Th2 cytokines. Immunity 2:271–279.

64. Cronin DC 2nd, Stack R, Fitch FW (1995) IL-4 producing CD8+ T-cell clones can provide B cell help. J Immunol 154:3118–3127.

65. Croft M, Carter L, Swain SL, Dutton RW (1994) Generation of polarized antigen-specific CD8 effector populations: reciprocal action of interleukin IL-4 and IL-12 in promoting type 2 versus type 1 cytokine profiles. J Exp Med 180:1715–1728.

66. Fong TAT, Mosmann TR (1990) Alloreactive CD8+ T-cell clones secrete the TH1 pattern of cytokines. J Immunol 144:1744–1752.

67. Sander B, Cardell S, Moller E (1991) Interleukin 4 and interferon gamma production in restimulated CD4+ and CD8+ cells indicates memory type responsiveness. Scand J Immunol 33:287–296.

68. Horvat B, Loukides JA, Anadan L, Brewer E, Flood PM (1991) Production of interleukin 2 and interleukin 4 by immune CD4−CD8+ and their role in the generation of antigen-specific cytotoxic T-cells. Eur J Immunol 21:1863–1871.

69. Taguchi T, Aicher WK, Fujihashi K, Yamamoto M, McGhee JR, Bluestone JA, Kiyono H (1991) Novel function for intestinal intraepithelial lymphocytes. Murine CD3+, gamma/delta TCR+ T-cells produce IFN-gamma and IL-5. J Immunol 147:3736–3744.

70. Riddell SR, Gilbert MJ, Greenberg PD (1993) CD8+ cytotoxic T-cell therapy of cytomegalovirus and HIV infection. Curr Opin Immunol 5:484–491.

71. Maggi E, Guidizi MG, Biagiotti R, Annunziato F, Manetti R, Piccinni MP, Parronchi P, Sampognaro S, Giannarini L, Zuccati G, et al. (1994) Th2-like CD8⁺ T-cells showing B cell helper function and reduced cytolytic activity in human immunodeficiency virus type 1 infection. J Exp Med 180:489–495.

72. Salgame P, Convit J, Bloom BR (1991) Immunological suppression by human CD8⁺ T-cells is receptor dependent and HLA-DQ restricted. Proc Natl Acad Sci USA 88:2598–2602.

73. Noble A, Staynov D, Kemeny DM (1993) Generation of rat Th2-like cells in vitro is IL-4 dependent and is inhibited by IFN-γ. Immunology 79:562–567.

74. Albina JE, Abate JA, Henry W Jr (1991) Nitric oxide production is required for murine resident peritoneal macrophages to suppress mitogen-stimulated T-cell proliferation. Role of IFN-gamma in the induction of the nitric oxide-synthesizing pathway. J Immunol 147:144–148.

75. Yamaguchi K, Mori A, Ohno H, Tagaya Y, Ishizaka K (1992) Requirement of certain epitope specificities of glycosylation inhibiting factor for the suppression of in vivo IgE and IgG antibody responses. Int Immunol 4:337–346.

14

Airway Wall Structure

Peter K. Jeffery, PhD, Mariusz J. Gizycki, MD, and Andrew V. Rogers, BSc

CONTENTS

INTRODUCTION

In man and other mammalian species, the upper and lower airways are lined by a continuous mucosal layer. It is the site at which immune responses are initiated by immuno-competent cells on recognition of foreign molecules, suitably processed by resident antigen- presenting cells (APC). In humans, subsequent exposure to the relevant allergen initiates immune reactions, which may become persistent. Immune reactions are designed as defense mechanisms that normally protect the body; however, inappropriate or misdirected responses may lead to damage of host tissues. Control is maintained by cell–cell signaling via the release of cytokines that have the potential to induce an allergic inflammatory response. At rest, approx 10,000 to 15,000 L of air, containing allergen and pollutants, moves daily over the nasal and tracheobronchial airway mucosal lining of the adult human lung. In the upper respiratory tract and proximal conducting airways of the lung the air is sampled, conditioned, and rendered free of many irritants and allergens before reaching the respiratory portion of the lung. The function of the conducting airways, in many respects, depends on the branching pattern and the dynamic interaction of structural, immuno-competent, and neural elements. Changes in the composition and integrity of airway-wall structural components may alter its effectiveness. A prerequisite to understanding the pathogenesis of allergic inflammatory disorders is an appreciation of normal airway structure and function. The present chapter focuses on cells that comprise the normal structure of the airway wall of the lower respiratory tract and considers briefly the cellular and structural variations that

From: *Allergy and Allergic Diseases: The New Mechanisms and Therapeutics*
Edited by: J. A. Denburg © Humana Press Inc., Totowa, NJ

occur in allergic disease, in particular, those that may lead to the process of airway-wall remodeling, a characteristic change in chronic asthma. After an introduction to the structural features of the upper and lower respiratory tract, the surface epithelium is considered in some detail, as is its supporting reticular basement membrane, followed by a consideration of the fibroblast, bronchial smooth muscle, bronchial vasculature, and mucosal nerves.

ANATOMIC FEATURES

The lining of the respiratory tract is continuous with both the skin and the lining of the alimentary tract, from which the lower respiratory tract develops *in utero*. The larynx is conventionally considered to mark the boundary between upper and lower portions of the respiratory tract: the upper extends from the external nares to the larynx, and the lower from the larynx to the visceral pleura. The upper respiratory tract consists of the nose and the pharynx; the former is divided into two nostrils by a median septum. The superior part of the nose is surrounded entirely by bone, and posteriorly it opens into the nasopharynx, which continues into the oro- and laryngopharynx. Each nasal cavity is wider anteriorly than posteriorly. On each lateral wall there are three turbinates. A system of air sinuses also drains into the upper respiratory tract. Lymphoid tissue in the upper respiratory tract comprises the nasopharyngeal and palatine tonsils. The former, termed adenoids, are a diffuse aggregate of lymphoid cells in the mucosa lining of the nasopharynx, covered by folds of predominantly pseudostratified epithelium. Two palatine tonsils are situated in the lateral walls of the oropharynx, covered by a stratified, squamous, nonkeratinizing epithelium invaginated to form deep crypts. Posterior to the pharynx are the larynx, the organ of speech, and the glottis, through which air enters into the lower respiratory tract and its tree of successively branching airways.

The larynx opens into the trachea, which enters the thorax and divides to form two main bronchi, one leading to each lung. The right and left lungs are lobed, occupy most of the thorax, are enclosed within the rib cage, and are enveloped by pleural membranes. Medially the lungs abut on the mediastinum (which includes the pericardium) and posteriorly they rest on the diaphragm. Airways and vessels meet at the hilum of the lung at a point where it connects to the mediastinum. The pattern of airway branching is described as one of asymmetrical dichotomy, and from trachea to alveolus there are 8–23 generations of airways, depending on the distance from the hilum to the pleural surface.

In the trachea, supportive cartilage is present in the form of irregular, sometimes branching, crescentic rings (16–20 in humans), all of which are incomplete dorsally; the dorsal gaps are bridged with fibrous tissue and bands of smooth muscle. Airways are designated by structure and position along a pathway (i.e., generation or order of division) (*1,2*). Designation of intrasegmental airways by size is regarded as unsatisfactory as the size of each division also varies with the phase of inspiration or expiration and the state of muscle contraction. Airways distal to the trachea that have supportive cartilage in their walls are, by definition, bronchi. In large bronchi, the cartilage plates are irregular in shape but are frequent enough to be found in any cut plane of the airway; however, in "small" bronchi cartilage is less abundant and may be absent in cross-sections. Those airways distal to the last cartilage plate are referred to as bronchioli. More peripheral bronchiolar divisions have a ciliated lining epithelium interrupted by occasional alveoli, and these are called respiratory bronchioli. The respiratory bronchiolus is the first peripheral site at which gaseous exchange occurs and is also where the ciliary escalator ends. The generation proximal to the first-order respiratory bronchiolus is called the terminal bronchiolus and is the last solely conductive airway. The acinus, the basic respiratory unit of the lung, is about 1 cm across and is formed by a single terminal bronchiolus with its succeeding branches of respiratory bronchioli (generally, three orders), two to nine orders of alve-

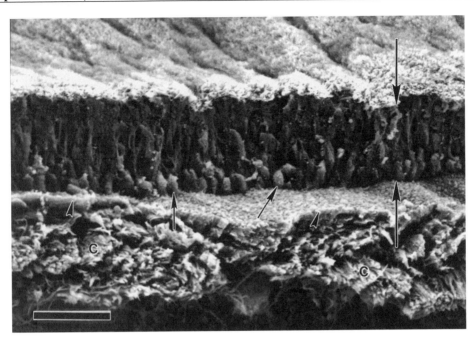

Fig. 1. Scanning electron micrograph (SEMG) of human bronchial mucosa showing the pseudostratified, columnar surface epithelium (large arrows) of mainly ciliated cells and basal cells (small arrows): both cell types attach to a reticular basement membrane (arrowheads). Beneath this there is interstitial collagen (C) in the subepithelium zone (scale bar = 50 μm).

olar ducts, and their alveolar sacs. The summed cross-sectional area for each generation of airways increases logarithmically; thus, at the periphery, the resistance to air flow is negligible *(1,2)*. With inspiration, the velocity of air entering the lungs falls rapidly due to the marked increase in total cross-sectional area of the more peripheral airways. The surface of the alveolar walls available to gas transfer is about 60–70 m^2, i.e., about half the area of a singles tennis court.

The more distal respiratory zone is kept free of allergens, pollutants, and infection by airway defense mechanisms that include nervous reflexes leading to bronchoconstriction and/or cough, ciliary activity, secretion of mucus, lysozyme, lactoferrin, and secretory immunoglobulin A (IgA), and cellular immune response and reactions.

The airway wall is comprised of a surface epithelium supported by a reticular basement membrane (Fig. 1) and a poorly defined subepithelial zone consisting of bronchial vessels, connective tissue (Fig. 2), and lymphatics that merges with a submucosal zone of mucus-secreting glands, cartilage, and/or bronchial smooth muscle; external to this there is a thin adventitial coat (Fig. 3).

SURFACE EPITHELIUM

Upper respiratory tract epithelium is comprised mainly of ciliated, pseudostratified, columnar cells, interspersed with mucus-secreting cells. However, the anterior nares are lined by stratified keratinizing squamous epithelium (*see* Figs. 1 and 2). Areas of nonkeratinizing squamous epithelium are found in the pharynx, whereas in the larynx, epithelium of this type is present on the epiglottis and the vocal chords. The stratified squamous epithelium covering the vocal cords gives way to one that is ciliated, pseudostratified, and columnar when the trachea

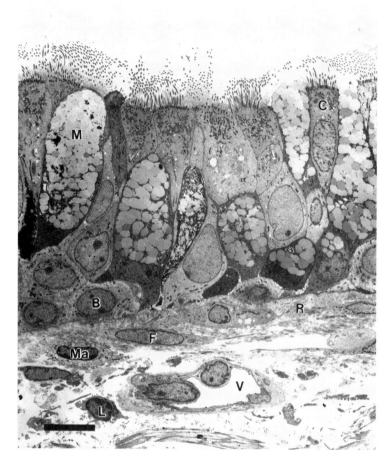

Fig. 2. Transmission electron micrograph (TEMG) demonstrates that the epithelium is made up of various cell types: mucous (M), ciliated (C), and basal (B) cells. The subepithelial zone beneath the reticular layer (R) contains many cell types: lymphocytes (L), mast cells (Ma), fibroblasts (F), and there is a small bronchial vessel (V) (scale bar = 10 μm).

is reached. The term "pseudostratified" refers to the appearance of more than one layer of cells and implies that all cells rest on the basement membrane but not all reach the airway lumen. However, basal cells may also play a role in attachment of superficial cells to the basal lamina by acting as a bridge between columnar cells and the epithelial basement membrane. Evans et al. *(3)* studied a number of species whose tracheal epithelia varied in thickness and concluded that the thicker the surface epithelium the greater the number and proportion of basal cells present and the greater the percentage of columnar-cell attachment to the basal cell. In humans, this appearance to the epithelium persists throughout the major bronchi, thereafter becoming simple cuboidal distally. In other species, the transition to simple cuboidal occurs more proximally: for example, in the specific pathogen-free rat, it is found at the hilum of the lung *(4)*. Mucus-secreting cells are found regularly in the tracheobronchial tree in humans but are sparse in bronchioli less than 1 mm in diameter *(5)*. Species differences exist: mucus-secreting cells are numerous in the trachea and bronchi of the guinea pig and cat, but few are found in these regions in the rat, mouse, hamster, or rabbit, whereas in the cat mucus-secreting cells are found additionally in the bronchioli *(6,7)*.

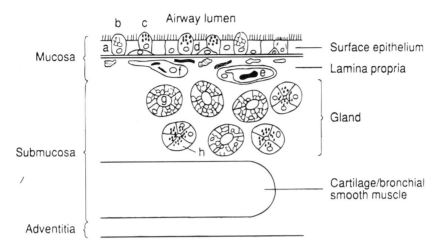

Fig. 3. Diagrammatic representation of the various layers present in a section through the bronchial wall: the mucosa, comprised of the epithelium and its supporting subepithelium, external to this is a sub-mucosal zone that contains mucus-secreting glands, cartilage and/or bronchial smooth muscle and the outermost layer, the thin adventitia. There are: ciliated (a), mucous (b), serous or nonciliated bronchiolar (Clara) (c), and basal (d) cells in the epithelium. Beneath there are bronchial vessels lined by endothelial cells (e), fibroblasts (f), and mucous (g) and serous acini (h) of the submucosal glands.

EPITHELIAL CELLS

A variety of cell types are recognized in airway surface epithelium *(4,8–10)*. There are at least eight morphologically distinct epithelial-cell types in the surface epithelium, determined by transmission electron microscopy (TEM). Many of the epithelial cells have overlapping functions (Table 1). In addition, cells involved in the immune response and its reactions may migrate across the epithelial basement membrane and remain within the epithelium or pass to the airway lumen *(11)*. The terminal processes of nerve fibers whose cell bodies are present external to the epithelium also cross the epithelial basement membrane and lie between and are enclosed by epithelial cells, in which they are thought to initiate airway reflexes such as bronchoconstriction and cough and also neurogenic inflammation *(12,13)*. The main cell types are considered in more detail below.

Ciliated Cells

Except for the alveoli, the ciliated cell is present throughout the lower respiratory tract. The ciliated cell apex has 200–300 cilia, each of which beats at 1000 times/min with its effective stroke generally in the rostral direction *(14)* (Fig. 4A,B). The cilia are thought to beat in a periciliary fluid layer of low viscosity, the origin of which is as yet unknown. Each cilium has a characteristic internal arrangement of microtubules responsible for their movement (Fig. 5, inset). Cilia move the overlying mucus only by their tips, the interaction of the ciliary tips and mucus being facilitated by minute terminal hooklets *(4)* (Fig. 5). Mucociliary transport is known to be reduced in asthma *(15)*. However, this is unlikely to result from a defect in the ciliary structure, as the ciliary beat frequency and mucociliary clearance can be increased by β-agonists *(15,16)*.

Mucous Cells

Mucous (or goblet) cells are normally present in the trachea and bronchi (major and sequential) and are only occasionally present in membranous bronchioli *(5)*. Mucous cells contain electron-lucent, confluent granules about 775 nm in diameter (*see* Fig. 2). The granules are

Table 1
Summary of Surface Epithelial and Associated Cell Types and Their Functions

Epithelial cells	Function(s)
Ciliated	Movement of mucus
	Secretion of a mucosubstance
	Control of periciliary fluid
	Secretion of cytokines
Mucous	Mucus-secreting (acidic)
	Absorptive
	Proliferative/bronchial stem cell
Serous	Mucus-secreting (neutral)
	Secretory piece (component)
	Secretion of periciliary fluid (?)
	Proliferative
Clara (nonciliated bronchioles)	Secretion of surfactant-hypophase
	Proliferative/bronchial stem cell
DCG/endocrine	Secretion of amines (5-HT)
(dense-core granulated)	Peptides (e.g., bombesin)
Basal	Proliferative/bronchial stem cell
Brush	Function unknown
Special-type	Function unknown
Indeterminate	Function unknown
Intraepithelial cells	
Dendritic	Antigen presentation
Lymphocyte	Immunoresponsive
Mast cell	Immunoreactive
Globular leukocyte	Transport of immunoglobulins
	Self-cure phenomenon
	Release of inflammatory mediators
Nerve	
NEB (neuroepithelial body)	Chemo/mechanoreceptor modulation:
	Growth
	Vessel and bronchial tone
	Mucosal secretion
Nerve terminals	Sensory:
	Bronchoconstriction
	Secretion
	Hyperpnea
	Motor:
	Ciliary rate
	Secretion
	Endocrine response

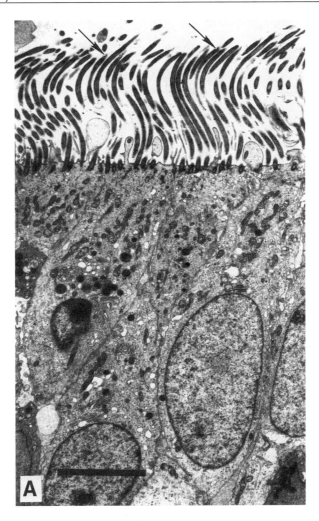

Fig. 4. (A) TEMG of surface epithelial ciliated cells. Cilia (arrows) beat synchronously to move mucus along the respiratory tract toward the laryngopharynx (scale bar = 5 μm).

thought to contain an acidic mucin; their acidity is owing to sialic acid or sulfate groups at terminal positions on the oligosaccharide side chains of the glycoprotein core *(17)*. The production of mucus of the required amount and viscoelasticity is important in the maintenance of mucociliary clearance. The degree of acidity may determine the viscoelastic profile of mucus and hence the ease with which it is transported by cilia and/or cough. The number of goblet cells increases in conditions of airway inflammation (e.g., chronic bronchitis) and experimentally, in the rat, following inhalation of sulfur dioxide *(18)* or tobacco smoke *(19–21)*. There is evidence that mucus-secreting cells are not merely "end" cells, but are capable of division *(22–25)*. In the human trachea, the normal mean density is estimated at about 6800 mucous cells/mm^2 of surface epithelium *(26)*. Productive cough is a characteristic feature of chronic bronchitis and is also frequently associated with an acute attack of asthma. Mucous-cell hyperplasia in the large airways and mucous-cell metaplasia in membranous bronchioles are characteristic changes in chronic bronchitis. Whether there is mucous metaplasia and hyperplasia in

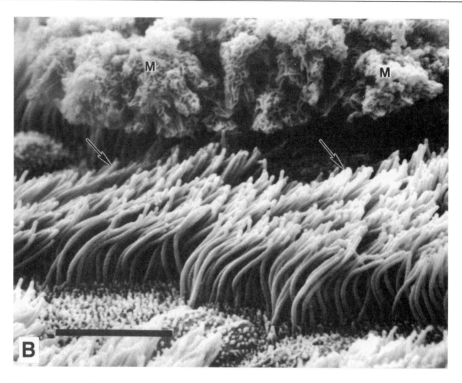

Fig. 4.(B) *(continued)* SEMG of the cilia (arrows) supporting a raft of mucus (M) by their tips (scale bar = 5 μm).

asthma remains to be established *(27)*. Its has been suggested that much of the mucus found in the peripheral airways in asthma may be secretions aspirated from the larger proximal airways. Only a proportion of the plugging of airways in asthma results from the mucus *per se;* the bulk results from an inflammatory exudate mixed with sloughed epithelial and inflammatory cells.

Serous Cells

In contrast to the mucous cell, two populations of cells with electron-dense secretory granules have been described in the human small airway: serous cell and Clara cell. These cells can be distinguished on the basis of granule size, the number of granules, and the area of the cell cytoplasm occupied by the granules. The serous cell of the human has discrete electron-dense granules 300 nm in diameter resembling the serous cells of submucosal glands *(28)* (Fig. 6). These resemble the serous cells of the surface epithelium described previously in the rat: the chemical composition of these secretory granules still requires characterization: they may contain a small-molecular-weight antiprotease (i.e., bronchial mucus proteinase inhibitor) *(29)*, lipid, and/or neutral glycoprotein. In the rat airway, this cell type may divide and is likely to have a stem-cell potential.

Clara (Nonciliated Bronchiolar) Cells

Clara cells have electron-dense granules about 200 nm in diameter (Fig. 7). The function of this cell has long been in dispute. It has been suggested that it produces bronchiolar surfactant *(30)*, a hypophase component of surfactant *(31)*, or a proteinase inhibitor *(32)*. Furthermore, it also has stem-cell multipotentiality, as following irritation or drug administration, both ciliated and mucous cells may develop from the Clara cell *(25,33)*.

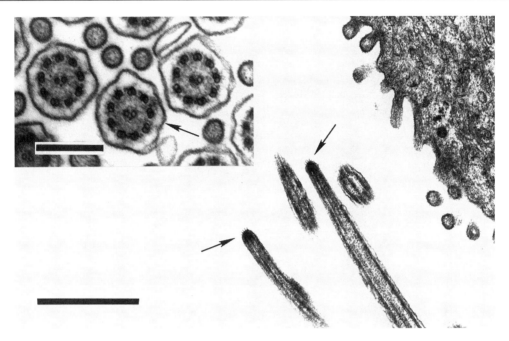

Fig. 5. TEMG of ciliary ultrastructure. The tip of each cilium possesses terminal hooklets (arrows) that facilitate the movement of mucus (scale bar = 1 μm). A cross section (see inset, arrow) through normal cilia shows the characteristic "nine (peripheral doublets) plus two (central single)" arrangement of microtubules (scale bar = 0.25 μm).

Dense-Core Granulated (DCG) Cells

DCG cells are present infrequently in the surface epithelium and are generally basal in position, but may have a thin cytoplasmic projection extending to the lumen. Clusters of such cells associated with intraepithelial nerves (i.e., neuroepithelial bodies) have also been described *(34)*. DCG cells have small (120 nm) spherical granules, with an electron-dense core surrounded by an electron-lucent halo (Fig. 8). They have been shown to contain biogenic amines *(35)* and peptides such as bombesin *(36)*, which may regulate smooth muscle of both blood vessels and bronchi, secretion by mucous cells, and/or ciliary activity.

Basal Cells

It is the presence of a basal-cell layer in the large bronchi and trachea that contributes to the pseudostratified appearance of the epithelium (Figs. 1 and 9). The basal cell has sparse electron-dense cytoplasm, often with bundles of tonofilaments shown by immunocytochemistry to be keratin *(37)*. Rather like the undifferentiated basal cells of the epidermis, the tracheobronchial basal cell is thought to be the main stem cell from which the more superficial mucus-secreting and ciliated cells derive *(38)*. In bronchioli, in which basal cells are sparse or absent, Clara cells appear to be able to perform the role of a stem cell *(33)*.

Airway surface epithelium is replaced slowly, as normally less than 1% of cells are in division at any one time. However, the mitotic index increases in response to irritation by noxious agents such as tobacco smoke *(23–25,39)* and also to β-adrenergic agents such as isoproterenol *(39)*. The mitotic index of the airway epithelium under conditions of allergic inflammation has not been studied extensively but there are indications of increased mitotic activity, presumably associated with areas of epithelial loss and healing in asthma *(40)*.

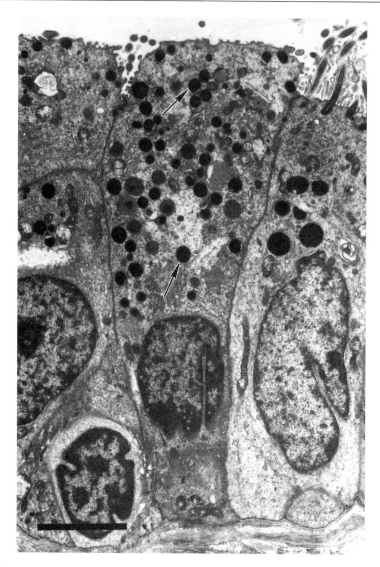

Fig. 6. TEMG of a human epithelial serous cell that contains in its cytoplasm large, discrete, electron-dense granules each with a circular outline (arrows) (scale bar = 2 μm).

Observations of areas of surface columnar cell loss in mild atopic asthma in which basal cells remain attached to the basal lamina *(27,41)* (*see* Epithelial Cells) have led to the proposal that columnar to basal cell attachment points form a potential cleavage plane that is particularly vulnerable to damage by the products of infiltrating inflammatory cells *(42)*.

Intraepithelial Migratory Cells

In addition to the structural cells of the epithelial surface, there are cells that migrate into and/or "home" to the epithelial layer at an early stage during fetal development or throughout life: many of these are considered to reside there for several months/years. These cells normally include mast cells (Fig. 10A), intraepithelial lymphocytes (IEL) (*see* Fig. 9), and dendritic cells (*see* Chapter 7).

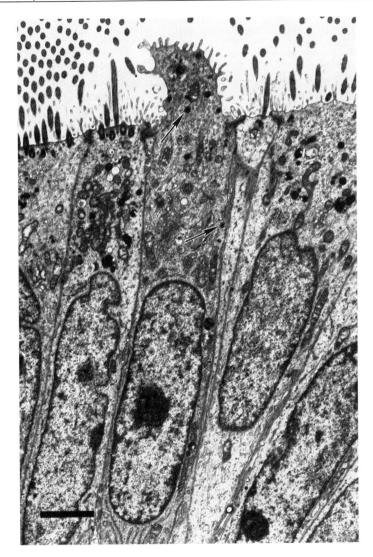

Fig. 7. TEMG of a human nonciliated bronchiolar (Clara) cell with its apex protruding into the airway lumen, whose cytoplasm contains a few small, ovoid granules (arrows) (scale bar = 2 μm).

Mast Cells

In humans, mast cells (MC) form up to 2% of surface epithelial cells, with a higher proportion found in smokers than in nonsmokers *(43)* *(see* Fig. 10A). Based on the differences in neutral protease composition, two distinct types of mature mast cell have been described *(44)*; (i) cells containing tryptase alone (MCT, also called mucosal MC) and (ii) those with tryptase and chymase (MCTC, known as connective tissue MC), the former requiring T-lymphocytes for maturation and proliferation *(45)*. More than 90% of mast cells found in the bronchial subepithelium comprise MCT, whereas MCTC are predominantly observed in the skin *(44,46)*. Intraepithelial MC may share some, but not all, of the morphological and functional characteristics of the subepithelial mast cell and release a variety of preformed and granule-derived mediators of inflammation, some of which may affect epithelial tight junction permeability (such as histamine, leukotrienes, prostaglandins, and platelet activating factor).

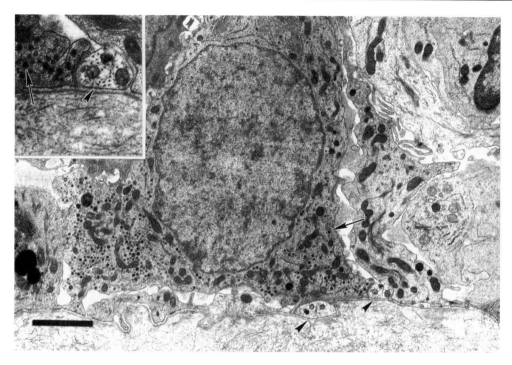

Fig. 8. TEMG of the basal portion of a dense-core granulated cell (D) with cytoplasmic electron-dense granules (arrow) each showing a characteristic electron-lucent halo (see inset). Intraepithelial nerve fibers (arrowheads) are present in close association with the plasma membrane of the cell (scale bar = 2 µm).

In the authors' experience, intraepithelial mast cells may appear to be apoptotic, as evidenced by chromatin condensation and nuclear electron-density (Fig. 10B). Mast cells with a morphology indicative of apoptosis have also been identified in the subepithelium, sometimes engulfed by macrophages. The function of so-called globular leukocytes described by Kent *(47)* and Jeffery and Reid *(4)* is unknown, but derivation from subepithelial mast cells has been suggested. Globular leukocytes are particularly frequent (in excess of 10% of nucleated cells counted in the trachea of laboratory rats) *(4)*, but have not yet been identified in humans.

Lymphocytes

Small, "resting" lymphocytes are present normally in adult and fetal human airway epithelium and can be identified by TEM as early as 16 wk of gestation *(48)*. A major function of IEL is to recognize "nonself" and to bring about, directly or indirectly, the removal of such molecules from the body *(see* Fig. 9). The IEL present in the airway epithelium may be either T- or B-cells. T-cell surface markers normally identified include CD3, CD4 (helper), and, predominantly, CD8 (suppressor/cytotoxic) markers. It is known that the numbers of IEL increase in smoker's chronic bronchitis and that the predominance of the CD8$^+$ phenotype is retained *(49)*. Because of factors such as the fragility of the surface epithelium in asthmatic subjects, there are no data for changes to the IEL CD4/CD8 subsets in asthma. However, the CD4 phenotype predominates in the subepithelial zone of atopic asthmatics, in which the allergic (i.e., T helper 2 [Th2]) profile of inflammation is characteristic *(50–52)*. In contrast, the CD8 phenotype predominates in smoker's chronic bronchitis, particularly when there is fixed airflow obstruction *(53)*. IEL recognize antigens as such only when they are expressed

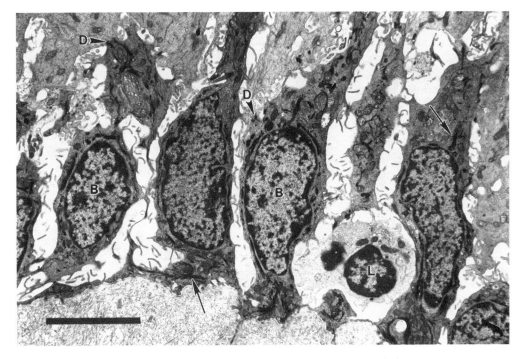

Fig. 9. TEMG of bronchial epithelial basal cells (B), which are thought to provide additional attachment sites via desmosomes (D) for the more superficial columnar cells. Bundles of "tonofilaments" (arrows) are present in the cytoplasm of the basal cells. Lymphocytes (L) may enter and reside within the epithelium (scale bar = 5 μm).

on the surface of APCs bound to surface molecules encoded by major histocompatibility complex (MHC) genes.

Dendritic Cells

Immunostimulation of naive resting T-lymphocytes is thought to require the initial presentation of antigen in association with class II MHC (Ia) molecules expressed by dendritic cells, which are present normally *(54)*. In tissue digests these cells are obtained in low density on percoll gradients and are nonadherent, nonphagocytic, Ia positive, and surface Ig negative. Also identified in airway digests is an endogenous macrophage population that, on balance, inhibits dendritic cell-induced T-lymphocyte activation in vitro. Accordingly, Holt and coworkers *(54,55)* suggest that induction of T-cell immunity is regulated in vivo by a balance of cell signals from resident dendritic and macrophage cell populations. By taking tangential sections of rat and human airway epithelium these authors have shown that virtually all Ia positive expression in noninflamed airways results from cells with characteristic dendritic morphology *(55,56;* also *see* Chapter 7). The surface density of these cells in the laboratory rat is estimated at between 50 and 600 cells/mm^2, the lowest number being present in the most peripheral airways. It is assumed that intraepithelial dendritic cells arrive initially via the airway wall vasculature in the form of precursor cells. Within the epithelium, dendritic cells are thought to mature under the influence of T-lymphocyte-derived cytokines (such as tumor necrosis factor [TNF] α, granulocyte-macrophage colony-stimulating factor [GM-CSF], interleukin [IL]-4, interferon [IFN] γ) *(57–61)*, in which they "sample, process, and store" inhaled antigen before migrating and homing to T-cell zones in the regional lymph nodes.

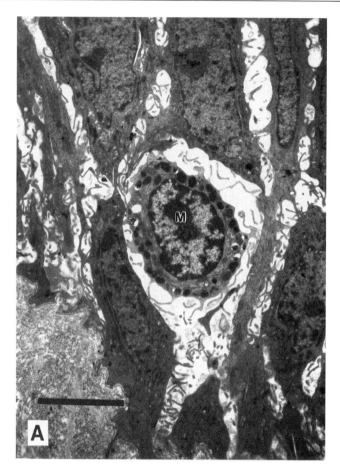

Fig. 10. (A) TEMG of a mast cell (M), a cell often found within the bronchial surface epithelium (scale bar = 5 µm).

The origin of dendritic cells is unclear. They may differentiate from myeloid precursors *(62)* and from human peripheral blood monocytes, via an early indeterminate monocyte-derived cell type that can further develop into either the dendritic phenotype or macrophage *(63,64)*. GM-CSF generally appears to be indispensable for the process of dendritic-cell differentiation. Despite the present lack of a commonly accepted nomenclature for dendritic cells, the criteria that can be used to define them in vitro include lack of CD14 and CD64 but expression of CD1a, accessory markers such as CD40, CD80, CD86, and MHC class II, as well as the ability to stimulate proliferation of allogenic T-cells in a mixed leukocyte reaction *(65,66)*. Processing of antigen by dendritic cells is required for initial stimulation of intra-epithelial T-cells, which leads to the production of "memory" (CD45RO[+]) T-cells. Re-exposure of "memory" T-cells to the same antigen presented by any Ia-bearing accessory cell then results in a much enhanced and specific response.

In addition to intraepithelial dendritic cells, Ia antigen can also be expressed by bronchial epithelial cells *(67,68)*, activated T-lymphocytes, B-lymphocytes, macrophages, and fibroblasts. The immunological sequelae of such stimulation may be T-cell anergy/tolerance or the development of hypersensitivity reactions with release of proinflammatory cytokines

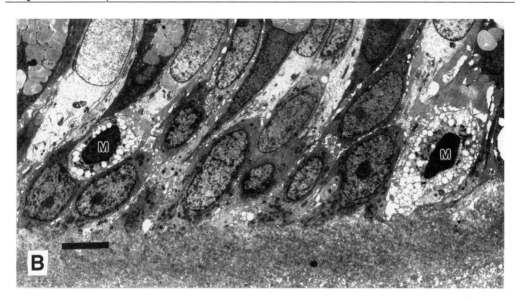

Fig. 10. *(continued)* **(B)** Surface epithelium showing intraepithelial mast cells (M); the mast cell on the right has a morphology suggesting apoptosis (scale bar = 5 μm).

(e.g., IL-4 and IL-5), effector-cell (e.g., eosinophil) recruitment, and release of toxins that may damage the airway mucosa.

EPITHELIAL PERMEABILITY AND FRAGILITY IN ASTHMA

Epithelial fragility is frequently reported in asthmatics; this results in loss, damage, and disruption of the epithelial layer *(27,41,69,70)* with an associated increased epithelial permeabilty *(71)*. The admixture of serum constituents and inflammatory and epithelial cells to epithelial-derived mucus probably contributes to the tenacity of the airway plugs that characterize a severe attack of asthma. The tight junction (zonula occludens) located at the apicolateral border of each epithelial cell normally selectively controls the transepithelial movement of macromolecules, ions, and water between cells. Tight junctions thereby form the first critical barrier that allergen must breach in order to interact with APCs, most of which lie at the base of the epithelium. The technique of freeze fracture demonstrates that tight junctional elements surround each cell as a complex pattern of strands and grooves (Fig. 11) *(72,73)*. Tight junctions are dynamic and readily alter their structure and function in response to local change *(74,75)*. The limited structural data available suggests that epithelial tight junctions are disrupted in asthma *(76,77)*; however further investigation is required. Recent studies have revealed the existence of a degree of homology between some allergens (i.e., the house dust mite allergen Der p1) and proteolytic enzymes *(78)*. Acute exposure to Der p1 has been shown to cause detachment of canine primary cultured cells from artificial and matrix protein substrata, to increase permeability in isolated sheets of bovine mucosa, and to cause epithelial damage in bovine bronchial segments *(79)*. These findings raise the intriguing possibility that local changes in airway epithelial permeability may be induced by the enzymatic activity of an allergen *(78,79)*. This may facilitate the passage of the allergen through the epithelium, and it may be that the surface epithelium of the asthmatic is more susceptible than normal to such proteolysis.

Cell–cell adhesion does not rely on the tight junction *per se*, but rather on adhering junctions such as desmosomes and cell surface adhesive molecules, including E-cadherin

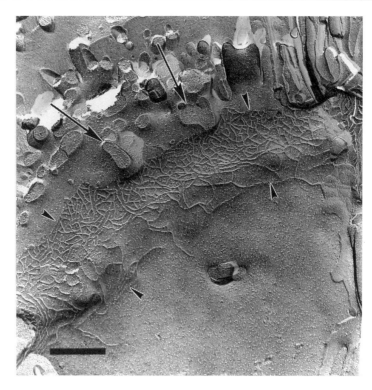

Fig. 11. TEMG of freeze-fracture replica of bronchial epithelial cell demonstrating the arrangement of the "tight junction" (arrowheads) present between surface cells: it consists of a belt of interlinking strands and grooves that surrounds the apico-lateral border of the cell. Fractured microvilli (arrows) are also shown at cell apex (scale bar = 0.5 μm). (Reproduced with permission from ref. *72*.)

(uvomolurin) *(80)*. Intercellular adhesion molecule 1 (ICAM-1) is another epithelial cell surface molecule reported to be upregulated in asthma *(81,82)* and is of importance in entrapping migrating inflammatory cells within the surface epithelium. Experimental blockade of ICAM-1 cell surface expression demonstrated the attenuation of the tissue eosinophilia of asthma *(83)*.

RETICULAR BASEMENT MEMBRANE

The epithelial basement membrane acts as an extracellular scaffold supporting the surface epithelium. It may also control the spatial interrelationship and status of differentiation of its overlying epithelial cells by its interaction with the cell cytoskeleton and by providing a variety of chemical signals *(84)*. The so-called "true" basement membrane consists of a lamina rara (lucida) and a lamina densa (basal lamina) each about 40–60 nm thick (below the 200-nm limit resolution of the light microscope) *(85–87)* (Fig. 12). The principal components are type-IV collagen, proteoglycans, laminin, entactin (nidogen), and fibronectin in both soluble and insoluble forms *(88–96)*. Its negative charge, owing to sulfate and carboxyl moieties, appears to determine, in part, its permeability and capacity for filtration. With respect to adult human airways, there is a characteristic additional reticular component beneath (external to) the basal lamina, the so-called lamina reticularis (also called the fibro-reticularis) (*see* Fig. 12), which is normally about 7–10 μm in thickness; this is absent in fetal airways. It is the lamina reticularis, *not* the basal lamina, that takes on a hyaline appearance in hematoxylin and eosin (H&E)

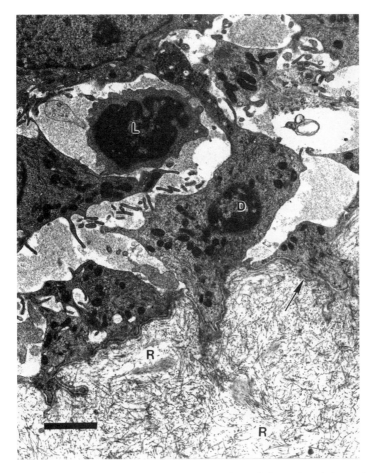

Fig. 12. TEMG showing the so-called "true basement membrane" (arrow) and the underlying reticular fibers of the lamina reticularis (R). Lymphocyte (L) and dense-core granulated cell (D) (scale bar = 2 μm).

stained sections and becomes *homogeneously* thickened in asthma (Fig. 13A). As a structural boundary it acts as a partial barrier to the passage of macromolecules and cells, although inflammatory cells have the capacity to secrete proteases that facilitate passage through the basement membrane and entry into the epithelium and eventually the airway lumen (Fig. 13B). Focal thickening of the reticular basement membrane may also be seen in bronchiectasis, tuberculosis, and chronic sinusitis *(97)*. Roche and colleagues *(98)* have referred to such thickening in asthma as "subepithelial fibrosis," which is present without apparent association with asthma severity, duration, degree of airway responsiveness, or extent of surface cell shedding. Roche and coworkers demonstrated by immunostaining that the lamina reticularis contained immunological determinants for collagen types III and V and for fibronectin. The underlying interstitial collagen reacted with antibodies to collagen types I, III, and V as well as fibronectin. These results indicate that the lamina reticularis and the interstitial collagen do have epitopes in common. However, their ultrastructural distinctiveness indicates fundamental differences in their chemical make-up. There is evidence that epithelia may secrete collagen in vitro and may contribute to the production of the basal lamina or even the reticular basement membrane. Studies of bronchial epithelial cells obtained from asthmatic subjects that allow the investigation of gene expression for collagens of various forms are now

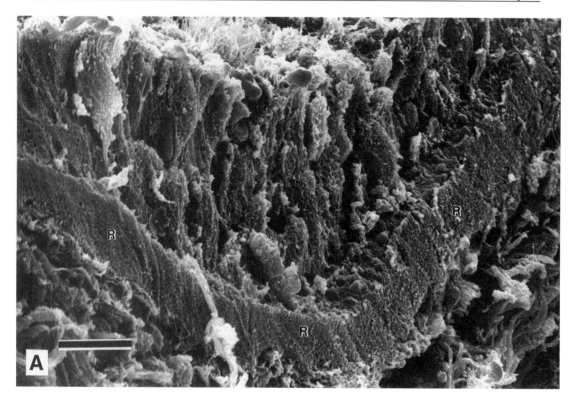

Fig. 13. (A) SEMG showing thickening of the lamina reticularis (R) in the bronchus of a patient with chronic late onset asthma (scale bar = 10 μm).

required to determine the origin of the thickened lamina reticularis in asthma. This important aspect of airway wall remodeling occurs very early on in allergic asthmatics and to a lesser extent in allergic individuals with no evidence of asthma. The extent of thickening (i.e., 2–7 μm) does not of itself contribute greatly to the overall increased wall thickness of asthma, but it may alter the dynamic properties of the airway wall during contractions and contribute to the hyperresponsiveness characteristics of asthma *(99)*.

FIBROBLASTS

Fibroblasts are ubiquitous in the airway wall and may constitute 30% of subepithelial cells in normal conditions and up to 50% of the total number of dispersed cells in chronic inflammatory or fibrotic conditions in lung interstitium *(100)*. Each fibroblast is usually spindle-shaped or bipolar, with a centrally placed mononucleus containing a nucleolus. Fibroblasts adjacent to the subepithelial reticular layer are usually aligned with it (Fig. 14). Fibroblasts are the major source of extracellular matrix (ECM), which includes interstitial collagen and elastin, which form the structural scaffold for interstitially located cells, whether residing in or migrating through subepithelial tissue. Following appropriate stimulation, fibroblasts increase synthetic activity, a change which may be associated with phenotypic alteration (*see* Myofibroblasts).

Transforming growth factor (TGF) β and platelet-derived growth factor (PDGF) influence the activity of fibroblasts and modulate their production of collagens, fibronectin, proteoglycans, integrins, as well as matrix-degrading enzymes (neutral metalloproteinases or matrixin proteases) such as elastases, collagenases, and gelatinases *(101)*. Fibroblasts can also synthe-

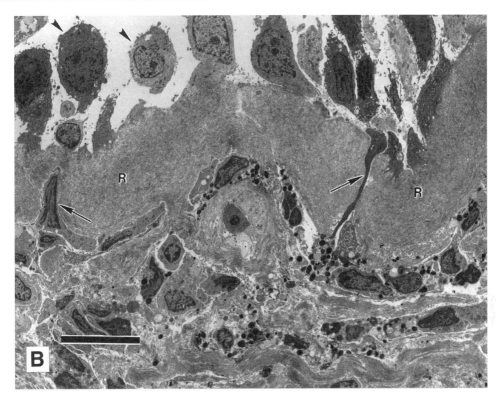

Fig. 13.(B) *(continued)* TEMG of bronchial tissue from an atopic asthmatic showing epithelial loss (arrowheads) and a thickened lamina reticularis (R). Inflammatory cells (arrows) crossing the lamina reticularis (scale bar = 10 μm).

size a number of proinflammatory mediators, particularly after stimulation by interleukin (IL)-1 and tumor necrosis factor (TNF) α. Stimulated fibroblasts appear to be a major source of prostaglandin E$_2$ *(102,103)*, which appears to help shift the balance of T-helper cells toward the Th2 (allergic) type of immune response *(104–106)*. Cytokines and growth factors that have been reported to be produced by fibroblasts include monocyte chemoattractant protein-1 *(107)*, insulin-like growth factors (IGF) *(108)*, macrophage inflammatory peptide 1α *(107)*, and granulocyte-macrophage colony-stimulating factor (GM-CSF) *(109,110)*. GM-CSF is of special interest because it may induce the accumulation of cells with a myofibroblast-like phenotype *(111)*.

MYOFIBROBLASTS

Myofibroblasts are a nonhomogeneous group of cells that share features of both fibroblasts and smooth muscle cells (Fig. 15). Myofibroblasts contain cytoplasmic bundles of contractile filaments whose ultrastructure is similar to that observed in the bronchial smooth muscle cell (*see* Bronchial Smooth Muscle). Their abundant dilated rough endoplasmic reticulum is indicative of increased synthesis of extracellular matrix. The nuclear outline is convoluted in cross section, an ultrastructural feature associated with cellular contraction *(112)*. In contrast to fibroblast, myofibroblasts may be partially invested by basement membrane, which is not, however, as extensive as that found in association with smooth muscle cells (*see* Bronchial Smooth Muscle). Cells with a myofibroblast-like morphology have been found

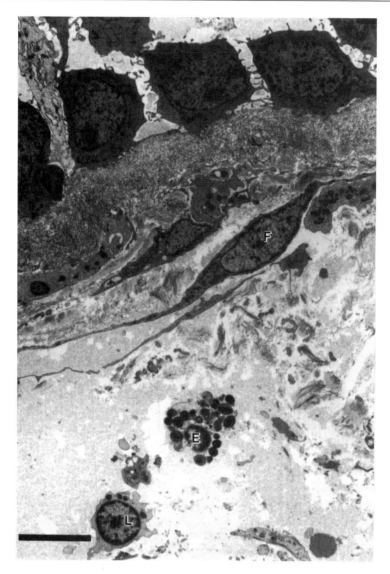

Fig. 14. TEMG of a typical, spindle-shaped fibroblast (F) observed in the subepithelium an atopic asthmatic airway. A lymphocyte (L) and an eosinophil (E) are also present (scale bar = 5 μm).

normally in a variety of organs such as intestine, uterus, spleen, liver, lymph nodes, and lung parenchyma. Pulmonary myofibroblasts were first described by Kapanci et al. *(113)* in the alveolar wall, hence the alternative terms alveolar myofibroblast and interstitial contractile cells of alveolar septa.

Roche et al. *(98)*, using electron microscopy and the immunohistochemical marker PR 2D3, known to be specific for molecules associated with the smooth muscle cell membrane, identified the myofibroblast-like phenotype in human conducting airways in close apposition to the reticular basement membrane. In the subepithelium of asthmatic subjects, myofibroblast number has been reported to be positively associated with the thickness of reticular basement membrane *(114)*. Our observations by transmission electron microscopy have confirmed the presence of myofibroblast-like cells beneath the airway epithelium and have demonstrated that

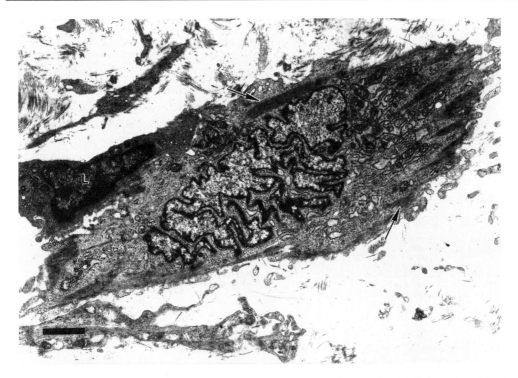

Fig. 15. TEMG of a myofibroblast, with adjacent lymphocyte (L), in the subepithelial matrix of the airway wall. Contractile filaments (arrows) can be observed at the periphery of the myofibroblast: there is also much dilated rough endoplasmic reticulum indicating both the contractile and secretory nature of this phenotype (scale bar = 2 μm).

their numbers increase within the 24 h following an allergen challenge. In unchallenged asthmatics, in whom the reticular basement membrane is thickened, this cell type constitutes less than two percent of the total number of subepithelial cells, and this increases approx 10-fold during the late-phase response to allergen, when there is also an increase in the number of activated eosinophils, as indicated by their degranulation *(115)*.

Although their origin is unclear, it has been suggested that the myofibroblast may be derived from one or all of three different cell types: fibroblasts, smooth muscle cells, and pericytes. Analysis of α smooth-muscle actin (αSMA) and the cytoplasmic intermediate filament proteins vimentin and desmin has shown that their occurrence varies in the myofibroblast population. Vimentin is characteristically present in cells of mesenchymal origin such as the fibroblast, whereas desmin and αSMA are associated with the smooth muscle cell phenotype. At least four myofibroblast phenotypes have been identified based on the immuno-localization of the cytoskeletal proteins desmin, vimentin, and αSMA within them: (1) cells positive only for vimentin (i.e., type V), (2) those positive for vimentin and αSMA (type VA), (3) those positive for vimentin and desmin (type VD), and (4) those positive for all three proteins (type VAD) *(116,117)*. Some myofibroblasts may also express a smooth muscle myosin heavy-chain protein *(117,118)*. Thus a heterogeneous population of myofibroblasts exists, indicative of their changing structure and form.

Under normal conditions, pulmonary myofibroblasts synthesize only the cytoplasmic isoform of actin. In the rat, most alveolar wall myofibroblasts stain for desmin, whereas in humans these cells are devoid of this intermediate filament *(119)*. However, myofibroblasts may express an α smooth muscle actin isoform in postcapillary pulmonary hypertension associated with fibrosis and septal thickening in humans *(120)* and in the areas of lung parenchymal damage caused by experimental bleomycin instillation in the rat *(121)*.

Myofibroblasts are activated in response to tissue injury and produce extracellular matrix components that contribute to the formation of scar tissue *(116,122)*. The presence of contractile fibres in myofibroblast suggests a role for these cells in tissue contraction, and this is evident from observations of granulation tissue formed during wound healing *(123)*. Experimentally, it has been found that the contractile filaments that appear during the early stages of healing disappear when the wound is closed *(124)*. This process of acquiring and then losing αSMA-rich contractile filaments, by myofibroblasts involved in wound healing, favors a fibroblast origin for this cell. In allergic inflammation in asthma, fibroblasts stimulated by proinflammatory cytokines develop a contractile phenotype and participate in a local process of tissue traction and contraction *(115)*. We suggest that such forms would likely be transient, unless there were repeated exposure to allergen, which would drive the process of differentiation in the direction of myofibroblast hyperplasia and possibly smooth muscle mass enlargement, a characteristic change in the airway wall seen in fatal asthma *(125)*.

An alternative explanation for the origin of the airway wall myofibroblast is that bronchial smooth muscle cells may dedifferentiate and adopt a secretory phenotype with increased amounts of Golgi, rough endoplasmic reticulum, and ribosomes, but retain contractile filaments. In this respect, there may be parallels with the alterations observed in experimentally induced atheroma *(126)*. For example, vascular smooth muscle cells seeded in culture modulate their phenotype with an increase in synthetic organelles *(127)* and a decrease in microfilament content, indicated by a decrease in the intensity of immunostaining for smooth muscle-specific contractile proteins *(128)*. It has been shown experimentally that endothelial and arterial injury induced by balloon catheter use stimulates quiescent vascular smooth muscle cells of the tunica media to dedifferentiate and form a synthetic phenotype that migrates to the tunica intima, in which redifferentiation into new vascular smooth muscle occurs *(129)*. This process is associated with the production of interstitial matrix by migrating smooth muscle cells. The capacity of vascular smooth muscle cells to leave locations in the tunica media and migrate depends on the production of metalloprotein enzymes that digest their attachment to the surrounding extracellular matrix. We have suggested that similar phenotypic changes may occur in bronchial asthma following repeated or prolonged exposure to allergen *(115)*. In support of this, bronchial smooth muscle appears capable of similar phenotypic alteration. In culture, growth factors such as fibroblast growth factor (FGF) *(130)*, PDGF *(131,132)*, and TGF *(133,134)* and also mast cell tryptase *(135)* stimulate these cells to undergo a sequence of morphological changes with increased mitogenic activity and the expression of intracellular organelles. It has been shown for vascular smooth muscle cells that an increased expression of connexin 43, a major gap junction (nexus) protein, is associated with the synthetic phenotype *(136)*. This increase in the number of gap junctions, also observed between myofibroblast during wound healing *(123)*, facilitates communication between muscle cells and influences their coordinated contraction.

Pericytes

Vascular pericytes (mesangial cells) have also been proposed as potential precursors of myofibroblasts *(118,137)*. Mesenchymal in origin, pericytes form an incomplete envelope around endothelial cells within the microvascular bed (Fig. 16). Based on microvascular location, there are at least three types of pericytes: precapillary, capillary, and postcapillary venular. Morphologically, they appear as pleomorphic cells with an elongated cell body, from which slender branches arise *(138,139)*. In vessels, endothelial cells and pericytes are

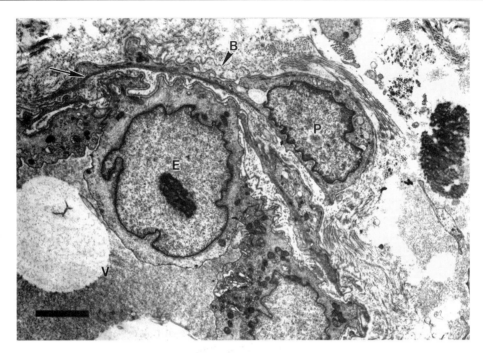

Fig. 16. TEMG of a bronchial vascular pericyte (P) with partial investment of basement membrane (B), which envelopes the vessel (V). The pericyte is a possible precursor of vascular smooth muscle and shares some features with the myofibroblast. Contractile filaments are present in the cytoplasm (arrow). Endothelial cell (E) (scale bar = 2 μm).

each surrounded by a basement membrane except for regions in direct contact with each other. The type of intracellular contractile protein in pericytes depends on their location. Most pericytes express αSMA and smooth-muscle myosin isoforms, as well as vimentin and/or desmin. Pericytes form extensive connections with endothelial cells through adhesive and gap junctions and interrelate functionally during the process of angiogenesis, which is thought to occur in asthma *(140)*. Several functions for the pericyte have been proposed: capillary contraction, regulation of permeability, maintenance of endothelial integrity (especially during inflammation), modulation of endothelial growth, and as a progenitor of pulmonary vascular smooth muscle in medial muscle extension in response to hypoxia. Experimental high-altitude hypoxia in rats induces progressive vascular remodeling with an increase in arterial-wall thickness and extension of muscle into the walls of smaller and more peripheral vessels *(141,142)*. Muscularization of nonmuscular arteries in response to hypoxia occurs when undifferentiated precursors for smooth-muscle cells, such as pericytes, proliferate and differentiate *(143)*. Sundberg et al. *(144)* investigated pericyte function during dermal injury and suggested that this cell may be responsible for the collagen synthesis and hypertrophic scarring observed in areas of vessel branching. These investigators demonstrated that pericytes are able to migrate out from the microvascular wall, i.e., during angiogenesis, and may serve as a precursor to collagen-producing fibroblast-like cells. It is also possible that pericyte-derived fibroblasts that inherit the potential to express αSMA may also have the potential to transform into the myofibroblasts characteristic of the late-phase response.

The literature suggests that in airway inflammatory disease, airway myofibroblasts may be derived from resident fibroblasts, bronchial smooth muscle, and/or vascular pericytes and that

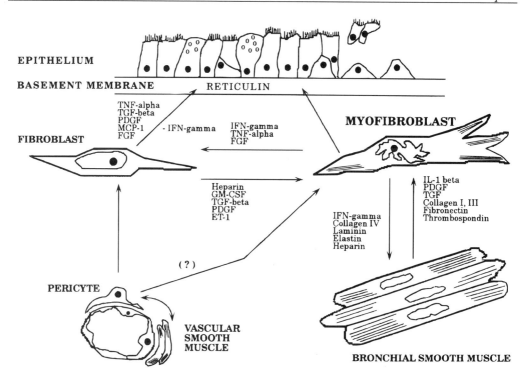

Fig. 17. Schema of the potential role of the myofibroblast and influencing factors in airway wall remodeling.

their alteration following chronic allergen stimulation may result in the enlargement of the bronchial smooth muscle mass that is characteristic of life-threatening asthma (Fig. 17).

BRONCHIAL SMOOTH MUSCLE

The anatomic arrangement of smooth muscle as opposing spirals (i.e., geodesic) around bronchi is thought to cause both airway constriction and shortening on contraction (Fig. 18) *(145)*. The amount of bronchial smooth muscle expressed as a proportion of the airway wall increases in asthma *(146,147)*. Enlarged blocks of bronchial muscle in the airway wall of asthmatics are characteristic of individuals who suffer a fatal attack *(125)* (Fig. 19). An increased amount of bronchial smooth muscle likely contributes not only to bronchial hyperresponsiveness but also to life-threatening attacks of asthma. This increase is thought to result from smooth-muscle hyperplasia (an increase in muscle-fiber number) rather than muscle-fiber hypertrophy (an increase in fiber size) *(148)*; however, it has been suggested that both processes may be involved, depending on which level of the bronchial tree is examined *(149)*. These findings require confirmation and further study.

Ultrastructural examination of smooth-muscle cells demonstrates the presence of a basement membrane surrounding each cell. Ninety percent of the cell cytoplasm is occupied by filaments of actin or myosin together with a small quantity of smooth endoplasmic reticulum, mitochondria, and lipid (Fig. 20) *(150)*. The contractile filaments are associated with electron-dense condensations; these dense bands provide structural support linking the contractile apparatus to the surrounding stroma. Caveolae, small stable invaginations of the cell surface, that are uniform in size and shape are another characteristic feature of the smooth-muscle cell. They are not involved

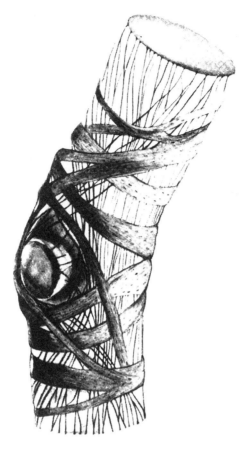

Fig. 18. Diagrammatic representation of the geodesic arrangement of bronchial smooth muscle around the bronchial wall, which on contraction likely causes both airway constriction and shortening. (Reproduced from ref. *145*.)

in the process of pinocytosis, but may have a role in calcium transport and cell volume control and act as stretch receptors to prevent cell deformation *(150)*. Species variation in the nature of muscle-to-muscle cell contact exist. Smooth-muscle fibers are separate in the airways of guinea pig and dog, while frequent connections of the nexus (gap-junction) type are seen in humans. The presence of a gap junction implies electrical as well as chemical coupling between cells and is similar to that found in muscle of the gastrointestinal tract. Cell–cell communication may also occur via release and local diffusion of cytokines and prostanoids. The number of gap junctions in human bronchi is estimated (in cross sections) at 2.5 per 100 muscle-cell profiles *(151)*. However, it is not known whether the expression of connexin 43, a major gap-junction protein of smooth muscle *(152)*, is altered during the process of bronchial smooth muscle mass enlargement in asthma. The origins and mechanisms of bronchial smooth muscle enlargement require much investigation, as this would seem to be a feature that distinguishes between the mild, symptomatic form of asthma and that which is severe and life-threatening.

BRONCHIAL VASCULATURE

The walls of the bronchi are richly supplied by systemic bronchial arteries derived from the descending aorta. Each airway, as it branches, is also closely accompanied by a branch of the

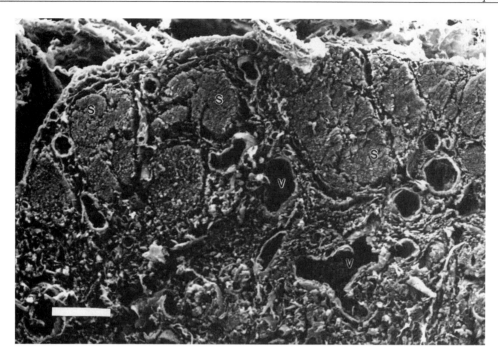

Fig. 19. SEMG of bronchial mucosa showing enlarged bronchial smooth muscle blocks (S) in fatal asthma. Dilated bronchial vessels (V) are also observed throughout the thickened wall (scale bar = 80 μm).

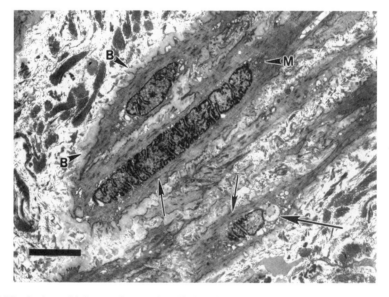

Fig. 20. TEMG of a bronchial smooth muscle cell showing the characteristic envelopment by basement membrane (B). Most of the cytoplasm has contractile filaments (small arrows) but there are also many mitochondria (M) and lipid (large arrow) (scale bar = 5 μm).

245.17.23

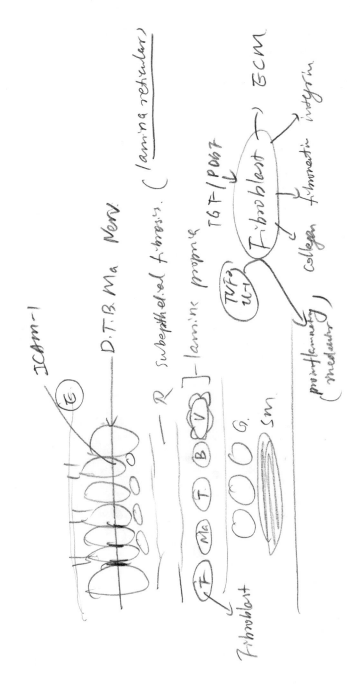

ICAM-1

Fibroblast

F Ma T B V G

D.T.B Ma Nerv

R subepithelial fibrosis. (lamina reticular)

R lamina propria

SM

proinflammatory mediator

TNFα
IL-1

Fibroblast

TGF/PDGF

collagen fibronectin

Fibroblast
fibronectin integrin

ECM

pulmonary artery. The bronchial vasculature has been relatively little studied, and its extensive subepithelial network and role in inflammation and wall thickening are only recently being appreciated *(153–155)*. In humans, the trachea receives systemic blood through branches of the inferior thyroid arteries, which anastomose with bronchial arteries. Most of the inflammatory cells recruited during allergic inflammation of the airway wall are derived from these bronchial vessels *(see* Fig. 2). The extent to which normal nasal and tracheobronchial mucosa is vascularized varies greatly between species *(155,156)*. Tracheobronchial vessels may act: (i) to supply heat and water to breath in order to lessen the effects of evaporation on the moist airway lining, (ii) as a reservoir for blood-borne mediators, and (iii) to decrease compliance and so stiffen the airway wall to minimize the adverse effects of cough. The role of tracheobronchial vessels probably differs greatly in each species, as complexity and vessel wall structure show much variation *(155)*. Innervation and the action of locally released mediators control blood flow through airway wall vessels. Mediators released as a result of mucosal inflammation or antigen–antibody reactions have marked effects on these vessels. Histamine, bradykinin, platelet activating factor, prostaglandins, substance P, and 5-hydroxytryptamine all cause vasodilatation in the dog *(157)*. The interacting effect of these mediators may be quite complex *(155)*. Some of these mediators may act directly on the vessels, whereas others stimulate sensory nerves to induce vasodilatation via the axonal reflex *(158,159)*. Cooling and the application of hypertonic saline to the tracheal mucosa cause vasodilatation *(160,161)*, and this response is of great interest in the context of cold- and exercise-induced asthma associated with bronchial hyperresponsiveness and hyperventilation *(162)*.

The contribution of bronchial vasculature to thickening/swelling of the airway wall in inflammatory disease has probably been underestimated, as vasodilation and congestion of these vessels are a feature of endobronchial challenge and fatal asthma *(see* Fig. 19). Corrosion casting and scanning electron microscopic techniques have demonstrated both a dense subepithelial capillary network and a deeper-lying system of venules, sinuses, or sinusoids in the airway wall. The subepithelial capillaries of the nose are fenestrated *(163)*, whereas in the tracheobronchial tree of healthy humans and many species such fenestration is reported to be confined to bronchial capillaries underlying neuroepithelial bodies and glands *(156,164)*. However, the bronchial capillaries of asthmatic subjects and normal rat, hamster, and guinea pig are fenestrated *(153,156,164)* and are likely to be more permeant to water flux and the exudation and oedema formation associated with inflammation. The sinusoids have been suggested to act as a "mucosal-capacitance" system in the nose that conditions inspired air *(164)*. The function of sinusoids in the lower airways is unclear. Congestion of tracheo-bronchial vessels may cause the airway wall to thicken, thus reducing airway diameter (estimated to be by three percent in the dog and sheep trachea) *(166)*. The effect of this congestion in smaller airways has not been quantified *(140)*.

In addition to the aforementioned functions, the endothelium of bronchial and pulmonary vessels controls the passage of fluid and cells between the intravascular compartment and the interstitial and epithelial compartments, in which the reaction to allergen occurs. The increased endothelial surface expression of cell adhesion molecules (CAMs) and specific interactions with ligands (integrins) on distinct intravascular inflammatory cells promote leukocyte diapedesis ("rolling," adhesion, and migration) into surrounding tissues. The time- and stimulus-dependent expression of CAMs and their ligands results from the release of cytokines and other mediators of inflammation, which allows for a controlled and relatively specific response to allergen or irritant. In this context, the IL-4-induced upregulation of the endothelial cell surface molecule VCAM (vascular CAM) results in the selective retention of eosinophils by interaction with its ligand VLA-4 (very late activation antigen-4), present on the surface of eosinophil but not neutrophils *(167,168)*.

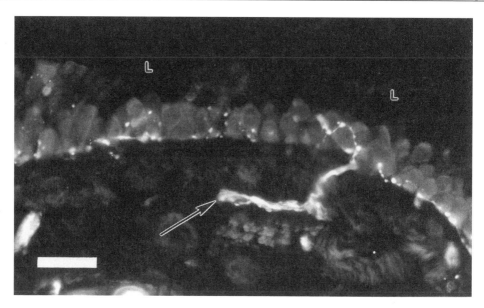

Fig. 21. Immunofluorescence of human airway mucosa stained with PGP 9.5 directed against neural elements: there is a nerve bundle (arrow) in the bronchial subepithelium that extends into the epithelium where it branches to run between epithelial cells toward the airway lumen (L) (scale = 10 μm).

NERVES

The early use of silver staining techniques showed a rich innervation to airway surface epithelium at all levels of airway in rat, mouse, cat, dog, chicken, rabbit, monkey, and man *(121,169)*. In humans, immunoreactivity for protein gene product (PGP)-9.5, a useful marker of neural elements, demonstrates large numbers of subepithelial nerves that penetrate the surface epithelium focally, branch and spread at the base of the epithelium and along the basement membrane, and then run superficially, extending between cells as far as the airway lumen (Fig. 21). Their concentration about the airway circumference varies greatly. It is estimated that there are about 2 nerve fibers per mm of length of surface epithelium in man *(170)*. Depending upon species and site, there is general agreement that substance P (SP)/neurokinin A (NKA) and calcitonin gene-related peptide (CGRP)-containing sensory nerves are found within and immediately below surface epithelium. Most animals have a moderate supply of SP-containing nerve fibers *(158,171)*; in contrast, in humans, SP positive fibers in surface epithelium are rarely detected by immunofluorescence. In vivo, SP is metabolized rapidly by neutral endopeptidase (NEP) (also called enkephalinase), localized to airway epithelium *(172)*. The tissue activity of NEP is an important determinant of tachykinin effectiveness. Reductions of NEP activity occur after respiratory-tract infections, cigaret smoke, ozone, and high doses of toluene diisocyanate *(173,174)*. CGRP is reported to be conspicuous within and beneath surface epithelium in animals, and its distribution resembles closely that of SP/NKA, supporting the concept of colocalization of CGRP and SP/NKA. In humans CGRP is rarely found in the nerves of surface epithelium, but it is conspicuous in intraepithelial neuroendocrine cells.

A number of electron-microscopic (EM) studies have shown unequivocally that nerve fibers do pierce the airway surface epithelial basement membrane and come to lie in apposition to a number of distinct epithelial cell types in various species *(12,169,175–187)* (Fig. 22). However, there appears to be great species variation in the morphology, distribution, and number of intraepithelial nerves in each succeeding airway generation. The observations of Laitinen *(187)*

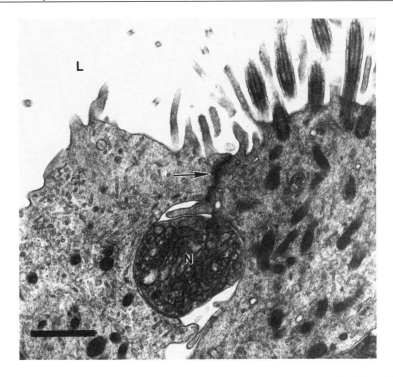

Fig. 22. TEMG of an intraepithelial nerve (N) between two epithelial cells, joined by a tight junction (arrow). The tight junction separates intraepithelial nerve from airway lumen (L) (scale = 1 μm).

and our own observations of bronchial biopsies obtained from normal healthy individuals show that intraepithelial nerve fibers are present in main-stem extrapulmonary bronchi and segmental airways, but in comparison with rat and cat, they are found infrequently. The intraepithelial endings are ideally placed to receive mechanical stimuli or those of allergen or irritant gases such as cigaret smoke, ammonia, sulfur dioxide, and ethyl ether and may also respond to inert (carbon) dust. The only barrier to the penetration of these substances is the tight junction (*see* above). Boucher *(179)* and Hulbert et al. *(188)* have shown in the guinea pig that the epithelial exclusion of horseradish peroxidase (HRP, mol wt 40,000) placed in the airway lumen can be overcome, experimentally, following exposure to cigaret smoke; the penetration of HRP past the tight junction has been observed by its subsequent accumulation around intraepithelial nerve fibers. Though circumstantial, it is likely that intraepithelial nerves are the morphological correlate of cough-irritant and airway C-fibers. It is likely that allergen that passes the barrier afforded by tight junction may stimulate these intraepithelial nerves, whose local reflexes give rise to the mucous secretion, vasodilatation, and the edema associated with neurogenic inflammation *(12,189,190)*. EM studies of the motor innervation of normal bronchial smooth muscle have not shown synaptic contact between nerve varicosities and muscle *(191)*. Whereas some nerve varicosities lie outside the muscle, others may share a common investment of basement membrane with muscle, but no synaptic specialization is observed (Fig. 23).

CONCLUSION

The structural cell types that make up the normal airway wall are many. Epithelial cells normally interact by contact and local production of cytokines to form an intact surface epithe-

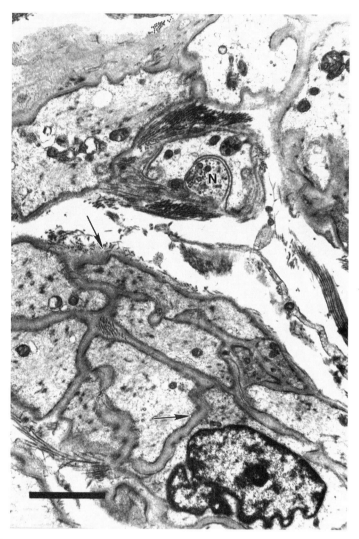

Fig. 23. TEMG of bronchial smooth muscle cells enveloped by basement membrane (arrows) and associated with a motor nerve varicosity (N). A specialized neuromuscular junction is not observed (scale = 2 μm).

lium, with barrier and secretory properties supported by a structurally and biochemically complex reticular basement membrane. Beneath, there is a matrix of connective tissue associated with migratory cells, vessels, mucus-secreting glands, bronchial smooth muscle, and nerves. In allergic inflammatory conditions such as asthma, the mucosal surface becomes fragile and there is an early thickening of its reticular basement membrane. Repeated exposure to allergen appears to induce an inflammatory response characterized by a selective eosinophilia and altered differentiation of fibroblasts and an associated increase in the numbers of myofibroblasts and the mass of bronchial smooth muscle; the last is a characteristic of fatal asthma. This chapter highlights the need for further research into the mechanisms of cell–cell interaction in the normal in order to understand better the changes that occur in allergic disease, particularly those that lead to the airway wall remodeling associated with symptoms and acute severe attacks of asthma.

REFERENCES

1. Horsefield K (1974) The relation between structure and function in the airways of the lung. Br J Dis Chest 68:145.
2. Horsefield K (1981) The structure of the tracheobronchial tree. In: Scadding JG, Cumming G, Thurlbeck WM, eds. Respiratory Medicine. Heinemann, London, p. 54.
3. Evans MJ, Plopper CG (1988) The role of basal cells in adhesion of columnar epithelium to airway basement membrane. Am Rev Respir Dis 138:481–483.
4. Jeffery PK, Reid L (1975) New observations of rat airway epithelium: a quantitative electron microscopic study. J Anat 120:295–320.
5. Lumsden AB, McLean A, Lamb D (1984) Goblet and Clara cells of human distal airways: evidence for smoking-induced changes in numbers. Thorax 39:844–853.
6. Jeffery PK (1983) Morphology of airway surface epithelial cells and glands. Am Rev Respir Dis 128:S14–S20.
7. Jeffery PK (1978) The structure and function of the mucus-secreting cells of cat and goose airway epithelium. In: Porter R, ed. Respiratory Tract Mucus, 56th CIBA Foundation Symposium. Elsevier/Excerpta Med, Amsterdam, pp. 5–24.
8. Jeffery PK (1995) Microscopic structure of normal lung. In: Brewis RAL, Gibson GJ, Geddes GM, eds. Respiratory Medicine. 2nd Ed. Bailliere Tindall, London/Toronto, pp. 54–72.
9. Jeffery PK, Corrin B (1984) Structural analysis of the respiratory tract. In: Bienenstock J, ed. Immunology of the Lung. McGraw-Hill, New York, pp. 1–27.
10. Breeze RG, Wheeldon EB (1977) The cells of the pulmonary airways. Am Rev Respir Dis 116:705–777.
11. McDermott MR, Befus AD, Bienenstock J (1982) The structural basis for immunity in the respiratory tract. Internat Rev Exp Path 23:47–112.
12. Jeffery PK (1986) Innervation of airway epithelium. In: Kay AB, ed. Asthma: Clinical Pharmacology and Therapeutic Progress. Blackwell, Oxford, pp. 376–392.
13. Jeffery PK (1994) Innervation of the airway mucosa: structure, function and changes in airway disease. In: Goldie R, et al., eds. Immunopharmacology of Epithelial Barriers. Academic, London, pp. 85–118.
14. Sleigh HA (1977) The nature and action of respiratory tract cilia. In: Brain JD, et al., eds. Respiratory Defense Mechanisms, Part 1. Dekker, New York.
15. Pavia D, Lopez-Vidriero MT, Clarke SW (1987) Mediators and mucociliary clearance in asthma. Bull Eur Physiopathol Respir 23Suppl. 10:89s–94s.
16. Mossberg B, Strandberg K, Phillipson K, Camner P (1976) Tracheobronchial clearance in bronchial asthma: response to beta-adrenoceptor stimulation. Scand J Respir Dis 57:119–128.
17. Carlstedt I, Sheehan JK (1984) Macromolecular properties and polymeric structure of mucus glycoproteins. In: Nugent J, O'Connor M, eds. Mucus and Mucosa, Ciba Foundation Symposium 109. Pitman, Bath, pp. 157–172.
18. Lamb D, Reid L (1968) Mitotic rates, goblet cell increase and histochemical changes in mucus in rat bronchial epithelium during exposure to SO_2. J Pathol Bacteriol 96:97–111.
19. Jones R, Bolduc P, Reid L (1972) Protection of rat bronchial epithelium against tobacco smoke. Br Med J 2:142–144.
20. Jeffery PK, Reid L (1981) The effect of tobacco smoke with or without phenylmethyloxadiazole (PMO) on rat bronchial epithelium: a light and electron microscopic study. J Pathol 133:341–359.
21. Jeffery PK (1990) Tobacco smoke-induced lung disease. In: Cohen RD, Lewis B, Alberti KGMM, Denman AM, eds. The Metabolic and Molecular Basis of Acquired Disease. Balliere Tindall, London, pp. 466–495.
22. McDowell EM, Trump BF (1983) Conceptual review: histogenesis of preneoplastic and neoplastic lesions in tracheobronchial epithelium. Surv Synth Path Res 2:235–279.
23. Ayers M, Jeffery PK (1982) Cell division and differentiation in the respiratory tract. In: Cumming G, Bonsignore G, eds. Cell Biology and the Lung. Plenum, New York, pp. 33–60.
24. Jeffery PK, Ayers M, Rogers DF (1982) The mechanisms and control of bronchial mucous cell hyperplasia. Chest 815:27S–29S.
25. Ayers M, Jeffery PK (1988) Proliferation and differentiation in adult mammalian airway epithelium: a review. Eur Respir J 1:58–80.
26. Ellefsen P, Tos M (1972) Goblet cells in the human trachea: quantitative studies of a pathological biopsy material. Arch Otolaryngol 95:547–555.

27. Jeffery PK, Wardlaw A, Nelson FC, Collins JV, Kay AB (1989) Bronchial biopsies in asthma: an ultra-structural quantification study and correlation with hyperreactivity. Am Rev Respir Dis 140:1745–1753.

28. Rogers AV, Dewar A, Corrin B, Jeffery PK (1993) Identification of serous-like cells in the surface epithelium of human bronchioles. Eur Respir J 6:498–504.

29. Willems LNA, Kramps JA, Jeffery PK, Dijkman JH (1988) Detection of antileukoprotease in the developing foetal lung. Thorax 43:784–786.

30. Niden AH (1980) Bronchiolar and large alveolar cell in pulmonary phospholipid metabolism. Science 158:1323–1324.

31. Gil J, Weibel E (1971) Extracellular lining of bronchioles after perfusion-fixation of rat lungs for electron microscopy. Anat Rec 169:185–200.

32. Sallenave JM, Silva A, Marsden ME, Ryle AP (1993) Secretion of mucus proteinase inhibitor and alefin by Clara cell and type II pneumocyte cell lines. Am J Resp Cell Mol Biol 8:126–133.

33. Evans MJ, Cabral-Anderson LJ, Freeman G (1978) Role of the Clara cell in renewal of bronchiolar epithelium. Lab Invest 38:648–655.

34. Lauweryns JM, Cokelaere M, Theunynck P (1972) Neuro-epithelial bodies in the respiratory mucosa of various mammals. Z Zellforsch Mikrosk Anatomy 135:569–592.

35. Lauweryns JM, De Bock V, Verhofstad AAJ, Steinbusch HWM (1982) Immunohistochemical localization of serotonin in intrapulmonary neuro-epithelial bodies. Cell Tiss Res 226:215–223.

36. Wharton J, Polak JM, Bloom SR, Ghatei MA, Solcia E, Brown MR, Pearse AG (1978) Bombesin-like immunoreactivity in the lung. Nature 273:769–770.

37. Schlegel R, Banko-Schlegel S, Pinkus GS (1980) Immunohistochemical localization of keratin in normal human tissues. Lab Invest 42:91–96.

38. Blenkinsopp WK (1967) Proliferation of respiratory tract epithelium in the rat. Exp Cell Res 46:144–154.

39. Bolduc P, Reid L (1978) The effect of isoprenaline and pilocarpine on mitotic index and goblet cell number in rat respiratory epithelium. Br J Exp Pathol 59:311–318.

40. Erjefalt JS, Erjefalt I, Sundler F, Persson CGA (1995) In vivo restitution of airway epithelium. Cell Tissue Res 281:305–316.

41. Beasley R, Roche W, Roberts JA, Holgate ST (1989) Cellular events in the bronchi in mild asthma and after bronchial provocation. Am Rev Respir Dis 139:806–817.

42. Montefort S, Roberts JA, Beasley R, Holgate ST, Roche WR (1992) The site of disruption of the bronchial epithelium in asthmatic and non-asthmatic subjects. Thorax 47:499–503.

43. Lamb D, Lumsden A (1982) Intra-epithelial mast cells in human airway epithelium: evidence for smoking-induced changes in their frequency. Thorax 37:334–342.

44. Irani AA, Bradford TR, Kepley CL, Schechter NM, Schwartz LB (1989) Detection of MC-T and MC-TC types of human mast cells by immunohistochemistry using new monoclonal anti-tryptase and anti-chymase antibodies. J Histochem Cytochem 37:1509–1515.

45. Razin E, Ihle JW, Seldin D, et al. (1984) Interleukin 3: a differentiation and growth factor for the mouse mast cell that contains chondroitin sulfate E proteoglycan. J Immunol 132:1479–1486.

46. Irani AA, Schechter NM, Craig SS, Deblois G, Schwartz LB (1986) Two types of human mast cells that have distinct neutral protease compositions. Proc Natl Acad Sci USA 83:4464–4468.

47. Kent JF (1966) Distribution and fine structure of globular leukocytes in respiratory and digestive tracts of the laboratory rat. Anat Rec 156:439–454.

48. Jeffery PK, Reid L (1977) The ultrastructure of the airway lining and its development. In: Hodson WA, ed. The Development of the Lung. Marcel Dekker, New York, pp. 87–134.

49. Fournier M, Lebargy F, Le Roy Ladurie F, Lenormand E, Pariente R (1989) Intraepithelial T-lymphocyte subsets in the airways of normal subjects and of patients with chronic bronchitis. Am Rev Respir Dis 140:737–742.

50. Corrigan CJ, Hartnell A, Kay AB (1988) T lymphocyte activation in acute severe asthma. Lancet, Vol 1:1129–1131.

51. Robinson DS, Hamid Q, Sun-Ying, Tsicopoulos A, Barhani J, Bentley AM, Corrigan CJ, Durham SR, Kay AB (1992) Predominant Th2-type bronchoalveolar lavage T lymphocyte popularity in atopic asthma. N Engl J Med 326:298–304.

52. De Carlo Massaro G (1989) Nonciliated bronchoepithelial (Clara) cells. In: Massaro D, ed. Lung Cell Biology. Markel Dekker, New York, pp. 81–107.

53. O'Shaughnessy TC, Ansari TW, Barnes NC, Jeffery PK (1995) T-cell markers in smokers' chronic bronchitis with and without airflow obstruction. Eur Respir J 8(Suppl. 19):493s.

54. Holt PG (1993) Regulation of antigen-presenting cell function(s) in lung and airway tissues. Eur Respir J 6:120–129.

55. Holt PG, Schon-Hegrad MA, Phillips MJ, McMenamin PG (1989) Ia-positive dendritic cells form a tightly meshed network within the human airway epithelium. Clin Exp Allergy 19:597–601.

56. Holt PG, Schon-Hegrad MA, Oliver J, Holt BJ, McMenamin PG (1990) A contiguous network of dendritic antigen-presenting cells within the respiratory epithelium. Int Arch Allergy Appl Immunol 91:155–159.

57. Caux C, Dezutter-Dambuyant C, Scmitt D, Banchereau J (1992) GM-CSF and TNF-α cooperate in the generation of dendritic Langerhans cells. Nature 360:258–261.

58. Kasinrerk W, Baumruker T, Majdic O, Knapp W, Stockinger H (1993) CD1 molecule expression on human monocytes induced by GM-CSF. J Immunol 150:579–584.

59. Steinbach F, Krause B, Thiele B (1995) Monocyte derived dendritic cells (MODC) present phenotype and functional activities of Langerhans cells/dendritic cells. Adv Exp Med Biol 378:151–153.

60. Xu H, Kramer M, Spengel HP, Peters JH (1995) Dendritic cells differentiated from human monocytes through a combination of IL-4, GM-CSF and IFN-τ exhibit phenotype and function of blood dendritic cells. Adv Exp Med Biol 378:75–78.

61. Peters JH, Ruppert J, Gieseler RK, Najar HM, Xu H (1991) Differentiation of human monocytes into CD14 negative accessory cells: do dendritic cells derive from the monocyte lineage? Pathobiology 59:122–126.

62. Reid CD, Stackpoole A, Meager A, Tikarpae J (1992) Interaction of TNF with GM-CSF and other cytokines in the regulation of dendritic cell growth in vitro from early bipotent CD34+ progenitors in human bone marrow. J Immunol 149:2681–2688.

63. Rossi G, Heveker N, Thiele B, Gelderblom H, Steinbach F (1992) Development of Langerhans cell phenotype from peripheral blood monocytes. Immunol Lett 31:189–197.

64. Peters JH, Ruhl S, Friedrichs D (1987) Veiled accessory cells deduced from monocytes. Immunobiology 176:154–166.

65. Steinbach F, Thiele B (1993) Monocyte-derived Langerhans cells from different species—morphological and functional characterization. Adv Exp Med Biol 239:213–218.

66. Peters JH, Gieseler R, Thiele B, Steinbach F (1996) Dendritic cells: from ontogenetic orphans to myelomonocytic descendants. Immunol Today 17:273–278.

67. Glanville AR, Tazelaar HD, Therodore J, et al. (1989) The distribution of mhc class I and II antigens on bronchial epithelium. Am Rev Respir Dis 139:330–334.

68. Natali PC, De Martino C, Quarawta V (1981) Expression of Ia-like antigens in normal human non-lymphoid tissues. Transplantation 31:75–78.

69. Dunnill MS (1960) The pathology of asthma, with special reference to changes in the bronchial mucosa. J Clin Pathol 13:27–33.

70. Laitinen LA, Heino M, Laitinen A, Kava T, Haahtela T (1985) Damage of the airway epithelium and bronchial reactivity in patients with asthma. Am Rev Respir Dis 131:599–606.

71. Ilowite JS, Bennett WD, Sheetz MS, Groth ML, Nierman DM (1989) Permeability of the bronchial mucosa to 99mTc DTPA in asthma. Am Rev Respir Dis 139:1139–1143.

72. Godfrey RWA, Severs NJ, Jeffery PK (1992) Freeze-fracture morphology and quantification of human bronchial epithelial tight junctions. Am J Respir Cell Molec Biol 6:453–458.

73. Schneeberger EE, Lynch RD (1992) Structure, function, and regulation of cellular tight junctions. J Appl Phys 262:L647–L661.

74. Faff O, Mitreiter R, Muckter H, Ben-Shaul Y, Bacher A (1988) Rapid formation of tight junctions in HT 29 human adenocarcinoma cells by hypertonic salt solutions. Exp Cell Res 177:60–72.

75. Madara JL (1988) Tight junction dynamics: is paracellular transport regulated. Cell 53:497–498.

76. Elia C, Bucca C, Rolla G, Scappaticci E, Cantino D (1988) A freeze-fracture study of tight junctions in human bronchial epithelium in normal, bronchitic and asthmatic subjects. J Submic Cytol Pathol 20:509–517.

77. Ohashi Y, Montojima S, Fukuda T, Makino S (1992) Airway hyperresponsiveness, increased intracellular spaces of bronchial epithelium, and increased infiltration of eosinophils and lymphocytes in bronchial mucosa in asthma. Am Rev Respir Dis 145:1469–1476.

78. Lake FR, Ward LD, Simpson PJ, Thompson PJ (1991) The group III allergens from house dust mite Dermatophagoides pteronyssinus is a trypsin-like enzyme. Immunobiology 87:1035–1042.

79. Herbert CA, King CM, Ring PC, Holgate ST, Stewart GA, Thompson PJ (1995) Augmentation of permeability in the bronchial epithelium by the house dust mite allergen, Der p1. Am J Respir Cell Mol Biol 129:369–378.

80. Takeichi M (1996) Cadherins: a molecular family important in selective cell-cell adhesion. Annu Rev Biochem 59:237–252.

81. Trigg CJ, Manolitsas ND, Wang J, Calderon MA, McAulay A, Jordan SE, Herdman MJ, Jhalli N, Duddle JM, Hamilton SA, Devalia JL, Davies RJ (1994) Placebo-controlled immunopathologic study of four months of inhaled corticosteroids in asthma. Am J Respir Crit Care Med 150:17–22.

82. Gosset P, Tillie-Leblond I, Janin A, Marquette CH, Copin MC, Wallaert B, Tonnel AB (1994) Increased expression of ELAM-1, ICAM-1, and VCAM-1 on bronchial biopsies from allergic asthmatic patients. Ann N Y Acad Sci 725:163–172.

83. Wegner CD, Gundel RH, Reilly P, Haynes N, Letts LG, Rothlein R (1990) Intercellular adhesion molecule-1 [ICAM-1] in the pathogenesis of asthma. Science 247:456–459.

84. Kleinman HK, Graf J, Iwamoto Y, Kitten GT, Ogle RC, Sasaki M, Yamada Y, Martin GR, Luckenbill-Edds L (1987) Role of basement membranes in cell differentiation. Ann N Y Acad Sci 513:134–145.

85. Merker HJ (1994) Morphology of the basement membrane. Microsc Res Tech 28:95–124.

86. Timpl R, Dziadek M (1986) Structure, development, and molecular biology of basement membranes. Int Rev Exp Pathol 29:1–112.

87. Scittny JC, Yurchenco PD (1989) Basement membranes: molecular organisation and function in development and disease. Curr Opin Cell Biol 1:983–988.

88. Ozawa M, Sato M, Muramatsu T (1983) Basement membrane glycoprotein laminin is an agglutin. J Biochem 94:479–485.

89. Laurie GW, Bing JT, Kleinman HK, Hassell JR, Aumailley M, Martin GR, Feldmann RJ (1986) Localization of binding sites for laminin, heparan sulfate proteoglycan and fibronectin on basement membrane (type IV) collagen. J Mol Biol 189:205–216.

90. Abrahamson DR (1986) Recent studies on the structure and pathology of basement membranes. J Pathol 149:257–278.

91. Timpl R (1989) Structure and biological activity of basement membrane proteins. Eur J Biochem 180:487–502.

92. Chung AE, Durkin ME (1990) Entactin: structure and function. Am J Resp Cell Mol Biol 3:275–282.

93. Martin GR, Timpl R (1987) Laminin and other basement membrane components. Ann Rev Cell Biol 3:57–85.

94. Dziadek M (1995) Role of laminin-nidogen complexes in basement membrane formation during embryonic development. Experientia 51:901–913.

95. Timpl R (1993) Proteoglycans of basement membrane. Experientia 49:417–428.

96. Kuhn K (1995) Basement membrane (type IV) collagen. Matrix Biology 14:439–445 (abstract).

97. Crepea SB, Harman JW (1955) The pathology of bronchial asthma. I. The significance of membrane changes in asthmatic and non-allergic pulmonary disease. J Allergy 26:453–460.

98. Roche WR, Beasley R, Williams JH, Holgate ST (1989) Subepithelial fibrosis in the bronchi of asthmatics. Lancet i:520–523.

99. Lambert RK (1991) Role of bronchial basement membrane in airway collapse. J Appl Physiol 71:666–673.

100. Rennard SI, Bitterman PB, Crystal RG (1984) Pathogenesis of the granulomatous lung disease. IV. Mechanisms of fibrosis. Am J Resp Crit Care Med 130:492–496.

101. Stetler-Stevenson WG (1996) Dynamics of matrix turnover during pathologic remodelling of the extracellular matrix. Am J Pathol 148:1345–1350.

102. Lin LL, Lin AY, DeWitt DL (1992) Interleukin-1 alpha induces the accumulation of cytosolic phospholipase A2 and the release of prostaglandin E2 in human fibroblasts. J Biol Chem 267:23451–23454.

103. Dayer JM, Beutler B, Cerami A (1985) Cachectin/tumor necrosis factor stimulates collagenases and prostaglandin E production by human synovial cells and dermal fibroblasts. J Exp Med 162:2163–2166.

104. Snijdewint FGM, Kalinsky P, Wierenga EA, Bos JD, Kapsenberg ML (1993) Prostaglandin E2 differentially modulates cytokine secretion profiles of human T-helper lymphocytes. J Immunol 150:5321–5329.

105. Roper RL, Conrad DH, Brown DM, Warner GL, Phipps RP (1990) Prostaglandin E2 promotes IL-4 induced IgE and IgG1 synthesis. J Immunol 145:2644–2651.

106. Betz M, Fox BS (1991) Prostaglandin E2 inhibits production of Th1 lymphokines but not of Th2 lymphokines. J Immunol 146:108–113.

107. Lukacs NW, Chensue SW, Smith RE, et al. (1994) Production of monocyte chemoattractant-1 (MCP-1) and macrophage inflammatory protein (MIP-1α) by inflammatory granuloma fibroblasts. Am J Pathol 144:711–718.

108. Stiles AD, D'Ercole AJ (1990) The insulin-like growth factors and the lung. Am J Resp Cell Mol Biol 3:93–100.
109. Zucali JR, Dinarello CA, Oblon DJ, Gross MA, Anderson L, Weiner RS (1986) Interleukin-1 stimulates fibroblasts to produce GM-CSF. J Clin Invest 77:1857–1863.
110. Vancheri C, Ohtoshi T, et al. (1991) Neutrophil differentiation by human upper airway fibroblast-derived granulocyte/macrophage colony stimulating factor (GM-CSF). Am J Resp Cell Mol Biol 4:11–17.
111. Rubbia-Brandt L, Sappino A, Gabbiani G (1991) Locally applied GM-CSF induces accumulation of alpha-smooth muscle actin containing fibroblasts. Virchows Arch B Cell Pathol 60:73–82.
112. Franke WW, Schinko W (1969) Nuclear shape in muscle cells. J Cell Biol 42:326–331.
113. Kapanci Y, Assimacopoulos A, Irle C, Zwahlen A, Gabbiani G (1974) "Contractile interstitial cells" in pulmonary alveolar septa: A possible role of ventilation/perfusion ratio? J Cell Biol 60:375–392.
114. Brewster CEP, Howarth PH, Djukanovic R, Wilson J, Holgate ST, Roche WR (1990) Myofibroblasts and subepithelial fibrosis in bronchial asthma. Am J Respir Cell Mol Biol 3:507–511.
115. Gizycki MJ, Adelroth E, Rogers AV, O'Byrne PM, Jeffery PK (1997) Myofibroblast involvement in the allergen induced late response in mild atopic asthma. Am J Respir Crit Care Med 16:664–673.
116. Skalli O, Schurch W, Seemayer T, Lagace R, Montandon D, Pittet B, Gabbiani G (1989) Myofibroblast from diverse pathologic settings are heterogenous in their content of actin isoforms and intermediate filament proteins. Lab Invest 60:275–285.
117. Schmitt-Graff A, Desmouliere A, Gabbiani G (1994) Heterogeneity of myofibroblast phenotypic features: an example of fibroblastic cell plasticity. Virchows Archiv 425:3–24.
118. Sappino AP, Schurch W, Gabbiani G (1990) Differentiation repertoire of fibroblast cells: expression of cytoskeletal proteins as markers of phenotypic modulation. Lab Invest 63:144–161.
119. Adler KB, Callahan LM, Evans JN (1986) Cellular alterations in the alveolar wall in bleomycin-induced lung fibrosis in rats: An ultrastructural morphometric study. Am J Resp Crit Care Med 133:1043–1048.
120. Kapanci Y, Burgan S, Pietra GG, Conne B, Gabbiani G (1990) Modulation of actin isoforms expression in alveolar myofibroblasts (contractile interstitial cells) during pulmonary hypertension. Am J Pathol 136:881–889.
121. Mitchell J, Woodcock-Mitchell J, Reynolds S, Low RB, Leslie KO, Adler K, Gabbiani G, Omar S (1989) Alpha smooth muscle actin in parenchymal cells of bleomycin-injured rat lung. Lab Invest 60:643–650.
122. Gabbiani G, Lous ML, Bailey AJ, Bazin S, Delaunay A (1976) Collagen and myofibroblasts of granulation tissue. A chemical, ultrastructural and immunologic study. Virchows Arch B Cell Pathol 21:133–145.
123. Gabbiani G, Chaponnier C, Huttner I (1978) Cytoplasmic filaments and gap junctions in epithelial cells and myofibroblasts during wound healing. J Cell Biol 76:561–568.
124. Darby I, Skalli O, Gabbiani G (1990) α-Smooth muscle actin is transiently expressed by myofibroblasts during experimental wound healing. Lab Invest 63:21–29.
125. Carroll N, Elliot A, Morton A, James A (1993) The structure of large and small airways in nonfatal and fatal asthma. Am Rev Respir Dis 147:405–410.
126. Severs NJ, Robenek H (1992) Constituents of the arterial wall and atherosclerotic plaque: an introduction to atherosclerosis. In: Cell Interactions in Atherosclerosis. Robenek H, Severs NJ, eds. CRC Press, Boca Raton, pp. 1–49.
127. Campbell GR, Chamley-Campbell JH, Burnstock G (1981) Differentiation and phenotypic modulation of arterial smooth muscle. In: Schwartz CJ, Werthessen NT, Wolf S, eds. Structure and Function of Circulation, vol. 3. Plenum, New York, pp. 357–399.
128. Thyberg J, Nilsson J, Palmberg L, Sjolund M (1985) Adult human arterial smooth muscle cells in primary culture: modulation from contractile to synthetic phenotype. Cell Tissue Res 239:501–513.
129. Okamoto E, Imataka K, Fujii J, Kuro M, Nakaharak K, Nishimura H, Yazaki Y, Nagai R (1992) Heterogeneity in smooth muscle cell populations in neointimas and the media of post-stenotic dilatation of rabbit carotid artery. Biochem Biophys Res Commun 185:459–464.
130. Kelleher MD, Schneider SD, Naureckas ET, Abe Mk, Jain M, Solvay J, Hershenson MB (1994) Responsiveness of bovine tracheal smooth muscle cells to various mitogens. Am J Resp Crit Care Med 149:A304 (abstract).
131. Hirst SJ, Barnes PJ, Twort CHC (1996) PDGF receptor expression and differential proliferation induced by PDGF isoforms in human cultured bronchial smooth muscle. Am J Physiol 270:L415–428.
132. Hirst SJ, Barnes PJ, Twort CHC (1994) Proliferation of human and rabbit smooth muscle in culture by platelet-derived growth factor isoforms. Am J Resp Crit Care Med 149:A303 (abstract).

133. Black PN, Young PG, Scott L, Merrolees MJ, Skinner SJM (1994) Is Transforming growth factor-beta an autocrine growth factor for airway smooth muscle? Am J Resp Crit Care Med 149:A302 (abstract).

134. Amento EP, Ehsani N, Palmer H, Libby P (1991) Cytokines and growth factors positively and negatively regulate interstitial collagen synthesis gene expression in human vascular smooth muscle cells. Arteriosclerosis Thromb 11:1223–1230.

135. Brown JK, Tyler CL, Jones CA, Ruoss SJ, Hartmann T, Caughey GH (1995) Tryptase, the dominant secretory granular protein in human mast cells, is a potent mitogen for cultured dog tracheal smooth muscle cells. Am J Resp Cell Mol Biol 13:227–236.

136. Rennick RE, Connat J-L, Burnstock G, Rothery S, Severs NJ, Green CR (1993) Expression of connexin 43 gap junctions between cultured vascular smooth muscle cells is dependent upon phenotype. Cell Tissue Res 271:323–332.

137. Skalli O, Pelte MF, Peclet MC, Gabbiani G, Gugliotta P, Bussolati G, Ravazzola M, Orci L (1989) Alpha smooth muscle actin, a differentiation marker of smooth muscle cells, is present in microfilamentous boundles of pericytes. J Histochem Cytochem 37:315.

138. Shepro D, Morel NML (1993) Pericyte physiology. FASEB J 7:1031–1038.

139. Diaz-Flores L, Gutierrez R, Varela H, Rencel N, Valladares F (1991) Microvascular pericytes: a review of their morphological and functional characteristics. Histol Histopath 6:269–286.

140. Charan NB, Baile EM, Paré PD (1997) Bronchial vascular congestion and angiogenesis. Eur Respir J 10:1173–1180.

141. Hislop A, Reid L (1976) New findings in pulmonary arteries of rats with hypoxia-induced hypertension. Br J Exp Path 57:542–554.

142. Langlebeb D, Jones RC, Aronovitz MJ, Hill NS, Ou L-C, Reid LM (1987) Pulmonary artery structural changes in two colonies of rats with different sensitivity to chronic hypoxia. Am J Pathol 1128:61–66.

143. Meyrick B, Reid L (1978) The effect of continued hypoxia on rat pulmonary arterial circulation: an ultrastructural study. Lab Invest 38:188–192.

144. Sundberg C, Ivarsson M, Rubin K (1996) Pericytes as collagen-producing cells in excessive dermal scarring. Lab Invest 74:452–466.

145. Miller (1937).

146. Dunnill MS, Massarella GR, Anderson JA (1969) A comparison of the quantitative anatomy of the bronchi in normal subjects, in status asthmaticus, in chronic bronchitis, and in emphysema. Thorax 24:176–179.

147. Jeffery PK (1992) Pathology of asthma. Br Med Bull 48:23–39.

148. Heard BE, Hossain S (1973) Hyperplasia of bronchial muscle in asthma. J Pathol 110:319–331.

149. Ebina M, Takahashi T, Chiba T, Motomiya M (1993) Cellular hypertrophy and hyperplasia of airway smooth muscle underlying bronchial asthma. Am J Resp Crit Care Med 148:720–726.

150. Gabella G (1994) Anatomy of airways smooth muscle. In: Reaburn D, Giembycz MA, eds. Airways Smooth Muscle: Structure, Innervation and Neurotransmission. Birkhauser Verlag, Basel, pp. 1–27.

151. Daniel EE, Triggle DJ (1993) Structure and function of airway smooth muscle. In: Middleton E Jr, Busse WW, Ellis EF, Reed CR, Yunginger JW, eds. Allergy: Principles and Practice. Mosby Year Book Co., St. Louis, MO, pp. 629–649.

152. Janssen L, Daniel EE (1994) Myogenic control of airways smooth muscle and cell-to-cell coupling. In: Raeburn D, Giembycz MA, eds. Airways Smooth Muscle: Development, and Regulation of Contractility. Birkhauser Verlag, Basel, pp. 101–136.

153. Laitinen A, Laitinen LA, Moss R, Widdicombe JG (1989) Organisation and structure of the tracheal and bronchial blood vessels in the dog. J Anat 165:133–140.

154. Laitinen LA, Robinson NP, Laitinen A, Widdicombe JG (1986) Relationship between tracheal mucosal thickness and vascular resistance in dogs. J Appl Physiol 61:2186–2194.

155. Widdicombe J (1993) New perspectives on basic mechanisms in lung disease: 4. Why are the airways so vascular? Thorax 48:290–295.

156. Laitinen LA, Laitinen A (1992) The bronchial circulation: Histology and electron microscopy. In: Butler J, ed. The Bronchial Circulation. Dekker, New York, pp. 79–98.

157. Laitinen LA, Laitinen A, Widdicombe J (1987) Effects of inflammatory and other mediators on airway vascular beds. Am Rev Respir Dis 135:S67–S70.

158. Lundberg JM, Lundblad C, Martling C, Saria A, St. Jarne P, Anggard A (1987) Coexistence of multiple peptides and classic transmitters in airway neurons: functional and pathophysiologic aspects. Am Rev Respir Dis 136:S16–S22.

159. Lundblad L (1984) Protective reflexes and vascular beds in the nasal mucosa elicited by activation of capsaicin sensitive substance P immunoreactive trigeminal neurons. Acta Physiol Scand (Suppl)529:1–42.

160. Deffebach ME, Salonen RO, Webber SE, Widdicombe JG (1991) Cold and hyperosmolar fluids in canine trachea: vascular and smooth muscle tone and albumin flux. J Appl Physiol 71:50–59.

161. Salonen RO, Webber SE, Deffebach ME, Widdicombe JG (1991) Tracheal vascular and smooth muscle responses to air temperature and humidity in dogs. J Appl Physiol 71:50–59.

162. McFadden ERJ (1990) Hypothesis: exercise-induced asthma as a vascular phenomenon. Lancet, 335:880–883.

163. Cauna N (1982) Blood and nerve supply of the nasal lining. In: Proctor DE, Anderson ID, eds. The Nose: Upper Airway Physiology and the Atmospheric Environment. Elsevier Biomedical, Amsterdam, pp. 45–69.

164. McDonald DM (1990) The ultrastructure and permeability of tracheobronchial blood vessels in health and disease. Eur Respir J 3:572–855.

165. Cole P (1988) Nasal airflow resistance. In: Mathew OP, Sant'Ambrogio G, eds. Respiratory Function of the Upper Airway. Dekker, New York, pp. 391–414.

166. Baile EM, Sotres-Vega A, Pare PD (1994) Airway blood flow and bronchovascular congestion in sheep. Eur Respir J 7:1300–1307.

167. Schleimer RP, Benenati SV, Friedman B, Bochner BS (1991) Do cytokines play a role in leukocyte recruitment and activation in the lungs? Am Rev Respir Dis 143:1169–1174.

168. Schleimer, Sterbinsky, Saiser, Bickel, Klunk, Tomoika, Newman, Luscinskas, Gimbrone, McIntyre, Bochner, (1992) IL-4 induces adherence of human eosinophils and basophils but not neutrophils to endothelial cells. J Immunol 148:1048–1092.

169. Jeffery PK (1982) Bronchial mucosa and its innervation. In: Cumming G, Bonsignore G, eds. Cell Biology and the Lung Plenum, New York, pp. 1–32.

170. Shipperbottom CA (1988) Histochemical studies of the autonomic innervation of "normal" and diseased human lung. Thesis submitted to the University of London for MPhil degree.

171. Uddman R, Sundler F (1987) Neuropeptides in the airways. Am Rev Respir Dis 136:S3–S8.

172. Dusser DJ, Umeno E, Graf PD, Djokic T, Borson DB, Nadel JA (1988) Airway neutral endopeptidase-like enzyme modulates tachykinin-induced bronchoconstriction in vivo. J Appl Physiol 65:2585–2591.

173. Dusser DJ, Djokic TD, Borson DB, Nadel JA (1989) Cigarette smoke induces bronchoconstrictor hyperresponsiveness to substance P and inactivates airway neutral endopeptidase in the guinea pig lung. Possible role of free radicals. J Clin Invest 84:900–906.

174. Barnes PJ (1992) Modulation of neurotransmission in airways. Physiol Rev 72:699–729.

175. Jeffery PK, Reid L (1973) Intraepithelial nerves in normal rat airways: a quantitative electron microscopic study. J Anat 114:33–45.

176. Hung KS (1976) Fine structure of tracheobronchial epithelial nerves of the cat. Anat Rec 185:85–91.

177. Das RM, Jeffery PK, Widdicombe JG (1978) The epithelial innervation of the lower respiratory tract of the cat. J Anat 126:123–131.

178. Fillenz M, Woods MJ (1970) Sensory innervation of airways. In: Porter R, ed. Breathing: Hering-Breuer Centenary Symposium. Ciba Foundation Symp., Amsterdam, pp. 101–109.

179. Boucher RC, Johnson J, Inoue S, Hulbert W, Hogg JC (1980) The effect of cigarette smoking on the permeability of guinea pig airways. Lab Invest 43:94–100.

180. Cook RD, King RS (1969) A neurite-receptor complex in the avian lung: electron microscopical observations. Experientia 25:1162–1164.

181. Cook RD, King RS (1969) Nerves of the avian lung: electron microscopy. J Anat 105:202–203.

182. King AS, McLelland J, Cook RD, King DZ, Walsh C (1974) The ultrastructure of afferent nerve endings in the avian lung. Resp Physiol 22:21–40.

183. Walsh C, McLelland J (1974) The ultrastructure of the avian extrapulmonary respiratory epithelium. Acta Anat 89:412–422.

184. Phipps RJ, Richardson PS, Corfield A, Gallagher JT, Jeffery PK, Kent PW, Passatore M (1977) A physiological biochemical and histological study of goose tracheal mucin and its secretion. Phil Trans Roy Soc (Lond) B, 279:513–543.

185. Rhodin J (1966) The ciliated cells. Ultrastructure and function of the human tracheal mucosa. Am Rev Respir Dis 93:1–15.

186. Lauweryns JM, Peuskens JC, Cokelaere M (1970) Argyrophil, fluorescent and granulated (peptide and amine producing?) AFG cells in human infant bronchial mucosa. Light and electron microscopic studies. Life Sci 9:1417–1429.

187. Laitinen A (1985) Ultrastructural organization of intraepithelial nerves in the human airway tract. Thorax 40:488–492.
188. Hulbert WC, Walker DC, Jackson A, Hogg JC (1981) Airway permeability to horseradish peroxidase in guinea pigs: the repair phase after injury by cigarette smoke. Am Rev Respir Dis 123:320–326.
189. McDonald DM (1987) Neurogenic inflammation in the respiratory tract: actions of sensory nerve mediators on blood vessels and epithelium of the airway mucosa. Am Rev Respir Dis 136:S65–S71.
190. McDonald DM (1988) Neurogenic inflammation in the rat trachea I. Changes in venules, leucocytes and epithelial cells. J Neurocytol 17:583–603.
191. Richardson JB, Ferguson CC (1979) Neuromuscular structure and function in the airways. Fed Proc 38:202–208.

15 Epithelium

Mary H. Perdue, PHD and Derek M. McKay, PHD

CONTENTS

INTRODUCTION

The epithelium is the critical cell layer at mucosal surfaces since it forms the boundary between the external environment and the body proper. This cell layer plays a major role in host defense since it serves as a barrier and secretes fluid, mucus, and antibodies that contribute to the elimination of antigens from the body. Over the past 15 y, many experimental studies have been published that provide insights into the role of epithelial cells in allergic diseases. It is now recognized that the functions of epithelia are regulated by nerves and altered by immune cell mediators and cytokines. New evidence suggests that stress increases epithelial permeability. Enhanced transepithelial uptake of antigens, infectious agents, and toxins may stimulate allergic reactions and/or inflammatory responses that cause epithelial injury.

Besides being a passive bystander in inflammatory reactions, it is now clear that the epithelium actively participates in immune responses and contributes to both innate and specific immunity. Epithelial cells can synthesize and release a variety of messenger molecules such as lipid metabolites, nitric oxide, proteolytic enzymes, and cytokines. These molecules provide protection against foreign invasion, signal the recruitment of immune/inflammatory cells, or modulate the effect of extracellular signals. Recent reports indicate that epithelial cells have the ability to process and present antigens to T-cells, stimulating their proliferation.

This chapter will provide an overview of the experimental evidence that illustrates the key roles of airway and intestinal epithelium in allergic disease. General epithelial functions will be described, and, where appropriate, specializations of epithelia in specific locations will be indicated.

STRUCTURAL CONSIDERATIONS

The epithelium has a strategic location in both the respiratory and gastrointestinal (GI) tracts, covering the mucosal surface. It may be a single cell thick, as in the gut, or pseudostratified (appearance of multicellular layer, with columnar cells bordering on the basement

From: *Allergy and Allergic Diseases: The New Mechanisms and Therapeutics*
Edited by: J. A. Denburg © Humana Press Inc., Totowa, NJ

membrane or on basal cells, some of which do not extend to the lumen), as in the airways. Epithelial cells are bound together at their apical borders by tight junctions, structures that connect membranes of adjacent cells. Tight junctions (zona occludens) are selectively permeable to ions and allow the passage of small molecules, but restrict the movement of macromolecules such as protein antigens, microbes, etc. *(1)*. Several proteins have been localized to the tight-junction region, such as cingulin, occludin, and zona occuldens 1 (ZO-1). Immunocytochemical staining for ZO-1 has been used to outline epithelial cells and demonstrate breaks that occur, for example, during infection *(2)*. Only recently has it become apparent that the permeability of tight junctions is regulated by neuro-immune factors, a finding that has important implications for normal physiology and the pathophysiology of allergic disease. Epithelial cells are also joined to each other by adhering junctions (zona adherens) and desmosomes (macula adherens). Desmosomes join columnar cells to basal cells; hemidesmosomes attach cells to the basal lamina. Gap junctions are also present and allow ions and intracellular messenger molecules to pass from cell to cell, a function that may be necessary for synchronization of cilia beating on airways epithelium.

Columnar Cells

The main cell type of the epithelial layer is the columnar cell (enterocyte in the gut, ciliated cell in the airways), which has properties of active transport for ions (and nutrients in the gut) against a concentration gradient and therefore plays a key role in regulation of water transport. This cell also secretes the mucosal antibody, secretory immunoglobulin A (IgA), via binding to its receptor (secretory component, SC) located in the basolateral cell membrane *(3,4)*. This complex of immunoglobulin (Ig) and SC is then transported across the cell and into the lumen, where it serves to inhibit antigen uptake. Columnar cells also express a low-affinity receptor for IgE *(5)* and therefore presumably can react directly to antigens, although such reactions have not yet been demonstrated. However, the expression of this receptor is enhanced in asthma *(6)* and food allergies *(5)*. Columnar epithelial cells have certain specializations depending on their location. In the GI tract, the apical membrane of the enterocyte contains numerous finger-like projections, or microvilli, that give the appearance of a brush border; this feature greatly increases the surface area available for absorption. In the airways, the apical membrane contains 200–300 cilia per cell that beat at ~1000 beats/min; this function is essential for mucociliary clearance.

Secretory Cells

Mucus-secreting goblet cells are prominent in epithelia at mucosal surfaces and play an important role in host defense, since mucus traps particles and antigens (in part by complexing with secreted antibodies) that are then removed by peristalsis or ciliated action. The amount of water in the mucus layer is critical, as demonstrated in cystic fibrosis, where disregulation of the cyclic adenosine monophosphate (cAMP)-regulated chloride channel by a mutated protein (the cystic fibrosis transmembrane regulator [CFTR]) results in less chloride, and therefore water, being secreted *(7)*. The consequence of this defect is a thick sticky mucus that cannot be propelled normally, resulting in persistent airway infection and intestinal dysfunction. Also interspersed in epithelia are cells that secrete peptide or amine mediators with paracrine or hormonal actions. These cells are referred to as dense core granulated (DCG) cells in the airways or enteroendocrine (EC) cells in the gut. These cells are closely associated with nerve fibers, and their secretory activity is regulated by nerves.

Specialized Cells

In addition to cells that are common in both epithelia, specialized cells are present in the respiratory and GI tracts. In the airways, these include the basal cells, thought to be progenitor and anchoring cells for columnar cells, serous cells that line serous glands, and Clara cells that produce surfactant or a hypophase component of surfactant. In the gut, the crypts of intestinal glands contain the progenitor cells and Paneth cells that secrete lysozyme and other antimicrobial proteins, called defensins *(8)*. In the lung, epithelial-derived molecules with antimicrobial actions include lysozyme, lactoferrin, and peroxidases, although the precise cells secreting these molecules have not been identified. Another difference in airways versus intestine is the presence of nerve profiles in airway epithelium *(9,10)*, which are almost never observed above the basement membrane in the gut. There is now evidence that epithelial cells can express messenger ribonucleic acid (mRNA) for nerve growth factor (NGF) *(11)*, a trophic factor necessary for nerve maintenance and neurite outgrowth, although the implication of this finding in terms of nerve extension into epithelia is not yet clear. However, NGF appears to be responsible for nerve remodeling and phenotypic changes in neurotransmitter content that occur during inflammation.

Immune Cells

Cells with immune properties are present within the epithelia. The most common of these are intraepithelial lymphocytes (IEL), which are located below the tight junctions of columnar cells. Compared with other lymphocytes, IEL have unique markers (including the $\gamma\delta$ T-cell receptor) and are relatively unreactive *(12,13)*. Other cells with immune/inflammatory properties (mast cells, neutrophils, macrophages) may also be present depending on the state of immune activation or sensitization of the individual. Dendritic cells have been identified below and within epithelia in both the lung and gut *(14,15)*. These cells with their long processes play a key role in antigen sampling and presentation *(16)*. Traffic of immune cells to specific locations in the mucosae or epithelium occurs during inflammation and is related to the expression of adhesion molecules on endothelial and epithelial cells *(17,18)*. In addition to adhesion factors (e.g., E-cadherin) expressed by epithelial cells, other epithelial molecules (interleukin [IL]-8, leucotriene B4 [LTB$_4$], etc.) may be responsible for localization of immune cells within the epithelium.

MODEL SYSTEMS

Animal Models of Hypersensitivity

Animal models have provided important information on the role of the epithelium in allergy. Typically, rodents or guinea pigs are sensitized to a protein by intraperitoneal or subcutaneous injection. Alternate sensitization strategies have used intraluminal (nasal/gut) or aerosol (lung) administration. Adjuvants may be injected simultaneously to promote IgE antibody production, the most common adjuvants being pertussis vaccine (or its active component, pertussis toxin) and/or alum. Guinea pigs can be sensitized to milk proteins by feeding cow's milk *(19)*. Animals such as dogs, sheep, and primates previously infected with *Ascaris suum* parasites respond to ascaris antigen challenge with symptoms of immediate hypersensitivity. Infection with nematode parasites in general (*Nippostrongylus brasiliensis* or *Trichinella spiralis*) results in sensitization. In such model systems, epithelial responses to antigen challenge have been demonstrated in response to local challenge in the airways or GI tract. In vivo experiments and Using chamber studies of ex vivo tissues from sensitized animals have provided considerable information on antigen-induced changes in epithelial physiology.

Culture Models

Epithelial cell lines and short-term cultures of primary isolates of epithelial cells have enabled investigators to examine the direct effects of neuro-immune mediators on epithelial

Table 1
Direct Effects of Cytokines on Epithelia[a]

Target function	Cytokine effector	Outcome
Chloride secretion	IL-4, IFN-γ, TNF-α	$\Downarrow$
	IL-1, IL-3	$\Uparrow$
Mucin secretion	IL-1β, IL-6, IFN-γ, TNF-α	$\Uparrow$
Cytokine production	IL-1, IL-1β, IL-2, IL-6, IFN-γ,	
	TNF-α, TGF-β	$\Uparrow$
ICAM-1 expression	IL-1β, IL-4, IFN-γ, TNF-α	$\Uparrow$
MHC II expression	IFN-γ, TNF-α	$\Uparrow$
	TGF-β_2	$\Downarrow$
Neutrophil chemotaxis, attachment	IL-1β, IL-8, IFN-γ, TNF-α	$\Uparrow$
Monocyte chemotaxis	MCP-1, RANTES	$\Uparrow$
Secretory component expression	IFN-γ	$\Uparrow$
Barrier function	IL-4, IFN-γ, TNF-α, HSF, IGF	$\Downarrow$
	TGF-β_2	$\Uparrow$
NO induction	IL-1β, IFN-γ, TNF-α	$\Uparrow$
Glutamine absorption	IFN-γ	$\Downarrow$
Cytostatic/cytotoxic effects	IFN-γ, TNF-α	$\Uparrow$

[a]Summary of studies employing intestinal or airways cell lines, isolated epithelial cells, or tissue segments. HSF, hepatocyte stimulating factor; IGF, insulin-like growth factor; NO, nitric oxide.

cells. Numerous neuro-immune mediators (cytokines, lipid metabolites, reactive oxygen species, nitric oxide, neuropeptides) have been shown to alter many aspects of epithelial function. The effects of cytokines are summarized in Table 1. In addition, investigations of pathogenic (toxin-producing, invasive and noninvasive) and commensal bacteria, bacterial products (lipopolysaccharide [LPS], toxins), and other microbes on epithelial permeability and secretion have utilized epithelial cell lines. Information from coculture studies of immune cells with epithelial monolayers has significantly expanded our understanding of the potential of various populations of immune cells alone or in combination to change epithelial-cell physiology. A synopsis of data from coculture studies is provided in a later Section.

FUNCTIONAL CONSIDERATIONS

In Vivo Studies

ION SECRETION

Antigen-induced secretions (ions, water, mucus, glandular secretions) that originate from the epithelium are commonly documented in allergy. For example, allergic rhinitis is associated with hypersecretion of fluid, and allergic reactions to food may result in diarrhea. Studies of the content, magnitude, and timing of the secretory response, particularly in animal models, has provided valuable insights into the mechanism of immediate hypersensitivity. The greatest detail is available on the intestinal response, however, similar changes have been documented in nasal and tracheal epithelium. Because mucus secretion is covered in another chapter, we will concentrate on changes in ion transport, particularly those responses that occur in immediate hypersensitivity.

Our early studies of the intestinal reaction showed that rats sensitized to ovalbumin (OVA) respond 2 wk later to in vivo intraluminal antigen challenge with reduced net absorption of ions

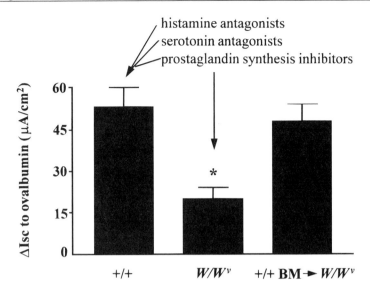

Fig. 1. Bar graph showing the change in secretory response (i.e., Isc) evoked by OVA challenge of Ussing-chambered segments of small intestine from sensitized normal mice (+/+), mast cell deficient mice (W/W^v), and W/W^v mice reconstituted with mast cells following transfer of bone-marrow precursors cells from +/+ littermates. The antigen response in normal mice was inhibited by histamine and serotonin antagonists and by inhibition of PG synthesis. Only PG inhibition reduced the secretory response in mast cell deficient mice (*, $p < 0.05$ compared to +/+; $n = 6$–12 mice).

and water *(20)*. This malabsorption was associated with secretion of histamine and evidence of mast cell activation. Isolated segments of small intestine studied in Ussing chambers indicated that active Cl⁻ secretion was the driving force for water secretion *(21)*. The secretory response (indicated by increased short-circuit current, Isc) began within minutes of adding antigen to the luminal surface of intestinal tissues from rodents sensitized to OVA *(22)*. Nerve blockade or depletion of sensory neuropeptides by capsaicin significantly reduced the Isc response in both rat gut and trachea *(22,23)*. Studies in genetic mutant mice *(24)* provided direct evidence for the role of mast cells as key effector cells in this model, since secretory responses were reduced to >30% in sensitized W/W^v (mast cell-deficient) mice compared to their congenic +/+ controls. In addition, responses were normalized in W/W^v mice that had their mast cell populations restored by adoptive transfer of bone marrow from normal mice (Fig. 1). We found that antigen-induced secretion was inhibited by antihistamines, serotonin antagonists, and neural blockade, but only in tissues from +/+ controls and not in tissues from W/W^v mice, suggesting that mast cell–nerve interactions regulated epithelial ion secretion. On the other hand, blockade of cyclooxygenase activity resulted in decreased responses in both types of mice. These studies implicated mast-cell products and neurotransmitters as the main mediators in the acute secretory response to antigen, with a small component from other cells and mediators.

Similar findings of antigen-induced altered ion transport have been described in the intestine and tracheal/bronchial epithelium from sensitized rodents or guinea pigs *(23,25–30)* (the mechanisms of water and mucus transport in the airways have recently been reviewed *(31,32)*). An additional feature of histamine release from mast cells in the respiratory tract can be the induction of the production of lymphocyte chemoattractant factor (LCF) by the epithelium and the subsequent recruitment of T-cells *(33)*. In human nasal epithelium, potential-difference changes were measured in response to pollen antigens in and out of season *(34)*, the abnormalities correlated with symptoms of rhinitis and were modified by inhibitors of activation of mast cells or their antagonists and/or nerve blockade or antagonism. Alterations in transport of both Na$^+$ and Cl$^-$ have been described *(35,36)*.

One important finding from such studies is the long-lived nature of the response. Pertussis toxin has been identified as the active ingredient in the pertussis vaccine adjuvant used to sensitized animals to various antigens *(37)*. Recombinant wild-type pertussis toxin injected into rats in nanogram quantities with OVA resulted in sensitization that lasted at least 8 mo, measured by antigen-induced changes in the electrophysiology of gut tissues; however, sensitization was short-lived (lasting only days) in rats injected with OVA alone *(38)*. Also, enzymatically inactive mutant pertussis toxin (owing to substitution of two amino acids) had no adjuvant effect in stimulating intestinal hypersensitivity. Pertussis toxin/OVA treatment also resulted in mast-cell hyperplasia and increased responsiveness to nerve stimulation, as well as the expected stimulation of IgE synthesis. Blood levels of IgE in individual animals did not correlate well with the magnitude of their secretory responses *(38)*. This is not surprising since it is known that circulating antibodies do not reflect IgE bound to tissue mast cells. In fact, the Sprague Dawley rats used in those studies are not "high-responder" rats in terms of IgE production compared, with other strains such as brown Norway rats *(37)*. This finding confirms that allergic reactions can occur in individuals with even relatively low reaginic antibody titres and indicates that circulating IgE is not necessarily a good indicator of sensitization. Other microbial products can act as adjuvants in hypersensitivity, including toxins from various bacteria (*Escherichia coli, Vibrio cholerae,* etc.) *(39,40)* and secreted products from nematode parasites (*Ascaris suum, Nippostrongylis brasiliensis, Trichinella spiralis*) *(41,42)*.

BARRIER FUNCTION

The epithelium barrier restricts the uptake of inhaled/ingested particles, microbes, and soluble antigens from the lumen. It is recognized that epithelial-cell injury/loss can occur during severe infections or as a result of immune reactions or the inflammatory response *(43–45)*. In this situation, host protection is diminished and normal physiology is altered. In addition, more subtle changes can occur that impair epithelial barrier function, often with no apparent morphological damage *(46)*. There is evidence that such changes play a role in allergy and may be present in sensitized individuals both before as well as after antigen challenge *(47)*. The fact that allergic reactions are manifested within minutes implies that intact macromolecular antigens can rapidly cross the epithelium to reach effector cells located below the tight junctions or in the subepithelial compartment.

Under normal circumstances, macromolecules are thought to be able to cross the epithelium at several sites. Particulate antigens and microbes are "sampled" by microfold M-cells that are located over lymphoid aggregates such as Peyer's patches in the gut, and are released intact into the lymphoid dome *(48–50)*. Once in the dome, antigens are taken up by professional antigen-presenting cells such as macrophages and are presented to T-cells to initiate the immune response. Although areas of epithelial-cell extrusion (such as the tips of intestinal villi) are thought to be additional sites of antigen uptake, no firm evidence has emerged to substantiate this hypothesis. Columnar epithelial cells themselves can transport soluble protein antigens, including those that bind to receptors and those that are taken up as a bystander effect of membrane recycling. Uptake occurs via endosomes that then coalesce with lysosomes; subsequently, most of the protein is degraded within these organelles *(51)*. However, some intact protein escapes degradation and is released intact into the mucosa, where it can activate local effector cells and/or enter the circulation. Endosomal transfer of intact antigen across normal epithelium takes at least 20 min. Tight junctions are thought to be impermeable to macromolecules *(1)*.

Extravasation is a common consequence of an allergic response resulting from increased endothelial permeability *(52,53)*. Less recognized is the alteration of epithelial permeability induced by antigen. It has clearly been shown in both the gut and lung that sloughing of epithelial cells occurs during severe anaphylactic reactions and in asthma *(44,54,55)*. In the rat, recent evidence suggests that the effect can be due to rat mast cell protease II (RCMP II) acting on elements of the basement membrane to release the cells *(56)*. Such major damage would certainly impair the epithelial barrier function. Similar effects have been described in asthma, for which mast cell proteases, eosinophil major basic protein or cationic protein, or neutrophil elastase may be responsible *(43,57–59)*. Also, mast cell-derived chymase has been found to cleave the glycocalyx of airways epithelial cells *(60)*, and both protective (sloughing of adhered micoorganisms) and pathological (formation of viscous hydrated gels) consequences have been postulated for this event. However, there are indications that permeability changes can occur without evidence of gross morphological injury and that antigen uptake can be regulated by neuro-immune factors. Furthermore, it has recently been reported that patients with bronchial asthma also display increased intestinal epithelial permeability, leading the authors to speculate that this disorder causes a general defect in the entire mucosal system *(61)*.

Recently, a number of groups have reported that transepithelial antigen uptake is regulated by nerves *(62–64)*, although debate has ensued over whether neural regulation is related to intracellular or paracellular transport, or both. In addition, it is not clear whether sensitization alters the rate or route of antigen uptake. We previously showed that intestinal epithelial permeability to the inert probe ^{51}Cr-ethylenediame tetra-acetic acid (EDTA) was ~50% greater in sensitized versus control rats and increased 20-fold when these rats were challenged with intraluminal antigen *(62)*. Neural blockade inhibited this dramatic rise and also inhibited uptake of the antigen itself. Other studies have suggested that both capsaicin treatment and atropine can inhibit epithelial permeability and transepithelial protein transport *(22,65,66)*, suggesting the involvement of neuropeptide (e.g., substance P) and cholinergic nerves in the regulation of this epithelial function. Recent preliminary reports indicate that neuropeptides such as neuropeptide Y can play an inhibitory role in allergic reactions *(67)*.

Studies to address the question of the route of transepithelial antigen transport have used electron microscopy to trace the uptake pathway of various proteins in normal and sensitized animals. Horseradish peroxidase (HRP) has been used as a model protein since its reaction product can be identified at the ultrastructural level; other groups have used immunogold-labelled proteins such as OVA. In our recent studies, we found that the rate of transport of HRP-containing endosomes across columnar epithelial cells was accelerated in sensitized rats *(68)*. In fact, in rats sensitized to HRP, the protein was visualized in the subepithelial space within 2 min after its addition to the luminal surface of intestine mounted in Ussing chambers. In contrast, in intestine from naive rats studied at 2 min, HRP was localized within endosomes only in the apical region of epithelial cells. The mechanism responsible for this enhanced antigen uptake is not clear. However, histamine and methacholine were shown to increase transepithelial transport of HPR across guinea pig tracheal epithelium *(69)*.

In concluding this section on epithelial barrier function, we would draw attention to the elegant studies by Persson and colleagues, who have developed an in vivo model to examine epithelial shedding and restitution (reviewed in ref. *70*). Following epithelial denudation in the guinea-pig trachea that does not damage the basement membrane or cause vascular damage, these workers have observed that the ciliated epithelium immediately lose their cilia and that goblet cells discharge their mucus. This is followed by flattening of the epithelial cells and migration to seal the "wound." The development of a new tight epithelium preceeds the proliferation of fibroblasts and the appearance of peptidergic nerve profiles in the epithelium. These researchers have also shown that the denudation–restitution process can be accompanied by plasma exudation and secretion, transepithelial migration of eosinophils into the lumen, and recruitment of neutrophils.

ROLE OF PSYCHOLOGICAL FACTORS ON THE EPITHELIUM

Several studies have shown that stress affects the epithelium. Gastric ulceration is the most obvious example of epithelial damage induced by cold restraint or water stress *(71)*. Johnson *(72)* showed that stress-induced activity of ornithine decarboxylase was involved in gastric epithelial injury. Convincing evidence also exists for the involvement of neuro-immune factors in stress-induced epithelial damage. Neural inhibition or antagonism of various transmitters inhibits stress-induced ulceration *(71,73)*. A role for mast cells has not been examined in stress ulcers, although mast cells have been shown to be important in ulceration following administration of noxious substances such as ethanol *(74)*. Pavlovian conditioning of mast-cell activation has been demonstrated in sensitized rats *(75)* and in humans with allergic rhinitis *(76)*. Emotions have also been implicated in symptom exacerbation in asthma *(77)*.

In addition, subtle changes in epithelial function that occur without obvious morphological abnormalities have been reported as a consequence of stress. Alterations in fluid and electrolyte absorption in humans and rats have been described *(78,79)*. We examined parameters of epithelial ion transport and permeability in intestinal mucosa from rats stressed by restraint ± cold and compared results with those in controls. We found that stress profoundly affected both functions, stimulating ion secretion and impairing the barrier function of the epithelium *(46)*. Importantly, stress increased protein flux across the epithelium and resulted in a larger number of HRP-containing endosomes within epithelial cells *(66)*. HRP was also visualized penetrating through epithelial tight junctions in jejunum from stressed rats. Our results suggest that stress, via the central nervous system and the release of acetylcholine, can cause epithelial dysfunction and enhance uptake of macromolecules. Stress may increase epithelial permeability, facilitating passage of protein antigens, including food antigens, microbial toxins/products, from the gut lumen that may lead to an immune/inflammatory response. Antigen-induced mast-cell activation with the release of mediators (e.g., histamine, prostaglandins, and cytokines) may further increase epithelial permeability and enhance pathophysiology. Exacerbation of symptoms in allergy and asthma may be related to stress-enhanced release of acetylcholine and neuropeptides that can induce priming of effector cells, lowering their threshold for allergic responses *(80)*.

Coculture Studies

Within the context of dynamic multifunctional tissues, where numerous intercellular signaling events occur, it is difficult to precisely assign a role to a particular cell type in any physiological or pathological reaction. A number of investigators have adopted a reductionistic strategy in which epithelial cells are cocultured with defined immune or stromal cell populations and the ability of the latter cell type to regulate epithelial physiology either tonically or following activation is determined (summarized in Table 2).

Employing a novel "sandwich" coculture model composed of confluent monolayers of the HCA-7 epithelial cell line and peritoneal cells (~14% mast cells) from rats sensitized to OVA, Baird et al. *(81)* showed that antigen challenge led to a transient increase in epithelial ion secretion. This antigen-evoked secretion did not occur in the absence of the peritoneal cells and was inhibited by the H_1 antagonist mepyramine, illustrating that the secretory response was histamine mediated. Studies conducted with the human colonic T84 epithelial cell line and fibroblasts have shown that fibroblasts can enhance the epithelial secretory responses to exogenous histamine, serotonin, bradykinin, and hydrogen peroxide via generation of prostaglandin E2, (PGE_2) *(82)*. In addition, fibroblast-derived growth factors increased epithelial (rat IEC-6 cell line and human HT-29 and Caco-2 cell lines) proliferation rates and enhanced epithelial restitution in vitro following injury by a transforming growth factor (TGF)-β dependent mechanism *(83)*. Conditioned media from cultures of fibroblasts isolated from patients with idiopathic

Table 2
Summary of Coculture Studies Showing Immune-Mediated Alteration of Epithelial Function

Immune cell	Immune stimulus	Epithelial cell type	Altered epithelial function
Mast cells	Antigen	HCA-7 Human colonocytes	Vectorial ion secretion
Neutrophils	IFN-γ	T84 Human colonocytes	fMLP-Induced neutrophil transmigration; decreased transepithelial resistance (TER)
	LPS/fMLP or PMA	T84 Cells	5′-AMP-Induced Cl$^-$ secretion
Eosinophils	GM-CSF	T84 Cells	PAF-Induced eosinophil transmigration
	GM-CSF or PMA	T84 Cells	5′-AMP-Induced Cl$^-$ secretion
Monocytes/macrophages	LPS	Isolates of rat distal lung	Decrease in TER and Na$^+$ transport; altered F-actin
	LPs/fMLP	T84 Cells	Decrease in TER and cAMP-elicited Cl$^-$ secretion; increased baseline Cl$^-$ secretion
T-cells	Coal dust	Rat type II pneumocytes	Increased synthesis of extracellular matrix
PBMC	Anti-CD3	T84 Cells	Decrease in TER, cAMP- and Ca$^+$-elicited Cl$^-$ secretion;
			Rearrangement and reduction in F-actin; increased permeability to probe molecules
	Cow's-milk protein	HT-29 Human colonocytes	Reduced barrier function
Mucosal-like T-cell	—	T84 Cells	Decrease in TER, cAMP- and Ca$^+$-elicited Cl$^-$ secretion

pulmonary fibrosis or rats treated with 75% O_2 and paraquat stimulated apoptosis and necrosis in the A549 human alveolar type II epithelial cell line and in rat alveolar cells *(84)*.

Neutrophil infiltration is one of the defining features of inflammation. In the gut, these cells can cross the epithelium and form crypt abscesses. Neutrophils derived from human blood were induced to cross T84 monolayers in response to chemotactic substances, such as the bacterial tripeptide f-Met-Leu-Phe (fMLP), placed on the luminal side of the epithelium *(85)*. Concomitant with the neutrophil translocation event there was a transient increase in epithelial permeability. This decreased barrier function appeared to be a consequence of the mechanical force generated by the neutrophils as they squeezed through the epithelial tight junctions and not to result from cytotoxic or degradative events caused by neutrophil release of proteases or reactive oxygen metabolites. This translocation event was enhanced by addition of interferon-γ (IFN-γ) *(86)*. Once in the gut lumen, the neutrophils caused epithelial Cl$^-$ secretion via the release of adenosine 5^1-monophosphate (5′-AMP) *(87)*. Therefore, these cells are likely to contribute to diarrhea.

Eosinophils also migrate into the intestinal lumen in a number of enteropathies, including parasitic infections, acute radiation enteritis, and eosinophilic proctocolitis. Similarly, eosinophil migration into the bronchial lumen plays a major role in allergic asthma pathophysiologic reactions. Coculture studies with eosinophils isolated from the blood of mildly atopic, but otherwise normal, individuals and T84 monolayers revealed that eosinophils exposed to granulocyte-macrophage colony-stimulating factor (GM-CSF) crossed the epithelium in response to platelet-activating factor (PAF), but not fMLP or the complement fragment C5a *(88)*. This epithelial transmigration event was accompanied by an increase in epithelial permeability and could be inhibited with monoclonal antibodies (MAbs) to CD11b, but not CD11a, very late activation antigen-4 (VLA-4), or intercellular adhesion molecule-1 (ICAM-1).

Macrophages are a major source of inflammatory mediators and are a key component in respiratory inflammatory problems such as asthma and in inflammatory bowel disease. Pseudopodia extensions from macrophages have been identified in the villus epithelial compartment of the guinea pig small intestine. Rat alveolar cells, a human bronchial epithelial cell line (BEAS-2B), and intestinal epithelial cells have been shown to synthesize RANTES and/or monocyte chemoattractant peptide 1 (MCP-1) *(89–91)*. This ability to recruit monocytes/macrophages implies a functional relationship. Yet few studies have examined the direct consequences of monocyte activation on epithelial physiology. Our recent studies demonstrated that coculture of fMLP+LPS-activated monocytes with T84 epithelial monolayers resulted in a significant increase in epithelial ion secretion and permeability (increased transepithelial flux of ^{51}Cr-EDTA) *(92)*. Subsequent investigation revealed that the increased baseline Isc resulted from active Cl$^-$ secretion and that the monocyte-induced epithelial abnormalities resulted, at least in part, from tumor necrosis factor α (TNF-α). These findings are complemented by the observation that LPS-activated macrophages from rat lung lavages decreased the barrier function of primary cultures of rat lung epithelium *(93)*. Coculture with activated monocytes also led to a drop in Isc, which resulted from a reduced capacity to vectorially transport Na$^+$. The authors present data to illustrate that the epithelial pathophysiology in this coculture model was L-arginine-dependent and therefore resulted from nitric oxide. Also, rat type II pulmonary epithelial cells showed increased deposition of extracellular-matrix (ECM) proteins when cocultured with alveolar macrophages and coal dust *(94)*. These findings were not reproduced by conditioned media from macrophage cultures, suggesting that macrophage-epithelial contact was required for this event or, if the enhanced ECM deposition resulted from a soluble mediator, that this mediator had a short half-life.

Regulation of T-cell activity is an essential element of the control of mucosal immune reactions. Studies in the early 1970s implicated T-cells in the change in villus-crypt architecture following allograft rejection or parasitic infection *(95)*. These and other studies with human fetal intestinal explants *(96)* and athymic rats *(97)* support the hypothesis that T-cells can influence epithelial function. Using peripheral-blood mononuclear cells (PBMC) cocultured with T84 cells, we have defined one pathway of T-cell-initiated epithelial dysfunction *(98)*. Following coculture with PBMC in which the T-cells (~75% of population) were activated by anti-CD3, epithelia displayed decreased barrier function and diminished secretory responses to the Ca^{2+} and cAMP chloride secretagogues carbachol and forskolin, respectively (Fig. 2). These abnormalities were associated with rearrangement of the epithelial cell F-actin and occurred in the absence of major cytotoxic effects. These alterations in epithelial function were mimicked by addition of conditioned media from anti-CD3-activated PBMC cultures. The strategic use of neutralizing antibodies to IFN-γ and TNF-α revealed that these changes in epithelial function were evoked by activated T-cells releasing IFN-γ, which in turn caused monocyte TNF-α production. In support of these findings, PBMC from cow's-milk allergic infants released significant amounts of TNF-α in response to cow's-milk protein and, when cocultured with monolayers of the human colonic HT-29 cell line, led to TNF-α-dependent increased epithelial permeability *(99)*. Also, cells of mucosal-like T-cell line, when cocultured with T84 cells, took up a basolateral, intraepithelial IEL-like position *(100)*. These cocultured epithelial monolayers showed decreased transepithelial resistance and diminished secretory responses to carbachol, forskolin, and vasoactive intestinal peptide, compared to naive T84 monolayers.

The above studies illustrate the value of a coculture approach to obtain specific data pertinent to our understanding of the regulation of epithelial function by immune activation. However, it would be remiss of us not to point out that many of these studies were conducted with epithelial cell lines that may not exactly mirror the function of their normal counterparts in vivo. Maximum advantage of this in vitro approach is achieved when such studies are integrated with data from animal models and clinical observations. To this end, we have presented preliminary data showing that anti-CD3-treated mice develop intestinal ion transport abnormalities reminiscent of those observed in the T84-PBMC coculture model *(101)*.

THE "ACTIVATED" EPITHELIUM

Thus far we have focused on the epithelium as a barrier and secretory cell layer that is passive in mucosal immune reactions, responding to neuro-immune mediators generated in the mucosa. However, evidence is accumulating that the epithelial cell can act as a sentinel to inform cells in the mucosa of events in the lumen and can actively participate in inflammatory/allergic reactions. Review of the literature on epithelial immunobiology is beyond the scope of this chapter, rather, we will briefly define the role that an "activated" epithelium can play in the regulation of immune activity by highlighting selected studies.

Cytokine and Mediator Production

Epithelial cells, irrespective of their site of origin (intestinal, airways, urogenital), are a significant source of cytokines (Table 3) *(102,103)*. For instance, airways epithelium produce chemokines *(89,91,104)*, growth factors *(104)*, and pleitrophic lymphokines and therefore are capable of attracting immune cells, prolonging their survival, and directing their function *(102)*. Epithelial cell lines or freshly isolated epithelial cells produce cytokines in response to a diverse variety of stimuli that can be derived from the lumen or the mucosa: inflammatory cytokines such as TNF-α; bacterial products such as LPS and cholera toxin; and infectious agents such as bacteria (*Salmonella dublin, Escherichia coli, Helicobacter pylori, Pseudomona aeruginosa*), protozoa (*Entamoeba histolytia*), and viruses (respiratory syncytial virus) *(105–107)*.

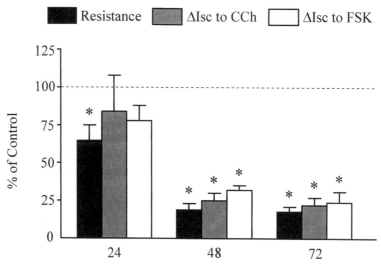

Co-culture of T84 monolayers with anti-CD3 activated
peripheral blood mononuclear cells (hours)

Fig. 2. Bar graph showing the reduction in epithelial (T84 monolayers) barrier function (resistance) and secretory function (changes in Isc evoked by serosally applied carbachol [CCh, 10^{-4} M, cholinergic agonist] and forskolin [FSK, 10^{-5} M, activates adenylate cyclase]) following coculture with PBMC (10^6) from healthy humans in which the T-cells had been specifically activated through the T-cell receptor/CD3 complex (data are presented as change in response relative to nontreated, time-matched naive monolayers; *, $p < 0.05$ compared to control; $n = 8$–12).

Epithelial-derived cytokines are bioactive. For instance, epithelial-derived interleukin-8 (IL-8) is chemotactic for neutrophils and increases their adhesion to HT-29 enterocytes via ICAM-1 and CD18 *(108)*. Recently, it was reported that mast-cell tryptase added to HT-29 cells caused an increase in their proliferation rate, IL-8 synthesis, and ICAM-1 expression *(109)*. Furthermore, TNF-α-stimulated A549 pulmonary epithelial cells were found to facilitate neutrophil chemotaxis via the release of IL-8 *(110)*. This communication is not unidirectional since neutrophil-derived elastase has been shown to evoke epithelial IL-8 synthesis *(111)*. Eosinophils also produce elastase, and a recent study has shown that these important inflammatory cells can be induced to degranulate in the presence of bronchial epithelial cells (BEAS-2B cells) *(112)*. Thus, coculture of eosinophils with epithelial cells treated with IL-5 and TNF-α, respectively, led to increased eosinophil-epithelial adhesion and eosinophil cationic protein (ECP) release. Indeed this epithelial-eosinophil interaction during inflammatory/allergic reactions is typified by the expression of eotaxin, a specific eosinophil chemoattractant. This chemokine is produced by epithelial (and endothelial) cells, and its expression has been shown to be upregulated in a guinea-pig model of allergic inflammation *(113)* and in tissues obtained from patients with inflammatory bowel disease *(114)*. Similarly, eotaxin mRNA expression is enhanced in respiratory (BEAS-2B) and colonic (Caco-2) epithelial cell lines in response to TNF-α and IFN-γ *(114)*. Once eosinophils have been recruited to the site of insult it has been shown that airways epithelium can promote their survival *(115)*. Thus, conditioned media from human bronchial epithelial cells can sustain the survival of eosinophils and neutrophils in vitro by the release of granulocyte colony-stimulating factor (G-CSF) and/or GM-CSF *(116)*.

While we hesitate to make generalizations, it appears that epithelial cytokine production is skewed in favor of proinflammatory cytokines (IL-1, IL-6, IL-8, TNF-α) *(105)* rather than

Table 3
Epithelial Cytokine Production[a]

Intestinal epithelium

IL-1α, IL-1β, IL-1 receptor antagonist, IL-6, IL-8, MCP-1, TNF-α
IGF-II, IGF binding proteins I-V, GM-CSF, NGF, TGF-α,
  TGF-β$_{1-3}$, eotaxin

Airways epithelium

IL-1, IL-6, IL-8, IL-11, eotaxin, GRO-α[b], GRO-γ, LCF,
  MCP-1, MCP-3, RANTES, TNF-α
CSF-1, G-CSF, GM-CSF, M-CSF, TGF-β

Urogenital tract epithelium

IL-1α, IL-6, IL-8, GRO-α
GM-CSF

---

[a]Summary of studies employing cell lines, isolated epithelial cells, and *in situ* hybridization on tissue sections to examine epithelial expression of cytokine mRNA and production of functional cytokines.

[b]GRO-α, growth-related oncogene.

---

those that regulate antibody production (e.g., IL-4). However, the epithelium also produces growth factors that are important in growth and repair *(83)*, such as TGF-β. Additionally, conditioned media from nasal epithelial cultures induced the development of monocytes from human HL-60 promyelocytic leukemia cells. Of note is the fact that epithelial cells from inflamed tissues, particularly nasal polyps, were a more potent stimulus for monocyte development than normal epithelium *(116)*. This finding is supported by recent data on cytokine gene expression and release from human nasal epithelium. Epithelial cells from nasal polyps released significantly more IL-8 and GM-CSF than those from healthy nasal mucosa. *(117)*.

In addition, receptors for IL-1, IL-2, and IL-6 have been identified on epithelial cells *(118,119)*, implying that epithelial-derived cytokines may have autocrine, in addition to paracrine, functions. Preliminary data have been presented showing that a human bronchial epithelial cell line can release soluble type I TNF receptors (sTNF-R1) in response to IL-1β *(120)*. Whether this represents a mechanism to attenuate the effects of TNF-α or to stabilize the cytokine and thus act as a biological reservoir for TNF-α is currently unknown.

Another group of proteins worthy of mention is the defensins. Defensins are small (30–35 amino acids) peptides that have a conserved heptacystine motif and were originally identified as an element of the nonoxidative, antimicrobial response of phagocytes. The defensins cryptins 1–5 were subsequently localized in murine Paneth cells, in which cryptin-1 was found to be the most abundant. Cryptin-1 can be released into the lumen and has antimicrobial activity against *Salmonella tryphimurium (8)*. Defensins 5 and 6 have now been localized to human Paneth cells *(121)*. Paneth cell degranulation, and thus defensin release, can be evoked by live or heat-treated bacteria and cholinergic stimulation. Consequently, the epithelium can generate an immediate defense response to infection or following instruction by enteric neurones.

Epithelial cells can synthesize lipid metabolites (Table 4), and this aspect of epithelial function was recently been reviewed *(122)*. Epithelial cells express both the constitutive and inducible form of nitric oxide (NO) synthase (NOS). Epithelial cells from bovine or fetal rat lung show increased NO production when exposed to conditioned media from macrophages, combinations of proinflammatory cytokines, or cytokines administered in combination with LPS *(123)*. Furthermore, NOS synthesis in response to LPS in the rat proximal small intestine is most evident in the villus cells *(124)*. The role of NO is controversial, with some investigators

Table 4
Lipid Metabolites Synthesized by Epithelial Cells

Intestinal epithelium
Arachidonic acid
LTB_4
PGE_2, $PGF_{2\alpha}$
PAF

Airways epithelium
LTB_4, LTC_4
PGD_2, PGE_2, $PGF_{2\alpha}$, PG6-keto-Fl_α
12-hydroxyeicosatetraenoic acid (12-HETE), 15-HETE

favoring a protective role in acute inflammation, in which NO helps maintain the mucosal barrier and exhibits anti-inflammatory properties *(125)*. For instance, NO has been implicated as a switch factor for the transition of primate renal epithelial cells (BSC-1) from a stationary to a locomotory state, and this has obvious implications for epithelial restitution *(126)*. Additionally, NO-induced increases in ciliary beat frequency on bovine lung epithelial cells is advantageous in clearing antigen *(127)*. In contrast, Barnes and Liew *(128)* have hypothesized that NO produced in the airways could potentiate inflammation by downregulating T-helper 1 (Th_1) cells, thus allowing an increase in Th_2 cells that produce IL-4 and IL-5, cytokines important in IgE synthesis and eosinophil recruitment, respectively. The epithelium has been identified as an important source of NO, with increased expression of inducible NOS (iNOS) being noted in biopsy specimens from 22 of 23 patients with asthma, and increased iNOS expression was observed in cultured human lung epithelial cells after exposure to TNF-α *(129)*. Also, increased iNOS has been correlated with decreased epithelial viability in the rat intestine *(124)*, and exposure of monolayers of the human Caco-2 cell line to various NO donors led to increased epithelial permeability. Similarly, evidence has been presented that IFN-γ-induced increased permeability of Caco-2 monolayers is mediated by the release of NO from the epithelium itself *(130)*. Finally, the role of epithelial-derived NO as a putative effector molecule in parasite killing should be acknowledged *(131)*.

Major Histocompatibility Class II (MHC II)
Expression and Antigen Presentation

It is clear that nonlymphoid/nonmonocytoid cells can express MHC II antigens when activated. Many of these cells (islet cells, basal keratinocytes) occur in a relatively antigen-free environment, and MHC II expression on these cells has been linked with autoimmune responses. This is not the case for epithelial cells. Epithelial cells from the small intestinal, respiratory, and female reproductive tracts constitutively express low levels of MHC II *(132)*. In the case of the intestine, it has been postulated that constitutive MHC II expression may be due to the juxtaposition of intraepithelial lymphocytes or lamina propria lymphocytes that produce IFN-γ. Independent of their tissue of origin, epithelial cells show increased MHC II expression during inflammation. For example, rats infected with parasitic enteric nematodes show increased epithelial staining for MHC II *(133)*, as does examination of intestinal biopsies from patients with inflammatory bowel disease (IBD) and nasal polyps, compared to noninflamed tissues *(116,134)*. In accordance with these findings, it has been shown that both IFN-γ and TNF-α can induce epithelial MHC II expression *(135)*.

Indeed, it has been hypothesized that increased MHC II staining on gut epithelium from IBD patients results not from an epithelial abnormality *per se*, but from increased exposure to IFN-γ. Thus, the constitutive expression of MHC II on epithelial cells would allow for constant antigen presentation, and the rate of this epithelial-T-cell interaction would be enhanced during immune activation and inflammatory reactions.

Epithelial antigen presentation in the gut is truly unconventional *(132,136)*. Foreign antigen coupled to epithelial MHC II selectively activates CD8$^+$ suppressor T-cells (in contrast to CD4$^+$ T-cells, which will be activated by professional antigen presenting cells), and whereas the T-cell-epithelial cell interaction is antigen-specific, the resultant suppressor activity is not antigen-specific. Many aspects of these events remain unclear, but it is feasible that in an environment of constant antigen (dietary, microflora) availability, it is biologically prudent not to evoke an active immune response against foreign, but nonnoxious substances. In contrast to this normal situation, enterocytes from inflamed or noninflamed gut regions from IBD patients have been found to present antigen to CD4$^+$ T-cells. This apparent intrinsic difference between IBD patients and those who do not develop this disorder may be a focal point in the etiology of these idiopathic inflammatory conditions. CD1 is described as a nonclassical MHC molecule that occurs in 4 configurations, CD1a–d. CD1d is largely restricted to epithelial cells and B-lymphocytes. CD1 is an epithelial ligand for the T-cell CD8 molecule, and recent studies suggest that an additional molecule on the epithelial surface, designated glycoprotein 180 (gp180) is important in mediating the CD1–CD8 association. In this way the epithelial cell may regulate IEL activity and extrathymic education and mechanisms of oral tolerance.

Adhesion-Molecule Expression

The majority of adhesion molecules have been grouped into one of three families: the immunoglobulin superfamily (ICAM, vascular cell adhesion molecule [VCAM], leucocyte function antigen 3 [LFA-3]); the integrins, heterodimers of α and β chains; and the selectins (L, E, and P). The role of these molecules in extravasation from the vasculature is the focus of extensive research, with less attention being paid to their role on epithelial cells. Human colonic epithelial cell lines (HT-29, T84) can be induced to express ICAM-1 (the ligand for ICAM-1 occurs on lymphocytes and monocytes/neutrophils) by exposure to IFN-γ or phorbol 12-myristate 13 acetate (PMA) *(137,138)*. Constitutive expression of LFA-3 (CD58) on HT-29 cells was not altered by these treatments. Similarly, LFA-3 can be detected on isolated human enterocytes. However, antibody blocking studies revealed that this antigen did not participate in T-cell-epithelial cell mixed lymphocyte reactions *(132)*. Furthermore, a recent immunocytochemical analysis failed to reveal the presence of ICAM-1 on the epithelium in large bowel sections from IBD patients or normal controls *(139)*. ICAM-1 expression has been demonstrated on airways epithelial cell lines and on in tissues from nonasthmatics and in asthmatics, where expression is increased *(18)*. In addition, ICAM-1 expression was induced on conjunctival epithelial cells within 30 min of exposure to allergen *(17)*. This remarkably rapid response has yet to be defined.

The functional correlate of expression of adhesion molecules on epithelial cells has lagged behind their demonstration. Nevertheless it seems likely that, having attracted immune cells to the site of an inflammatory reaction by the release of chemokines, the expression of adhesion molecules would facilitate migration into the lumen or immobilize them *in situ*. The additional intriguing possibility that these molecules are viral receptors has been postulated. Thus, human rhinovirus can bind to ICAM-1, and one can postulate a disease scenario for this association (Fig. 3). Epithelial cells can also express the CD21 antigen, a known receptor for the Epstein-Barr virus.

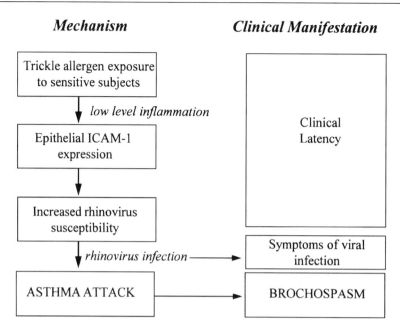

Fig. 3. Hypothetical schema in which continued exposure of allergen in small amounts could lead to increased epithelial expression of the ICAM-1, the receptor for rhinovirus. Subsequent rhinovirus infection could then evoke the clinical symptomatology of airways hyperresponsiveness and asthma.

Epithelial-Derived Relaxing Factors (EpDRFs)

Airways epithelium from several mammalian species has been reported to reduce airways smooth muscle contractile responses to exogenous stimuli such as acetylcholine, histamine, and serotonin *(44)*. Whereas some investigators suggest that these events result from removal of the epithelium, which acts as a physical restraint to contraction or as a diffusion barrier to agonist uptake or is involved in enzymatic degradation of agonists, others favor the release of soluble mediators, EpDRFs. Evidence supports all of the hypotheses, including the latter. For instance, O'Byrne et al. *(140)* reported reduced contraction of smooth muscle when the airways mucosa was attached to or juxtaposed to canine trachelis. The nature of an EpDRF is controversial. It is clear that if such a molecule is liberated from the epithelium, it has short-lived biological activity. Furthermore, airways allergic responses and chronic inflammatory diseases are characterized by "patchy" epithelial exfoliation. Consequently, it is tempting to postulate that the airways hyperresponsiveness observed during these conditions results from loss of the beneficial EpDRF. However, it has not been possible to test this postulate in humans, and data from animal studies are equivocal. Compelling evidence exists for epithelial-induced smooth muscle relaxation by release of PGE_2 and endopeptidase degradation of tachykinins, such as substance P, which are known bronchoconstrictors. The mechanism by which the epithelium can influence smooth contractility requires clarification; nevertheless, it is clear that the epithelium is important in controlling the pathophysiology of airways allergic and inflammatory reactions. In addition, the epithelium may exert an anti-inflammatory influence by producing neutral endopeptidases that can degrade the proinflammatory neuropeptide, substance P *(141)*.

In concluding this section, we would draw the readers attention to a small number of reports suggesting that epithelial cells can inhibit or potentiate T-cell proliferation by a mechanism/ mediator that remains to be identified *(142,143)*.

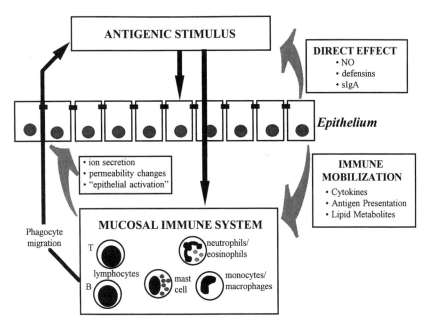

Fig. 4. Conceptual schema in which the epithelial lining of mucosal surfaces is highlighted not only as an effector cell in immune (allergic/inflammatory) reactions but also as a cell that has the potential to combat infectious agents directly, or indirectly by initiating/enhancing the immune response.

Thus, there is ample evidence illustrating that epithelial cells play a pivotal role in inflammatory and allergic events at mucosal surfaces and are an integral component in both the afferent and efferent arms of the host immune response to antigen (Fig. 4).

CONCLUDING REMARKS

The purpose of the host response to antigens is to eliminate invading substances, a goal usually accomplished with minimal damage to host tissue. Thus, an acute inflammatory response is, by and large, a physiological defense mechanism essential for host survival. However, if this response becomes dysregulated, the outcome can be chronic inflammatory disorders that are severely debilitating and may be fatal. We have focused on the role of the epithelium as both an effector cell and a cell capable of reacting to and modulating immune reactions. It is by considering all of the cellular components in mucosal tissues and defining their interrelationships that novel and specific pharmacological therapies to combat a variety of inflammatory disorders can be formulated. A more comprehensive understanding of the role of epithelial cells in allergic/inflammatory reactions is likely to highlight these cells as a rational target for therapeutic intervention.

ACKNOWLEDGMENTS

Studies conducted in the authors' laboratories were funded by grants from the Medical Research Council of Canada, the Crohn's and Colitis Foundation of Canada, Astra-Pharma Draco, and the J. P. Bickell Foundation (Canada).

REFERENCES

1. Madara JL (1989) Loosening tight junctions—lessons from the intestine. J Clin Invest 83:1089–1094.
2. Philpott DJ, McKay DM, Sherman P, Perdue MH (1996) Infection of T84 cells with enteropathogenic *Escherichia coli* alters barrier and transport functions. Am J Physiol 270:G634–G645.
3. Kiyono H, Taguchi T, Aicher WK, Beagley KW, Fujihashi K, Eldridge JH, McGhee JR (1990) Immunoregulatory confluence: T cells, Fc receptors and cytokines for IgA immune responses. Int Rev Immunol 6:263–273.
4. Brandtzaeg P, Halstensen TS, Huitfeldt HS, Krajci P, Kvale D, Scott H, Thrane PS (1992) Epithelial expression of HLA, secretory component (Poly-Ig receptor), and adhesion molecules in the human alimentary tract. Ann NY Acad Sci 664:157–179.
5. Kaiserlian D, Lachaux A, Grosjean I, Graber P, Bonnefoy JY (1993) Intestinal epithelial cells express the CD23/Fcε/RII molecule—enhanced expression in enteropathies. Immunology 80:90–95.
6. Cambell AM, Vignola AM, Chanez P, Godard P, Bousquet J (1994) Low-affinity receptor for IgE on human bronchial epithelial cells in asthma. Immunity 82:506–508.
7. Field M, Semrad CE (1993) Toxigenic diarrheas, congenital diarrheas, and cystic fibrosis—disorders of intestinal ion transport. Ann Rev Physiol 55:631–655.
8. Selsted ME, Miller SI, Henschen AH, Ouellette AJ (1992) Enteric defensins: antibiotic peptide components of intestinal host defense. J Cell Biol 118:929–936.
9. Spits BJ, Bretschneider F, Hendriksen EGJ, Kuper CF (1993) Ultrastructure of free nerve endings in respiratory and squamous epithelium on the rat nasal septum. Cell Tiss Res 274:329–335.
10. Laitinen A (1985) Ultrastructural organization of intraepithelial nerves in the human airway tract. Thorax 40:488–492.
11. Varilek GW, Neil GA, Bishop WP, Lin J, Pantazis NJ (1995) Nerve growth factor synthesis by intestinal epithelial cells. Am J Physiol 269:G445–G452.
12. Poussier P, Julius M (1994) Intestinal intraepithelial lymphocytes: the plot thickens. J Exp Med 180:1185–1189.
13. Camerini V, Panwala C, Kronenberg M (1993) Regional specialization of the mucosal immune system. J Immunol 151:1765–1776.
14. Schon-Hegrad MA, Oliver J, McMenamin PG, Holt PG (1991) Studies on the density, distribution and surface phenotype of intraepeithelial class II major histocompatibility complex antigen (Ia)-bearing dendritic cells in the conducting airways. J Exp Med 173:1345–1356.
15. Maric I, Holt PG, Perdue MH, Bienenstock J (1996) Class II MHC antigen (Ia)-bearing dendritic cells in the epithelium of the rat. J Immunol 156:1408–1414.
16. Liu LM, MacPherson GG (1993) Antigen acquisition by dendritic cells: intestinal dendritic cells acquire antigen administered orally and can prime naive T cells *in vivo*. J Exp Med 177:1299–1307.
17. Ciprandi G, Buscaglia S, Pesce GP, Villaggio B, Bagnasco M, Canonica GW (1993) Allergic subjects express intercellular adhesion molecule-1 (ICAM-1 or CD54) on epithelial cells of conjunctiva after allergen challenge. J Allergy Clin Immunol 91:783–792.
18. Canonica GW, Ciprandi G, Pesce GP, Buscaglia S, Paolieri F, Bagnasco M (1995) ICAM-1 on epithelial cells in allergic subjects: a hallmark of allergic inflammation. Inter. Arch Allergy Appl Immunol 107:99–102.
19. Heyman M, Andriantsoa M, Crain-Denoyelle AM, Desjeux JF (1990) Effect of oral or parenteral sensitization to cow's milk on mucosal permeability in guinea pigs. Int Arch Allergy Appl Immunol 92:242–246.
20. Perdue MH, Chung M, Gall DG (1984) The effect of intestinal anaphylaxis on gut function in the rat. Gastroenterology 86:391–397.
21. Perdue MH, Gall DG (1986) Intestinal anaphylaxis in the rat jejunal response to in vitro antigen exposure. Am J Physiol 250:G427–G431.
22. Crowe SE, Sestini P, Perdue MH (1990) Allergic reactions of rat jejunal mucosa. Ion transport responses to luminal antigen and inflammatory mediators. Gastroenterology 99:74–82.
23. Sestini P, Bienenstock J, Crowe SE, Marshall JS, Stead RH, Kakuta Y, Perdue MH (1990) Ion transport in rat tracheal epithelium in vitro: role of capsaicin-sensitive nerves in allergic reactions. Am Rev Resp Dis 141:393–397.
24. Perdue MH, Masson S, Wershil BK, Galli SJ (1991) Role of mast cells in ion transport abnormalities associated with intestinal anaphylaxis. Correction of the diminished secretory response in genetically mast cell-deficient W/W^v mice by bone marrow transplantation. J Clin Invest 87:687–693.

25. Larsen GL, Fame TM, Renz H, Loader JE, Graves J, Hill M, Gelfand EW (1994) Increased acetylcholine released in tracheas from allergen-exposed IgE-immune mice. Am J Physiol 266:L263–L270.

26. Russell DA, Castro GA (1985) Anaphylactic-like reaction of small intestinal epithelium in parasitized guinea pigs. Immunology 54:573–579.

27. Castro GA, Harari Y, Russell D (1987) Mediators of anaphylaxis-induced ion transport changes in small intestine. Am J Physiol 253:G540–G548.

28. Javed NH, Barrett KE, Wang YZ, Bidinger J, Cooke HJ (1994) Enhanced tissue responsiveness in colonic ion transport of cow's milk-sensitized guinea pigs. Agents Actions 41:25–31.

29. Rothberg KG, Hitchcock M (1982) *In vitro* biosynthesis of cyclooxygenase metabolites in ovalbumin-sensitized and control lungs of guinea pigs. Biochem Pharm 31:2381–2388.

30. Matsuse T, Thomson RJ, Chen X, Salari H, Schellenberg RR (1991) Capsaicin inhibits airway hyper-responsiveness but not lipoxygenase activity or eosinophilia after repeated aerosolized antigen in guinea pigs. Am Rev Resp Dis 144:368–372.

31. Matthay MA, Folkesson HG, Verkman AS (1996) Salt and water transport across alveolar and distal airway epithelium in the adult lung. Am J Physiol 270:L487–L503.

32. Widdicombe J (1995) Relationships among the composition of mucus, epithelial lining liquid and adhesion of microorganisms. Am J Respir Crit Care Med 151:2088–2093.

33. Bellini A, Yoshimura H, Vittori E, Marini M, Mattoli S (1993) Bronchial epithelial cells of patients with asthma release chemoattractant factors from T cells. J Allergy Clin Immunol 92:41–424.

34. Suzumura E, Takeuchi K (1992) Antigen reduces nasal transepithelial electric potential differences and alters ion transport in allergic rhinitis *in vivo*. Acta Otolaryngol (Stockholm) 112:552–558.

35. Phipps RJ, Denas SM, Wanner A (1983) Antigen stimulates glycoprotein secretion and alters ion fluxes in sheep trachea. J Appl Physiol 55:1593–1602.

36. Knowles MR, Buntin WH, Bromberg PA, Gatzy JT, Boucher RC (1982) Measurements of transepithelial electric potential difference in the trachea and bronchi of human subjects in vivo. Am Rev Respir Dis 126:108–112.

37. Jarrett EEE, Hall E, Karlsson T, Bennich H (1980) Adjuvants in the induction and enhancement of rat IgE responses. Clin Exp Immunol 39:183–189.

38. Kosecka U, Marshall JS, Crowe SE, Bienenstock J, Perdue MH (1994) Pertussis toxin stimulates hypersensitivity and enhances nerve-mediated antigen uptake in rat intestine. Am J Physiol 267:G745–G753.

39. Snider DP, Marshall JS, Perdue MH, Liang H (1994) Production of IgE antibody and allergic sensitization of intestinal and peripheral tissues following oral immunization with protein antigen and cholera toxin. J Immunol 153:647–657.

40. Levy DA, Dorat A, Pinel AM, Normier G, Dussourd L, D'Hinterland DB (1989) Relationship between bacteria and IgE. Int Arch Allergy Appl Immunol 88:237–239.

41. Finkelmann FD, Pearce EJ, Urban JF, Sher A (1991) Regulation and biological function of helminth-induced cytokine responses. Immunol Today 12:62–65.

42. Scott P, Pearce E, Cheever AW, Coffman RL, Sher A (1989) Role of cytokines and CD4;pl T-cell subsets in the regulation of parasite immunity and disease. Immunol Rev 112:161–182.

43. Montefort S, Herbert CA, Robinson C, Holgate ST (1992) The bronchial epithelium as a target for inflammatory attack in asthma. Clin Exp Allergy 22:511–520.

44. O'Byrne PM, Adelroth E (1994) Airway epithelial inflammation and its functional consequences. In: Goldie R, ed. Immunopharmacology of Epithelial Barriers. Academic, London, pp. 147–157.

45. O'Byrne PM (1991) The airway epithelium in asthma. In: Farmer S, ed. Lung Biology in Health and Disease. Marcel Dekker, New York, pp. 171–186.

46. Saunders PR, Kosecka U, McKay DM, Perdue MH (1994) Acute stressors stimulate ion secretion and increase epithelial permeability in rat intestine. Am J Physiol 267:G794–G799.

47. Crowe SE, Perdue MH (1992) Gastrointestinal food hypersensitivity: basic mechanisms of pathophysiology. Gastroenterology 103:1075–1095.

48. Neutra MR, Phillips TL, Mayer EL, Fishkind DJ (1987) Transport of membrane-bound macromolecules by M-cells in follicle associated epithelium of rabbit Peyer's patch. Cell Tiss Res 247:537–546.

49. Clark MA, Jepson MA, Simmons NL, Hirst BH (1994) Preferential interaction of *Salmonella typhimurium* with mouse Peyer's patch M cells. Res Microbiol 145:543–552.

50. Smith MW, Thomas NW, Jenkins PG, Miller NGA, Cremaschi D, Porta C (1995) Selective transport of microparticles across Peyer's patch follicle-associated M cells from mice and rats. Exp Physiol 80:735–743.

51. Sanderson IR, Walker WA (1993) Uptake and transport of macromolecules by the intestine—possible role in clinical disorders (an update). Gastroenterology 104:622–639.
52. Kowalski ML, Kaliner MA (1988) Neurogenic inflammation, vascular permeability, and mast cells. J Immunol 140:3905–3911.
53. Gustafsson B, Persson CGA (1992) Allergen-induced mucosal exudation of plasma into rat ileum and its inhibition by budesonide. Scand J Gastroenterol 27:587–593.
54. Perdue MH, Forstner JF, Roomi NW, Gall DG (1984) Epithelial response to intestinal anaphylaxis in rats: goblet cell secretion and enterocyte damage. Am J Physiol 247:G632–G637.
55. D'Inca R, Ramage JK, Hunt RH, Perdue MH (1990) Antigen-induced mucosal damage and restitution in the small intestine of the immunized rat. Int Arch Allergy Appl Immunol 91:270–277.
56. Scudamore CL, Pennington AM, Thornton E, McMillan L, Newlands GFJ, Miller HRP (1995) Basal secretion and anaphylactic release of rat mast cell protease-II (RMCP-II) from *ex vivo* perfused rat jejunum: translocation of RMCP-II into the gut lumen and its relation to mucosal histology. Gut 37:235–241.
57. Marshall JS, Bienenstock J (1994) The role of mast cells in inflammatory reactions of the airways, skin and intestine. Curr Opin Immunol 6:853–859.
58. Fujisawa T, Kephart GM, Gleich GJ (1989) Neutrophils and eosinophils in chronic allergic inflammation in the respiratory tract. In: Sluiter HJ, Van der Lende, eds. Bronchitis IV. Van Gorcum, Aspen, pp. 210–221.
59. Jeffery PK, Wardlaw AJ, Nelson FC, Collins JV, Kay AB (1989) Bronchial biopsies in asthma—an ultrastructural, quantitative study and correlation with hyperreactivity. Am Rev Respir Dis 140:1745–1753.
60. Nadel JA (1992) Biologic effects of mast cell enzymes. Am Rev Respir Dis 145:S37–S41.
61. Benard A, Desreumeaux P, Huglo D, Hoorelbeke A, Tonnel A-B, Wallaert B (1996) Increased intestinal permeability in bronchial asthma. J Allergy Clin Immunol 97:1173–1178.
62. Crowe SE, Soda K, Stanisz AM, Perdue MH (1993) Intestinal permeability in allergic rats: nerve involvement in antigen-induced changes. Am J Physiol 264:G617–G623.
63. Kimm MH, Curtis GH, Hardin JA, Gall DG (1994) Transport of bovine serum albumin across rat jejunum: the role of the enteric nervous system. Am J Physiol 266:G186–G193.
64. Heyman M, Ducroc R, Desjeux J-F, Morgat JL (1982) Horseradish peroxidase transport across adult rabbit jejunum in vitro. Am J Physiol 242:G558–G564.
65. Sestini P, Dolovich M, Vancheri C, Stead RH, Marshall JS, Perdue M, Gauldie J, Bienenstock J (1989) Antigen-induced lung solute clearance in rats is dependent on capsaicin-sensitive nerves. Am Rev Respir Dis 139:401–406.
66. Saunders PR, Kiliaan AJ, Groot JA, Bijlsma PB, Taminiau JA, Perdue MH (1995) Stress-enhanced epithelial permeability to antigenic proteins is mediated by cholinergic mechanisms and occurs via both transcellular and paracellular pathways. Gastroenterology 108:A911 (abstract).
67. McKay DM, Berin MC, Fondacaro J, Perdue MH (1996) Effects of neuropeptide Y and substance P on antigen-induced ion secretion in rat jejunum. Am J Physiol 271:G987–992.
68. Berin MC, Kiliaan AJ, Groot JA, Taminiau JA, Perdue MH (1995) Transepithelial antigen transport occurs via endosomes in <2 min in intestine of sensitized rats. Can J Gastoenterol 10:39A (abstract).
69. Nocka K, Majumder S, Chabot B, Ray P, Cervone M, Berstein A, Besmer P (1989) Expression of *c-kit* gene products in known cellular targets of *W* mutant mice. Genes and Dev 3:816–826.
70. Persson CG (1996) Epithelial cells: barrier functions and shedding-restitution mechanisms. Am J Respir Crit Care Med 153:S9–S10.
71. Glavin GB (1980) Restraint ulcer: history, current research and future implications. Brain Res Bull 5:51–58.
72. Wang J, Johnson LR (1989) Induction of gastric and duodenal mucosal ornithine decarboxylase during stress. Am J Physiol 257:G259–G265.
73. Hernandez DE (1990) The role of brain peptides in the pathogenesis of experimental stress gastric ulcers. Ann NY Acad Sci 597:1–29.
74. Galli SJ, Wershil BK, Bose R, Walker PA, Szabo S (1987) Ethanol-induced acute gastric injury in mast cell-deficient and congenic normal mice. Evidence that mast cells can augment the area of damage. Am J Pathol 128:131–140.
75. MacQueen G, Marshall J, Perdue M, Siegel S, Bienenstock J (1989) Pavlovian conditioning of rat mucosal mast cells to secrete rat mast cell protease II. Science 243:83–85.
76. Gauci M, Husband AJ, Saxarra H, King MG (1994) Pavlovian conditioning of nasal tryptase release in human subjects with allergic rhinitis. Physiol Behav 55:1–3.

77. Isenberg SA, Lehrer PM, Hochron S (1992) The effects of suggestion and emotional arousal on pulmonary function in asthma: a review and hypothesis regarding vagal mediation. Psychosom Med 54:192–216.

78. Empey LR, Fedorak RN (1989) Effect of misoprostol in preventing stress-induced intestinal fluid secretion in rats. Prostagland Leukol Essent Fatty Acids 38:43–48.

79. Barclay GR, Turnberg LA (1988) Effect of cold-induced pain on salt and water transport in the human jejunum. Gastroenterology 94:994–998.

80. McKay DM, Bienenstock J (1994) The interaction between mast cells and nerves in the gastrointestinal tract. Immunol Today 15:533–538.

81. Baird AW, Cuthbert AW, MacVinish LJ (1987) Type 1 hypersensitivity reactions in reconstructed tissues using syngeneic cell types. Br J Pharmacol 91:857–869.

82. Berschneider HM, Powell DW (1992) Fibroblasts modulate intestinal secretory response to inflammatory mediators. J Clin Invest 89:484–489.

83. Dignass AU, Podolsky DK (1993) Cytokine modulation of intestinal epithelial cell restitution: central role of transforming growth factor-β. Gastroenterology 105:1323–1332.

84. Uhal BD, Joshi I, True AL, Mundle S, Raza A, Pardo A, Selman M (1995) Fibroblasts isolated after fibrotic lung injury induce apoptosis of alveolar epithelial cell *in vitro*. Am J Physiol 269:L819–L928.

85. Parkos CA, Delp C, Arnaout MA, Madara JL (1991) Neutrophil migration across a cultured intestinal epithelium. J Clin Invest 88:1605–1612.

86. Colgan SP, Parkos CA, Delp C, Arnaout MA, Madara JL (1993) Neutrophil migration across cultured intestinal epithelial monolayers is modulated by epithelial exposure to IFN-γ in a highly polarized fashion. J Cell Biol 120:785–798.

87. Madara JL, Patapoff TW, Gillece-Castro B, Colgan SP, Parkos CA, Delp C, Mrsny RJ (1993) 5′-Adenosine monophosphate is the neutrophil-derived paracrine factor that elicits chloride secretion from T84 intestinal epithelial cell monolayers. J Clin Invest 91:2320–2325.

88. Resnick MB, Colgan SP, Parkos CA, Delparcher C, McGuirk D, Weller PF, Madara JL (1995) Human eosinophils migrate across an intestinal epithelium in response to platelet-activating factor. Gastroenterology 108:409–416.

89. Stellato C, Beck LA, Gorgone GA, Proud D, Schall TJ, Ono SJ, Lichtenstein LM, Schleiner RP (1995) Expression of the chemokine RANTES by a human bronchial epithelial cell line. Modulation by cytokines and glucocorticoids. J Immunol 155:410–418.

90. Reinecker H-C, Loh EY, Ringler DJ, Mehta A, Rombeau JL, MacDermott RP (1995) Monocyte-chemoattractant protein 1 gene expression in intestinal epithelial cells and inflammatory bowel disease mucosa. Gastroenterology 108:40–50.

91. Paine R, Rolfe MW, Standiford TJ, Burdick MD, Rollins BJ, Strieter RM (1993) MCP-1 expression by rat type II alveolar epithelial cells in primary culture. J Immunol 150:4561–4570.

92. Kovarik G, McKay DM, Perdue MH (1995) Activated monocytes/macrophages stimulate ion secretion of T84 epithelium and impair its barrier function. Gastroenterology 108:A298 (Abstract).

93. Compeau CG, Rotstein OD, Tohda H, Marunaka Y, Rafii B, Slutsky AS, O'Brodovich H (1994) Endotoxin-stimulated alveolar macrophages impair lung epithelial Na$^+$ transport by an L-Arg-dependent mechanism. Am J Physiol 266:C1330–C1341.

94. Lee Y-C, Rannels DE (1996) Alveolar macrophages modulate the epithelial cell response to coal dust in vitro. Am J Physiol 270:L123–L132.

95. Ferguson A (1976) Models of intestinal hypersensitivity. Clin Gastroenterol 5:271–288.

96. Lionetti P, Breese E, Braegger CP, Murch SH, Taylor J, MacDonald TT (1993) T-cell activation can induce either mucosal destruction or adaptation in cultured human fetal small intestine. Gastroenterology 105:373–381.

97. D'Inca R, Ernst P, Hunt RH, Perdue MH (1992) Role of T lymphocytes in intestinal mucosal injury. Inflammatory changes in athymic nude rats. Dig Dis Sci 37:33–39.

98. McKay DM, Croitoru K, Perdue MH (1996) T cell-monocyte interactions regulate epithelial physiology in a co-culture model of inflammation. Am J Physiol 270:C418–C428.

99. Heyman M, Darmon N, Dupont C, Dugas B, Hirribaren A, Desjeux JF, Blaton MA (1994) Mononuclear cells from infants allergic to cow's milk secrete tumor necrosis factor alpha, altering intestinal function. Gastroenterology 106:1514–1523.

100. Kaoutzani P, Colgan SP, Cepek KL, Burkard PG, Carlson S, Delp-Archer C, Brenner MB, Madara JL (1994) Reconstitution of cultured intestinal epithelial monolayers with a mucosal-derived T-lymphocyte cell line. J Clin Invest 94:788–796.

101. McKay DM, Croitoru K (1996) Specific T cell activation in vivo causes epithelial ion transport abnormalities in the intestine of Balb/c mice. Gastroenterology 110:A346 (Abstract).

102. Levine SJ (1995) Bronchial epithelial cell-cytokine interactions in airways inflammation. J Invest Med 43:241–249.

103. Stadnyk A (1994) Cytokine production by epithelial cells. FASEB J 8:1041–1047.

104. Cromwell O, Hamid Q, Corrigan CJ, Barkans J, Meng Q, Collins PD, Kay AB (1992) Expression and generation of interleukin-8, IL-6 and granulocyte-macrophage colony-stimulating factor by bronchial epithelial cells and enhancement by IL-1β and tumour necrosis factor-α. Immunology 77:330–337.

105. Jung HC, Eckmann L, Yang S, Panja A, Fierer J, Morzycka-Wroblewska E, Kagnoff MF (1995) A distinct array of proinflammatory cytokines is expressed in human colon epithelial cells in response to bacterial invasion. J Clin Invest 95:55–65.

106. DiMango E, Zar HJ, Bryan R, Prince A (1995) Diverse *Pseudomonas aeruginosa* gene products stimulate respiratory epithelial cells to produce interleukin-8. J Clin Invest 96:2204–2210.

107. Noah TL, Becker S (1993) Respiratory syncytial virus-induced cytokine production by a human bronchial epithelial cell line. Am J Physiol 265:L472–L478.

108. Kelly CP, Keates S, Siegenberg D, Linevsky JK, Pothoulakis C, Brady H (1994) IL-8 secretion and neutrophil activation by HT-29 colonic epithelial cells. Am J Physiol 267:G991–G997.

109. Cairns JA, Walls AF (1996) Mast cell tryptase is a mitogen for epithelial cells. Stimulation of IL-8 production and intracellular adhesion molecule-1 expression. J Immunol 156:275–283.

110. Smart SJ, Casale TB (1994) Pulmonary epithelial cells facilitate TNFα-induced neutrophil chemotaxis. A role for cytokine networking. J Immunol 152:4087–4094.

111. Nakamura H, Yoshimura K, McElvaney NG, Crystal RG (1992) Neutrophil elastase in respiratory epithelial lining fluid in individuals with cystic fibrosis induces IL-8 gene expression in a human bronchial epithelial cell line. J Clin Invest 89:1478–1484.

112. Takafugi S, Ohtoshi T, Takizawa H, Tadokoro K, Ito K (1996) Eosinophil degranulation in the presence of bronchial epithelial cells. J Immunol 156:3980–3985.

113. Jose PJ, Griffiths-Johnson DA, Collins PD, Walsh DT, Moqbel R, Totty NF, Truong O, Hsuan JJ, Williams TJ (1994) Eotaxin: a potent eosinophil chemoattractant cytokine detected in a guinea pig model of allergic airways inflammation. J Exp Med 179:881–887.

114. Gracia-Zepeda EA, Rothenberg ME, Ownbey RT, Celestin J, Leder P, Luster AD (1996) Human eotaxin is a specific chemoattractant for eosinophils and provides a new mechanism to explain tissue eosinophilia. Nature Genetics 2:449–456.

115. Cox G, Ohtoshi T, Vancheri C, Denburg JA, Dolovich J, Gauldie J, Jordana M (1991) Promotion of eosinophil survival by human bronchial epithelial cells and its modulation by steroids. Am J Respir Cell Mol Biol 4:525–531.

116. Jordana M, Clancy R, Dolovich J, Denberg J (1992) Effector role of the epithelium in inflammation. Ann N Y Acad Sci 664:181–189.

117. Mullol J, Xaubet A, Gaya A, Roca-Ferrer J, Lopez E, Fernandez JC, Fernandez MD, Picado C (195) Cytokine gene expression and release from epithelial cells. A comparison study between healthy nasal mucosa and nasal polyps. Clin Exp Allergy 25:607–615.

118. Takizawa H, Ohtoshi T, Yamashita N, Oka T, Ito K (1996) Interleulin 6 receptor expression on human bronchial cells: regulation by IL-1 and IL-6. Am J Physiol 270:L346–L352.

119. Ciacci C, Mahida YR, Dignass A, Koizumi M, Podolsky DK (1993) Functional Interleukin-2 receptors on intestinal epithelial cells. J Clin Invest 92:527–532.

120. Logun C, Shelhamer JH, Chopra DP, Rhim JS, Levine SJ (1994) Corticosteroids down-regulate PMA-induced release of the type I (p55) soluble TNF receptor from a human bronchial epithelial cell line. Am J Respir Cell Crit Care Med 149:A990.

121. Jones DE, Bevins CL (1993) Defensin-6 messenger RNA in human Paneth cells—implications for antimicrobial peptides in host defense of the human bowel. FEBS Lett 315:187–192.

122. Perdue MH, McKay DM (1994) Integrative immunophysiology in the intestinal mucosa. Am J Physiology 267:G151–G165.

123. Gutierrez HH, Pitt BR, Schwarz M, Watkins SC, Lowenstein C, Caniggia I, Chumley P, Freeman BA (1995) Pulmonary alveolar epithelial inducible NO synthase gene expression: regulation by inflammatory mediators. Am J Physiol 268:L501–L508.

124. Tepperman BL, Brown JF, Whittle BJR (1993) Nitric oxide synthase induction and intestinal epithelial cell viability in rats. Am J Physiol 265:G214–G218.

125. Alcian I, Kubes P (1996) A critical role for nitric oxide in intestinal barrier function and dysfunction. Am J Physiol 270:G225–G237.
126. Nori E, Peresleni T, Srivastava N, Weber P, Bahou WF, Peunova N, Goligorsky MS (1996) Nitric oxide is necessary for a switch from stationary to locomoting phenotype in epithelial cells. Am J Physiol 270:C794–C802.
127. Jain B, Rubinstein I, Robbins RA, Sisson JH (1995) TNFα and IL-1β upregulate nitric-oxide dependent cilliary motility in bovine airway epithelium. Am J Physiol 268:L911–L917.
128. Barnes PJ, Liew FY (1995) Nitriic oxide and asthmatic inflammation. Immunol Today, 130:128–130.
129. Hamid Q, Springall DR, Riveros-Moreno V, Chanez P, Howarth P, Redington A, Bousquet J, Godard P, Holgate S, Polak JM (1993) Induction of nitric oxide synthase in asthma Lancet 342:1510–1513.
130. Unno N, Menconi MJ, Smith M, Fink MP (1995) Nitric oxide mediates interferon-γ-induced hyperpermeability in cultured human intestinal epithelial monolayers. Crit Care Med 23:1170–1176.
131. Oswald IP, Wynn TA, Sher A, James SL (1994) NO as an effector molecule of parasite killing: modulation of its synthesis by cytokines. Comp. Biochem Physiol 108C:11–18.
132. Mayer L, Panja A, Li Y, Siden E, Pizzimenti A, Gerardi F, Chandswang N (1992) Unique features of antigen presentation in the intestine. Ann N Y Acad Sci 664:39–46.
133. Masson SD, Perdue MH (1990) Changes in distribution of Ia antigen on epithelium of the jejunum and ileum in rats infected with *Nippostrongylus brasiliensis*. Clin Immunol Immunopathol 57:83–95.
134. Mayer L, Eisenhardt D, Salomon P, Bauer W, Plous R, Piccinini L (1991) Expression of class II molecules on intestinal epithelial cells in humans. Differences between normal and inflammatory bowel disease. Gastroenterology 100:3–12.
135. Sturgess RP, Hooper LB, Spencer J, Hung CH, Nelufer JM, Ciclitira PJ (1992) Effects of interferon-γ and tumour necrosis factor-α on epithelial HLA class-II expression on jejunal mucosal biopsy specimens cultured in vitro. Scand J Gastroenterol 27:907–911.
136. Bland PW, Kambarage DM (1991) Antigen handling by the epithelium and lamina propria macrophages. Gastroenterol Clin N Am 20:577–596.
137. Kvale D, Krajci P, Brandtzaeg P (1992) Expression and regulation of adhesion molecules ICAM-1 (CD54) and LFA-3 (CD58) in human intestinal epithelial cell lines. Scand J Immunol 35:669–676.
138. Kaiserlian D, Rigal D, Abello J, Revillard J-P (1991) Expression, function and regulation of the intercellular adhesion molecule-1 (ICAM-1) on human intestinal epithelial cell lines. Eur J Immunol 21:2415–2421.
139. Bloom S, Simmons D, Jewell DP (1995) Adhesion molecules intercellular adhesion molecule-1 (ICAM-1), ICAM-3 and B7 are not expressed by epithelium in normal or inflamed colon. Clin Exp Immunol 101:157–163.
140. Manning PJ, Jones GL, Otis J, Daniel EE, O'Byrne PM (1990) The inhibitory influence of tracheal mucosa mounted in close proximity to canine trachealis. Eur J Pharm 178:85–89.
141. Nadel JA (1992) Regulation of neurogenic inflammation by neutral endopeptidase. Am Rev Respir Dis 145:S48–S52.
142. Pang G, Clancy R, Saunders H (1990) Dual mechanisms of inhibition of the immune response by enterocytes isolated from the rat intestine. Immunol Cell Biol 68:387–396.
143. Li X-C, Almawi W, Jevnikar A, Tucker J, Zhong R, Grant D (1995) Allogenic lymphocyte proliferation stimulated by small intestine-derived epithelial cells. Transplantation 60:82–89.

III INFLAMMATION: *MOLECULAR ASPECTS*

16

Proinflammatory Cytokines in Allergic Disease

Daniel L. Hamilos, MD

CONTENTS

INTRODUCTION

Amid the complex regulatory network of cytokines that produce the phenotype of allergic inflammation, there are processes that depend heavily on the participation of cytokines that are not specific to the allergic process. An example of this is the role of proinflammatory cytokines in allergic inflammation. These cytokines can be produced by allergen-specific or immunoglobulin E (IgE)-dependent mechanisms, and they play a key role in allergic inflammation. Similarly, many of the small-molecular-weight chemokines participate in allergic inflammation. The chemokines are of great interest because of their potent and selective chemoattractant properties, which make them likely candidates for regulating cellular influx into sites of allergic inflammation.

The allergic "cascade" involves all inflammatory events and other processes (such as structural changes in epithelium, smooth muscle, and the lamina propria) that occur subsequent to the initiation of IgE-mediated immediate allergic reactions. The cascade of events has been most easily studied by performing allergen challenge studies on allergic subjects. Most of what are considered "inflammatory" events occur several hours after allergen exposure and

From: *Allergy and Allergic Diseases: The New Mechanisms and Therapeutics*
Edited by: J. A. Denburg © Humana Press Inc., Totowa, NJ

comprise elements of the allergic late-phase response. Even within the late-phase response, there is a progression of inflammatory events, and attempts to understand this progression have lead to important advances in our understanding of allergic inflammation and its sensitivity to pharmacologic suppression. Another approach to studying allergic inflammation has been to isolate individual cellular components, cytokines, or inflammatory mediators and thereby attempt to understand their role in the process. Both approaches have provided valuable insight and helped to identify critical regulatory elements in the allergic inflammatory cascade. For the most part, immunopathologic studies of natural allergen exposure in airway mucosa have confirmed the findings of allergen challenge studies, but they have also shown that there are chronic effects, such as epithelial-cell changes and stromal remodeling, that have yet to be studied in the allergen challenge models.

This chapter summarizes current knowledge regarding the special role of proinflammatory cytokines and chemokines in promoting allergic inflammation. The chapter begins with a summary of the individual cytokines and cells known to produce them in allergic inflammation and then discusses their putative role in the pathophysiologic chain of events. The chapter also discusses their potential role in perpetuation of chronic allergic inflammation.

THE CONTRIBUTION OF PROINFLAMMATORY CYTOKINES TO ALLERGIC INFLAMMATION

Granulocyte-Macrophage Colony-Stimulating Factor (GM-CSF)

GM-CSF is hematopoietic growth factor that acts at a somewhat later stage of myeloid progenitor cell than interleukin (IL)-3 to promote the maturation of granulocytes, macrophages, and eosinophils. GM-CSF is produced by numerous cell types, including mononuclear phagocytes, T-lymphocytes, mast cells, endothelial cells, fibroblasts, eosinophils and epithelial cells *(1)*. GM-CSF is produced by T-lymphocytes of both the T-helper 1 (Th1) and T-helper 2 (Th2) phenotype. In addition, activated eosinophils have been shown to produce abundant GM-CSF messenger ribonucleic acid (mRNA) *(2,3)*.

Much of the interest in GM-CSF in allergic disease has stemmed from its production by Th2 T lymphocytes at sites of chronic allergic inflammation and its effects on eosinophil activation and survival. Activated CD4[+] T lymphocytes expressing mRNA for the Th2 cytokines IL-4, IL-3, IL-5, and GM-CSF have been demonstrated to infiltrate sites of allergen challenge in allergic subjects in the skin *(4,5)*, nose *(6–8)*, and lungs *(9,10)*. Similarly, CD3[+] T-lymphocytes expressing these cytokines have been demonstrated in subjects with perennial allergic rhinitis *(11)*, allergic asthma *(12,13)*, atopic dermatitis *(14)*, and allergic subjects with chronic hyperplastic sinusitis and nasal polyps *(15,16)*.

GM-CSF activates eosinophils to become hypodense and have increased functional properties, including enhanced respiratory burst activity, augmentation of leukotriene C4 (LTC_4), production, enhanced expression of CD18 and CD11b, enhanced CD18-mediated adhesion *(17,18)*, and enhanced responses to other chemoattractants *(19)*. In addition, GM-CSF markedly prolongs eosinophil survival by interrupting the normal apoptotic process *(20–22)*.

GM-CSF also exerts other effects on neutrophils, monocytes, and eosinophils that contribute to local inflammatory responses. These include enhancement of neutrophil LTB_4 production (via augmentation of 5-lipoxygenase enzyme synthesis) *(23)*, superoxide generation *(24)*, and production of IL-8 *(25)*. Along with other proinflammatory cytokines, GM-CSF potentiates monocyte/macrophage phagocytosis *(26)* and at least partially accounts for increased monocyte survival through decreased apoptosis at sites of chronic allergic inflammation *(27)*.

Adenoviral vectors have been used to generate mice that overexpress GM-CSF in a tissue-specific manner in the lungs *(1)*. These mice develop marked pulmonary accumulation of eosinophils and macrophages, macrophage granulomas, and irreversible lung fibrosis. These effects are distinct from those seen with other cytokine transgenic mice. For instance, IL-5 overexpression in the lungs induces eosinophilia but not macrophage granulomas or fibrosis. The eosinophil and macrophage accumulation in GM-CSF-overexpressed mice may be the result of effects on monocyte survival, proliferation, and differentiation into macrophages *(1)*.

After allergen challenge of allergic asthmatics, a small percentage of alveolar macrophages isolated from bronchoalveolar lavage express GM-CSF mRNA *(28)*. Immunohistochemical staining of endobronchial biopsies has revealed staining for GM-CSF in the bronchial epithelium in asthmatics but not in normal controls *(29)*. GM-CSF protein levels are markedly increased in bronchoalveolar lavage 24 h after allergen challenge *(28)*. GM-CSF is one of the predominant eosinophil survival-enhancing activities in the peripheral blood of asthmatics but not normal control subjects *(30)*. GM-CSF protein levels are also increased in bronchoalveolar lavage from both symptomatic and asymptomatic asthmatics *(31)*. Cultured explants of nasal polyp epithelium from allergic subjects have also been shown to produce abundant quantities of GM-CSF, whereas explants from normal subjects do not *(32)*. Production of GM-CSF by airway epithelial and stromal cells may be an important stimulus for persistent mucosal inflammation in asthma and chronic hyperplastic sinusitis with nasal polyposis (*see* the Structural Cells).

Tumor Necrosis Factor α *(TNFα)*

TNFα may be one of the most important proinflammatory cytokines in allergic inflammation. It is synthesized and stored preformed, along with IL-4, IL-5, and IL-6, in mast cell granules *(33–35)*. This provides a ready source of TNFα for rapid release after allergen-induced mast cell triggering. Highly purified mast cells from human lung produce TNF mRNA and release TNFα bioactivity on activation with anti-IgE *(36)*. In addition, human lung fragments challenged in vitro with anti-IgE induce both mast cells and macrophages to express TNFα mRNA *(37)*.

The existence of a preformed source of TNFα is probably of critical importance during allergen-induced inflammation, since it has been demonstrated that TNFα-inducible endothelial E-selectin and intercellular adhesion molecule (ICAM)-1 are upregulated within 6 h of allergen challenge, i.e., before significant T-lymphocyte infiltration and cytokine mRNA production are seen. In combination with IL-4, TNFα also causes the selective upregulation of endothelial vascular cell adhesion molecule (VCAM)-1, which is likely to account, in part, for the selective accumulation of eosinophils and lymphocytes at tissue sites 24–48 h after allergen challenge *(38–40)*.

Whereas the mast cell may be an important source of preformed TNF-α, other cell types have been shown to produce it in allergic disease. Alveolar macrophages from allergic asthmatics spontaneously produce increased TNFα and IL-6 (but little IL-1β), and this production can be enhanced in vitro by exposure to allergen or anti-IgE-antibody *(41,42)*. These effects are further augmented by interferon (IFN) γ *(41)*. Similarly, bronchoalveolar lavage leukocytes from asthmatics have been shown to release TNF-α *(43)*. In chronic allergic inflammation, potential sources include the mast cell, T-lymphocytes (both Th1 and Th2), monocytes, and eosinophils *(44)*. The contribution of each to TNF-α production is unknown; however, each has been shown to have the capacity to produce TNF-α mRNA and protein. In nasal polyps, eosinophils and monocytes, along with mast cells, appear to be the major sources *(44)*.

A mouse model of shistosomal egg antigen-induced airway inflammation has been used to investigate the role of TNFα in leukocyte recruitment *(45)*. In this model, which has been shown to be a Th2-type IL-4-dependent response *(46)*, intratracheal instillation of allergen leads to neutrophil infiltration peaking at 8 h and eosinophil infiltration peaking at 48 h. TNF-α protein has bee shown to be produced in the lungs of allergen-challenged mice. Both the early neutrophil and the late eosinophil infiltration were shown to be abrogated by pretreatment with intratracheal instillation of a soluble TNFα receptor linked to an antibody Fc component (sTNFr-:Fc) that neutralized TNFα activity in vivo. Eosinophil infiltration was nearly completely abrogated at 48 h by sTNFr-:Fc treatment 24 h after allergen challenge. Similarly, Wershil and colleagues *(47)* showed that anti-TNF-α antibody reduced IgE and mast cell dependent leukocyte infiltration in allergen sensitized mice. These animal studies suggest that the sustained production of TNF-α may be a key factor in perpetuation of chronic allergic inflammation.

IL-1

IL-1 is a multifunctional cytokine that has been detected in increased amounts in association with allergic disease. Its effects are predominantly proinflammatory, including supporting T-cell activation and local accumulation and activation of neutrophils *(48)*. The latter effect is, in part, mediated by the induction of ICAM-1, E-selectin, and VCAM-1 on vascular endothelial cells *(49–52)*. Low concentrations of IL-1α induce production of GM-CSF, IL-6, and IL-8 in bronchial epithelial cells from normal subjects in vitro *(53)*. Since GM-CSF, IL-8, and IL-6 mRNA and protein are produced in asthmatic bronchial epithelial cells *(54)*, this provides further evidence for the involvement of IL-1 in asthma.

There is debate over the mechanism of release of IL-1 from cells. IL-1α and IL-1β represent two distinct gene products with distinct protein sequences, but both species bind the same receptor and have essentially the same biologic activities. A large amount of IL-1 accumulates in the cytoplasm of certain cells, such as monocytes. Most IL-1 detected in biological fluids is in the form of IL-1β. In allergic inflammation, tissue and alveolar macrophages and infiltrating monocytes are the predominant sources of IL-1. Based primarily on in vitro studies, other cells, including T-cells (both Th1 and Th2), eosinophils, and mast cells, may also contribute to IL-1 production in allergic inflammation.

Alveolar macrophages from asthmatic and normal subjects express a low-affinity receptor for IgE (FcεRII), also known as the CD23 determinant. Alveolar macrophages isolated by bronchoalveolar lavage from allergic asthmatics show increased CD23 expression and a hypodense "activated" phenotype *(55)*. Blood monocytes and alveolar macrophages from allergic subjects can be induced with IgE-immune complexes to produce IL-1β and TNFα protein *(56)*. This effect is mediated through crosslinking of surface FcεRII-type receptors (CD23 epitope). Kinetic studies have indicated that IL-1 mRNA is upregulated within 30 min and is maximal after 2 h of incubation with IgE-immune complexes *(56)*.

Allergen challenge studies in allergic rhinitis and asthma have consistently reported upregulation of proinflammatory cytokines in lavage fluid. Results differ, however, in these two diseases. In allergic rhinitis, allergen challenge was associated with an increase in nasal lavage neutrophils and eosinophils and an increase in IL-1 and IL-6 protein in lavage *(57)*. In contrast, TNFα protein levels were not increased. Increased IL-1β but not IL-6 has also been found in subjects with allergic rhinitis *(58)*.

In contrast, alveolar macrophages studied after allergen bronchial challenge were shown to produce TNF and IL-6 but not IL-1β *(59)*. This is curious, since significant elevations of IL-1β, TNF-α, and IL-6 have been detected in bronchoalveolar lavage fluid of symptomatic versus asymptomatic asthmatics *(60)*. It is possible that these disparate results reflect differences in timing of release of TNF, IL-6, and IL-1β.

The importance of IL-1 in allergen-induced late asthmatic responses was tested in a guinea pig model of allergen-induced asthma *(61)*. Pretreatment of guinea pigs with IL-1 receptor antagonist protein (IRAP) had no effect on the cellular components of the late asthmatic reaction (LAR) but attenuated the LAR in terms of pulmonary resistance. IRAP was also shown to inhibit allergen-stimulated IgE production and production of IL-6, TNF-α, and soluble CD23 (cleaved FcεRII) but not IL-1β in cultured peripheral-blood mononuclear cells *(62)*.

IL-6

Like IL-1, IL-6 is a multifunctional cytokine with prominent proinflammatory properties. Of relevance to allergic disease, IL-6 induces B-cell differentiation and has also been shown to be essential for IgE antibody production *(63)*. The latter effect is now known to be owing to the capacity of IL-6 to upregulate expression of the CD40 glycoprotein on B lymphocytes. Engagement of B-cell CD40 with its ligand (CD40 ligand) on helper T-cells delivers an obligate activation signal to the B-cell for isotype switching *(64)*.

The principal cellular source of IL-6 is the tissue macrophage or blood monocyte. Activated T-cells of both the Th1 and Th2 types also produce IL-6, and IL-6 production has also been detected in asthmatic airway epithelium *(54)* and in normal epithelial cells after stimulation with IL-1α *(53)*. As previously mentioned, alveolar macrophages from asthmatics spontaneously produce increased amounts of TNFα and IL-6, and this production can be enhanced in vitro by exposure to allergen or anti-IgE antibody *(41)*. These effects are further augmented by IFNγ *(41)*. Increased production of IL-6 along with either IL-1 or TNFα in allergen challenge studies *(57,59)* and during asthma exacerbations *(60,65,66)* have already been discussed.

PROINFLAMMATORY EFFECTS OF
CHEMOKINES IN ALLERGIC INFLAMMATION

Allergic inflammation is associated with increased production of both C-C and C-X-C chemokines. They are produced by multiple cell types, including epithelial cells and other structural cells and infiltrating inflammatory cells. Their differential capacity to chemoattract neutrophils, lymphocytes, monocytes, basophils, and eosinophils make them ideal candidates for regulating the complex kinetics of cellular infiltration seen in allergic inflammation.

A great deal of attention has focused on the C-C chemokines in allergic inflammation because of their chemotactic effects on eosinophils. The C-C chemokines also chemoattract monocytes, T-lymphocytes, natural killer cells, and basophils *(67)*. The C-C chemokines are a highly interrelated group with a complex pattern of cross-interaction with cellular receptors (Table 1). The mechanisms controlling their production within allergic tissues, including the epithelium, remain unknown. Certain of the C-C chemokines, including RANTES, MIP-1α, and MIP-1β, also increase the adhesion properties of the cells that they chemoattract *(67)*. It has also been proposed that the chemokines may function primarily as scaffolding molecules by virtue of electrostatic interactions with negatively charged extracellular proteoglycan molecules to create an immobilized chemotactic gradient. In a similar manner, the chemokine may be sequestered in a solid phase on the surface of endothelial cells and thereby be in a location to trap leukocytes that are normally rolling along the intravascular endothelial surface *(67)*. In this paradigm, the chemokine directly stimulates increased leukocyte adhesiveness, thereby facilitating firm attachment to the intravascular endothelium, and then functions as an immobilized chemoattractant gradient to facilitate leukocyte movement through the extracellular matrix.

RANTES

RANTES is a member of the C-C chemokine family and a potent chemoattractant factor for eosinophils, T lymphocytes, basophils, natural killer cells, and monocyte/macrophages *(67,68)*. A variety of cell types have been reported to produce RANTES, including T-lymphocytes, platelets, fibroblasts, macrophages, endothelial cells, and eosinophils *(67)*. Recent reports also suggest that human airway mucosa may be an important source of RANTES, thereby contributing to eosinophil recruitment *(69,70)*.

RANTES is believed to be important in eosinophil recruitment in allergic disease. In a study by Ying et al. *(71)*, the C-C chemokines monocyte chemotactic protein (MCP)-3 and RANTES were shown to be elaborated at sites of allergen challenge in allergic subjects. MCP-3 mRNA peaked within the first 6 h and progressively declined over 24–48 h. In contrast, RANTES mRNA was detectable at 6 h but peaked at 24 h and declined only slightly at 48 h. The kinetics of MCP-3 mRNA most closely paralleled the influx of MBP[+] and EG2[+] eosinophils. The kinetics of appearance of RANTES mRNA paralleled the influx of CD3[+], CD4[+], and CD8[+] T-lymphocytes, suggesting that T-cells may be the principal source of RANTES during the late-phase response. Thus, MCP-3 and RANTES may act sequentially to promote eosinophil, lymphocyte, and monocyte migration during the allergic late-phase response. The cellular sources of MCP-3 during allergic responses are not known, although several cell types have been shown to produce it in vitro (see Table 1).

In nasal polyps, we have found that RANTES mRNA[+] cells are increased in both allergic and nonallergic subjects, suggesting that RANTES may also be important in nonallergic eosinophilic inflammation *(72)*.

MCP-1, MCP-2, and MCP-3

MCP-1, MCP-2, and MCP-3 are highly homologous at the level of gene composition and amino acid sequence. These three C-C chemokines also cross-desensitize each other and RANTES at the level of the cell receptor *(73–75)*. All three are chemotactic for monocytes, T-lymphocytes, natural killer (NK) cells, eosinophils, and basophils *(67)*. The potency of MCP-3 for eosinophil chemotaxis is approximately equal to that of RANTES *(76)*.

MCP-3 expression in nasal epithelial cells is both constitutive and inducible by TNFα *(77)*. As mentioned above, MCP-3 was shown to be elaborated at sites of allergen challenge in allergic subjects, peaking within the first 6 h and progressively declining over 24–48 h *(71)*.

MIP-1α, MIP-1β

MIP-1α is produced primarily by monocytes. Cross-desensitization has been observed between MIP-1α, MIP-1β, and RANTES *(75)*, and the cellular responses to these chemokines are similar but not identical *(75)*. Production of MIP-1α by monocytes can be induced by several proinflammatory cytokines. Furthermore, production is increased on contact with endothelial cells, which may function to upregulate the process of transendothelial migration of cells *(78,79)*. The interaction of leukocytes with endothelial cells may also activate intracellular signals for leukocyte production of chemokines, such as MIP-1α *(80)*.

Using the mouse model of schistosomal egg antigen-induced pulmonary eosinophilia, Lukacs et al. *(81)* demonstrated an increase in MIP-1α mRNA and protein in the lungs 8 h after allergen challenge. MIP-1α protein expression was associated with airway epithelial cells and macrophages and later with recruited mononuclear cells and eosinophils. Pretreatment of the mice with neutralizing MIP-1α antibody prior to allergen challenge significantly reduced the recruitment of eosinophils but not the early recruitment of neutrophils into the airways.

Table 1
The C-C Chemokine Family in Humans: Cellular Sources,
Activities, Interrelationships

Chemokine	Cellular sources	Chemotactic effect	Chemokine receptor sharing	References
RANTES	Activated T-cells Memory T-cells NK cells Epithelial cells	Eosinophils T lymphocytes	MIP-1α MIP-1β MCP-1, -2, -3	67,75,120, 159,160

MCP-1	Bronchial
	  epithelial cells
	Alveolar
	  macrophages
	Endothelial
	  cells
	T-cells
	NK cells
		Monocytes
		Eosinophils
		CD4$^+$, CD8$^+$
		T-cells
		NK cells
		Basophils
		Mast cells
			MCP-2, -3	73–76,
				161–165,167

MCP-2	(See MCP-1)	(See MCP-1)	MCP-1, -3	
MCP-3	(See MCP-1)	(See MCP-1)	MCP-1, -2	
MIP-1α	Monocytes	Naive T-cells B-cells NK cells	RANTES MIP-1β MCP-1, -2, -3	75,160
MIP-1β	Monoyctes	Naive T-cells B-cells NK cells?	RANTES MIP-1α MCP-1, -2, -3	75
Eotaxin	Epithelial cells	Eosinophils	Unknown	83,84

There have been relatively few studies examining the presence of MIP-1α or MIP-1β in human allergic disease, although an increase in MIP-1α has been reported after nasal allergen challenge (82).

Eotaxin

Eotaxin is one of the most recently cloned members of the C-C chemokine family that has been shown to be highly potent and selective in eosinophil chemotaxis, with relatively little activity for monocytes or lymphocytes (83,84). Eotaxin induces a selective infiltration of eosinophils when injected into the lungs or skin of guinea pigs (83). The guinea pig eotaxin gene has significant sequence homology to other C-C chemokines, and it is constitutively expressed in various guinea pig tissues, including the lungs and gastrointestinal tract (83,84). Allergen challenge of ovalbumin-sensitized guinea pig airways leads to a rapid and significant increase in eotaxin mRNA within 3 h by Northern blot analysis with a return to baseline by 6 h (83). Analogously, eotaxin bioactivity in the allergen-challenged guinea pig bronchoalveolar lavage (BAL) peaked at 3–6 h and declined to low levels at 24 h (84). It is unclear how the kinetics of eotaxin mRNA and protein production correlate with eosinophil influx in the lungs, however. Preliminary work suggests that eotaxin production may be predominantly epithelial in origin.

IL-8

In general, less attention has been given to the role of C-X-C chemokines in allergic disease, since they are primarily chemoattractive for neutrophils. However, certain chemokines of this family, such as IL-8, are produced in large quantity by epithelial cells, such as the lung epithelium, in response to a variety of stimuli, including allergen exposure *(62)*. IL-8 may be important in the early part of the late-phase allergic response, in which neutrophil infiltration predominates *(85)*. IL-8 might also exert significant proinflammatory effects during the latter portion of the late-phase response, when mononuclear cell, T-cell, and eosinophil infiltration occur. Some investigators have found IL-8 to be chemotactic for unprimed human eosinophils *(86)*, whereas others have reported that eosinophils respond to IL-8 only after priming with IL-5 (10^{-11} *M*) *(87)*. However, after priming with IL-5, the response of eosinophils to IL-8 is similar in magnitude and concentration to the response to RANTES *(87)*.

Studies of human nasal challenge with recombinant human IL-8 (10^{-7} *M*) in both allergic and nonallergic subjects showed a marked increase in nasal neutrophilia but essentially no eosinophilia *(88)*. Similarly, repeated intranasal administration of IL-8 to guinea pigs over a 3-wk period resulted in significant bronchoalveolar lavage neutrophilia but not eosinophilia *(89)*.

IL-8 protein has been detected in airway epithelium of chronic asthmatic subjects, suggesting that it may be produced continually and therefore serve as a contributing factor to sustained airway inflammation and eosinophilia *(85)*. Epithelial cells are an important cellular source of IL-8 in asthma *(85,90)*. Many other cell types produce it, including monocytes, endothelial cells, lymphocytes, fibroblasts, keratinocytes, and hepatocytes *(90,91)*. Eosinophils and GM-CSF-stimulated neutrophils may be other cellular sources of IL-8 in allergic inflammation *(25,92)*.

SUMMARY OF CELLULAR SOURCES OF PROINFLAMMATORY CYTOKINES AND CHEMOKINES IN ALLERGIC INFLAMMATION

Mast Cells

Mast cells are a probable source of proinflammatory cytokines during allergic inflammation. The initial observation of cytokine production by mast cells came from studies of virally transfected murine cell lines *(93)*. Subsequently, cultured human mast cells from bone marrow and later mature cutaneous mast cells were shown to possess TNF-α mRNA *(94–98)*. At least some of this activity was demonstrated to be associated with cytoplasmic granules *(99)*. Using very thin (2-μm) glycol methacrylate sections of tissue, Bradding and colleagues *(33,100)* demonstrated increased mast cell-associated immunoreactivity for IL-4, and later IL-5 and IL-6, in allergic rhinitis. Similarly, IL-6 was detected in nasal mucosal biopsies of normal and allergic rhinitis subjects, and nearly 100% of the immunoreactivity was localized to mast cells. However, IL-6 does not appear to be increased in mast cells of allergic rhinitis patients. Using analogous techniques, Bradding and colleagues have examined normal and asthmatic airways and found that the majority of cells positive for IL-4, IL-5, IL-6, and TNF-α are mast cells *(34)*. A sevenfold increase in the number of mast cells staining for TNF-α was observed in asthmatic biopsies *(34)*. Human skin mast cells have also been reported to produce TNF-α mRNA and protein *(101)*.

In addition to the storage of cytokines in mast cell granules, activation of mast cells through the FcεRI receptor leads to production of mRNA for multiple cytokine species, including IL-1α, IL-3, IL-4, IL-5, IL-6, GM-CSF, IFN-γ, IL-13, and TNF-α and certain chemokines *(35,99,102,103)*. Mast cell production of cytokines has been demonstrated at sites of allergic inflammation *(11)*. In addition, Klein et al. *(104)* demonstrated that human foreskin mast cells generated a cytokine with TNF-α activity in response to IgE-dependent signaling.

Table 2
Cytokines of Relevance to Allergic Disease

Cytokines produced by Th2 T-lymphocytes	Cytokines that promote the development of Th2 T-lymphocytes	Cytokines that promote Th1 T-lymphocyte development	Cytokines that upregulate vascular adhesion molecules
IL-4	IL-4	IL-12	TNF-α
IL-5	IL-10	IFN-γ	(ICAM-1, E-selectin,
IL-3			VCAM-1)
GM-CSF			IL-1β
IL-10			(ICAM-1, E-selectin,
IL-6			VCAM-1)
			IL-4, IL-13
IL-13			(VCAM-1)

Th2 T-Lymphocytes

Allergen-specific T lymphocytes produce a characteristic Th2 cytokine profile, including IL-4, IL-5, IL-3, and GM-CSF, at sites of allergic inflammation *(4–16)* as summarized in Table 2. Minimal IFN-γ is produced in allergen-specific clones. The relative contribution of Th2 T lymphocytes to the production of GM-CSF at sites of allergic inflammation is difficult to estimate, given the multiplicity of cells that produce it.

Eosinophils

Activated eosinophils isolated from peripheral blood or from allergic tissues are a source of multiple cytokines, including TNF-α, IL-1α, IL-6, IL-8, GM-CSF, and MIP-1α *(105,106)*. In addition, eosinophils have recently been shown to release the chemokine RANTES and lymphocyte chemoattractant factor (LCF) *(107)*. Of particular interest has been the demonstration that a large percentage of eosinophils in nasal polyps produce TNF-α mRNA *(44)*. Since our own studies *(72)* and the animal studies of Lukacs et al. *(45)* suggest that TNF-α may play a key role in the induction and maintainence of VCAM-1 expression, this suggests that production of TNF-α by eosinophils may provide a positive-feedback loop for eosinophil infiltration. Also of special interest is the demonstration that eosinophils at sites of allergic inflammation produce immunoreactive GM-CSF *(2,3,31)*. GM-CSF may be the most important autocrine growth factor and activating factor for eosinophils in allergic tissues.

Monocytes/Macrophages

In allergic tissues, tissue and alveolar macrophages and infiltrating monocytes are the predominant sources of IL-1 and IL-6 and a major source of TNF-α *(44)*. Alveolar macrophages and monocytes from asthmatic and normal subjects show increased expression of the low-affinity FcεRII receptor CD23 *(110)*, and cross-linking of this receptor with IgE immune complexes induces the production of IL-1β and TNF-α protein *(56)*. Alveolar macrophages isolated by bronchoalveolar lavage from allergic asthmatics show increased CD23 expression and a hypodense "activated" phenotype *(55,56)*. IL-1 mRNA is upregulated within 30 min of receptor cross-linking and is maximal after 2 h of incubation *(56)*. Similarly, Gosset et al. *(41)* showed that alveolar macrophages from allergic asthmatics spontaneously produced increased

TNFα and IL-6, and this production could be enhanced in vitro by exposure to allergen or anti-IgE-antibody. The production of proinflammatory cytokines by monocytes or macrophages in allergic disease differs by location (*see* IL-1).

Structural Cells

The production of cytokines by structural cells and eosinophils at sites of allergic inflammation represents an important amplification step promoting chronic allergic inflammation. Structural cells, such as epithelial cells, fibroblasts, and myofibroblasts, are induced to produce cytokines apparently in response to inflammatory signals. The cytokines produced by these cells have been elucidated in cultured explants and in diseased tissues *(111–113)*.

The nasal and airway epithelium are important targets for proinflammatory cytokines and eosinophil-mediated tissue injury in allergic disease. The cytokines IL-1β and TNFα induce expression of ICAM-1 on primary human tracheal epithelial cells *(114)*, which appears to be critical for intraepithelial migration of eosinophils in allergen-challenged primates *(115,116)*. IFNγ has also been shown to induce ICAM-1 expression and enhance T-lymphocyte adhesion to human tracheal epithelium *(117)*.

The epithelium is also a potentially important source of proinflammatory cytokines in allergic disease. Cultured nasal epithelial cells from allergic subjects produce fourfold greater quantities of GM-CSF than normal nasal epithelial cells and increased amounts of IL-6 and IL-8 *(113)*. Similarly, airway epithelium from asthmatic subjects has been shown by reverse transcriptase-polymerase chain reaction (RT-PCR) to produce IL-6, IL-8, and GM-CSF mRNA *(118)* and immunoreactive GM-CSF *(29,119)*. Production of GM-CSF by airway epithelial cells may contribute to the sustained airway eosinophilia in asthma, and its suppression by inhaled steroids is associated with decreased airway eosinophilia and bronchial hyperreactivity *(29)*.

The epithelium is also an important source of chemokines in allergic disease. Using immunohistochemistry or mRNA probes to study asthmatic airways or nasal polyp biopsies, the epithelium has been shown to be a source of IL-8 *(85)*, MCP-1 *(77)*, RANTES *(120)*, LCF *(121)*, and possibly eotaxin.

ROLE OF CYTOKINES AND CHEMOKINES IN RECRUITMENT OF EOSINOPHILS AT SITES OF ALLERGIC INFLAMMATION

The recruitment of eosinophils into sites of allergen exposure, which peaks at 24–48 h, is a complex process. At least four components of the process can be discerned, including (*see* Fig. 1):

1. The systemic stimulus for eosinophilopoiesis and release of mature eosinophils from the marrow compartment;
2. Upregulation of endothelial cell adhesion molecules;
3. Eosinophil chemoattraction/transendothelial migration; and
4. The elaboration of cytokines that prolong eosinophil survival at the tissue site.

Eosinophilia in asthma has been shown to be associated with increased serum levels of IL-5 and GM-CSF *(30)*. The most likely source of these cytokines is Th2 T lymphocytes activated by allergen at the tissue site. In addition to promoting the release of mature eosinophils from the marrow, IL-5 also primes eosinophils for transendothelial migration *(122,166)* and response to C-C chemokines *(123)*. The importance of the eosinophilopoietic stimulus has been demonstrated in animals in which it has been shown that systematically administered

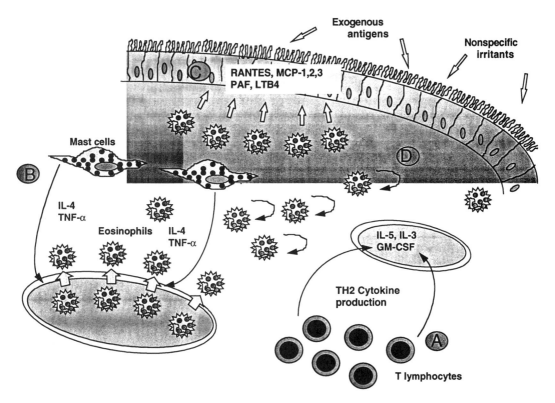

Fig. 1. Recruitment of eosinophils into sites of allergic inflammation. (A) Eosinophilopoiesis and release of mature eosinophils from the marrow compartment is caused by production of TH2 cytokines IL-5, IL-3, and GM-CSF. (B) Transendothelial migration of eosinophils is dependent on interaction with endothelial cellular adhesion molecules ICAM-1, E-selectin, and VCAM-1. Studies of eosinophil migration through endothelial monolayers suggest that all three cellular adhesion molecules are utilized, and all three are upregulated at sites of allergic inflammation. Cytokines, which promote adhesion molecule expression, such as IL-4 and TNF-α, are probably released within minutes of allergen challenge, since these cytokines are stored preformed in mast cell granules. (C) Several members of the C-C chemokine family function as potent chemoattractant factors for eosinophils, T-lymphocytes, basophils, and other cell types. The cellular sources of C-C chemokines during allergic responses are probably multiple and include inflammatory cells and epithelial cells. (D) Eosinophils at sites of allergic inflammation produce multiple cytokines, including GM-CSF which may be the most important autocrine growth factor and activating factor for eosinophils in allergic tissues.

IL-5 markedly augments the cutaneous eosinophil accumulation in response to eotaxin, whereas intradermally injected IL-5 fails to produce eosinophilia *(124)*.

Eosinophil recruitment requires transendothelial migration that is dependent on interaction with the endothelial cellular adhesion molecules ICAM-1, E-selectin, and VCAM-1. Studies of eosinophil migration through endothelial monolayers suggest that all three cellular adhesion molecules are utilized, and all three are upregulated at sites of allergic inflammation *(108,125–129)*. Pretreatment of primates with anti-ICAM-1 or anti-VCAM-1 antibody inhibits eosinophil recruitment into sites of allergen challenge *(115,116,130–133)*.

Certain cytokines also serve as potent chemoattractants for eosinophils and/or neutrophils. There are important differences between eosinophils and neutrophils in their response to these substances *(134,135)*. The cytokines IL-2 and lymphocyte chemoattractant factor (LCF or

IL-16) are highly potent eosinophil chemoattractants, whereas GM-CSF, IL-3, and IL-5 are relatively weak. IL-4 has no significant chemoattractant effect on eosinophils. The significance of cytokines such as IL-2 and LCF at sites of allergic inflammation is uncertain, since these cytokines are not produced in tissues until T-cell infiltration occurs. The C-C chemokines have received the greatest attention as selective eosinophil chemoattractants. They are elaborated within 3 h after allergen challenge by mononuclear cells and airway epithelial cells. As previously mentioned, IL-8 may also promote eosinophil chemotaxis, and this action is enhanced by eosinophil priming with IL-5 *(87)*. The stimuli leading to the production of chemokines in allergic inflammation are largely unknown.

Eosinophils induced to become hypodense also manifest prolonged survival in vitro and in vivo *(20,22,136)*. Eosinophils require IL-5 for survival, proliferation, and effector functions *(105)*. Prolongation of eosinophil survival by GM-CSF, IL-3, and IL-5 is associated with inhibition of the normal process of apoptosis, and this effect is abrogated by transforming growth factor (TGF)-β *(105)*. Eosinophil activation is also associated with autocrine production of GM-CSF and IL-3 *(2,3,31,137)*. Binding to extracellular matrix fibronectin also prolongs eosinophil survival possibly owing to the autocrine production of GM-CSF *(138)*.

CYTOKINE AND CHEMOKINE INVOLVEMENT IN CELLULAR ADHESION MOLECULE EXPRESSION, LEUKOCYTE ADHESION, AND TRANSENDOTHELIAL MIGRATION

The emigration of leukocytes from the intravascular space to tissue sites of allergic inflammation represents a complex interplay of adhesive ligand interactions, upregulation of cellular adhesion molecule expression, changes in avidity of adhesion molecules, shedding of ligands from the cell surface, and response of the leukocyte to chemoattractant factors (reviewed in refs. *139* and *140*). Cytokines and chemokines play key roles in regulating these processes. In allergic disease, most studies have focused on eosinophil and lymphocyte migration through vascular endothelium. Neutrophils accumulate at tissue sites within the first 6–8 h after allergen challenge *(141)* but are relatively sparse at later time points, and they are typically not increased during ongoing natural allergen exposure *(13,108,142)*.

Expression of endothelial ICAM-1 and E-selectin are most prominently induced in vitro by TNFα and IL-1β *(49–52,109,143,144)*. Expression of endothelial VCAM-1, which promotes the selective recruitment of eosinophils at sites of allergic inflammation *(49,145,146)*, is also induced in vitro by TNFα and to a lesser extent IL-1β *(49,50)*. VCAM-1 is also selectively upregulated, though to a lesser extent than by TNFα or IL-1, by the Th2 cytokines IL-4 and IL-13 *(40,147,148)*. This selective upregulation is also markedly potentiated by either TNF-α or IL-1β *(38–40,147)*. Hence, at least four cytokines work in combination to upregulate VCAM-1 at sites of allergic inflammation. The kinetics of expression of VCAM-1 on cultured human vascular endothelial cells (HUVEC) are relatively rapid with IL-1 (with a peak at 4 h) and relatively slow with IL-4 or IL-13 (with a peak at 16 h) *(147)*.

Studies of adhesion molecule expression in endobronchial or nasal biopsies obtained from allergic subjects before and after allergen challenge have yielded conflicting results. Bentley et al. *(125)* did not find a significant increase in tissue staining for ICAM-1, E-selectin, or VCAM-1 24 h after allergen bronchial challenge. This may reflect a lack of induction of these molecules or baseline upregulation owing to ongoing inflammation. Other studies have reported upregulation of VCAM-1, ICAM-1, and E-selectin in chronic asthma *(129,149)* and nasal polyposis *(150)*. Montefort et al. *(108)* found increased mucosal expression of ICAM-1 and VCAM-1 but not E-selectin in nasal biopsies from subjects with perennial allergic rhinitis. Lee et al. *(151)* found increased expression of VCAM-1 and E-selectin in lamina propria vessels 24 h after nasal allergen challenge, and the percentage of vessels expressing VCAM-1 correlated with the number of eosinophils present. In this study, ICAM-1 was found to be expressed in normal controls and allergic subjects prior to allergen challenge. Increased ICAM-1 expression on nasal epithelium is also a characteristic feature of allergic inflammation which persists even when other features of inflammation are relatively minimal *(152–154)*.

The role of adhesion molecules in allergen-induced eosinophil recruitment has also been studied in vivo in animals using anti-adhesion molecule blocking monoclonal antibodies. In monkeys, Wegner et al. *(115,116,130)* showed that anti-ICAM-1 antibody but not anti-E-selectin antibody blocked airway hyperreactivity and bronchoalveolar eosinophilia after allergen challenge *(131)*. In allergen-sensitized guinea pigs and sheep, anti-VLA-4 (very late activation antigen-4) monoclonal antibody (MAb) blocked allergen-induced increased bronchial hyperreactivity and bronchoalveolar lavage eosinophilia *(132,133)*.

To date, there has been little investigation of the potential of chemokines to upregulate endothelial adhesion molecules.

SUMMARY OF CELLS AND CYTOKINES INVOLVED IN ALLERGIC INFLAMMATION

In the mildest form of allergic disease, allergen exposure is intermittent, and the inflammatory response within the target tissue has time to resolve prior to a subsequent exposure to allergen. Hence, the target tissue shows little or no evidence of an inflammatory cell infiltrate and essentially no cytokine production. In the absence of sustained allergen exposure, allergic inflammation and local cytokine production probably subside within a few days.

Most of our knowledge of the allergic cytokine cascade comes from biopsy and lavage studies performed on mildly allergic subjects 6–24 h after allergen challenge. The timing of these studies corresponds to the early and intermediate points during late-phase allergic responses. Allergic subjects generally show minimal evidence of inflammation and low basal levels of T-lymphocyte or eosinophil infiltration and low levels of Th2 cytokine production in the target organ in placebo-challenged sites. Studies in the skin *(5)*, lungs *(9)*, and nasal mucosa *(6)* have yielded similar results.

Cytokines such as IL-4, IL-5, IL-6, and TNF-α are probably released within minutes of allergen challenge, since these cytokines are stored preformed in mast cell granules. In contrast, macrophages, B-cells, and T-cells do not store appreciable preformed TNFα bioactivity *(99)*. Allergen-triggered mast cell release of TNFα promotes the rapid upregulation of endothelial adhesion molecules, including ICAM-1, P- and E-selectin, and VCAM-1. Animal experiments suggest a pivotal role for TNF-α in leukocyte recruitment at sites of allergen challenge *(45,47)*. The concurrent release of preformed IL-4 further promotes the selective upregulation of VCAM-1 and creates a cytokine milieu favoring Th2 T lymphocyte development. Allergen crosslinking of IgE via FcεRI on mast cells also induces de novo synthesis of multiple cytokine mRNA species *(35,99,102,103)*. IL-1 release, mediated primarily by FcεRII-dependent activation of macrophages and monocytes, also occurs within hours of allergen exposure *(56)*. Its roles in the generation of allergic inflammation are overlapping with those of TNF-α.

The mechanism whereby CD4[+] Th2 T lymphocytes infiltrate sites of allergen exposure has not been carefully studied. It has been speculated that VLA-4/VCAM-1-mediated adhesion may play a role in this process *(130)*. Allergen-induced activation of CD4[+] T lymphocytes may upregulate VLA-4 expression or VLA-4 avidity for VCAM-1, thereby promoting their selective accumulation at sites of allergic inflammation. Local accumulation is also enhanced by elaboration of the C-C chemokines and LCF (IL-16), which promote T lymphocyte chemotaxis *(67,155)*.

By mechanisms that are still unknown, allergen triggering also results in epithelial cytokine and chemokine production. These effects are most likely indirect, since bronchial epithelial cells do not bind IgE but produce TNF-α after anti-IgE triggering of lung explants in vitro *(156)*. In vitro evidence suggests a role for IL-1 and possibly TNFα in inducing epithelial cytokine and chemokine production. As previously discussed, nasal and airway epithelium produce abnormal quantities of GM-CSF, IL-6, IL-8, and several chemokines in allergic subjects.

The late phase of the allergic response typically begins 3–6 h after allergen exposure and is heralded by the appearance of infiltrating inflammatory cells. Neutrophils appear within this time frame, probably promoted by upregulation of the vascular adhesion molecules ICAM-1 and E-selectin and epithelial-cell production of C-X-C chemokines. A critical feature of this process involves the production of cytokines and chemokines that promote mast cell mediator release, activation of eosinophils, and influx of inflammatory cells. Beyond the first few hours, the inflammatory cells are mostly monocytes, lymphocytes, eosinophils, and metachromatic cells. These leukocytes accumulate in response to upregulation of the adhesion molecules ICAM-1 and VCAM-1 and the local production of several C-C chemokines. Each of these cell types is induced to produce cytokines at the site. The predominant cytokines are the Th2 cytokines and the proinflammatory cytokines TNF-α, IL-1, and IL-6. Consequences of the persistence of late-phase allergic inflammation are the development of structural and functional changes in allergic tissues, including subepithelial fibrosis and hyperplastic tissue formation and the development of bronchial hyperreactivity (reviewed in ref. *157*).

Jordana, Denburg, and colleagues *(32,111,112,158)* have hypothesized that cytokine production by structural airway cells, such as epithelial cells and fibroblasts, represents a key factor in the perpetuation of chronic allergic inflammation. This process may become independent of allergen sensitization and therefore self-sustaining. The mechanism of this nonallergic form of chronic allergic inflammation, however, remains unknown. Once the tissue becomes deranged, it can probably be triggered by a variety of noxious stimuli, such as air pollutants or viral infection.

Nasal polyps obtained from subjects with chronic hyperplastic sinusitis (CHS/NP) have served as a useful model for studying chronic allergic inflammation. The polyp mucosa typically shows a chronic mononuclear cell infiltration with increased numbers of eosinophils, metachromatic cells, and T-lymphocytes *(15)*. The profile of cytokine mRNA species present in nasal polyps depends on the allergic status of the patient *(16)*. Approximately 50% of patients with CHS/NP have no evidence of IgE-mediated allergy despite prominent nasal polyp eosinophilia. In the subjects with positive allergy skin tests ("allergic CHS/NP"), there is evidence for increased expression of the Th2 cytokine profile, including IL-4, IL-5, IL-3, GM-CSF, and IL-13 *(15,16,72)*. In contrast, the cytokine profile of the "nonallergic CHS/NP" subjects shows increased expression of IL-3, GM-CSF, and IFN-γ *(15,16)*. Both allergic and nonallergic CHS/NP polyps show increased expression of TNF-α and IL-1β mRNA[+] cells and endothelial VCAM-1 *(72)*. In contrast to allergen challenge studies *(5,6,9)*, the density of Th2 mRNA-positive cells in allergic CHS/NP polyps does not correlate with the density of tissue eosinophils. This is consistent with a chronic "buildup" of eosinophilic inflammation that may be independent of allergen. Furthermore, the eosinophilia may be a reflection of cytokine production by infiltrating inflammatory cells, including eosinophils, that have been shown to produce GM-CSF, TNF-α, and possibly IL-3 in nasal polyps *(3,44)*. Hence, in chronic allergic inflammation, the density of tissue eosinophilia may be less dependent on influx and more dependent on local chemokine and cytokine production, which promotes their retention in the tissue and prolongs their survival.

A striking relationship has been found between the density of endothelial VCAM-1 expression and the density of TNF mRNA[+] cells in nasal polyps *(72)*. This is consistent with animal studies showing TNF-α to be a major cytokine controlling allergen-induced inflammatory cell infiltration (45). This raises the possibility that TNF-α may be necessary to sustain eosinophilia in chronic allergic inflammation. Other investigators have found that nasal polyp epithelium is an important source of GM-CSF, and increased numbers of RANTES mRNA[+] inflammatory cells have also been found in nasal polyps (72). Thus, we speculate that as allergic inflammation becomes more chronic, epithelial cells, eosinophils, and other inflammatory cells become more prominent contributors to local cytokine and chemokine production.

SUMMARY

We have only begun to unravel the complexities of cytokine/chemokine elaboration and its effects in chronic allergic inflammation (Tables 1 and 2). Many cytokines and chemokines other than those discussed above undoubtedly also participate. The interplay between allergen, mast cells, inflammatory cells, and structural cells needs further study. More and more evidence is accumulating to implicate structural cells, such as epithelial cells as important contributors to cytokine and chemokine production in chronic allergic inflammation. In the chronic state, their production may be independent of allergen and driven by as yet undefined stimuli.

REFERENCES

1. Xing Z, Braciak T, Ohkawara Y, Sallenave J, Foley R, Sime P, Jordana M, Graham F, Gauldie J (1996) Gene transfer for cytokine functional studies in the lung: the multifunctional role of GM-CSF in pulmonary inflammation. J Leukocyte Biol 59:481–488.
2. Moqbel R, Hamid Q, Ying S, Barkans J, Hartnell A, Tsicopoulos A, Wardlaw AJ, Kay AB (1991) Expression of mRNA and immunoreactivity for the granulocyte/macrophage colony-stimulating factor in activated human eosinophils. J Exp Med 174:749–752.
3. Ohno I, Lea R, Rinotto S, Marshall J, Denburg J, Dolovich J, Gauldie J, Jordana M (1991) Granulocyte/macrophage colony-stimulating factor (GM-CSF) gene expression by eosinophils in nasal polyposis. Am J Respir Cell Mol Biol 5:505–510.
4. Gaga M, Frew AJ, Varney VA, Kay AB (1991) Eosinophil accumulation and T-lymphocyte infiltration in allergen-induced late phase skin reactions and classical delayed-type hypersensitivity. J Immunol 147:816–22.
5. Kay AB, Ying VS, Varney M, Gaga SR, Durham R, Moqbel R, Wardlaw AJ, Hamid QA (1991) Messenger RNA expression of cytokine gene cluster, IL-3, IL-4, IL-5 and GM-CSF in allergen-induced late phase cutaneous reactions in atopic subjects. J Exp Med 173:775–778.
6. Durham SR, Ying S, Varney VA, Jacobson MR, Sudderick RM, Mackay IS, Kay AB, Hamid QA (1992) Cytokine messenger RNA expression for IL-3, IL-4, IL-5, and granulocyte/macrophage-colony-stimulating factor in the nasal mucosa after local allergen provocation: relationship to tissue eosinophilia. J Immunol 148:2390–2394.
7. Varney V, Jaconsen M, Sudderick R, Robinson D, Irani A, Schwartz L, Mackay I, Kay A, Durham S (1992) Immunohistology of the nasal mucosa following allergen-induced rhinitis. Am Rev Respir Dis 146:170–176.
8. Ying S, Durham SR, Barkans J, et al. (1993) T cells are the principal source of interleukin-5 mRNA in allergen-induced rhinitis. Am J Respir Cell Mol Biol 9:356–360.
9. Bentley AM, Meng Q, Robinson DS, et al. (1993) Increases in activated T lymphocytes, eosinophils and cytokine mRNA expression for interleukin-5 and granulocyte/macrophage colony-stimulating factor in bronchial biopsies after allergen inhalation challenge in atopic asthmatics. Am J Respir Cell Mol Biol 8:35–42.
10. Hamid W, Azzawi M, Ying S, Moqbel R, Wardlaw AJ, Corrigan CJ, Bradley B, Durham SD, Collins JV, Jeffery PK, et al. (1991) Interleukin-5 in mRNA mucosal bronchial biopsies from asthmatic subjects. Int Arch Allergy Immunol 94:169–170.
11. Ying S, Durham SR, Jacobson MR, Rak S, Masuyama K, Lowhagen O, Kay AB, Hamid QA (1994) T lymphocytes and mast cells express messenger RNA for interleukin-4 in the nasal mucosa in allergen-induced rhinitis. Immunology 82:200–206.

12. Hamid Q, Azzawi M, Ying S, et al. (1991) Expression of mRNA for interleukin-5 in mucosal bronchial biopsies from asthma. J Clin Invest 87:1541–1546.
13. Robinson DS, Hamid Q, Ying S, et al. (1992) Predominant TH2-line bronchoalveolar T-lymphocyte population in atopic asthma. N Engl J Med 326:298–304.
14. Hamid Q, Boguniewicz M, Leung DY (1994) Differential in situ cytokine gene expression in acute versus chronic atopic dermatitis. J Clin Invest 94:870–876.
15. Hamilos DL, Leung DYM, Wood R, et al. (1993) Chronic hyperplastic sinusitis: association of tissue eosinophilia with mRNA expression of granulocyte-macrophage colony-stimulating factor and interleukin-3. J Allergy Clin Immunol 92:39–48.
16. Hamilos DL, Leung DYM, Wood R, Cunningham L, Bean DK, Yasruel Z, Schotman E, Hamid Q (1995) Evidence for distinct cytokine expression in allergic versus nonallergic chronic sinusitis. J Allergy Clin Immunol 96:537–544.
17. Nagata M, Sedgwick J, Busse W (1995) Differential effects of granulocyte-macrophage colony-stimulating factor on eosinophil and neutrophil superoxide anion generation. J Immunol 155 (10):4948–4954.
18. Sedgwick J, Quan S, Calhoun W, Busse W (1995) Effect of interleukin-5 and granulocyte-macrophage colony stimulating factor on in vitro eosinophil function: comparison with airway eosinophils. J Allergy Clin Immunol 96(3):375–385.
19. Resnick M, Weller P (1993) Mechanisms of eosinophil recruitment. Am J Respir Cell Biol 8:349–355.
20. Owen W Jr, Rothenberg ME, Silberstein DS, Gasson JC, Stenens RL, Austen KF, Soberman RJ (1987) Regulation of human eosinophil viability, density and function by granulocyte macrophage colony-stimulating factor in the presence of 3T3 fibroblasts. J Exp Med 166:129.
21. Rothenberg MW, Owen WF, et al. (1987) Eosinophils co-cultured with endothelial cells have increased survival and functional properties. Science 137:645–647.
22. Rothenberg MW, Owen WF, et al. (1988) Human eosinophils have prolonged survival, enhanced functional properties and become hypodense when exposed to human interleukin-3. J Clin Invest 81:1986–1992.
23. Stankova J, Rola-Plexzczinski M, Dubois C (1995) Granulocyte-macrophage colony-stimulating factor increases 5-lipoxygenase gene transcription and protein expression in human neutrophils. Blood 85:3719–3726.
24. Ottonello L, Morone M, Dapino P, Dallegri F (1995) Cyclic AMP-elevating agents down-regulate the oxidative burst induced by granulocyte-macrophage colony-stimulating factor (GM-CSF) in adherent neutrophils. Clin Exp Immunol 101:502–506.
25. McCain R, Dessypris E, Christman J (1993) Granulocyte/macrophage colony-stimulating factor stimulates human polymorphonuclear leukocytes to produce interleukin-8 in vitro. Am J Respir Cell Mol Biol 8:28–34.
26. Ren Y, Savill J (1995) Proinflammatory cytokines potentiate thrombospondin-mediated phagocytosis of neutrophils undergoing apoptosis. J Immunol 154:2366–2374.
27. Bratton D, Hamid Q, Boguniewicz M, Doherty D, Kailey J, Leung D (1995) Granulocyte macrophage colony-stimulating factor contributes to enhanced monocyte survival in chronic atopic dermatitis. J Clin Invest 95:211–218.
28. Broide DH, Firestein GS (1991) Endobronchial allergen challenge in asthma: demonstration of cellular source of granulocyte macrophage colony-stimulating factor by in situ hybridization. J Clin Invest 88:1048–1053.
29. Sousa AR, Poston RN, Lane SJ, Nakhosteen JA, Lee TH (1993) Detection of GM-CSF in asthmatic bronchial epithelium and decrease by inhaled corticosteroids. Am Rev Respir Dis 147:1557–1561.
30. Walker C, Virchow JC, Bruijnzeel PLB, Blaser K (1991) T cell subsets and their soluble products regulate eosinophilia in allergic and non allergic asthma. J Immunol 146:1829–1835.
31. Broide DH, Paine MM, Firestein GS (1992) Eosinophils express interleukin 5 and granulocyte macrophage-colony stimulating factor mRNA at sites of allergic inflammation in asthmatics. J Clin Invest 80:1414–1424.
32. Jordana M, Vancheri C, Ohtoshi T, et al. (1989) Hemopoietic function of the micro environment in chronic airway inflammation. Agents Actions 28:85–95.
33. Bradding P, Feather IH, Howarth PH, Mueller R, Roberts JA, Britten K, Bews JPA, Hunt TC, Okayama Y, Heusser CH, Bullock GR, Church MK, Holgate ST (1992) Interleukin-4 is localized to and released by human mast cells. J Exp Med 176:1381–1386.

34. Bradding P, Roberts JA, Britten KM, Montefort S, Djukanovic R, Howarth PH, Holgate ST (1994) Interleukins (IL)-4, -5, -6 and TNF α in normal and asthmatic airways: evidence for the human mast cell as an important source of these cytokines. Am Rev Respir Cell Mol Biol 10:471–480.

35. Okayama Y, Petit-Frere C, Kassel O, Semper A, Quint D, Tunon-de-Lara MJ, Bradding P, Holgate ST, Church MK (1995) Ig-E-dependent expression of mRNA for IL-4 and IL-5 in human lung mast cells. J Immunol 155:1796–1808.

36. Gordon JR, Post T, Schulman ES, Galli SJ (1991) Characterization of mouse mast cell TNF-α induction in vitro and cells containing TNF-α. FASEB J 5:A1009.

37. Ohkawara Y, Yamauchi K, Tanno Y, et al. (1992) Human lung mast cells and pulmonary macrophages produce tumor necrosis factor-α in sensitized lung tissue after IgE receptor triggering. Am J Respir Cell Mol Biol 7:385–392.

38. Schleimer RP, Sterbinsky SA, Kaiser J, Bickel C, Klunk D, Tomioka K, Newman W, Luscinskas FW, Gimbrone MJ, McIntyre BW, Bochner BS (1992) Interleukin-4 induces adherence of human eosinophils and basophils but not neutrophils to endothelium: association with expression of VCAM-1. J Immunol 148:1086–1092.

39. Moser R, Fehr J, Bruijnzeel PLB (1992) IL-4 controls the selective endothelium-driven transmigration of eosinophils from allergic individuals. J Immunol 149:1432–1438.

40. Iademarco MF, Barks JL, Dean DC (1995) Regulation of vascular cell adhesion molecule-1 expression by IL-4 and TNF-α in cultured endothelial cells. J Clin Invest 95:264–271.

41. Gosset P, Tsicopoulis A, Wallaert B, Joseph M, Capron A, Tonnel AB (1992) Tumor necrosis factor-α and interleukin-6 production by human mononuclear phagocytes from allergic asthmatics after IgE-dependent stimulation. Am Rev Respir Dis 146:768–774.

42. Gosset P, Lassalle P, Tonnell AB, et al. (1988) Production of an IL-1 inhibitory factor by human alveolar macrophages from normal subjects and allergic asthmatic subjects. Am Rev Resp Dis 138:40–46.

43. Cembryznska-Nowak M, Szklarz E, Inglot AD, Teodoczyk-Injeyan JA (1993) Elevated release of tumor mecrosis factor-α interferon-γ by bronchoalveolar leukocytes from patients with bronchial asthma. Am Rev Respir Dis 147:291.

44. Finotto S, Ohno I, Marshall JS, Gauldie J, Denburg JA, Dolovich J, Clark DA, Jordana M (1994) TNF-α production by eosinophils in upper airways inflammation (nasal polyposis). J Immunol 153:2278–2289.

45. Lukacs NW, Strieter RM, Chenuse SW, Widmer M, Kunkel SL (1995) TNF-α mediates recruitment of neutrophils and eosinophils during airway inflammation. J Immunol 154:5411–5417.

46. Lukacs NW, Streieter RM, Chensue SW, Kunkel SL (1994) Interleukin-4-dependent pulmonary eosinophil infiltration in a murine model of asthma. Am J Respir Cell Mol Biol 10:526–532.

47. Wershil BK, Wang ZS, Gordon JR, Galli SJ (1991) Recruitment of neutrophils during IgE-depednent cutaneous late phase responses in the mouse is mast cell dependent: partial inhibition of the reaction with antiserum against tumor necrosis factor-α. J Clin Invest 87:446–453.

48. Moser R, Schleiffenbaum B, Groscurth P, Fehr J (1989) Interleukin 1 and tumor necrosis factor stimulate human vascular endothelial cells to promote transendothelial neutrophil passage. J Clin Invest 83:444.

49. Bochner BS, Luskinskas FW, Gimbrone MA, et al. (1991) Adhesion of human basophils, eosinophils, and neutrophils to interleukin-1-activated human vascular endothelial cells: Contribution of endothelial cell adhesion molecules. J Exp Med 173:1553–1556.

50. Bochner BS, Undem BJ, Lichtenstein LM (1994) Immunological aspects of allergic asthma. Annu Rev Immunol 12:295–335.

51. Wellicome SM, Thornhill MH, Pitzalis C, et al. (1990) A monoclonal antibody that detects a novel antigen on endothelial cells that is induced by tumor necrosis factor, IL-1, or lipopolysaccharide. J Immunol 144:2558–2565.

52. Groves RW, Ross E, Barker JNWN, et al. (1992) Effect of in-vivo interleukin-1 on adhesion molecule expression in normal human skin. J Invest Dermatol 98:384–387.

53. Marini M, Soloperto M, Mezzetti M, Fasoli A, Mattoli S (1991) Interleukin-1 binds to specific receptors on human bronchial epithelial cells and upregulates granulocyte/macrophage colony-stimulating factor synthesis and release. Am J Respir Cell Mol Biol 4:519–524.

54. Marini M, Vittori E, Hollemborg J, Mattoli S (1992) Expression of the potent inflammatory cytokines, granulocyte-macrophage-colony-stimulating factor and interleukin-6 and interleukin-8, in bronchial epithelial cells of patients with asthma. J Allergy Clin Immunol 89:1001–1009.

55. Tomita K, Tanigawa T, Yajima H, Fukutani K, Matsumoto Y, Tanaka Y, Sasaki T (1995) Identification and characterization of monocyte subpopulations from patients with bronchial asthma. J Allergy Clin Immunol 96:230–238.

56. Borish L, Mascali JJ, Rosenwasser LJ (1991) IgE-dependent cytokine production by human peripheral blood mononuclear phagocytes. J Immunol 146:63–67.

57. Gosset P, Malaquin F, Delneste Y, Wallaert B, Carpon A, Joseph M, Tonnell A-B (1993) Interleukin-6 and interleukin-1α production is associated with antigen-induced late nasal response. J Allergy Clin Immunol 92:878–890.

58. Linden M, Greiff L, Andersson M, Svensson C, Akerlund A, Bendes M, Andersson E, Persson CGA (1995) Nasal cytokines in common cold and allergic rhinitis. Clin Exp Allergy 25:166–172.

59. Gosset P, Tsicopoulos A, Wallaert B, Vannimenus C, Joseph M, Tonnel AB, Capron A (1991) Increased secretion of tumor necrosis factor alpha and interleukin-6 by alveolar macrophages consecutive to the development of the late asthmatic reaction. J Allergy Clin Immunol 88:561–571.

60. Broide DH, Lotz M, Cuomo AJ, Coburn DA, Federman EC, Wasserman SI (1992) Cytokines in symptomatic asthma airways. J Allergy Clin Immunol 89:958–967.

61. Okada S, Inoue H, Yamauchi K, Iijima H, Ohkawara Y, Takishima T, Shirato K (1995) Potential role of interleukin-1 in allergen-induced late asthmatic reactions in guinea pigs: suppressive effect of interleukin-1 receptor antagonist on late asthmatic reaction. J Allergy Clin Immunol 95:1236–1245.

62. Sim TC, Grant JA, Hilsmeier KA, Fuquda Y, Alam R (1994) Proinflammatory cytokines in nasal secretions of allergic subjects after antigen challenge. Am J Resp Crit Care Med 149:339–344.

63. Vercelli D, Jabara HH, Arai K, Yokota T, Geha RS (1989) Endogenous interleukin 6 plays an obligatory role in interleukin 4-dependent human IgE synthesis. Eur J Immunol 19:1419–1424.

64. Shapira SK, Vercelli D, Jabara HH, Fu SM, Geha RS (1992) Molecular analysis of the induction of immunoglobulin E synthesis in human B cells by interleukin 4 and engagement of CD40 antigen. J Exp Med 175:289–292.

65. Fahy JV, Kim KW, Liu J, Boushey HA (1995) Prominent neutrophilic inflammation in sputum from subjects with asthma exacerbation. J Allergy Clin Immunol 95:843–852.

66. Yokoyama A, Kohno N, Fujina S, Hamada H, Inque Y, Fujioka S, Ishida S, Hiwada K (1995) Circulating interleukin-6 levels in patients with bronchial asthma. Am J Respir Crit Care Med 151:1354–1358.

67. Schall TJ, Bacon KB (1994) Chemokines, leukocyte trafficking and inflammation. Current Opin Immunol 6:865–873.

68. Alam R, Stafford S, Forsythe P, et al. (1993) RANTES is a chemotactic and activating factor for human eosinophils. J Immunol 150:3442–3447.

69. Davies RJ, Wang JH, Trigg CJ, Devalia JL (1995) Expression of granulocyte/macrophage-colony-stimulating factor, interleukin-8 and RANTES in the bronchial epithelium of mild asthmatics is down-regulated by inhaled beclomethasone dipropionate. Int Arch Allergy Immunol 107:428–429.

70. Stellato C, Beck LA, Gorgone GA, Proud D, Schall TJ, Ono SJ, Lichtenstein LM, Schleimer RP (1995) Expression of the chemokine RANTES by a human bronchial epithelial cell line. Modulation by cytokines and glucocorticoids. J Immunol 155:410–418.

71. Ying S, Tabora-Barata L, Meng Q, Humbert M, Kay AB (1995) The kinetics of allergen-induced transcription of messenger RNA for monocyte chemotactic protein-3 and RANTES in the skin of human atopic subjects: relationship to eosinophil, T cell and macrophage recruitment. J Exp Med 181:2153–2159.

72. Hamilos DL, Leung DYM, Wood R, Bean DK, Song YL, Schotman E, Hamid Q (1996) Eosinophil infiltration in nonallergic chronic hyperplastic sinusitis with nasal polyposis (CHS/NP) is associated with endothelial VCAM-1 upregulation and expression of TNF-α. Am J Respir Cell Mol Biol 15:443–450.

73. Noso N, Proost P, Van Damme J, Schroder JM (1994) Human monocyte chemotactic proteins-2 and 3 (MCP-2 and MCP-3) attract human eosinophils and desensitize the chemotactic responses towards RANTES. Biochem Biophys Res Communs 200:1470–1476.

74. Loetscher P, Seitz M, Clark-Lewis I, Baggiolini M, Moser B (1994) Monocyte chemotactic proteins MCP-1, MCP-2 and MCP-3 are major attractants for human CD4[+] and CD8[+] T lymphocytes. FASEB J 8:1055–1060.

75. Uguccioni M, D'Apuzzo M, Loetscher M, Dewald B, Baggiolini M (1995) Actions of the chemotactic cytokines MCP-1, MCP-2, MCP-3, RANTES, MIP-1 alpha and MIP-1 beta on human monocytes. Eur J Immunol 25:64–68.

76. Dahinden CA, Geiser T, Brunner T, von Tschamer V, Caput D, Ferrara P, Minty A, Baggiolini M (1994) Monocyte chemotactic protein 3 is a most effective basophil- and eosinophil-activating chemokine. J Exp Med 179:751–756.

77. Becker S, Quay J, Koren HS, Haskill JS (1994) Constitutive and stimulated MCP-1, GRO alpha, beta, and gamma expression in human airway epithelium and bronchoalveolar macrophages. Am J Physiology 266(Pt 1):L278–L286.

78. Lukacs NW, Kunkel SL, Allen R, Evanoff HL, Shaklee CL, Cherman JS, Burdick MD, Strieter RM (1995) Stimulus and cell-specific expression of C-X-C and C-C chemokines by pulmonary stromal cell populations. Am J Physiology 268(Pt 1):L856–L861.

79. Lukacs NW, Streiter RM, Elner V, Evanoff HL, Burdick MD, Kunkel SL (1995) Production of chemokines, interleukin-8 and monocyte chemoattractant protein-1 during monocyte:endothelial cell interactions. Blood 86:2757–2773.

80. Lukacs NW (1994) Intercellular adhesion molecule-1 mediates the expression of monocyte-derived MIP-1 alpha during monocyte-endothelial cell interactions. Blood 83:1174–1178.

81. Lukacs NW, Streiter RM, Shaklee CL, Chensue SW, Kunkel SL (1995) Macrophage inflammatory protein-1 influences eosinophil recruitment in antigen-specific airway inflammation. Eur J Immunol 25:245–251.

82. Sim TC, Reece LM, Hilsmeier KA, Grant JA, Alam R (1995) Secretion of chemokines and other cytokines in allergen-induced nasal responses: inhibition by topical steroid treatment. Am J Respir Crit Care Med 152:927–933.

83. Rothenburg ME, Luster AD, Lilly CM, Drazen JM, Leder P (1995) Constitutive and allergen-induced expression of eotaxin mRNA in the guinea pig lung. J Exp Med 181:1211–1216.

84. Jose PJ, Griffiths-Johnson DA, Collins PD, Walsh DT, Moqbel R, Totty NF, Truong O, Hsuan JJ, Williams TJ (1994) Eotaxin: a potent eosinophil chemoattractant cytokine detected in a guinea pig model of allergic airways inflammation. J Exp Med 179:881–887.

85. Holgate ST (1993) Asthma: past, present and future. Eur Respir J 6:1507–1520.

86. Erger A, Casale T (1995) Interleukin-8 is a potent mediator of eosinophil chemotaxis through endothelium and epithelium. Am J Physiol 268(Pt 1):L117–L122.

87. Schweizer R, Welmers B, Raaijmakers J, Zanen P, Lammers J, Koenderman L (1994) RANTES- and interleukin-8-induced responses in normal human eosinophils: effects of priming with interleukin-5. Blood 83:3697–704.

88. Douglass J, Dhami D, Gurr C, Bulpitt M, Shute J, Howarth P, Lindley I, Church M, Holgate S (1994) Influence of interleukin-8 challenge in the nasal mucosa in atopic and nonatopic subjects. Am J Respir Crit Care Med 150:1108–1113.

89. Xiu Q, Fujimura M, Nomura M, Saito M, Matsuda T, Akao N, Kondo K, Matsushima K (1995) Bronchial hyperresponsiveness and airway neutrophil accumulation induced by interleukin-8 and the effect of the thromboxane A2 antagonist S-1452 in guinea-pigs. Clin Exper Allergy 25:51–59.

90. Wang J, Trigg C, Devalia J, Jordan S, Davies R (1994) Effect of inhaled beclomethasone dipropionate on expression of proinflammatory cytokines and activated eosinophils in the bronchial epithelium of patients with mild asthma. J Allergy Clin Immunol 94(Pt 1):1025–1034.

91. Leonard EJ, Yoshimura T (1990) Neutrophil attractant/activation protein-1 (NAP-1 [interleukin-8]). Am J Respir Cell Mol Biol 2:479–486.

92. Miyamasu M, Hirai K, Takahashi Y, Iida M, Yamaguchi M, Koshino T, Takaishi T, Morita Y, Ohta K, Kasahara T (1995) Chemotactic agonists induce cytokine generation in eosinophils. J Immunol 154:1339–1349.

93. Chung SW, Wong PMC, Shen-Ong G, Ruscetti S, Ishizaka T, Eaves CJ (1986) Production of granulocyte-macrophage colony-stimulating factor by Abelson virus-induced tumorigenic mast cell lines. Blood 68:1074–1081.

94. Gordon JR, Galli SJ (1991) Release of preformed and newly synthesized tumor necrosis factor alpha (TNF-α)/cachectin by mouse mast cells stimulated by the FceRI. A mechanism of the sustained action of mast cell-derived TNF-α during IgE-dependent biological responses. J Exp Med 174:103–107.

95. Steffen M, Abboud M, Potter GK, Yung YP, Moore MAS (1989) Presence of tumor necrosis factor or a related factor in human basophils/mast cells. Immunology 66:445–450.

96. Klein LM, Lavker RM, Matis WL, Murphy GF (1989) Degranulation of human mast cells induces an endothelial antigen central to leukocyte adhesion. Proc Natl Acad Sci USA 86:8972–8976.

97. Walsh LJ, Trinchieri G, Waldorf HA, Whitaker D, Murphy GF (1991) Human dermal mast cells contain and release tumor necrosis factor alpha, which induces endothelial leukocyte adhesion molecule 1. Proc Natl Acad Sci USA 88:4220–4224.

98. Benyon RC, Bissonnette EY, Befus AD (1991) Tumor necrosis factor-alpha dependent cytotoxicity of human skin mast cells is enhanced by anti-IgE antibodies. J Immunol 147:2253–2258.

99. Gordon JR, Galli SJ (1990) Mast cells as a source of both preformed and immunologically inducible TNF-α/cachectin. Nature 346:274–276.

100. Bradding P, Feather IH, Wilson S, et al. (1993) Immunolocalization of cytokines in the nasal mucosa of normal and perennial rhinitic subjects. J Immunol 151:3852–3865.

101. Walsh LJ, Trinchieri G, Waldorf HA, Whitaker D, Murphy GF (1991) Human dermal mast cells contain and release tumor necrosis factor alpha, which induces endothelial leukocyte adhesion molecule-1. Proc Natl Acad Sci USA 88:4220–4224.

102. Burd PR, Thompson WC, Max EE, and Mills FC (1995) Activated mast cells produce interleukin 13. J Exp Med 181:1373–1830.

103. Galli SJ, Gordon JR, Wershil BK (1991) Cytokine production by mast cells and basophils. Current Opin Immunol 3:865–873.

104. Klein LM, Lavker RM, Matis WL, Murphy GF (1989) Degranulation of human mast cells induces an endothelial antigen central to leukocyte adhesion. Proc Natl Acad Sci USA 86:8972–8976.

105. Broide DH (1995) α4 integrin-induced cytokine production and eosinophil function. Springer Semin Immunopathol 16:405–415.

106. Costa JJ, Matossian K, Resnick MB, Beil WJ, Wong DTW, Gordon JR (1993) Human eosinophils can express the cytokines tumor necrosis factor-α and macrophage inflammatory protein-1α. J Clin Invest 91:2673.

107. Lim KG, Wan HC, Resnick M, Wong DT, Cruikshank WW, Kornfeld H, Center DM, Weller PF (1995) Human eosinophils release the lymphocyte and eosinophil active cytokines, RANTES and lymphocyte chemoattractant factor. Int Arch Allergy Immunol 107:342.

108. Montefort S, Feather IH, Wilson SJ, Haskard DO, Lee TH, Holgate ST, Howarts PH (1992) The expression of leukocyte-endothelial adhesion molecules is increased in perennial allergic rhinitis. Am J Respir Cell Mol Biol 7:393–398.

109. Schleimer RP, Rutledge BK (1986) Cultured human vascular endothelial cells acquire adhesiveness for leukocytes following stimulation with interleukin-1, endotoxin, and tumor-promoting phorbol esters. J Immunol 136:649–654.

110. Joseph M, Tonnel A-B, Torpier G, Capron A (1983) Involvement of immunoglobulin E in the secretory processes of alveolar macrophages from asthmatic patients. J Clin Invest 71:221–230.

111. Denburg JA, Gauldie J, Dolovich J, Ohtoshi T, Cox G, Jordana M (1991) Structural cell-derived cytokines in allergic inflammation. Int Arch Allergy Appl Immunol 94:127–132.

112. Dolovich J, Ohtoshi T, Jordana M, Gauldie J, Denburg J (1990) Nasal polyps: local inductive microenvironment in the pathogenesis of the inflammation. In: Mygind N, Pipkorm U, Ridah L, eds., Rhinitis and Asthma. Munksgaard, Copenhagen, pp. 233–241.

113. Ohnishi M, Rhuno J, Bienenstock J, Dolovich J, Denburg JA (1989) Hematopoietic growth factor production by cultured cells of human nasal polyp epithelial scrapings: kinetics, cell source, and relationship to clinical status. J Allergy Clin Immunol 83:1091–1100.

114. Tosi MF, Stark JM, Smith CW, Hamedani A, Gruenert DC, Infeld MD (1992) Induction of ICAM-1 expression on human airway epithelial cells by inflammatory cytokines: effects on neutrophil-epithelial cell adhesion. Am J Respir Cell Mol Biol 7:214–221.

115. Wegner CD, Gundel RH, Reilly P, Haynes N, Letts LG, Rothlein R (1990) Intercellular adhesion molecule-1 (ICAM-1) in the pathogenesis of asthma. Science 247:456–459.

116. Gundel RH, Wegner CD, Torcellini CA, Letts LG (1992) The role of intercellular adhesion molecule-1 in chronic airway inflammation. Clin Exp Allergy 22:569.

117. Nakajima S, Look DC, Roswit WT, Bragdon MJ, Holtzman MJ (1994) Selective differences in vascular endothelial versus airway epithelial T cell adhesion mechanisms. Am J Physiol 267:L422–L432.

118. Marini M, Vittori E, Hollemborg J, Mottoli S (1992) Expression of the potent inflammatory cytokines, granulocyte-macrophage-colony-stimulating factor, interleukin-6 and interleukin-8, in bronchial epithelial cells of patients with asthma. J Allergy Clin Immunol 89:1001–1009.

119. Soloperto M, Mattoso VL, Fasioli A, Mattoli S (1991) A chronical epithelial cell derived factor in asthma that promotes eosinophil action and survival as GM-CSF. Am J Physiol 260:L530–L538.

120. Kwon OJ, Jose PJ, Robbins RA, Schall TJ, Williams TJ, Barnes PJ (1995) Glucocorticoid inhibition of RANTES expression in human lung epithelial cells. Am J Respir Cell Mol Biol 12:488–496.

121. Belini A, Yoshimura H, Vittori E, Marini M, Mattoli S (1993) Bronchial epithelial cells of patients with asthma release chemoattractant factors for T lymphocytes. J Allergy Clin Immunol 92:412–424.

122. Coeffier E, Joseph D, Vargaftig BB (1994) Role of interleukin-5 in enhanced migration of eosinophils from airways of immunized guinea-pigs. Br J Pharmacol 113:749–756.

123. Schweizer RC, Welmers BA, Raaijmakers JA, Zanen P, Lammers JW, Koenderman L (1994) RANTES-and interleukin-8-induced responses in normal human eosinophils: effects of priming with interleukin-5. Blood 83:3697–3704.
124. Collins PD, Marleau S, Griffiths-Johnson DA, Jose PJ, Williams TJ (1995) Cooperation between interleukin-5 and the chemokine eotaxin to induce eosinophil accumulation in vivo. J Exp Med 182:1169–1174.
125. Bentley AM, Durham SR, Robinson DS, Menz G, Storz C, Cromwell O, Kay AB, Wardlaw AJ (1993) Allergens, IgE, mediators and inflammatory mechanisms. Expression of endothelial and leukocyte adhesion molecules intercellular adhesion molecule-1, E-selectin, and vascular cell adhesion molecule-1 in the bronchial mucosa in steady-state and allergen-induced asthma. J Allergy Clin Imunol 92:857–868.
126. Montefort S, Feather IH, Wilson SJ, Haskard DO, Lee TH, Holgate ST, Howarth PH (1992) The expression of leukocyte-endothelial adhesion molecules is increased in perennial allergic rhinitis. Am J Respir Cell Mol Biol 7:393–398.
127. Weller PF, Rand TH, Goelz SE, Chi-Rosso G, Lobb RR (1991) Human eosinophil adherance to vascular endothelium mediated binding to vascular cell adhesion molecule 1 and endothelial leukocyte adhesion molecule 1. Proc Natl Acad Sci. USA 88:7430.
128. Ebisawa M, Bochner BS, Georas SN, Schleimer RP (1992) Eosinophil transendothelial migration induced by cytokines. I. Role of endothelial and eosinophil adhesion molecules in IL-1β-induced transendothelial migration. J Immunol 149:4021–4028.
129. Ohkawara Y, Yamauchi K, Maruyama N, Hoshi H, Ohno I, Honma M, Tanno Y, Tamura G, Shirato K, Ohtani H (1995) In situ expression of the cell adhesion molecules in bronchial tissues from asthmatics with air flow limitation: in vivo evidence of VCAM-1/VLA-4 interaction in selective eosinophil infiltration. Am J Respir Cell Mol Biol 12:4–12.
130. Nakajima H, Sano H, Nishimura T, Yoshida S, Iwamoto I (1994) Role of vascular cell adhesion molecule 1/very late activation antigen 4 and intercellular adhesion molecule 1/lymphocyte function-associated antigen 1 in antigen-induced eosinophil and T cell recruitment into the tissue. J Exp Med 179:1145.
131. Gundel RH, Wegner CD, Torcellini CA, Clarke CC, Haynes N, Rothlein R, Smith CW, Letts LG (1991) Endothelial leukocyte adhesion molecule-1 mediates antigen-induced acute airway inflammation and late-phase airway obstruction in monkeys. J Clin Invest 88:1407–1411.
132. Abraham WM, Sielczak MW, Ahmed A, et al. (1994) α₄-integrins mediate antigen-induced late bronchial responses and prolonged airway hyperresponsiveness in sheep. J Clin Invest 93:776–787.
133. Pretolani M, et al. (1994) Antibody to VLA-4 prevents antigen-induced bronchial hyperreactivity and cellular infiltration in the guinea pig airways. J Exp Med 180:795–805.
134. Rand TH, Silberstein DS, Kornfeld H, Weller PF (1991) Human eosinophils express functional interleukin-2 receptors, J Clin Invest 88:825–832.
135. Rand TH, Cruikshank WW, Center DM, Weller PF (1991) CD4-mediated stimulation of human eosinophils: Lymphocyte chemoattractant factor and other CD4-binding ligands elicit eosinophil migration. J Exp Med 173:1521–1528.
136. Lopez AF, Sanderson CJ, Gamble JR, Campbell HD, Young IG, Vadas MA (1988) Recombinant human interleukin-5 is a selective activator of human eosinophil function. J Exp Med 167:219–224.
137. Kita H, Ohnishe T, Okubo Y, Weiler J, Abrams JS, Gleich GJ (1991) GM-CSF and IL-3 release from human peripheral blood eosinophils and neutrophils. J Exp Med 174:745–748.
138. Anwar ARE, Walsh GM, Moqbel RM, Kay AB, Wardlaw AJ (1993) Adhesion to fibronectin prolongs eosinophil survival. J Exp Med 177:839–843.
139. Baroody FM, Lee BJ, Lim MC, Bochner BS (1995) Implicating adhesion molecules in nasal allergic inflammation. Eur Arch Otorhinolaryngol 252(Suppl 1):S50–S58.
140. Butcher E (1991) Leukocyte-endothelial cell recognition: three (or more) steps to specificity and diversity. Cell 67:1033–1036.
141. Montefort S, Gratziou C, Goulding D, Polosa R, Haskard DO, Howarth PH, Holgate ST, Carroll MP (1994) Bronchial biopsy evidence for leukocyte infiltration and upregulation of leukocyte-endothelial cell adhesion molecules 6 hours after local allergen challenge of sensitized asthmatic airways. J Clin Invest 93:1411–1421.
142. Bentley A, Jacobson M, Cumberworth V, Barkans J, Moqbel R, Schwartz L, Irani A, Kay A, Durham S (1992) Immunohistology of the nasal mucosa in seasonal allergic rhinitis: increase in activated eosinophils and epithelial mast cells. J Allergy Clin Immunol 89:877–883.

143. Moser R, Schleiffenbaum B, Groscurth P, Fehr J (1989) Interleukin 1 and tumor necrosis factor stimulate human vascular endothelial cells to promote transendothelial neutrophil passage. J Clin Invest 83:444–455.

144. Luscinskas FW, Cybulsky MI, Kiely J-M, Peckins CS, Davis VM, Gimbrone MA Jr (1991) Cytokine-activated human endothelial monolayers support enhanced neutrophil transmigration via a mechanism involving both endothelial-leukocyte adhesion molecule-1 and intracellular adhesion molecule-1. J Immunol 146:1617–1625.

145. Walsh GM, Mermod J-J, Hartness A, Kay AB, Wardlaw AJ (1991) Human eosinophil, but not neutrophil, adherence to IL-1-stimulated human unbilical vascular endothelial cells is $\alpha4\beta1$ (very late antigen-4) dependent. J Immunol 146:3419–3423.

146. Dobrina A, Menegazzi R, Carlos TM, et al. (1991) Mechanisms of eosinophil adherence to cultures of vascular endothelial cells. Eosinophils bind to the cytokine-induced endothelial ligand vascular adhesion-1 via the very late activation antigen-4 integrin receptor. J Clin Invest 88:20–26.

147. Bochner BS, Klunk DA, Sterbinsky SA, Coffman RL, and Schleimer RP (1995) IL-13 selectively induces vascular cell adhesion molecule-1 expression in human endothelial cells. J Immunol 154:799–803.

148. Sironi M, Sciacca FL, Matteucci C, Conni M, Vecchi A, Bernasconi S, Minty A, Caput D, Ferrara P, Colotta F, Mantovani A (1994) Regulation of endothelial and mesothelial cell function by interleukin-13: Selective induction of vascular cell adhesion molecule-1 and amplification of interleukin-6 production. Blood 84:1913–1921.

149. Montefort S, Roche WR, Howarth PH, Djukanovic R, Gratziou C, Carroll M, Smith L, Britten KM, Haskard D, Lee TH, Holgate ST. Intercellular adhesion molecule-1 (ICAM-1) and endothelial leukocyte adhesion molecule-1 (ELAM-1) expression in the bronchial mucosa of normal and asthmatic subjects. Eur Respir J 5:815–823.

150. Jahnsen FL, Haraldsen G, Aanesen JP, Haye R, Brandtzaeg P (1995) Eosinophil infiltration is related to increased expression of vascular cell adhesion molecule-1 in nasal polyps. Am J Respir Mol Cell Biol 12:624–632.

151. Lee B-J, Naclerio RM, Bochner BS, Taylor RM, Lim MC, Baroody FM (1994) Nasal challenge with allergen upregulates the local expression of vascular endothelial adhesion molecules. J Allergy Clin Immunol 94:1006–1016.

152. Ciprandi G, Pronzato C, Ricca V, Passalacqua G, Bagnasco M, Canonica GW (1994) Allergen-specific challenge induces intercellular adhesion molecule 1 (ICAM-1 or CD54) on nasal epithelial cells in allergic subjects. Relationships with early and late inflammatory phenomenon. Am J Respir Crit Care Med 150:1653–1659.

153. Ciprandi G, Buscaglia S, Pesce GP, Pronzato C, Ricca V, Parmiani S, Bagnasco M, Canonica GW (1995) Miminal persistent inflammation is present at mucosal level in asymptomatic rhinitic patients with allergy due to mites. J Allergy Clin Immunol 96:971–979.

154. Canonica GW, Ciprandi G, Pesce GP, Buscaglia S, Paolieri F, Bagnasco M (1995) ICAM-1 on epithelial cells in allergic subjects: a hallmark of allergic inflammation. Int Arch Allergy Clin Immunol 107:99.

155. Berman JS, Weller PF (1992) Airways eosinophils and lymphocytes in asthma. Birds of a feather? Am Rev Respir Dis 145:1246–1248.

156. Ohkawara Y, Yamauchi K, Tanno Y, et al. (1992) Human lung mast cells and pulmonary macrophages produce tumor necrosis factor-α in sensitized lung tissue after IgE receptor triggering. Am J Respir Cell Mol Biol 7:385–392.

157. Leff AT (1994) Inflammatory mediation of airway hyperresponsiveness by granulocytes. The case for the eosinophil. Chest 106:1202–1208.

158. Otsuka H, Dolovich J, Richardson M, Bienenstock J, Denburg JA (1987) Metachromatic cell progenitors and specific growth and differentiation factors in human nasal mucosa and polyps. Am Rev Respir Dis 136:710–717.

159. Combadiere C, Ahuja SK, Murphy PM (1995) Cloning and functional expression of a human eosinophil CC chemokine receptor. J Biol Chem. 270:16,491–16,494.

160. Conlon K, Lloyd A, Chattopadhyay U, Lukacs N, Kunkel S, Schall T, Taub D, Morimoto C, Osborne J, Oppenheim J, et al. (1995) CD8+ and CD45RA+ human peripheral blood lymphocytes are potent sources of macrophage inflammatory protein 1 alpha, interleukin-8 and RANTES. Eur J Immunol 25:751–756.

161. Allavena P, Bianchi G, Zhou D, van Damme J, Jilek P, Sozzani S, Mantovani A (1994) Induction of natural killer cell migration by monocyte chemotactic protein-1, -2 and -3. Eur J Immunol 24:3233–3236.

162. Brieland JK, Flory CM, Jones ML, Miller GR, Remick DG, Warren JS, Fantone JC (1995) Regulation of monocyte chemoattractant protein-1 gene expression and secretion in rat pulmonary alveolar macrophages by lipopolysaccharide, tumor necrosis factor-alpha, and interleukin-1 beta. Am J Respir Cell Mol Biol 12:104–109.

163. Brown Z, Garritsen ME, Carley WW, Streiter RM, Kunkel SL, Westwick J (1994) Chemokine gene expression and secretion by cytokine-activated human microvascular endothelial cells. Differential regulation of monocyte chemoattractant protein-1 and interleukin-8 in response to interferon-gamma. Am J Pathol 145:913–921.

164. Minty A, Chalon P, Guillemot JC, Kaghad M, Liauzun P, Magazin M, Miloux B, Minty C, Ramond P, Vita N, et al. (1993) Molecular cloning of the MCP-3 chemokine gene and regulation of its expression. Eur Cytokine Network 4:99–100.

165. Proost P (1995) Chemical synthesis, purification and folding of the human monocyte chemotactic proteins MCP-2 and MCP-3 into biologically active chemokines. Cytokine 7:97–104.

166. Moser R, Fehr J, Olgiati L, Bruijnzeel PL (1992) Migration of primed human eosinophils across cytokine-activated endothelial cell monolayers. Blood 79:2937–2945.

167. Taub DD, Proost P, Murphy WJ, Anver M, Longo DL, van Damme J, Oppenheim JJ (1995) Monocyte chemotactic protein-1 (MCP-1), -2, and -3 are chemotactic for human T lymphocytes. J Clin Invest 95:1370–1376.

17

Hemopoietic Cytokines
Function, Receptor, and Signal Transduction

Hirokazu Kurata, MD
and Ken-ichi Arai, MD, PhD

GENERAL ASPECTS

Pleiotropism, Redundancy, and Modification

Cytokines regulate proliferation, differentiation, and function of cells in the immune as well as the hematopoietic systems *(1–3)*. They interact with more than one type of cell, have multiple biological activities, and act in synergistic or antagonistic manner with each other. Conversely, a single cell has receptors for multiple cytokines and is influenced by the cross talk of multiple cytokine networks. A single cytokine can act as both a positive and a negative signal, depending on the nature of the target cells. Furthermore, the effects of a cytokine are modified by multiple other cytokines.

The intercellular network between T-cells, B-cells, and hemopoietic cells can be exerted at both inducer and effector stages. The former includes the coordinated regulation of the expression of cytokines in the producer cells, and the latter corresponds the interaction of cytokines with receptors and signaling components in the target cells. Through these interactions, cytokine signals are enhanced, modified, or attenuated, and the allergic and inflammatory responses are controlled.

Constitutive and Inducible Hematopoiesis

All hemopoietic cells are produced continuously from self-renewing pluripotent hematopoietic stem cells in the bone marrow microenvironment (Fig. 1). These stem cells are usually in the resting G0 state but can be mobilized into a proliferative state under precise control mechanisms without immunological stimuli (constitutive hematopoiesis) *(1)* (Fig. 2). The developing hemopoietic cells are found in association with a complex stromal network containing

From: *Allergy and Allergic Diseases: The New Mechanisms and Therapeutics*
Edited by: J. A. Denburg © Humana Press Inc., Totowa, NJ

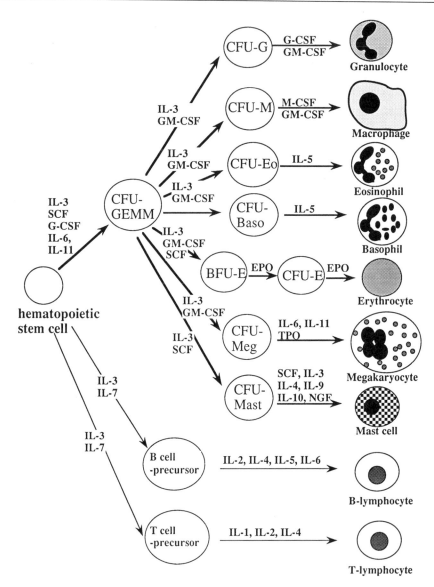

Fig. 1. Role of cytokines in the development of myeloid and lymphoid cells from multipotent hemopoietic stem cells. CFU, colony-forming unit; BFU, burst-forming unit.

macrophages, endothelial cells, fibroblasts, and adipocytes. Stromal cells may influence the growth and differentiation of pluripotent stem cells and committed progenitor cells, positively or negatively, through the production of cytokines or direct cell–cell interaction. In contrast, in inflammation, in which T-cells and macrophages play a major role, hematopoiesis is stimulated or regulated by the combination of multiple cytokines (inducible hematopoiesis) *(1)*.

Self-Renewal and Lineage-Commitment of Hemopoietic Stem Cells

The self-renewal and differentiation of hemopoietic stem cells and progenitors appear to be stochastic processes *(4)*, while survival and proliferation of the cells is regulated by cytokines (Fig. 1).

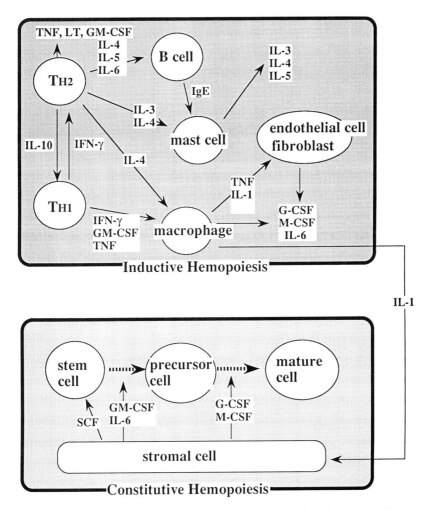

Fig. 2. Constitutive and inductive hemopoiesis. Constitutive hemopoiesis is supported by cytokines and cell–cell contact of stromal cells, whereas inductive hemopoiesis is stimulated by T-cells, macrophages, mast cells, and others during inflammatory responses.

The role of cytokines in lineage-commitment and proliferation was examined by the forced expression of human GM-CSF (granulocyte-macrophage colony-stimulating factor) receptor under the control of a universal (major histocompatibility complex [MHC]-class I) promoter using a transgenic mouse system *(5)*. The transgenic receptors were expressed in all the lineages and developmental stages of hemopoietic cells. The colony assay revealed that the proliferation of not only differentiated cells but also earlier progenitor cells, such as blast colony and granulocyte/erythrocyte/macrophage/megakaryocyte colony-forming unit (CFU-GEMM), was stimulated through the transgenic receptors, but that the lineage commitment of the progenitors was not significantly affected. Ogawa *(4)* classified cytokines based on their effects on different stages of target cells (Fig. 3); early-acting lineage-nonspecific factors, intermediate-acting lineage-nonspecific factors (interleukin-3 [IL-3], GM-CSF, IL-4), late-acting lineage-specific factors (erythropoietin [Epo], macrophage-CSF [M-CSF], IL-5, granulocyte-CSF [G-CSF], and thrombopoietin [Tpo]), and inhibitory cytokines (interferons [IFNs], tumor necrosis factor-α [TNF-α], transforming growth factor-β

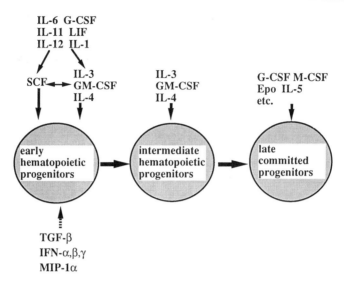

Fig. 3. Role of cytokines in the development of hemopoietic progenitors. Hemopoietic progenitors are differentially supported by several groups of cytokines *(4)*.

[TGF-β], and macrophage inhibitory protein-1α [MIP-1α]). The early-acting lineage nonspecific factors are classified into three subgroups: IL-3, GM-CSF, and IL-4; stem cell factor (SCF); IL-6, G-CSF, IL-11, leukemia inhibitory factor (LIF), and IL-12. Cytokines in different subgroups act synergistically in support of dormant murine hematopoietic progenitors *(4)*. The molecular mechanisms of their synergism remain to be clarified on the basis of analyses of signal transduction pathways.

INTERACTION BETWEEN CYTOKINE-PRODUCING CELLS AND EFFECTOR CELLS

Two Types of T Helper (Th) Cells (Th1 and Th2)

Two types of T-helper cell clones have been recognized in the murine system based on the pattern of cytokine production *(1,3,6)*. Th-1 cells produce IL-2 and IFN-γ, but do not produce IL-4, IL-5, or IL-10. In contrast, Th-2 cells produce IL-4, IL-5, and IL-10 but not IL-2 or IFN-γ. Both types produce IL-3 and GM-CSF, and they are derived from Th0 cells, which have the capacity to produce both Th1- and Th2-type cytokines. In contrast to murine T-cell clones, human T-cell clones seemed to produce cytokines in a manner similar to Th0 cells, including IL-2, IFN-γ, IL-3, GM-CSF, IL-4, IL-5, and IL-10. However, the human counterpart of the murine Th1 subset was demonstrated among T-cell clones derived from patients with inflammatory diseases *(7)*, whereas that of Th2 was established from allergic patients *(8)*.

Neutrophils, Eosinophils, and Macrophages

Four cytokines, including IL-3, GM-CSF, G-CSF, and M-CSF, stimulate production of neutrophils and macrophages from their precursor cells. Among them, G-CSF specifically acts on the neutrophil lineage, while M-CSF acts on the monocyte/macrophage lineage of cells. These cytokines also activate neutrophil functions, such as chemotaxis, phagocytosis, superoxide production, and tumoricidal activity *(9)*. GM-CSF, IL-3, and M-CSF activate macrophage functions, including phagocytosis, tumoricidal activity, antigen presentation, and cytokine production. Prostaglandin E_2 (PGE_2) secreted by macrophages is supposed to suppress macrophage functions and terminate the inflammatory response *(10)*.

Furthermore, in addition to IL-3 and GM-CSF, growth, differentiation, and functions of eosinophils are strongly stimulated by IL-5.

Stromal and Endothelial Cells

Stromal cells have been considered to be a group of nonhemopoietic cells organized into a hemopoietic microenvironment supporting hemopoiesis *(11)*. In vitro long-term bone marrow culture systems require absolutely the establishment of stromal cell layers for myelopoiesis *(12)* and lymphopoiesis *(13)*. Stromal cells regulate growth and differentiation of hematopoietic progenitors through direct cell–cell interactions, extracellular matrices, and secreted soluble mediators, such as GM-CSF, M-CSF, SCF, IL-6, and IL-7. In contrast, stromal cells are influenced by cytokines produced by hemopoietic cells, such as IL-1, TNF, and GM-CSF *(11)*.

REGULATION OF CYTOKINE GENES IN T-CELLS

Clusters of Cytokine Genes

Many cytokine genes are clustered in limited regions of a chromosome, suggesting that they have evolved from a set of common ancestral genes. For example, GM-CSF, IL-3, IL-4, IL-5, M-CSF, and M-CSF receptor (c-*fms*) genes are located on human chromosome 5 or mouse chromosome 11. The IL-3 gene is composed of 5 exons and 4 introns, whereas the GM-CSF, IL-4, and IL-5 genes are composed of 4 exons and 3 introns. Among these, IL-3 and GM-CSF are only 9 kb apart in humans (14 kb in mice), while IL-4 and IL-5 are clustered within a several hundred kilobase region. The expression of these cytokines in T-cells requires two signals, such as those induced by TPA and A23187.

Common Motifs of the Upstream Sequences of Cytokine Genes

IL-3 and GM-CSF are expressed in a coordinated fashion. Their 5′ flanking regions share two homologous deoxyribonucleic acid (DNA) motifs, CLE1 (5′-GGAGATTCCCA-3′) and CLE2 (5′-TCAGGTA-3′) *(14,15)*. CLE1 is relatively well conserved among cytokines, whereas CLE2 is not necessarily found in other cytokines. Downstream of CLE2 is a GC box motif, similar to the recognition site of transcription factor Sp1. Furthermore, the 5′ sequence of the GM-CSF gene has another CLE sequence, CLE0. Transfection experiments have established that both the CLE2/GC-box and CLE0 sequences of the mGM-CSF promoter are essential for transcriptional activation in response to PMA/A23187. The CLE2/GC-box is recognized by *NF-GM2*, indistinguishable from *NF-κB*, while CLE0 is recognized by two factors, AP1 and an NF-AT-like molecule. The presence of these sequences in other genes may be the basis for the coordinated induction of these genes during T-cell activation: CLE0-like sequences in promoters of IL-3, IL-4, and IL-5, and NF-AT sites in a promoter of IL-2.

STRUCTURES AND COMPOSITION OF CYTOKINE RECEPTORS

Cytokine Receptor Superfamilies

Recently, several genes encoding cytokine receptors have been isolated mainly by using expression cloning protocol. Based on the similarity of the extracellular amino acid sequences, they are classified into several distinct families *(16,17)* (Fig. 4): hemopoietic cytokine receptors (class 1), IFN-α/β and IFN-γ receptors (class 2), TNF and nerve growth factor (NGF)

A

Class 1
Hematopoietic Cytokine Receptor family

GMRα	IL-2Rβ	KH97	gp130	LIFR	IL-6R
IL-3Rα	IL-2Rγ	(βc)	G-CSFR		(CNTFR)
IL-5Rα	IL-4R	AIC2A			
	IL-7R	AIC2B			
	IL-9R	Mpl			
	EpoR				
	PRLR				
	GHR				

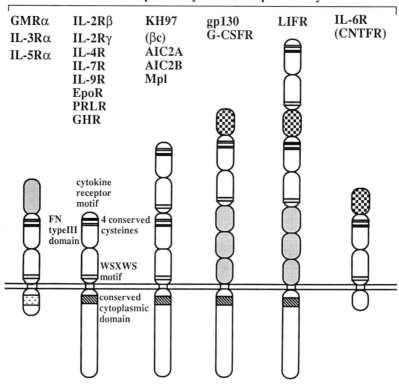

cytokine
receptor
motif

FN
typeIII
domain

4 conserved
cysteines

WSXWS
motif

conserved
cytoplasmic
domain

B

Class 2		Class 3				Class 4
IFN R family		TNF/NGF R family				Ig-like R family
IFNγR	IFNα/βR	CD30	TNFR	TNFR	Fas	IL-1R
IL-10R			(p75)	(p55)		type I
			NGFR	CD40		type II
			CD27			

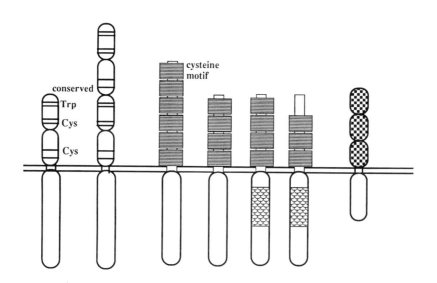

conserved
Trp
Cys

Cys

cysteine
motif

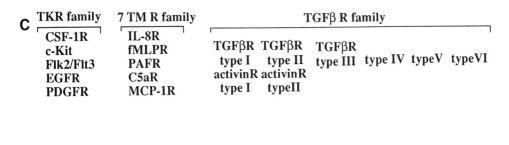

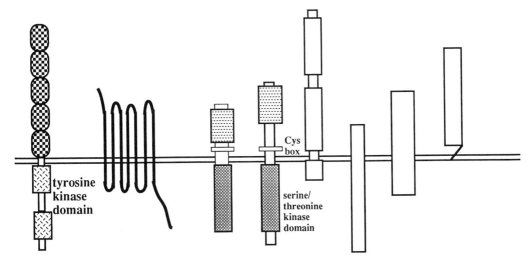

Fig. 4. Structure and common motifs of cytokine receptor families. Hemopoietic cytokine receptor family (class 1), interferon receptor family (class 2), TNF/NGF receptor family (class 3), immunoglobulin-like receptor (IL-1R) family (class 4), tyrosine kinase-type receptor (TKR) family, seven-transmembrane (7 TM)-receptor family, and TGFβ receptor family.

receptors, Fas, and CD40 (class 3), and immunoglobulin-like receptors (class 4), such as IL-1Rs. Other structurally distinct receptor families include the tyrosine kinase receptor family, the TGF-β receptor family, and seven-transmembrane-receptor family, etc.

Common Sequence Motifs of a Cytokine Receptor Superfamily

Members of the hemopoietic cytokine receptor (class 1 cytokine receptor) family have a typical structure, in the extracellular domain, consisting of 210 amino acid residues homologous to the fibronectin type-III domain. The domain has conserved motifs, such as $C-X_{9-20}-C-X-W-X_{22-36}-C-X_{8-25}-C$ (X is a nonconserved amino acid residue) in the N-terminal and W-S-X-W-S in the C-terminal portion *(16,17)*. This group of receptors includes the receptors for the IL-2 receptor β-subunit (IL-2Rβ), IL-3 receptor α-subunit (IL-3Rα), GM-CSF-Rα, IL-5Rα, common β-subunit (for IL-3, GM-CSF, and IL-5; $β_c$), IL-4R, IL-6Rα, glycoprotein 130 (gp130) (IL-6Rβ), IL-7R, erythropoietin receptor (EpoR), and G-CSFR.

To form high-affinity receptors, some of them form homodimers (G-CSFR, EpoR, TpoR, IL-4R), while others form heterodimers sharing common signaling subunits (GM-CSFR/IL-3R/IL-5R, IL-2R/IL-7R/IL-9R/IL-13R/IL-15R, IL-6R/IL-11R/LIFR/OSMR/CNTFR [LIF, OSM, and CNTF are defined below]) (Fig. 5).

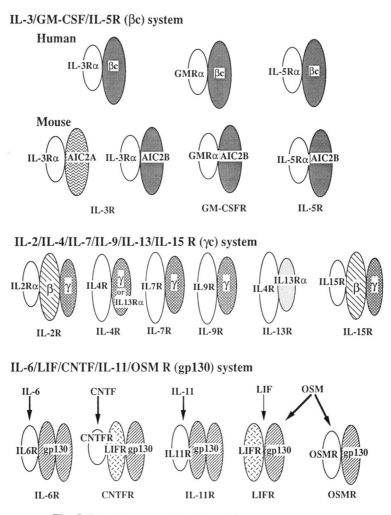

Fig. 5. Subunit composition of cytokine receptor systems.

GM-CSFR/IL-3R/IL-5R (Common β) Family

The high-affinity receptors for GM-CSF, IL-3, and IL-5 are composed of two distinct subunits, α and β. The α-subunits are specific for each cytokine and bind each ligand with low affinity, whereas the β-subunit ($β_c$) is common to these three cytokines and critical for signal transduction. In the human system only one $β_c$ molecule (KH97) has been cloned, whereas in the murine system there are two homologous β molecules. Of these, one (AIC2B; $β_c$) is common for three cytokines, but the other (AIC2A; $β_{IL-3}$) is only used by IL-3. In human hemopoietic cells, cross-competition for binding to the high-affinity receptors occurs between these three cytokines, whereas no such competition occurs in the murine system.

IL-2R/IL-4R/IL-7R/IL-9R/IL-13R/IL-15R (Common γ) Family

The IL-2 receptor consists of three subunits, α-, β-, and γ-chains. Combination of α and $γ_c$, β and $γ_c$, or all three subunits, but not of α- and β-subunits can deliver proliferative signals *(18)*. The $γ_c$-chain is shared by IL-2R, IL-4R, IL-7R, IL-9R, and IL-15R, whereas the β-chain is shared by IL-2R and IL-15R. IL-13 shares many biological functions with IL-4, but γ_c does not seem to be a component of IL-13R. An experiment with anti-γ_c antibody and truncated γ_c *(19,20)* suggested that there are two types of IL-4R, one is composed of IL-4Rα and γ_c and the other is composed of IL-4Rα and a second γ-subunit (γ_c'), which is shared by IL-4R and IL-13R. Recently the low-affinity IL-13Rα-subunit was cloned *(21)* and was shown to be a component of not only high-affinity IL-13R but also IL-4R, suggesting that the IL-13Rα-subunit is the second γ-subunit, γ_c'.

IL-6R / LIFR / OSMR / CNTFR / IL-11R / IL-12R (gp130) Family

IL-6, leukemia inhibitory factor (LIF), ciliary neurotrophic factor (CNTF), and oncostatin M (OSM) constitute a functionally related subfamily with similar effects on various tissues. In this receptor system, gp130 is shared by all the receptors except for IL-12R. gp130 alone does not bind any ligand, but forms high-affinity receptors with each α-chain. The binding of ligands/α-chains complexes induces disulfide-linked homodimerization of gp130 or heterodimerization of gp130 and LIFR, a closely related homolog of gp130 *(22)*. The activated IL-6 receptor complex contains a gp130 homodimer, whereas CNTF and LIF receptor complexes contain LIFR-gp130 heterodimers *(23–25)*. For LIFR, LIF directly binds to LIFR, and the binding induces the heterodimerization of LIFR and gp130 *(25)*. The dimerization triggers the activation of receptor-associated Janus kinases (JAKs).

The cytoplasmic region of IL-6R is dispensable for this signaling, and soluble IL-6R with IL-6 can deliver the signal. Like IL-6R, CNTFR has no cytoplasmic region and binds to the cell membrane via a glycosyl-phosphatidylinositol linker *(26)*. IL-12 consists of covalently bound p35 and p40 subunits that are closely homologous to IL-6 and IL-6R, respectively. IL-12 binds its specific receptor IL-12R, which is closely related to gp130 *(27)*. However, in contrast to gp130, IL-12R dimerization/oligomerization is ligand-independent, and it requires an unidentified subunit for the formation of a high-affinity IL-12R.

Other Receptors (EpoR, G-CSFR, TpoR)

Receptors for Epo, G-CSF, and Tpo are single classes of high-affinity receptors present on erythroid, neutrophilic, and magakaryocytic cells, respectively. Furthermore, prolactin and growth-hormone (GH) receptors are included in this receptor subfamily. The crystal structure of the GH–GH receptor complex revealed that a GH receptor homodimer is stabilized not only by ligand–receptor interaction but also through intermolecular interaction between the membrane-proximal domains of each receptor *(28)*.

Two activating mutations of EpoR were isolated: one is a single point mutation with substitution of arginine to cysteine within the extracellular domain, leading to disulfide-linked dimerization and constitutive, ligand-independent activation and tumorigenicity *(29,30)*. A homologous dimer interface domain exists in TpoR, and substitution of cysteines for specific amino acids within the region resulted in constitutive activation and tumorigenicity *(31)*. The other activating mutation of EpoR is a deletion of C-terminal 42 amino acids, resulting in hypersensitivity to Epo *(29)*.

TpoR was a homolog of myeloproliferative leukemia virus envelope protein (v-*mpl*) *(32)* but was shown to be a receptor specific for megakaryocyte proliferation and differentiation *(33)*. Gene disruption of c-*mpl* (TpoR) resulted in not only severe thrombocytopenia and marked decrease in bone marrow megakaryocyte precursors but also reduced numbers of primitive pluripotent progenitor cells *(34,35)*.

The extracellular domain of G-CSFR consists of an immunoglobulin (Ig)-like domain, a common motif in a type I cytokine receptor, and a contactin-like domain, and the overall structure is homologous to that of gp130. In the cytoplasmic domain of G-CSFR, the N-terminal region of G-CSFR, corresponding to box1 of gp130 or the serine-rich region of the IL-2Rβ chain, is sufficient for growth signal transduction, whereas both N-terminal and C-terminal regions are required for differentiation, as evidenced by myeloperoxidase and leukocyte elastase gene expression *(36)*.

Targeted Disruption of Cytokines and Cytokine Receptor Genes

Gene targeting experiments of cytokines and cytokine receptors have revealed the specific and nonredundant functions of some components, whereas others show redundant and overlapping functions.

Mice lacking the β_c gene show pulmonary proteinosis-like diseases *(37)*, as do GM-CSF-deficient mice *(38,39)*. These diseases are ascribed to decreased pulmonary macrophages. They also show decreased levels of eosinophils and absence of eosinophilia in response to parasite infection but exhibit no marked abnormalities in hematopoiesis. β_{IL-3}-deficient mice are almost normal, as IL-3 signals are transduced through the complex of IL-3Rα and β_c subunits.

IL-5-deficent mice revealed almost normal T- and B-cell function, including CD5+ B-cells, but do not become eosinophilic in response to parasite infection *(40)*. In IL-6-deficient mice, the infection of viruses and Listeria becomes fatal, T-cell-dependent antibody response against viruses is decreased, and decreased levels of acute phase responses occur after tissue injury or infection *(41)*.

Mice lacking gp130 do not survive, because they show a hypoplastic ventricular myocardium and decreased numbers of pluripotent and committed hematopoietic progenitors in the liver, as well as mature cells. This suggests that gp130 signals are crucial for myocardial development (as a component of the cardiotropin I receptor) and hematopoiesis (as a component of receptors for IL-6, LIF, IL-11, and others) *(42)*.

SIGNAL TRANSDUCTION BY CYTOKINE RECEPTORS

Signal Transduction Pathways

Cytokine signaling is initiated following the ligand binding and dimerization of two signaling receptor subunits *(2,22,43–47)*. After dimerization, the tyrosine kinases associated with the signaling subunits are brought into proximity and transphosphorylate each other, leading to activation of the kinases. Subsequently, the receptor subunits become tyrosine-phosphorylated and then attract intracellular signaling components, such as signal transducers and activators of transcription (STAT), phospholipase C-γ (PLC-γ), phosphatidylinositol 3′ (PI3) kinase, phosphatases, Shc, and Vav (Fig. 6). Through interaction with these components, cytokine receptors can activate multiple signaling cascades, including the protein tyrosine kinase cascade (JAK/STAT and others), the *myc* activation cascade, the Ras/Raf/MAP (mitogen-activated protein) kinase cascade, the protein kinase (PKC) cascade, and others. Furthermore, cross talk between different signaling cascades enables a cell to integrate information from multiple signals that it receives.

JAK/STAT Pathway

Although hemopoietic cytokine superfamily receptors have no catalytic domains in the cytoplasmic regions, they all induce protein tyrosine phosphorylation. The fact that transfer of oncogene tyrosine kinases (v-*src*, v-*abl*, v-*fms*) or treatment with sodium vanadate can replace cytokines suggests the significance of tyrosine kinases in signal transduction. Several candidates for tyrosine kinases coupling the cytokine receptors have been reported, such as *src, lyn,*

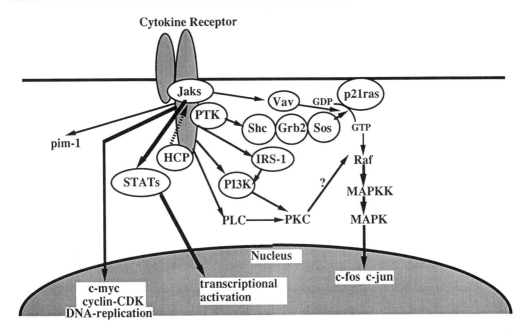

Fig. 6. Signaling pathways through cytokine receptor. Activation of cytokine receptors induces the signals to Ras pathway, *myc* pathway, JAK/STAT pathway, and so on. PI3 kinase (PI3K) and HCP are also activated.

fes/fps. IL-2Rβ is associated with p56^{lck} in peripheral blood lymphocytes *(48,49)* and with *fyn (50)* and *lyn (51)* in BAF-B03-derived cells. Several other tyrosine kinases, such as Btk *(52)*, Fes *(53)*, and Tec *(54)*, have been reported to be associated with cytokine receptors. However, the significance of such tyrosine kinases in receptor signaling had not been established.

Recently, a novel family of tyrosine kinases termed Janus kinases were found to mediate interferon signaling, and these pathways have been reported to be shared by several cytokines. The four known JAKS (JAK1, JAK2, JAK3, and TYK2) *(55,56)* bind to specific cytokine receptors. Studies involving complementation of genetic defects in cell lines unresponsive to interferon (IFN)-α/β and interferon-γ *(57–59)* showed that JAK1 and TYK2 are essential for the IFN-α/β response, whereas JAK1 and JAK2 are essential for the IFN-γ response. Subsequently, the association of the Janus family kinases with receptor subfamilies and their critical roles in cytokine signaling have been clarified with immunoprecipitation or dominant-negative mutants of JAKs *(60–72)* (Table 1). Generally, JAK1, JAK3 and TYK2 bind in combination with receptors of the same family, whereas JAK2 binds to receptors alone *(45)*. Receptors of β$_c$, GH, and receptor tyrosine kinase subfamilies associate with JAK2 alone. Receptors of the γ$_c$ subfamily utilize both JAK1 and JAK3, whereas receptors of the gp130 subfamily use combinations of JAK1, JAK2, and TYK2. Receptors for IFN-α/β (and IL-10) associate with JAK1 and TYK2, whereas the receptor for IFN-γ associates with JAK1 and JAK2, which is supposed to correlate with the functional differences between the IFNs.

JAKs bind to the membrane-proximal regions of receptors, constitutively or induced by ligand binding. After ligand binding, JAKs transphosphorylate and activate each other and then phosphorylate receptor subunits, creating docking sites for src-homology 2 (SH2)-containing signaling components, such as Shc, p85 of PI3 kinase, hematopoietic cell phosphatases (HCP), IRS-1, 4PS, Vav, Syp, and STAT family proteins *(73,74)*. JAK3 is

Table 1
JAKs and STATs in Cytokine Signaling

Cytokine	Activated JAK	Activated STAT
Common β family		
IL-3/GM-CSF/IL-5	JAK2	Stat5, Stat6
Growth hormone family		
Epo/GH/PRL	JAK2	Stat5
Tpo	JAK2	Stat3, Stat5
Receptor tyrosine kinase family		
EGF/PDGF/CSF-1	JAK2	Stat1, Stat3, Stat5
Common γ family		
IL-2/IL-15	JAK1, JAK3	Stat3, Stat5
IL-7	JAK1, JAK3	Stat5
IL-4/IL-13	JAK1, JAK3	Stat6
gp130 family		
IL-6/LIF/CNTF/OSM	JAK1, JAK2, TYK2	Stat1, Stat3
IL-12	JAK2, TYK2	Stat4, Stat3
G-CSF	JAK2	Stat3
Interferone family		
IFN-α, -β	JAK1, TYK2	Stat1, Stat2, Stat3
IFN-γ	JAK1, JAK2	Stat1
IL-10	JAK1, TYK2	Stat1, Stat3

selectively associated with the carboxy-terminal region of the γ_c chain, whereas JAK2 is linked to the "serine-rich" region of the IL-2Rβc chain *(75)*. Mutant mice lacking JAK3 show profound reduction in and severe dysfunction of both T- and B-cells, similar to severe combined immunodeficiency disease (SCID) *(76,77)*. Analyses of SCID patients showed that, whereas the γ_c chain mutation is the cause of X-linked SCID, the JAK3 mutation is one of the causes of autosomal SCID *(78,79)*.

Functions of STAT Family Proteins

STAT family proteins were first identified as DNA-binding proteins in IFN-regulated gene expression *(80–82)*. They are activated through phosphorylation by JAKs, form homo- or heterodimers, and translocate into nuclei. They share a conserved SH2 domain that is required for the recruitment to activated receptor complexes, the interaction with JAKs, and the dimerization and binding to DNA. Their activation correlates with mitogenesis, independent of the Ras pathway.

The differential activation of STAT family proteins by cytokine receptors seems to result not from the differential use of JAK kinases but from the selective recruitment of STAT proteins *(44,46,83–92)* (Table 1). Generally, Stat1 and Stat2 are activated by IFN signals and are critical for innate immunity *(84)*. In contrast, Stat4 and Stat6 are critical for acquired immunity, and are stimulated by IL-12 and IL-4, respectively *(84)*. Stat3 and Stat5 may be critical for cell proliferation in response to inflammatory cytokines *(84)*.

STATs seem not to be involved in proliferative responses, because mutant receptors that activate JAKs without activation of STATs can deliver mitogenic signals *(93–95)*. In contrast, STATs may be involved in functional activation or cellular differentiation.

Ras/Raf/MAP Kinase Pathways

p21ras is one of the small molecular weight guanine nucleotide binding proteins, and the switch from the guanosine 5'-triphosphate (GTP)-bound to the guanosine 5'-diphosphate (GDP)-bound form occurs in response to various cytokines. IL-2, IL-3, and GM-CSF, but not IL-4, increase GTP-bound p21ras *(96)*. This conversion is mediated through the intrinsic GTPase activity of Ras and by the nucleotide exchange factors, such as Sos and Vav.

When receptors are activated, Shc, an SH2-containing adaptor protein, binds to the receptors, becomes tyrosine-phosphorylated, and then binds to the SH2 domain of Grb2. In tyrosine kinase-type receptors, such as epidermal growth factor receptor (EGFR) and platelet-derived growth factor receptor (PDGFR), Grb2 binds to the receptors via its SH2 domain. Then the complex of Shc and Grb2 recruits Sos to its substrate Ras and induces the nucleotide exchange of Ras, resulting in the active form of Ras, Ras-GTP. Vav is composed of an SH2 domain, two SH3 domains, a cysteine-rich region, and a guanine nucleotide exchange activity region and is expressed only in hemopoietic cells. In response to cytokines, such as GM-CSF, IL-3, and SCF, it binds to receptors with the SH2 domain and is tyrosine-phosphorylated by JAKs *(97)*.

Activation of Ras leads to the activation of the downstream molecules, such as serine/threonine kinase Raf, MAP kinase kinase, and MAP kinase, resulting in the induction of c-*fos*/c-*jun*. Ras pathway activation has recently been shown to be necessary for full activation of STAT, whose tyrosine is phosphorylated by JAKs and serine is phosphorylated by MAP kinases *(98)*.

Protein Kinase C

(PKC), Phosphatases, PI3 Kinases, and Other Pathways PKC is activated in response to several cytokines, such as IL-2, IL-3, and GM-CSF *(99)*. Growth factor receptors, such as PDGFR, activate PKC through activation of PLC *(100)*. It hydrolyzes PI and results in the formation of inositol (1,4,5)-triphosphate (IP_3) and mobilization of Ca^{2+}, both of which synergize to activate PKC. Thereafter, hydrolysis of PC leads to extended activation of PKC. However, the exact mechanism of PKC by cytokines remains to be clarified.

PI3 kinase becomes associated with tyrosine-phosphorylated receptors with an SH2 domain and becomes activated *(101)*. PI3 kinase is supposed to activate several downstream targets, including PKC, Ras, Rac, MAP kinase, Jun kinase (JNK), and PLC, and to be involved in cellular functions, such as the respiratory burst and leukotriene release and survival *(102)*.

Hematopoietic cell protein tyrosine phosphatase (HCP; SH-PTP1) is expressed predominantly in hematopoietic cells and functions as a negative regulator, whereas SH-PTP2 is ubiquitously expressed and is a positive regulator *(103)*. HCP binds to several cytokine receptors via the SH2 domain and dephosphorylates JAK2 *(101)*. Mice with mutant HCP genes (motheaten) show multiple hematological abnormalities, including accumulation of macrophages and granulocytes in the organs and autoimmune diseases *(104)*.

Functional Domains of Cytokine Receptors

The membrane proximal domains containing the box1 and box2 regions have been reported to be required for the association with JAKs *(62,63,66,105)*.

Studies with deletion mutants have revealed that the β_c subunit contains two regions responsible for the growth signal and the Ras pathway signal, respectively *(101,106–108)*. The former is proximal to the membrane (455–517) and contains the box1 consensus sequence, and is essential for growth, binding, and activation of JAK2, leading to activation of Stat5 *(63,90)*, and activation of *myc* and *pim-1*. The latter region (626–763) is significant for activation of the Ras pathway (activation of Shc, Ras, Raf-1, MAP kinase, $p70^{S6K}$, c-*fos*, and c-*jun*) *(101,106,108)*. Furthermore, the tyrosine residue at 577 is essential for Shc phosphorylation, and the coexistence of Tyr577 and the C-terminal region is necessary for full activation of c-*fos* promoter *(108)*. Although the cytoplasmic regions of the IL-6Rα or CNTFRα subunits are dispensable, that of the GM-CSFRα subunit is essential for signaling *(109–111)*.

Similarly, G-CSFR, as mentioned above, contains a membrane-proximal region required for proliferation and a membrane-distal region required for cell differentiation *(36)*. Furthermore, the membrane-proximal region of EpoR is sufficient for signaling and binds JAK2, Stat5, and Vav, whereas the C-terminal region binds HCP, p85-PI3 kinase, Shc, PLC-γ, and Syp and acts as a negative-regulatory domain *(44,112)*.

In the IL-2R system, the membrane-proximal (serine-rich) region of the IL-2Rβ-subunit is essential for binding and activation of JAK1 and Syk and proliferation, whereas the acidic region of the β-subunit is necessary for binding of Lck, and the membrane-distal region is necessary for Stat5 binding *(75,113)*. The cytoplasmic region of the IL-2Rγ-subunit is also critical for activation of JAK3, which phosphorylates Stat5 in cooperation with JAK1 and is involved in c-*myc* and c-*fos* induction *(46,114)*.

CONCLUSION: SPECIFICITY AND REDUNDANCY OF CYTOKINE SIGNALS AND REGULATION OF THE IMMUNE SYSTEM

The specificity and redundancy of cytokine signals have been clarified on the basis of molecular components transducing cytokine signals. A single receptor may couple to multiple signal transduction systems, whereas multiple receptor signals may converge into the same signal transduction pathway via common transducers or effectors, such as Ras/Raf/MAP kinases, PKC, and *myc*. Furthermore, in contrast to the extracellular regions in the hemopoietic cytokine receptors, the intracellular regions have few common motifs, suggesting that those regions offer the specificity for their signals.

Therefore, the redundancy of cytokine signals can be explained by the existence of shared receptor subunits; common signaling components, and common target molecules or genes. In contrast, the specificity and pleiotropy may be explained by tissue- or stage-specific expression of receptor subunits, different cytoplasmic region structures of cytokine receptors that recruit and activate different combinations of JAKs, other protein kinases, and signaling molecules, including STATs; different sets of signaling molecules present in different cells; and different signaling machinery, including the states of chromosomes.

The system of hemopoietic cytokines provides an excellent model to study the cell–cell communication and the control of proliferation, differentiation, and functional activation of multiple effector and target cells. The exact principles regulating the specificity, pleiotropy, and plasticity will be clarified on the basis of molecular and cellular biology, and the results will prove useful in elucidation of the pathophysiology of allergic and autoimmune diseases and development of new approaches for their treatment.

ACKNOWLEDGMENTS

The authors thank A. E. Koch (Northwestern University, Chicago) for valuable discussion.

REFERENCES

1. Arai K, Lee F, Miyajima A, Miyatake S, Arai N, Yotoka T (1990) Cytokines: coordinators of immune and inflammatory responses. Ann Rev Biochem 59:783–836.

2. Miyajima A, Kitamura T, Harada N, Yokota T, Arai K (1992) Cytokine receptors and signal transduction. Ann Rev Immunol 10:295–331.

3. Miyajima A, Miyatake S, Schreurs J, de Vries J, Arai N, Yokota T, Arai K (1988) Coordinate regulation of immune and inflammatory responses by T cell-derived lymphokines. FASEB 2:2462–2473.

4. Ogawa M (1993) Differentiation and proliferation of hematopoietic stem cells. Blood 81:2844–2853.

5. Nishijima I, Nakahata T, Hirabayashi Y, Inoue T, Kurata H, Miyajima A, Hayashi N, Iwakura Y, Arai K, Yokota T (1995) A human GM-CSF receptor expressed in transgenic mice stimulates proliferation and differentiation of hemopoietic progenitors to all lineages in response to human GM-CSF. Mol Biol Cell 6:495–508.

6. Mosmann TR, Coffman RL (1989) Th1 and Th2 cells: different patterns of lymphokine secretion lead to different functional properties. Annu Rev Immunol 7:145–173.

7. Yssel H, Shanafelt MC, Soderberg C, Schneider PV, Anzola J, Peltz G (1991) *Borrelia burgdorferi* activates a T helper type 1-like T cell subset in Lyme arthritis. J Exp Med 174:593–601.

8. Yssel H, Johnson KE, Schneider PV, Wideman J, Terr A, Kastelein R, de Vries JE (1992) T cell activation-inducing epitopes of the house dust mite allergen Der p I. J Immunol 148:738–745.

9. Kurata H, Yokota T, Miyajima A, Arai K (1994) GM-CSF receptor: structure, function, and signal transduction. Adv Cell Mol Biol Membranes Organelles 3:111–155.

10. Heidenreich S, Gong JH, Schmidt A, Nain M, Gemsa D (1989) Macrophage activation by granulocyte/macrophage colony-stimulating factor. Priming for enhanced release of tumor necrosis factor-alpha and prostaglandin E2. J Immunol 143:1198–1205.

11. Dorshkind K (1990) Regulation of hemopoiesis by bone marrow stromal cells and their products. Annu Rev Immunol 8:111–137.

12. Dexter TM, Allan TG, Lajtha LG (1977) Conditions controlling the proliferation of haemopoietic stem cells *in vitro*. J Cell Physiol 91:335–344.

13. Whitlock CA, Witte ON (1982) Long-term culture of B lymphocytes and their precursors from murine bone marrow. Proc Natl Acad Sci USA 79:3608–3612.

14. Miyatake S, Seiki M, Yoshida M, Arai K (1988) T-cell activation signals and human T-cell leukemia virus type I-encoded p40[tax] protein activate the mouse granulocyte-macrophage colony-stimulating factor gene through a common DNA element. Mol Cell Biol 8:5581–5587.

15. Miyatake S, Shlomai J, Arai K, Arai N (1991) Characterization of the mouse granulocyte-macrophage colony-stimulating factor (GM-CSF) gene promoter: nuclear factors that interact with an element shared by three lymphokine genes—those for GM-CSF, interleukin-4 (IL-4), and IL-5. Mol Cell Biol 11:5894–5901.

16. Bazan JF (1990) Structural design and molecular evolution of a cytokine receptor superfamily. Proc Natl Acad Sci USA 87:6934–6938.

17. Bazan F (1990) Haemopoietic receptors and helical cytokines. Immunol Today 11:350–354.

18. Taniguchi T, Minami Y (1993) The IL-2/IL-2 receptor system: a current overview. Cell 73:5–8.

19. Zurawski SM, Vega F Jr, Huyghe B, Zurawski G (1993) Receptors for interleukin-13 and interleukin-4 are complex and share a novel component that functions in signal transduction. EMBO J 12:2663–2670.

20. He YW, Malek TR (1995) The IL-2 receptor γ_c chain does not function as a subunit shared by the IL-4 and IL-13 receptors. J Immunol 155:9–12.

21. Hilton DJ, Zhang JG, Metcalf D, Alexander WS, Nicola N, Willson TA (1996) Cloning and characterization of a binding subunit of the intereulkin 13 receptor that is a component of the interleukin 4 receptor. Proc Natl Acad Sci USA 93:497–501.

22. Kishimoto T, Taga T, Akira S (1994) Cytokine signal transduction. Cell 76:253–262.

23. Ip NY, Nye SH, Boulton TG, Davis S, Taga T, Li Y, Birren SJ, Yasukawa K, Kishimoto T, Anderson DJ, Stahl N, Yancopoulos GD (1992) CNTF and LIF act on neuronal cells via shared signaling pathways that involve the IL-6 signal transducing receptor component gp130. Cell 69:1121–1132.

24. Murakami M, Hibi M, Nakagawa N, Nakagawa T, Yasukawa K, Yamanishi K, Taga T, Kishimoto T (1993) IL-6-induced homodimerization of gp130 and associated activation of a tyrosine kinase. Science 260:1808–1810.

25. Davis S, Aldrich TH, Stahl N, Pan L, Taga T, Kishimoto T, Ip NY, Yancopoulos GD (1993) LIFRβ and gp130 as heterodimerizing signal transducers of the tripartite CNTF receptor. Science 260:1805–1808.

26. Davis S, Aldrich TH, Ip NY, Stahl N, Scherer S, Farruggella T, DiStefano PS, Curtis R, Panayatatos N, Gascan H, Chevalier S, Yancopoulos GD (1993) Released form of CNTF receptor a component as a soluble mediator of CNTF responses. Science 259:1736–1739.

27. Chua AO, Chizzonite R, Desai BB, Truitt TP, Nunes P, Minetti LJ, Warrier RR, Presky DH, Levine JF, Gately MK, Bubler U (1994) Expression cloning of a human IL-12 receptor component. J Immunol 153:128–136.

28. de Vos AM, Uitsh M, Kossiakoff AA (1992) Human growth hormone and extracellular domain of its receptor: crystal structure of the complex. Science 255:306–312.

29. Yoshimura A, Longmore G, Lodish H (1990) Point mutation in the exocytoplasmic domain of the erythropoietin receptor resulting in hormone-independent activation and tumorigenicity. Nature 348:647–649.

30. Watowich SS, Yoshimura A, Longmore GD, Hilton DJ, Yoshimura Y, Lodish HF (1992) Homodimerization and constitutive activation of the erythropoietin receptor. Proc Natl Acad Sci USA 89:2140–2144.

31. Alexander WS, Metcalf D, Dunn AR (1995) Point mutations within a dimer interface homology domain of *c-Mpl* induce constitutive receptor activity and tumorigenicity. EMBO J 14:5569–5578.

32. Souyri M, Vigon I, Penciolelli JF, Heard JM, Tambourin P, Wendling F (1990) A putative truncated cytokine receptor gene transduced by the myeloproliferative leukemia virus immortalizes hematopoietic progenitors. Cell 63:1137–1147.

33. Bartley TD, Bogenberger J, Hunt P, Li YS, Lu HS, et al. (1994) Identification and cloning of a megakaryocyte growth and development factor that is a ligand for the cytokine receptor Mpl. Cell 77:1117–1124.

34. Gurney AL, Carver-Moore K, de Sauvage FJ, Moore MW (1994) Thrombocytopenia in *c-mpl*-deficient mice. Science 265:1445–1447.

35. Alexander WS, Roberts AW, Nicola NA, Metcalf D (1996) Deficiencies in progenitor cells of multiple hematopoietic lineages and defective megakaryopoiesis in mice lacking the thrombopoietin receptor *c-Mpl*. Blood 87:2162–2170.

36. Fukunaga R, Ishizaka-Ikeda E, Nagata S (1993) Growth and differentiation signals mediated by different regions in the cytoplasmic domain of granulocyte colony-stimulating factor receptor. Cell 74:1079–1087.

37. Nishinakamura R, Nakayama N, Hirabayashi Y, Inoue T, Aud D, McNeil T, Azuma S, Yoshida S, Toyoda Y, Arai K, Miyajima A, Murray R (1995) Mice deficient for the IL-3/GM-CSF/IL-5 β_c receptor exhibit lung pathology and impaired immune response, while βIL-3 receptor-deficient mice are normal. Immunity 2:211–222.

38. Dranoff G, Crawford AD, Sadelain M, Ream B, Rashid A, Bronson RT, Dickersin GR, Bachurski CJ, Mark EL, Whitsett JA, Mulligan RC (1994) Involvement of granulocyte-macrophage colony-stimulating factor in pulmonary homeostasis. Science 264:713–716.

39. Stanley E, Lieschke GJ, Grail D, Metcalf D, Hodgson G, Gall JA, Maher DW, Cebon J, Sinickas V, Dunn AR (1994) Granulocyte/macrophage colony-stimulating factor-deficient mice show no major perturbation of hematopoiesis but develop a characteristic pulmonary pathology. Proc. Natl. Acad. Sci. USA 91:5592–5596.

40. Kopf M, Brombacher F, Hodgkin PD, Ramsay AJ, Milbourne EA, Dai WJ, Ovington KS, Behn CA, Kohler G, Young IG, Matthaei KI (1996) IL-5-deficient mice have a developmental defect in CD5$^+$ B-1 cells and lack eosinophilia but have normal antibody and cytotoxic T cell responses. Immunity 4:15–24.

41. Kopf M, Baumann H, Freer G, Freudenberg M, Lamers M, Kishimoto T, Zinkernagel R, Bluethmann H, Kohler G (1994) Impaired immune and acute-phase responses in interleukin-6-deficient mice. Nature 368:339–342.

42. Yoshida K, Taga T, Saito M, Suematsu S, Kumanogoh A, Tanaka T, Fujiwara H, Hirata M, Yamagami T, Nakahata T, Hirabayashi T, Yoneda Y, Tanaka K, Wang WZ, Mori C, Shiota K, Yoshida N, Kishimoto T (1996) Targeted disruption of gp130, a common signal transducer for the interleukin 6 family of cytokines, leads to myocardial and hematological disorders. Proc Natl Acad Sci USA 93:407–411.

43. Schindler C, Darnell JE (1995) Transcriptional responses to polypeptide ligands: The JAK-STAT pathway. Annu Rev Biochem 64:621–651.

44. Ihle JN (1995) Cytokine receptor signalling. Nature 377:591–594.

45. Ihle JN, Witthuhn BA, Quelle FW, Yamamoto K, Silvennoinen O (1995) Signaling through the hematopoietic cytokine receptors. Annu Rev Immunol 13:369–398.

46. Taniguchi T (1995) Cytokine signaling through nonreceptor protein tyrosine kinases. Science 268:251–255.

47. Heldin CH (1995) Dimerization of cell surface receptors in signal transduction. Cell 80:213–223.

48. Hatakeyama M, Kono T, Kobayashi N, Kawahara A, Levin SD, Perlmutter RM, Taniguchi T (1991) Interaction of the IL-2 receptor with the src-family kinase p56^{lck}: identification of novel intermolecular association. Science 252:1523–1528.

49. Horak ID, Gress RE, Lucas PJ, Horak EM, Waldmann TA, Bolen JB (1991) T-lymphocyte interleukin 2-dependent tyrosine protein kinase signal transduction involves the activation of p56^{lck}. Proc Natl Acad Sci USA 88:1996–2000.

50. Kobayashi N (1993) Functional coupling of the src-family protein tyrosine kinases p59^{fyn} and p53/56^{lyn} with the interleukin 2 receptor: implications for redundancy and pleiotropism in cytokine signal transduction. Proc Natl Acad Sci USA 90:4201–4205.

51. Torigoe T, Saragovi HU, Reed JC (1992) Interleukin 2 regulates the activity of the *lyn* protein-tyrosine kinase in a B-cell line. Proc Natl Acad Sci USA 89:2674–2678.

52. Sato S, Katagiri T, Takaki S, Kikuchi Y, Hitoshi Y, Yonehara S, Tsukada S, Kitamura D, Watanabe T, Witte O, Takatsu K (1994) IL-5 receptor-mediated tyrosine phosphorylation of SH2/SH3-containing proteins and activation of Bruton's tyrosine and Janus 2 kinases. J Exp Med 180:2101–2111.

53. Hanazono Y, Chiba S, Sasaki K, Mano H, Miyajima A, Arai K, Hirai H (1993) *c-fps/fes* protein-tyrosine kinase is implicated in a signaling pathway triggered by granulocyte-macrophage colony-stimulating factor and interleukin-3. EMBO J 12:1641–1646.

54. Mano H, Yamashita Y, Sato K, Yazaki Y, Hirai H (1995) *Tec* protein-tyrosine kinase is involved in interleukin-3 signaling pathway. Blood 85:343–350.

55. Wilks AF (1989) Two putative protein-tyrosine kinases identified by application of the polymerase chain reaction. Proc Natl Acad Sci USA 86:1603–1607.

56. Wilks AF, Harpur AG, Kurban RR, Ralph SJ, Zurcher G, Ziemiecki A (1991) Two novel protein-tyrosine kinases, each with a second phosphotransferase-related catalytic domain, define a new class of protein kinase. Mol Cell Biol 11:2057–2065.

57. Velazquez L, Fellous M, Stark GR, Pellegrini S (1992) A protein tyrosine kinase in the interferon alpha/beta signaling pathway. Cell 70:313–322.

58. Muller M, Briscoe J, Laxton C, Guschin D, Ziemiecki A, Silvennoinen O, Harpur AG, Pellegrini S, Wilks AF, Ihle JN, Stark GR, Kerr IM (1993) The protein tyrosine kinase Jak1 complements defects in interferon-α/β and -γ signal transduction. Nature 366:129–135.

59. Watling D, Guschin D, Muller M, Silvennoinen O, Witthuhn BA, Quelle FW, Rogers NC, Schinler C, Stark GR, Ihle JN, Kerr IM (1993) Complementation by the protein tyrosine kinase JAK2 of a mutant cell line defective in the interferon-γ signal transduction pathway. Nature 366:166–170.

60. Witthuhn BA, Silvennoinen O, Miura O, Lai KS, Cwik C, Liu ET, Ihle JN (1994) Involvement of the JAK3 Janus kinase in IL-2 and IL-4 signalling in lymphoid and myeloid cells. Nature 370:153–157.

61. Johnston JA, Kawamura M, Kirken R, Chen Y, Blake TB, Shibuya K, Ortaldo JR, McVicar DW, O'Shea JJ (1994) Phosphorylation and activation of the JAK3 Janus kinase in response to IL-2. Nature 370:151–153.

62. Witthuhn B, Quelle FW, Silvennoinen O, Yi T, Tang B, Miura O, Ihle JN (1993) JAK2 associates with the erythropoietin receptor and is tyrosine phosphorylated and activated following EPO stimulation. Cell 74:227–236.

63. Quelle FW, Sato N, Witthuhn BA, Inhorn RC, Eder M, Miyajima A, Griffin JD, Ihle JN (1994) JAK2 associates with the β$_c$ chain of the receptor for granulocyte-macrophage colony-stimulating factor, and its activation requires the membrane-proximal region. Mol Cell Biol 14:4335–4341.

64. Silvennoinen O, Witthuhn B, Quelle FW, Cleveland JL, Yi T, Ihle JN (1993) Structure of the JAK2 protein tyrosine kinase and its role in IL-3 signal transduction. Proc Natl Acad Sci USA 90:8429–8433.

65. Stahl N, Boulton TG, Farruggella TJ, Ip NY, Davis S, Witthuhn BA, Quelle FW, Silvennoinen O, Barbieri G, Pellegrini S, Ihle JN, Zhong Z, Yancopoulos GD (1994) Association and activation of Jak-Tyk kinases by CNTF-LIF-OSM-IL-6 beta receptor components. Science 263:92–95.

66. Narazaki M, Witthuhn BA, Yoshida K, Silvennoinen O, Yasukawa K, Ihle JN, Kishimoto T, Taga T (1994) Activation of JAK2 kinase mediated by the IL-6 signal transducer, gp130. Proc Natl Acad Sci USA 91:2285–2289.

67. Luttichken C, Wegenka UM, Yuan J, Buschman J, Schindler C, Ziemiecki A, Harpur AG, Wilks AF, Yasukawa K, Taga T, Kishimoto T, Barbieri G, Pellegrini S, Sendtner M, Heinrich PC, Horn F (1994) Transcription factor APRF and JAK1 kinase associate with interleukin-6 receptor signal transducer, gp130, and are tyrosine phosphorylated in response to interleukin-6. Science 263:89–92.

68. Argetsinger LS, Campbell GS, Yang X, Witthuhn BA, Silvennoinen O, Ihle JN, Carter-Su C (1993) Identification of JAK2 as a growth hormone receptor-associated tyrosine kinase. Cell 74:237–244.

69. Nicholson SE, Oates AC, Harpur AG, Ziemiecki A, Wilks AF, Layton JE (1994) Tyrosine kinase JAK1 is associated with the granulocyte-colony-stimulating factor receptor and both become tyrosine-phosphorylated after receptor activation. Proc Natl Acad Sci USA 91:2985–2988.

70. Campbell GS, Argentsinger LS, Ihle JN, Kelly PA, Rillema JA, Carter-Su C (1994) Activation of JAK2 tyrosine kinase by prolactin receptors in *Nb2* cells and mouse mammary gland explants. Proc Natl Acad Sci USA 91:5232–5236.

71. Rui H, Kirken RA, Farrar WL (1994) Activation of receptor-associated tyrosine kinase JAK2 by prolactin. J Biol Chem 269:5364–5368.

72. Winston LA, Hunter T (1995) JAK2, *Ras*, and *Raf* are required for activation of extracellular signal-regulated kinase/mitogen-activated protein kinase by growth hormone. J Biol Chem 270: 30,837–30,840.

73. Ihle JN, Kerr IM (1995) Jaks and Stats in signaling by the cytokine receptor superfamily. Trends Genet 11:69–74.

74. Ihle JN, Witthuhn BA, Quelle FW, Yamamoto K, Thierfelder WE, Kreider B, Silvennoinen O (1994) Signaling by the cytokine receptor superfamily: JAKs and STATs. Trends Biochem Sci 19:222–227.

75. Miyazaki T, Kawahara A, Fujii H, Nakagawa Y, Minami Y, Liu ZJ, Oishi I, Silvennoinen O, Witthuhn BA, Ihle JN, Taniguchi T (1994) Functional activation of Jak1 and Jak3 by selective association with IL-2 receptor subunits. Science 266:1045–1047.

76. Thomis DC, Gurniak CB, Tivol E, Sharpe AH, Berg LJ (1995) Defects in B lymphocyte maturation and T lymphocyte activation in mice lacking Jak3. Science 270:794–797.

77. Nosaka T, van Deursen JMA, Tripp RA, Thierfelder WE, Witthuhn BA, McMickle AP, Doherty PC, Grosveld GC, Ihle JN (1995) Defective lymphoid development in mice lacking Jak3. Science 270:800–802.

78. Russell SM, Tayebi N, Nakajima H, Riedy MC, Roberts JL, Aman MJ, Migone TS, Noguchi M, Market ML, Buckley RH, O'Shea JJ, Leonard WL (1995) Mutation of Jak3 in a patient with SCID: essential role in Jak3 in lymphoid development. Science 270:797–800.

79. Macchi P, Villa A, Giliani S, Sacco MG, Frattini A, Porta F, Ugazio AG, Johnston JA, Candotti F, O'Shea JJ, Vezzoni P, Nortarangelo LD (1995) Mutations of Jak-3 gene in patients with aytosomal severe combined immune deficiency (SCID). Nature 377:65–68.

80. Fu XY (1992) A transcription factor with SH2 and SH3 domains is directly activated by an interferon α-induced cytoplasmic protein tyrosine kinase(s). Cell 70:323–335.

81. Shuai K, Schindler C, Prezioso VR, Darnell JE (1992) Activation of transcription by IFN-γ: tyrosine phosphorylation of a 91-kD DNA binding protein. Science 258:1808–1812.

82. Muller M, Laxton C, Briscoe J, Schindler C, Improta T, Darnell JE, Stark GR, Kerr IM (1993) Complementation of a mutant cell line: central role of the 91 kDa polypeptide of ISGF3 in the interferon-α and -γ signal transduction pathways. EMBO J 12:4221–4228.

83. Ivashikiv LB (1995) Cytokines and STATs: how can signals achieve specificity? Immunity 3:1–4.

84. Ihle JN (1996) STATs: signal transducers and activators of transcription. Cell 84:331–334.

85. Gouilleux F, Pallard C, Dusanter-Fourt I, Wakao H, Haldosen LA, Norstedt G, Levy D, Groner B (1995) Prolactin, growth hormone, erythropoietin and granulocyte-macrophage colony stimulating factor induce MGF-Stat5 DNA binding activity. EMBO J 14:2005–2013.

86. Hou J, Schindler U, Henzel WJ, Wong SC, McKnight SL (1995) Identification and purification of human Stat proteins activated in response to interleukin-2. Immunity 2:321–329.

87. Larner AC, David M, Feldman GM, Igarashi K, Hackett RH, Webb DSA, Sweitzer SM, Petricoin EF, Finbloom DS (1993) Tyrosine phosphorylation of DNA binding proteins by multiple cytokines. Science 261:1730–1733.

88. Rothman P, Kreider B, Azam M, Levy D, Wegenka U, Eilers A, Decker T, Horn F, Kashieva H, Ihle J, Schindler C (1994) Cytokine and growth factors signal through tyrosine phosphorylation of a family of related transcription factors. Immunity 1:457–468.

89. Zhong Z, Wen Z, Darnell JE (1994) Stat3: A Stat family member activated by tyrosine phosphorylation in response to epidermal growth factor and interleukin-6. Science 264:95–98.

90. Mui AL, Wakao H, O'Farrell AM, Harada N, Miyajima A (1995) Interleukin-3, granulocyte-macrophage colony stimulating factor and interleukin-5 transduce signals through two STAT5 homologs. EMBO J 14:1166–1175.

91. Azam M, Erdjument-Bromage H, Kreider BL, Xia M, Quelle F, Basu R, Saris C, Tempst P, Ihle JN, Schindler C (1995) Interleukin-3 signals through multiple isoforms of Stat5. EMBO J 14:1402–1411.

92. Yamanaka Y, Nakajima K, Fukuda T, Hibi M, Hirano T (1996) Differentiation and growth arrest signals are generated through the cytoplasmic region of gp130 that is essential for Stat3 activation. EMBO J 15:1557–1565.

93. Quelle FW, Shimoda K, Thierfelder W, Fischer C, Kim A, Ruben SM, Cleveland JL, Pierce JH, Keegan AD, Nelms K, Paul WE, Ihle JN (1995) Cloning of murine Stat6 and human Stat6, Stat proteins that are tyrosine phosphorylated in responses to IL-4 and IL-3 but are not required for mitogenesis. Mol Cell Biol 15:3336–3343.

94. Stahl N, Farruggella TJ, Boulton TG, Zhong Z, Darnell JE, Yancopoulos GD (1995) Choice of STATs and other substrates specified by modular tyrosine-based motifs in cytokine receptors. Science 267: 1349–1353.

95. Fujii H, Nakagawa Y, Schindler U, Kawahara A, Mori H, Gouilleux F, Groner B, Ihle JN, Minami Y, Miyazaki T, Taniguchi T (1995) Activation of Stat5 by interelukin 2 requires a carboxyl-terminal region of the interleukin 2 receptor β chain but is not essential for the proliferative signal transmission. Proc Natl Acad Sci USA 92:5482–5486.

96. Satoh T, Nakafuku M, Miyajima A, Kaziro Y (1991) Involvement of *ras* in signal transduction pathways from interleukin-2, interleukin-3, and granulocyte-macrophage colony stimulating factor, but not from interleukin-4. Proc Natl Acad Sci USA 88:3314–3318.

97. Matsuguchi T, Inhorn RC, Carlesso N, Xu G, Drucker B, Griffin JD (1995) Tyrosine phosphorylation of p95^{Vav} in myeloid cells is regulated by GM-CSF, IL-3 and Steel factor and is constitutively increased by p210$^{BCR/ABL}$. EMBO J 14:257–265.

98. David M, Ill EP, Benjamin C, Pine R, Weber MJ, Larner A (1995) Requirement for MAP kinase (ERK2) activity in interferon α- and interferon β-stimulated gene expression through STAT proteins. Science 269:1721–1723.

99. Duronio V, Nip L, Pelch SL (1989) Interleukin 3 stimulates phosphatidylcholine turnover in a mast/megakaryocyte cell line. Biochem Biophys Res Commun 164:804–808.

100. Nishizuka Y (1992) Intracellular signaling by hydrolysis of phospholipids and activation of protein kinase C. Science 258:607–613.

101. Sato N, Sakamaki K, Terada N, Arai K, Miyajima A (1993) Signal transduction by the high-affinity GM-CSF receptor: two distinct cytoplasmic regions of the common β subunit responsible for different signaling. EMBO J 12:4181–4189.

102. Ward SG, June CH, Olive D (1996) PI 3-kinase: a pivotal pathway in T-cell activation? Immunol Today 17:187–197.

103. Kingmuller U, Lorenz U, Cantley LC, Neel BG, Lodish HF (1995) Specific recruitment of SH-PTP1 to the erythropoietin receptor causes inactivation of JAK2 and termination of proliferative signals. Cell 80:729–738.

104. Schultz LD, Schweitzer PA, Rajan TV, Yi T, Ihle JN, Matthews RJ, Thomas ML, Beier DR (1993) Mutations at the murine *motheaten* locus are within the hematopoietic cell protein-phosphatase (*Hcph*) gene. Cell 73:1445–1454.

105. DaSilva L, Howard OMZ, Rui H, Kirken RA, Farrar WL (1994) Growth signalling and JAK2 association mediated by membrane-proximal cytoplasmic regions of prolactin receptors. J Biol Chem 269:267–270.

106. Sakamaki K, Miyajima I, Kitamura T, Miyajima A (1992) Critical cytoplasmic domains of the common β subunit of the human GM-CSF, IL-3 and IL-5 receptors for growth signal transduction and tyrosine phosphorylation. EMBO J 11:3541–3549.

107. Watanabe S, Muto A, Yokota T, Miyajima A, Arai K (1993) Differential regulation of early response genes and cell proliferation through the human granulocyte macrophage colony-stimulating factor receptor: selective activation of the *c-fos* promoter by genistein. Mol Biol Cell 4:983–992.

108. Itoh T, Muto A, Watanabe S, Miyajima A, Yokota T, Arai K (1996) Granulocyte-macrophage colony stimulating factor provokes *RAS* activation and transcription of *c-fos* through different modes of signaling. J Biol Chem 271:7587–7592.

109. Muto A, Watanabe S, Itoh T, Miyajima A, Yokota T, Arai K (1995) Roles of the cytoplasmic domains of the α and β subunits of human granulocyte-macrophage colony stimulating factor receptor. J Allergy Clin Immunol 96:1100–1114.

110. Polotskaya A, Zhao Y, Lilly ML, Kraft AS (1993) A critical role for the cytoplasmic domain of the granulocyte-macrophage colony-stimulating factor a receptor in mediating cell growth. Cell Growth Diff 4:523–531.

111. Weiss M, Yokoyama C, Shikama Y, Naugle C, Druker B, Sieff CA (1993) Human granulocyte-macrophage colony-stimulating factor receptor signal transduction requires the proximal cytoplasmic domains of the α and β subunits. Blood 82:3298–3306.

112. D'Andrea AD, Yoshimura A, Youssoufian H, Zon LI, Koo JW, Lodish HF (1991) The cytoplasmic region of the erythropoietin receptor contains nonoverlapping positive and negative growth-regulatory domains. Mol Cell Biol 11:1980–1987.

113. Hatakeyama M, Kono T, Kobayashi N, Kawahara A, Levin SD, Perlmutter RM, Taniguchi T (1991) Interaction of IL-2 receptor with the src-family kinase p56[lck]: identification of novel intermolecular association. Science 252:1523–1528.

114. Kawahara A, Minami Y, Miyazaki T, Ihle JN, Taniguchi T (1995) Critical role of the interleukin 2 (IL-2) receptor γ-chain-associated Jak3 in the IL-2-induced *c-fos* and *c-myc*, but not bel-2, gene induction. Proc Natl Acad Sci USA 92:8724–8728.

18 Adhesion Receptors in Allergic Disease

Andrew Wardlaw, FRCP, PhD

CONTENTS

INTRODUCTION

The inflammatory process in allergic disease is characterized by a distinct pattern of leukocyte accumulation, in particular increased numbers of activated eosinophils, T-lymphocytes, and monocytes with a relative paucity of neutrophils. Leukocyte migration through endothelium has been shown to be a staged process in which the cells are initially lightly tethered to the endothelium under flow conditions and roll along its surface. This is followed by cell activation, thought to be mediated by a soluble chemotactic stimulus that allows a firmer bond to develop between the leucocyte and the endothelial cell, which results in successful adhesion and transmigration (Fig. 1) *(1)*. The steps occur in series so that each is essential for transmigration to occur. This means that selectivity can be introduced at each of the steps, resulting in considerable diversity in the pattern of signals at any one inflammatory site. It also means that migration can be modulated at each of the steps, offering a range of targets for pharmacological inhibition.

The receptors and mediators involved in leukocyte migration have, to a large extent, been characterized (Figs. 2 and 3). Selectins and their counterreceptors as well as $\alpha 4$ integrins are thought to mediate the initial attachment and rolling step, a number of chemotactic mediators have been implicated in the activation step, and $\beta 2$ and $\alpha 4$ integrins expressed on leukocytes binding to their endothelial adhesion counterreceptors belonging to the immunoglobulin superfamily are implicated in the firmer adhesion step *(2)*. Once through the endothelium, leukocytes interact via integrins with proteins of the extracellular matrix and with cells resident in the tissue such as fibroblasts, epithelial cells, and smooth muscle cells. Interaction with matrix proteins can have a profound effect on cellular function, leading to activation, prolonged survival, and mediator synthesis. There is an extensive body of work on the basic biology of adhesion molecules, and this area will be covered only briefly in the first part of the chapter. A number of studies have attempted to interpret the biology of adhesion receptors in the context of allergic disease. This work will be covered in the second half of the chapter.

From: *Allergy and Allergic Diseases: The New Mechanisms and Therapeutics*
Edited by: J. A. Denburg © Humana Press Inc., Totowa, NJ

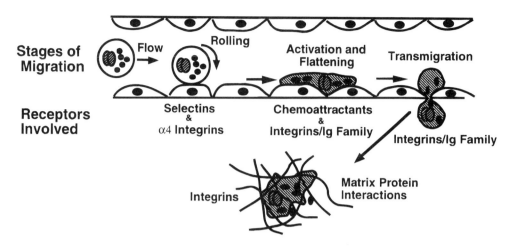

Fig. 1. Schematic outline of the stages involved in leukocyte migration and the adhesion receptor families involved.

STRUCTURE AND FUNCTION OF LEUCOCYTE ADHESION RECEPTORS

Selectins and Their Counterstructures

THE SELECTINS

The selectins consist of three type 1 glycoprotein membrane receptors (GMPs), L-selectin, P-selectin (formerly GMP-140), and E-selectin (formerly endothelial leucocyte adhesion molecule [ELAM]-1) *(3)*. E- and P-selectin are expressed on endothelium, whereas L-selectin is expressed by all leukocytes. P-selectin is also expressed on platelets. Whereas E-selectin expression is induced on endothelial cells as a result of cytokine-stimulated gene transcription and new protein synthesis *(4)*, P-selectin is stored in cytoplasmic Weibel-Palade bodies and translocated within minutes to the cell surface after stimulation of the endothelium by a variety of mediators, including thrombin, LTC_4, and histamine *(5)*. More prolonged expression is induced by interleukin (IL)-3, and IL-4 has also been recently shown to induce messenger ribonucleic acid (mRNA) expression and upregulate lumenal expression of P-selectin on cultured endothelial cells for prolonged periods *(6,7)*. L-selectin is constitutively expressed and shed on cell activation as a result of cleavage with an unidentified cell membrane-associated metalloproteinase *(8)*. The selectins have a common structure characterized by an N-terminal calcium-dependent (C-type) lectin domain that binds sugars consisting of a family of sialylated fucosylated glycosaminoglycans typified by the carbohydrate moiety sialyl Lewis X *(9)*. Sialylation and fucosylation appear necessary for function. Adjacent to the lectin domain are an epithelial growth factor (EGF)-like domain and a variable number of repeated units related to complement binding proteins such as decay accelerating factor (DAF). L-selectin has two repeat units, E-selectin 6 and P-selectin 9. Knockout mice have helped to define selectin function. Whereas an E-selectin knock-out mouse was normal with no obvious immunodeficiency, both P- and L-selectin knock-out mice had impaired neutrophil rolling and delayed recruitment of neutrophils to inflammatory lesions. The L-selectin knockout also had atrophy of peripheral lymph nodes *(10)*. A dual E- and P-selectin knockout mouse was profoundly immunodeficient and also had unexpected defects in hematopoiesis *(11)*. These studies have generally confirmed the role of selectins in mediating rolling interactions and demonstrated the overlap in their functions.

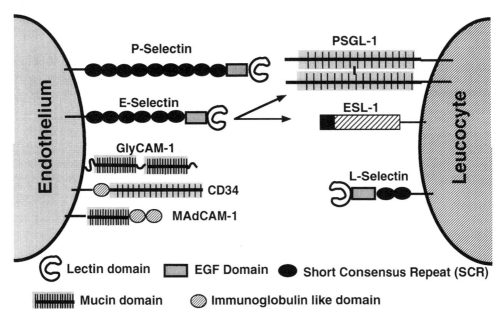

Fig. 2. Schematic representation of the structure of the selectins and their ligands.

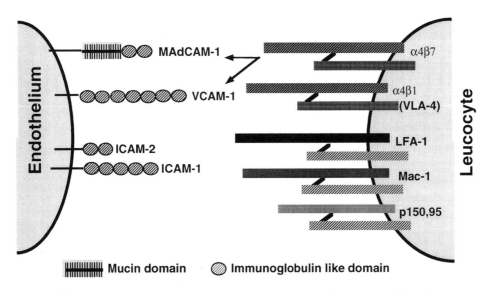

Fig. 3. Schematic representation of the structure of the integrins and their ligand.

SELECTIN COUNTERSTRUCTURES

Although the adhesion function of the selectins requires binding through sugars, the peptide backbone on which the sugars are presented is important in providing increased specificity and affinity of binding. Three ligands for L-selectin have been identified: glycosylated cell adhesion molecule-1 (GlyCAM-1) and a glycoform of CD34, which are ligands on lymph node high endothelial venules, and mouse mucosal addressin cell adhesion molecule (MAdCAM)-1. GlyCAM-1 does not have a transmembrane region and appears to be a secreted molecule

(12,13,14). CD34 is a heavily O-glycosylated transmembrane receptor with a mucin like structure. It is expressed widely on endothelial cells as well as hemopoietic stem cells.

P-selectin binds P-selectin glycoprotein-1 (PSGL-1) *(15)*. PSGL-1 is a mucin-like transmembrane protein that is a homodimer of 220 kDa. PSGL-1 also binds E-selectin, though with a lower affinity than P-selectin. It appears that E-selectin primarily binds through a sugar linkage, whereas P-selectin, in addition to a carbohydrate determinant, binds to sulfated tyrosine residues contained in N-terminal 20 amino acids *(16)*.

E-selectin, like P-selectin, recognizes an $\alpha(2–3)$ sialylated α 1(1–3) fucosylated lactosaminoglycan moiety that includes sialyl Lewis X. One molecule that carries this epitope is the cutaneous lymphocyte antigen (CLA) recognized by the monoclonal antibody (MAb)HECA 452. CLA binds E-selectin and recognizes a distinct subset of peripheral blood T-lymphocytes that home to the skin. E-selectin in this context is working as a skin vascular addressin for T-lymphocytes *(17)*. Whereas a majority of peripheral blood T cells express PSGL-1, only about 15% bind P-selectin, emphasising that subtle modifications of the selectin ligands can alter their functional capacity *(18)*. The mouse neutrophil E-selectin ligand (ESL-1) has recently been identified as a variant of a receptor for fibroblast growth factor *(19)*. L-selectin has also been shown to present carbohydrate ligands to E- and P-selectin *(20)*.

Integrins

Integrins are a superfamily of α,β, heterodimeric, type-1 transmembrane glycoproteins, noncovalently expressed on the cell surface *(21)*. Three main subfamilies of integrins were defined based on a common β-chain combining with a number of α-chains. Thus the $\beta1$ integrin family consisted of a single β-chain (CD29) combining with 6 α-chains (CD49a–f, $\alpha_{1–6}/\beta1$) to form the very late activation (VLA) family. The $\beta2$ integrin family (leucocyte integrins; CD18/CD11a–c; lymphocyte function associated antigen-1 (LFA-1), macrophage antigen-1 (Mac-1), p150,95; $\alpha_L/\beta1$, $\alpha_M/\beta1$, $\alpha_X/\beta1$) and the $\beta3$ family (cytoadhesins glycoprotein (gp)IIb/IIIa, CD41/CD61; vitronectin receptor; $\alpha_V\beta3$, CD51/CD61). Since that original classification, it has become apparent that the association between α- and β-chains is not as restricted as once thought. In addition a number of new α- and β-chains have been characterized, giving the integrin family another level of complexity.

$\beta2$ (Leukocyte) Integrins

There are four members of the leukocyte integrins. Mac-1 (CR3), LFA-1, and p150,95 were identified some years ago. The fourth member has only recently been characterized, and its role in leukocyte function is still uncertain, although it is widely expressed and appears to bind intercellular adhesion molecule (ICAM)-3 *(22)*. LFA-1 is expressed by virtually all leukocytes *(23)*, and Mac-1 is expressed by myeloid cells, large granular lymphocytes and a subset of B-cells *(24)*. p150,95 is expressed on macrophages and is a marker for hairy cell leukemia. It is only weakly expressed on peripheral blood neutrophils and eosinophils. The importance of the leukocyte integrins was underlined by the description of leukocyte adhesion deficiency (LAD), a life threatening immunodeficiency disease resulting from lack of expression of the $\beta2$ integrins by all leukocytes as a result of mutations in the β-chain *(25)*. Mac-1 appears to have an extensive range of binding activities. It binds the "inactivated" opsonic C3b (iC3b) component *(26)*. Neutrophils can also bind fibrinogen and heparin through Mac-1, and Mac-1 can bind Leishmania gp63 *(24,27)*. Another binding site on Mac-1 is "lectin-like" and binds to various ligands such as unopsonized rabbit erythrocytes, baker's yeast particles, and its capsule extract zymosan. In addition, Mac-1 is responsible for neutrophil binding to unstimulated vascular endothelium and plastic and glass surfaces and neutrophil aggregation *(28,29)*. The ligands for these binding activities have not been clearly defined.

OTHER LEUKOCYTE-EXPRESSED INTEGRINS

Other members of the integrin superfamily are variably expressed by peripheral blood leu-kocytes. Expression depends on the state of cell activation, particularly with lymphocytes. Of the $\beta3$ integrins only $\alpha IIb/\beta3$ appears to be expressed by platelets and megakaryocytes. $\alpha V\beta3$ is well expressed by tissue macrophages, in which it has been shown to mediate phagocytosis of apoptotic granulocytes [30]. Most members of the $\beta1$ integrin family bind to extracellular matrix proteins. An exception is $\alpha4$ integrin, which, as well as binding fibronectin, also binds vascular cell adhesion molecule (VCAM)-1 [31]. In addition $\alpha4\beta7$ binds the endothelial lym-phocyte homing receptor MAdCAM-1, and $\alpha E\beta7$, expressed by epithelial T-lymphocytes, binds E-cadherin [32]. $\alpha4\beta7$ is expressed by lymphocytes, eosinophils, and natural killer (NK) cells but not by neutrophils or monocytes [33].

It has recently been shown that, like the selectins, both $\alpha4\beta1$ binding to VCAM-1 and $\alpha4\beta7$ binding to MAdCAM-1 and VCAM-1 can participate in rolling interactions and arrest of leukocytes under conditions of flow [34,35].

Immunoglobulin Family Members

INTERCELLULAR ADHESION MOLECULES 1–3

ICAM-1 is a widely expressed 76–114-kDa heavily glycosylated single-chain transmem-brane receptor with a peptide backbone of 55 kDa, the variable molecular weight resulting from different degrees of glycosylation [36]. ICAM-1 contains five immunoglobulin (Ig)-like domains [37]. As well as binding LFA-1 and Mac-1 [38,39], ICAM-1 is also a receptor for *Plamodium falciparum* [40] and the major group of rhinovirus [41,42]. Its function appears to be regulated largely by increased expression, although dimerization also increases affinity of binding to LFA-1 [43]. Expression is increased on most cell types by a number of cytokines, including IL-1, tumor necrosis factor (TNF), and interferon (IFN-γ) [44]. Increased expression in vitro on human umbilical vein endothelial cells (HUVEC) is protein synthesis-dependent and generally detectable after about 4 h and maximal by 24 h. ICAM-1 has been implicated in a large number of cellular functions, including leukocyte migration, lymphocyte homing cyto-toxic T-lymphocyte (CTL) and large granular lymphocyte cytotoxicity, antigen presentation, and thymocyte maturation.

Two other ICAMs have been characterized. ICAM-2 is a 60,000-kDa single-chain trans-membrane receptor with a peptide backbone of 31 kDa. ICAM-2 has two Ig-like domains that are most homologous (35%) to the two amino-terminal domains of ICAM-1 [45]. ICAM-2 is constitutively expressed on vascular endothelial cells, and expression is not increased by cytokine activation. It is also expressed on lymphocytes, monocytes, and platelets but not neu-trophils [46]. ICAM-3 is a highly glycosylated protein of 124 kDa with five Ig domains that is well-expressed on all leukocytes, including neutrophils, but not endothelial cells [47].

VASCULAR CELL ADHESION MOLECULE-1

VCAM-1 is expressed by endothelial cells as well as fibroblasts and dendritic cells. Its expression is induced on HUVEC by TNF-α and IL-1 with a time course similar to ICAM-1. Both IL-4 and IL-13 selectively upregulate VCAM-1 expression [48,49]. VCAM-1 binds to VLA-4 [30]. This pathway has subsequently been shown to be important in monocyte, lym-phocyte, eosinophil, and basophil adhesion to HUVEC [50–55]. Neutrophils do not express VLA-4 [56] or bind to VCAM-1.

MUCOSAL ADDRESSIN CELL ADHESION MOLECULE-1

A recent addition to the Ig-like adhesion receptor family is the mucosal vascular addressin MAdCAM-1. Originally identified in mice, a human homolog has now been isolated [57]. It is preferentially expressed on high endothelial venules (HEVs) in Peyers patches and mesenteric lymph nodes. Mouse MAdCAM-1 has two N-terminal Ig domains, most closely related to VCAM-1 and ICAM-1, that bind $\alpha 4\beta 7$, followed by a mucin-like domain that can bind L-selectin. Closest to the membrane is an Ig domain related to the third domain of IgA_1 (58). The human receptor appears to lack the mucin-like domain. MAdCAM was originally identified as being involved in lymphocyte homing in mice. Its role in human leukocyte migration has not been defined.

PLATELET ENDOTHELIAL CELL ADHESION MOLECULE (PECAM)

PECAM (CD31) is composed of six extracellular domains (59). It is expressed on platelets, leukocytes, and endothelial cells (60). The exact role of PECAM in leukocyte emigration is unclear although MAbs against domains 1 and 2 of both leukocyte and endothelially expressed PECAM inhibit transmigration through the endothelial junction. In addition, antibodies against domain 6 do not block migration through the endothelium but prevent migration through the basement membrane, suggesting that PECAM interacts with matrix protein to allow its degradation, so mediating leukocyte traffic (61).

THE ROLE OF ADHESION RECEPTORS
IN ALLERGIC INFLAMMATION

Expression of Adhesion Receptors in Allergic Inflammation

Adhesion molecule function is controlled in a number of ways, including increased expression as with E- and P-selectin, ICAM-1, and VCAM-1, shedding as with L-selectin, and conformational changes in the binding affinity of the receptor as seen with many integrins. A number of groups have studied expression of E-selectin, ICAM-1, and VCAM-1 in biopsies of allergic tissues largely using immunohistochemistry. Biopsies of skin, nasal mucosa, and endobronchial mucosa have been investigated. P-selectin expression has been less widely studied, partly because of the difficulty in distinguishing between intracellular and lumenal staining. These studies are detailed in Tables 1 and 2.

The use of immunohistochemistry to study adhesion receptor expression can only ever be semiquantitative. In addition, several studies have only assessed the number of positive blood vessels and not the intensity of staining. Most studies have only used one monoclonal antibody for each adhesion receptor. This relies heavily on the specificity and effectiveness of that antibody. For example, in one instance a widely used anti-E-selectin antibody was later found to crossreact with P-selectin. Two types of studies have been undertaken: allergen challenge and clinical disease.

ALLERGEN CHALLENGE STUDIES

Findings have generally been consistent with observations in cytokine stimulated HUVECs. In the skin, low background expression of ICAM-1 is seen with absent expression of E-selectin and VCAM-1. After allergen challenge, increased endothelial expression of E-selectin and ICAM-1 has been observed in three studies. In one study by Leung et al. (63) the increased E-selectin expression was demonstrated to result from generation of TNF-α and IL-1. VCAM-1 expression was weak. E-selectin expression in the skin is of particular interest in view of its potential role as a skin homing receptor (*see* the T-Lymphocytes section). Smith et al. (77) found increased P-selectin expression up to 1 h after skin challenge with neuropeptides.

In the airway Montefort et al. (65) found increased expression of ICAM-1 and E-selectin 6 h after local allergen challenge with no increase in VCAM-1 expression. However at 24 h in the study by Bentley et al. (64) there was a trend toward increased VCAM-1 expression (significance was lost through one outlier) with a good correlation between VCAM-1

Table 1
Endothelial Expression of Adhesion Proteins in Allergic Inflammation

Tissue	Principal findings
Allergen challenge	
Skin (62)	Increased endothelial expression of ICAM-1 and E-selectin 6 h after allergen challenge.
Skin (63)	Increased expression of E-selectin as a result of TNF-α and IL-1 release
Bronchus (64)	Correlation between increased numbers of eosinophils and VCAM-1 expression at 24 h
Bronchus (65)	Increased expression of ICAM-1 and E-selectin 6 h after local allergen challenge (VCAM-1 expression not increased)
Skin (66)	Lumenal P-selectin expression 1 h after challenge dissipated by 6 h. Increased E-selectin expression at 6 h
Nose (67)	Increase from 9 to 26% in the number of blood vessels expressing VCAM-1 and an increase in E-selectin but not ICAM-1 24 h after challenge
Clinical disease	
Atopic asthma (68)	No increase in E-selectin, ICAM-1, or VCAM-1 expression observed
Atopic and nonatopic asthma (64)	No increase in E-selectin, ICAM-1, or VCAM-1 in atopic asthma. Significant increase in E-selectin and ICAM-1 in intrinsic asthma. High background expression
Asthma (69)	Increased expression of E-selectin, ICAM-1, and VCAM-1 in six asthmatics compared to six normal controls
Atopic and nonatopic asthma (70)	Increased expression of ICAM-1, VCAM-1, and E-selection in atopic asthma but not nonatopic asthma compared with controls. Low background expression
Atopic asthma (71)	Increased expression of VCAM-1 in patients with detectable IL-4 in BAL fluid compared with controls and asthmatics without IL-4 in BAL fluid. Correlation between eosinphil counts and VCAM-1 expression
Perennial rhinitis (72)	Increased expression of VCAM-1 and ICAM-1, although VCAM-1 weak
Nasal polyp (73)	Strong expression of ICAM-1 and P-selectin. Weak expression of VCAM-1.
Nasal polyp (74)	Increased expression of VCAM-1 compared to normal nasal tissue. 5% of blood vessels stained strongly. Correlation between VCAM-1 expression and eosinophil numbers
Atopic dermatitis (75)	Increased expression of E-selectin, VCAM-1, and ICAM-1.
Toluene diisocyamate asthma (76)	No increase in endothelial expression of ICAM-1 or E-selectin

Table 2
Summary of Endothelial Adhesion Receptor Expression
in Allergic Inflammatory Responses[a]

Model /organ	Endothelial adhesion receptor			
(number of studies)	*P-selectin (lumenal)*	*E-selectin*	*ICAM-1*	*VCAM-1*
Allergen challenge				
Skin (3)	+ (1 h)	+ (6 h)	+ (6 h)	– (6 h)
Upper airway (1)	NR	+ (24 h)	– (24 h)	+ (24 h)
Lower airway (2)	NR	+ (6 h)	+ (6 h)	+ (24 h)
Clinical disease				
Eczema (1)	NR	+	+	+
Rhinitis (1)	NR	–	+	+
Polyps (2)	+	–	+	+/–
Atopic asthma (5)	NR	+/–	+/–	+/–
Nonatopic asthma (2)	NR	+/–	+/–	–
TDI asthma (1)	NR	–	–	NR

[a]+: increased expression reported; –: no increase in expression reported; +/–: studies differ in results; NR: not reported: MAdCAM-1 expression has not been reported.

expression and eosinophil infiltration. One study by Lee et al. *(67)*, reported as an abstract, has investigated nasal allergen challenge. They found an increase in E-selectin and VCAM-1 but not ICAM-1.

STUDIES OF CLINICAL DISEASE

One study has reported adhesion receptor expession in atopic dermatitis and found increased endothelial expression of ICAM-1, E-selectin, and VCAM-1. Results in asthma have been more variable. Montefort et al. *(68)* were unable to detect changes in adhesion receptor expression in atopic asthma, and in a study of atopic and nonatopic asthma Bentley et al. *(64)* could only detect a modest increase in ICAM-1 and E-selectin expression in their nonatopic asthmatics with relatively high background expression. In contrast Gosset et al. *(70)* found low background expression in normal subjects and could detect increases in adhesion molecule expression in atopic but not nonatopic asthmatics. Ohkawara et al. *(69)* agreed with these findings in six atopic asthmatics, but Fukuda et al. *(71)* detected no increase in ICAM-1 or E-selectin staining over controls. However, the E-selectin antibody they used crossreacts with P-selectin. This group did, however, find an increase in VCAM-1 expression, which correlated with eosinophil counts but only in those subjects with detectable IL-4 in the broncoalveolar lavage (BAL) fluid. In the upper airway, generally weak expression of VCAM-1 has been observed, although increased over normal controls in both perennial rhintis and nasal polyps. In nasal polyps good staining for ICAM-1 and lumenal P-selectin has been observed by Symon et al. *(73)*. In clinical disease it is therefore difficult to be dogmatic about the pattern of endothelial adhesion receptor staining. Whereas there is a tendency toward increased expression of ICAM-1, E-selectin, and VCAM-1, this may reflect a bias toward publication of positive data. The general trend is toward the finding of increased expression of VCAM-1; however, the findings are not yet conclusive.

ICAM-1 expression on epithelial cells has also been studied. A number of groups have demonstrated increased ICAM-1 on bronchial epithelium in asthma *(64,78,79)*. The expression was generally on the basal part of the epithelium adjacent to the basement membrane, and the degree of expression in the study by Vignola et al. *(78)* correlated with clinical indices of disease. In addition, Ciprandi et al. *(80,81)* have demonstrated induction of ICAM-1 within 30 min of allergen challenge on both nasal and conjunctival epithelium. This is considerably faster than the rate at which expression is induced in HUVEC. The role of ICAM-1 as a receptor for the major group of rhinoviruses means that the epithelium in asthmatics may be more vulnerable to viral infection. Expression of CD44, a receptor for the matrix protein hyaluronate, is increased on the bronchial epithelium in asthma, although it is also found on normal epithelium.

SOLUBLE ADHESION MOLECULES

Several adhesion molecules can be detected in soluble form circulating in the plasma. Raised concentrations of circulating adhesion molecules have been detected in a number of diseases *(82)*. Montefort et al. *(83)* found that concentrations of E-selectin, ICAM-1, and VCAM-1 were not elevated in stable asthma, but there was a significant increase compared with normal controls in concentrations of soluble E (sE)-selectin and sICAM-1 in patients with acute severe asthma. However, concentrations of these molecules did not correlate with disease severity and were therefore not thought useful in clinical management. In another study of 45 atopic and nonatopic asthmatics serum concentrations of sICAM-1, sE-selectin, and sVCAM-1 were increased during "asthma attacks" when compared with stable periods *(84,85)*. Concentrations of sICAM-1 and sE-selectin were increased in severe atopic dermatitis but did not fall after successful treatment with UVA-1 therapy *(86)*. Modest increases in concentrations of sICAM-1 and sE-selectin have also been detected in BAL fluid after segmental allergen challenge *(87,88)*. Zangrilli et al. *(89)* measured sVCAM-1 concentrations in BAL fluid 24 h after segmental allergen challenge in 27 ragweed allergic asthmatics and 18 atopic nonasthmatics. A marked increase in sVCAM-1 concentrations was observed in BAL fluid, which correlated with increased numbers of eosinophils and concentrations of IL-4 and IL-5. Most of the increase occurred in the late responders *(89)*.

Role of Adhesion Receptors in Leukocyte Function in Allergic Disease

EOSINOPHILS: SELECTIN INTERACTIONS

The mechanisms involved in eosinophil and basophil recruitment have recently been reviewed *(90,91)*. Eosinophil adhesion to cytokine-stimulated cultured HUVEC has been shown to be inhibited by blocking MAbs against E-selectin and L-selectin *(52,92)*. Eosinophils express L-selectin in similar amounts to neutrophils, and like neutrophils L-selectin is shed on eosinophil activation *(93,94)*. Eosinophils can also bind to P-selectin *(95)*. Eosinophil binding to E- and P-selectin does not appear to be affected by the state of activation of the cells. Although superficially eosinophils appear similar in their selectin interactions to neutrophils, there are potentially important differences. Whereas neutrophils express sialyl Lewis (sLewis), eosinophils express relatively little of this sugar moiety. In addition neutrophils bound more avidly than eosinophils to purified E-selectin *(96)*. The pattern of inhibition of eosinophil adhesion to HUVEC by a panel of L-selectin antibodies was different between eosinophils and neutrophils *(97)*.

We have previously reported a study in which we used the frozen section, Stamper-Woodruff assay to investigate eosinophil adhesion to nasal polyp endothelium *(73)*. We found that eosinophil adhesion was mediated largely by endothelial P-selectin, which was constitutively expressed in this chronic inflammatory model. More recently we have compared neutrophil binding in the same assay. A striking finding was that eosinophils bound with much greater avidity to the polyp blood vessels that neutrophils (Fig. 4). However the profile of adhesion receptors used by the two cell types was broadly similar, with over 80% inhibition

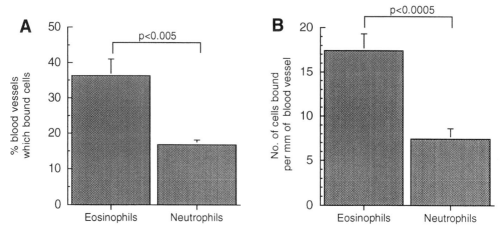

Fig. 4. In the frozen-section assay, eosinophils bind in greater numbers to nasal polyp endothelium than neutrophils.

of adhesion by antibodies against P-selectin and PSGL-1. To try to explain this observation we hypothesized that there may be differences in the eosinophil and neutrophil P-selectin ligands. The eosinophil P-selectin ligand, characterized using a P-selectin-IgG chimera and a rabbit antiserum against PSGL-1, appeared to be a structural isoform of PSGL-1 that migrated in sodium dodecyl sulfate (SDS) gels with a calculated molecular weight about 10 kDa higher than neutrophil PSGL-1. In agreement with Wein et al. *(95)*, we have found that under static conditions eosinophils and neutrophils bind to purified sP-selectin coated on tissue culture plates with the same avidity. However, in collaboration with Dr. Michael Lawrence of the University of Virginia, we have compared eosinophil and neutrophil binding to purified P-selectin under flow condition and were able to demonstrate that in the 5 subjects studied eosinophils bound to P-selectin with greater avidity than neutrophils. Using a monoclonal antibody PSL-275 from the Genetics Institute, we were able to demonstrate increased, expression of PSGL-1 by eosinophils compared to neutrophils, and sequencing of the complementary deoxyribonucleic acid (cDNA) and genomic clone of eosinophil PSGL-1 revealed that eosinophils express the 15-decapeptide form of PSGL-1 compared to the 16-decapeptide form expressed by neutrophils. There are therefore several differences in structure and expression between eosinophil and neutrophil PSGL-1 that could account for the functional difference in binding to P-selectin *(97)*.

EOSINOPHILS: INTEGRIN INTERACTIONS

Eosinophil adhesion to unstimulated HUVEC is enhanced about twofold by stimulation with platelet-activating factor (PAF), IL-5, and other eosinophil active inflammatory mediators, and this enhancement is almost totally inhibited by MAbs to the leukocyte integrin Mac-1 binding to an as yet unidentified endothelial ligand *(98–100)*. Compared to adhesion to unstimulated HUVEC, eosinophil adhesion to TNF-α- or IL-1-stimulated HUVEC under static condition is markedly increased, and this enhancement can be inhibited by MAbs against ICAM-1 and VCAM-1 on the endothelium and LFA-1, Mac-1, and VLA-4 on the leucocyte *(51–54)*. Eosinophil transmigration through HUVEC was increased by cytokine stimulation of the endothelium, and eosinophils from allergic donors showed an increased migration capacity consistent with the concept that eosinophils from subjects with allergic disease are activated *(101)*. Similarly, in vitro culture of peripheral blood eosinophils from normal donors with GM-CSF, IL-3, and IL-5 increased their migration capacity. The receptors that mediate transmigration of eosinophils through IL-1- or TNF-α-stimulated HUVEC appear to be primarily the leukocyte integrins LFA-1 and Mac-1 on the eosinophil binding to ICAM-1 and possibly other as yet unidentified ligands on the endothelium *(102)*. Antibodies against VLA-4 and VCAM-1 did not inhibit IL-1-stimulated transmigration. In contrast, eosinophil migration through IL-4-stimulated HUVEC was partly inhibited by anti-VLA-4 antibodies as well as antibodies against the leukocyte integrins *(103)*. The hypothesis that VLA-4/VCAM-1 could be a selective pathway of adhesion was strengthened, as discussed above, by the observation that IL-4 and the closely related IL-13 selectively induced expression of VCAM-1 on HUVEC. In our nasal polyp Stamper-Woodruff assay, no inhibition was seen with anti-VLA-4 or anti-α4β7, and in this situation the integrin component of adhesion appears to be mediated largely by the CD18 integrins.

EOSINOPHILS: ADHESION TO EXTRACELLULAR MATRIX

After migration through the endothelium the eosinophil comes into contact with the proteins of the extracellular matrix. Tissue eosinophils have an activated phenotype. They express activation receptors such as CD69 *(104)*, generate mRNA for a number of cytokines that do not appear to be generated by normal peripheral blood eosinophils *(105)*, express the secreted form of ECP as recognized by the MAb EG2 *(106)*, and have increased expression of CD11b and loss of expression of L-selectin *(107,108)*. The mechanism of eosinophil activation is not well understood. Interaction with the extracellular matrix can result in "outside in" signaling through integrin receptors, leading to eosinophil priming and mediator release. Dri et al. *(109)* found that the nature of the surface influenced the amount of superoxide produced with, for example, endothelial cells inhibiting superoxide production and fibrinogen priming eosinophils for enhanced superoxide generation after stimulation with N-formyl-methionyl-leukyl-phenylalanine (fMLP). Anwar et al. *(110)* demonstrated enhancement of calcium ionophore-stimulated leukotriene C4 generation by eosinophils adhering to fibronectin when compared with bovine serum albumin (BSA) coated surfaces, and Neeley et al. *(111)* have reported that VLA-4-mediated interaction with fibronectin resulted in increased fMLP-induced eosinophil degranulation. In contrast, Kita et al. *(112)* found that adherence to fibronectin and laminin inhibited eosinophil-derived neurotoxin (EDN) release stimulated by PAF, C5a, and IL-5 but not by PMA. The secretogogue used is obviously important in determining the effects of matrix proteins on eosinophil degranulation. When eosinophils were cultured for several days on plasma fibronectin, they had increased survival compared to eosinophils cultured on BSA or plastic as a result of autocrine generation of granulocyte-macrophage colony-stimulating factor (GM-CSF) and IL-3. Cytokine release and survival was inhibited by anti-VLA-4 MAb *(113)*. We have extended these observations to show that tissue fibronectin is considerably more effective than plasma fibronectin at supporting eosinophil survival *(114)*. This is consistent with the idea that survival is a result of triggering through α4/β1 (VLA-4), as tissue fibronectin contains more of the alternatively spliced 111CS region that contains the binding site for VLA-4 *(115)*. Activated eosinophils can also adhere to fibronectin through α4β7 *(116)*. Eosinophils can adhere to laminin through α6β1 *(117)*, and laminin also promotes eosinophil survival *(118)*. Eosinophil survival on matrix proteins is potently inhibited by glucocorticoids possibly by inhibiting autocrine synthesis of GM-CSF *(119)*.

T-LYMPHOCYTES

A central function of lymphocytes is their ability to recirculate from the blood into the lymphoid organs and back to blood in search of antigen. Lymphocyte recirculation is controlled by the interaction between adhesion receptors on lymphocytes (homing receptors) and their counterreceptors (addressins) on vascular endothelium. Thus the peripheral lymph node (PLN), T-lymphocyte homing receptor was defined as L-selectin, and the gut mucosal homing receptor was characterized as $\alpha 4\beta 7$. CD44 and LFA-1 appear to act as accessory adhesion receptors that strengthen the adhesive process without controlling selectivity of attachment *(120)*. An important observation was that a carbohydrate antigen on the surface of a subset of T-cells called the cutaneous lymphocyte antigen (CLA), which is thought to be related to sLewis X in structure, was a ligand for E-selectin. It was suggested that E-selectin was preferentially expressed in skin inflammation compared to other sites, in which it acted as a skin lymphocyte homing receptor *(121)*. Whereas CLA +ve T-cells constitute only a small subset of peripheral blood lymphocytes, almost all skin T-cells are CLA +ve. In contrast, T-lymphocytes in BAL fluid from asthmatics were largely CLA–ve *(122)*. Interestingly, caesin-reactive T-cells from patients with milk-induced eczema had higher expression of CLA than candida albicans-reactive T cells from the same patients or caesin-reactive T-cells from nonatopic controls *(123)*.

Furthermore, when house dust mite (HDM)-sensitive patients with asthma and atopic dermatitis were compared, the HDM-responsive T-cells from the eczema patients, but not from the asthma group, were in the CLA +ve T-cell subset *(124)*. Thus, there is increasing evidence that T-cell homing is relevant to human disease. This could explain why some HDM patients develop atopic dermatitis and others asthma. The mechanism by which allergen-reactive T cells in atopic dermatitis are confined to the CLA+ve population is not clear.

The lung homing receptor for T cells, if it exists, has not been defined. Limited studies of BAL T cells have been performed in terms of their homing capacity. BAL T-cells in normal subjects as well as asthmatics are mostly memory cells and express CD69. Increased numbers of CD25 positive T cells are seen in BAL fluid in asthma *(125)*. T cells in BAL fluid from allergen-challenged mice were L-selectin–ve and expressed increased amounts of VLA-4, although a variable pattern of adhesion receptor expression was observed on these cells *(126)*. BAL T cells from normal subjects contained increased numbers of cells expressing the epithelial homing receptor $\alpha E\beta 7$.

Mast Cells and Basophils

Possibly because they are seen as tissue-dwelling cells, mast cell adhesion interactions have been relatively little studied. Human skin and lung mast cells have been shown to express VLA-3, -4, and -5, through which they spontanously adhered to laminin and fibronectin. They did not express VLA-1, -2, or -6 and did not adhere to collagen type 1 or IV *(127,128)*.

Basophils express L-selectin, which is shed on activation, and have a more neutrophil- than eosinophil-like pattern of sialyl Lewis X expression. The expression of PSGL-1 on basophils has not been reported. Antibodies against E-selectin inhibit adhesion of basophils to cytokine-activated HUVEC. Like eosinophils, basophils express VLA-4 and can bind to VCAM-1 *(52)*. Crosslinking of basophil $\beta 1$ integrin receptors from asthmatic but not nonasthmatic donors resulted in histamine release *(129)*.

In Vivo Studies of Adhesion Receptor Antagonists in Models of Allergic Inflammation

An MAb against L-selectin (as well as $\alpha 4$) partially inhibited rolling of human eosinophils on rabbit mesentery venular endothelium in vivo, as shown by intravital microscopy *(130)*. The late response to ascaris challenge in a wild caught cyanomologous monkey model, which was neutrophil-dependent, was inhibited by anti-E-selectin *(131)*.

In a multiple antigen challenge version of the cyanomolgous monkey model, anti-ICAM was effective at inhibiting an airway eosinophilia that developed in association with increased bronchial hyperresponsiveness (BHR) *(132)*. In the same model, anti-Mac-1 MAb inhibited the development of BHR and reduced the levels of eosinophil cationic protein (ECP) in the BAL fluid, but did not inhibit the airway eosinophilia *(133)*. In a sheep model of allergen challenge the anti-VLA-4 MAb HP1/2 (which blocks both α4β and α4β7) was able to inhibit the late response to allergen challenge and the development of BHR when given both intravenously and by inhalation, again without affecting recruitment of eosinophils *(134)*. In a rat model, anti-VLA-4, -Mac-1, and -LFA-1 were all able to inhibit the early and late response to ovalbumin challenge but had no obvious effect on leucocyte recruitment into the lung, although this was measured 8 h after challenge, before any major cellular recruitment into the lung occurred *(135)*. The mechanism by which the antibodies inhibited the response to antigen challenge in this study is therefore not clear.

In guinea pigs the anti-VLA-4 MAb HP1/2 inhibited the migration of eosinophils into the skin both after injection of chemotactic factors and after passive cutaneous anaphylaxis *(136)*. Similarly HP1/2 was able to inhibit migration of eosinophils into the airway submucosa in sensitized, ovalbumin-challenged guinea pigs. The allergen challenge-induced increase in BHR was also prevented, as was the increase in the concentration of erythropoiesis (EPO) in BAL fluid *(137)*. In sensitized mice, anti-VLA-4 MAb inhibited eosinophil and T-cell infiltration into the trachea after ovalbumin challenge *(138)*. Anti-VCAM-1 MAb was also effective, and VCAM-1 expression was strongly induced by antigen challenge. Neither the VCAM-1 expression nor the eosinophil infiltration was IL-4-dependent. Unlike the monkey model, anti-ICAM-1 and anti-LFA-1 MAbs were ineffective at inhibiting eosinophil migration. Lastly, aerosolized anti-VLA-4 MAb inhibited allergen-induced BAL eosinophilia and BHR in rabbits sensitized to HDM *(139)*. These studies point to an important role for VLA-4, Mac-1, ICAM-1, and possibly VCAM-1 in eosinophil recruitment and activation in allergic inflammation and offer the possibility that suitably designed adhesion receptor antagonists may be therapeutically effective.

SUMMARY AND CONCLUSIONS

Considerable progress has been made in our understanding of the molecular mechanisms involved in leukocyte adhesion interactions. Migration through endothelium is a staged process with each stage offering a level of control over the cell specificity and degree of migration. This also offers a wide range of targets for pharmacological intervention. Although the structure and function of the receptors involved in leukocyte migration have been well characterized, the contribution each makes to the pattern of leucocyte accumulation in disease and in particular in allergic disease has still not been completely defined, although a number of interesting observations have been made (summarized in Table 3). There is evidence from in vitro studies using HUVEC, expression studies in allergic tissue, and in vivo studies in animal models for an important role for VLA-4/VCAM in mediating eosinophil transmigration through endothelium and into tissue. VLA-4 is attractive as a target because of its lack of expression on neutrophils. It is possible that VLA-4 may also mediate attachment to blood vessels under flow conditions. However our work has suggested a potential role for P-selectin in mediating the initial tethering step. Relatively little work has been undertaken on T-lymphocyte and monocyte adhesion interactions in allergic disease, although the suggestion that CLA +ve T-cells have an important role in atopic dermatitis but not asthma makes this an interesting area of further study. Conclusive results are likely to need selec-

Table 3
Summary of the Role of Adhesion Receptors in Allergic Disease

Receptor	Specific and principal role in allergic disease (key references)
Selectins	
P-selectin	Expression upregulated by IL-3 and IL-4 (6,7)
	Constitutively expressed on lumenal surface of nasal polyp endothelium (73)
	Eosinophils bind more avidly than neutrophils (97)
E-selectin	Endothelial expression upregulated after allergen challenge in vivo (63,64)
	Lymphocyte addressin in the skin (121)
	Neutrophils bind more avidly than eosinophils in vitro (95)
L-selectin	No special role in allergic disease defined at present
Integrins	
β2 integrins	Major family of receptors involved in endothelial transmigration of all leucocytes
α4β1/α4β7	Alternate transmigration pathway available to all leucocytes other than neutrophils (50–55)
	MAb against α4 inhibited eosinophil and lymphocyte tissue accumulation in nonhuman allergen challenge models (139)
α$_v$β3	Important in macrophage recognition of senescent eosinophils and neutrophils (30)
Immunoglobulin family CAMs	
ICAM-1	Widespread expression in inflamed tissue (including epithelum) in allergic diseases with a range of functions defined in vitro
	No clearly defined specific function in allergic disease other than as a receptor for rhinovirus (41)
	Anti-ICAM MAb-inhibited eosinophil transmigration and development of BHR in primate model of asthma (132)
ICAM-2 and -3	No defined role in allergic disease
VCAM-1	Endothelial expression upregulated in vitro by IL-4 (48,49)
	Ligand for VLA-4 and therefore involved in VLA-4 mediated transmigration
PECAM	Important in mediating transmigration through endothelial basement membrane
	No specific role in allergic disease yet defined

tive antagonists. Results using monoclonal antibodies in a number of animal models already offer the hope that this approach may be successful. The development of drugs that can be tested in the clinic are awaited with considerable interest.

REFERENCES

1. Springer TA (1994) Traffic signals for lymphocyte re-circulation and leukocyte emigration: the multi-step paradigm. Cell 76:310.
2. Bevilacqua MP (1993) Endothelial leukocyte adhesion molecules. Annu Rev Immunol 11:767–804.
3. Rosen SD (1993) Cell surface lectins in the immune system. Semin Immunol 5:237–247.
4. Bevilacqua MP, Pober JS, Mendrick DL, Cotran RS, Gimbrone MA (1987) Identification of an inducible endothelial leukocyte adhesion molecule ELAM-1. Proc Natl Acad Sci USA 84:9238–9242.
5. Geng JG, Bevilacqua MP, Moore KL, McIntyre TM, Prescott SM, Kim JM, Bliss GA, Zimmerman GA, McEver RP (1990) Rapid neutrophil adhesion to activated endothelium mediated by GMP-140. Nature 343:757–760.
6. Khew-Goodall Y, Butcher CM, Litwin MS, Newlands S, Korpelainen EI, Noack LM, Berndt MC, Lopez AF, Gamble JR, Vadas MA (1996) Chronic expression of P-selectin on endothelial cells stimulated by the T cell cytokine interleukin 3. Blood 87:1432–1438.
7. Yao L, Pan J, Setiadi H, Patel KD, McEver RP (1996) Interleukin 4 or oncostatin induces a prolonged increase in P-selectin mRNA and protein in human endothelial cells. J Exp Med 184:81–92.
8. Kishimoto TK, Jutila MA, Butcher EC (1990) Identification of a human peripheral lymph node homing receptor; a rapidly down regulated adhesion molecule. Proc Natl Acad Sci USA 87:2244–2248.
9. Springer TA, Lasky LA (1991) Sticky sugars for selectins. Nature 349:425–434.
10. Ley K, Tedder TF (1995) Leukocyte interactions with vascular endothelium. New insights into selectin mediated attachment and rolling. J Immunol 155:525–528.
11. Frenette PS, Mayadas TN, Rayburn H, Hynes RO, Wagner DD (1996) Susceptibility to infection and altered hematopoiesis in mice deficient in both P and E-selectins. Cell 84:563–574.
12. Lasky LA, Singer MS, Dowbenko D, et al. (1992) An endothelial ligand for L-selectin is a novel mucin like molecule. Cell 69:927–938.
13. Baumheuter S, Singer MS, Henzel W, Hemmerich S, Renz H, Rosen SD, Lasky LA (1993) Binding of L-selectin to the vascular sialomucin CD34. Science 262:436–438.
14. Berg EL, McEvoy LM, Berlin C, Bargatze RF, Butcher EC (1993) L-selectin mediated lymphocyte rolling on MAdCAM-1. Nature 366:695–698.
15. Sako D, Chang XJ, Barone KM (1993) Expression cloning of a functional glycoprotein ligand for P-selectin. Cell 75:1179.
16. Sako D, Comess KM, Barone KM, Camphausen RT, Cumming DA, Shaw GD (1995) A sulfated peptide segment at the amino terminus of PSGL-1 is critical for P-selectin binding. Cell 83:323–331.
17. Berg EL, Yoshin T, Rott LS (1991) The cutaneous lymphocyte antigen is a skin lymphocyte homing receptor for the vascular lectin endothelial cell-leukocyte adhesion molecule 1. J Exp Med 174: 1461–1466.
18. Alon R, Rossiter H, Wang X, Springer TA, Kupper TS (1994) Distinct cell surface ligands mediate T-lymphocyte attachment and rolling on P and E-selectin under physiological flow. J Cell Biol 127:1485–1495.
19. Steegmaler M, Levinovitz A, Isenmann S, Borges E, Lenter M, Kocher HP, Kleuser B, Vestweber D (1995) The E-selectin ligand ESL-1 is a variant of a receptor for fibroblast growth factor. Nature 373:615–620.
20. Picker LJ, Warnock RA, Burns AR, Doerschuk CM, Berg EL, Butcher EC (1991) The neutrophil selectin LECAM-1 presents carbohydrate ligands to the vascular selectins ELAM-1 and GMP-140. Cell 66:921–933.
21. Hynes RO (1992) Integrins: versatility, modulation and signalling in cell adhesion. Cell 69:11–25.
22. Hogg H, Berlin C (1995) Structure and function of adhesion receptors in leukocyte trafficking. Immunol Today 16:327–330.
23. Krensky AM, Sanchez-Madrid F, Robbins E, Nagy J, Springer TA, Burakoff SJ (1983) The functional significance, distribution and structure of LFA-1, LFA-2, and LFA-3: cell surface antigens associated with CTL-target interactions. J Immunol 131:611–616.
24. Arnaout MA, Colten HR (1984) Complement C3 receptors: structure and function. Mol Immunol 21:1191–1199.
25. Anderson DC, Springer TA (1987) Leukocyte adhesion deficiency: an inherited defect in the Mac-1, LFA-1 and p150,95 glycoproteins. Annu Rev Med 38:175–194.

26. Beller DI, Springer TA, Schreiber RD (1982) Anti-Mac-1 selectivity inhibits the mouse and human type three complement receptor. J Exp Med 156:1006–1009.

27. Russell DG, Wright SD (1988) Complement receptor type 3 (CR3) binds to an arg-gly-asp containing region of the major surface glycoprotein, gp63, of Leishmania promastigotes. J Exp Med 168:279–292.

28. Anderson DC, Miller LJ, Schmalsteig FC, Rothlein R, Springer TA (1986) Contributions of the Mac-1 glycoprotein family to adherence-dependent granulocytic functions: structure-function assessments employing sub-unit specific monoclonal antibodies. J Immunol 137:15–27.

29. Wallis WJ, Hickstein DD, Schwartz BR, June CH, Ochs HD, Beatty PG, Klebanoff SJ, Harlan JM (1986) Monoclonal antibody-defined functional epitopes on the adhesion promoting glycoprotein complex (Cdw18) of human neutrophils. Blood 67:1007–1013.

30. Savill J, Dransfield I, Hogg N, Haslett C (1990) Vitronectin receptor-mediated phagocytosis of cells undergoing apoptosis. Nature (Lond) 343:170–173.

31. Elices MJ, Osbourn L, Takada Y, et al. (1990) VCAM-1 on activated endothelium interacts with the leukocyte integrin VLA-4 at a site distinct from the VLA-4/fibronectin binding site. Cell 60:577–584.

32. Cepek KL, Shaw SK, Parker CM, Russell GJ, Morrow JS, Rimm DL, Brenner MB (1994) Adhesion between epithelial cells and T lymphocytes mediated by E-cadherin and the $\alpha E\beta 7$ integrin. Nature 372:190–193.

33. Erle DJ, Briskin MJ, Butcher ED, Garcia-Pardo A, Lazarovits AI, Tidswell M (1994) Expression and function of the MAdCAM-1 receptor integrin $\alpha 4/\beta 7$ on human leukocytes. J Immunol 153:517–528.

34. Berlin C, Bargatze RF, Campbell JJ, von Adrian UH, Szabo MC, Hasslen SR, Nelson EL, Berg EL, Ferlandsen SL, Butcher EC (1995) $\alpha 4$ integrin mediates lymphocyte attachment and rolling under physiologic flow. Cell 80:413–422.

35. Kassner AR, Carr MW, Finger EB, Hemler ME, Springer TA (1995) The integrin VLA-4 supports tethering and rolling in flow on VCAM-1. J Cell Biol 128:1243–1253.

36. Dustin ML, Rothlein R, Bhan AK, Dinarello CA, Springer TA (1986) Induction by IL-1 and interferon-gamma: tissue distribution, biochemistry and function of natural adherence molecule (ICAM-1). J Immunol 137:245–254

37. Simmons D, Makgoba MW, Seed B (1988) ICAM-1 an adhesion ligand of LFA-1 is homologous to the neural cell adhesion molecule NCAM. Nature 331:624–627

38. Makgoba MW, Sanders ME, Ginther GE, et al. (1988) ICAM-1 a ligand for LFA-1 dependent adhesion of B, T and myeloid cells. Nature 331:86–88.

39. Diamond MS, Staunton DE, de Fougerolles AR, Stacker SA, Garcia-Aguilar J, Hibbs ML, Springer TA (1990) ICAM-1 (CD54): a counter-receptor for Mac-1 (CD11b/CD18). J Cell Biol 111, 3129–3139.

40. Berendt AR, Simmons DL, Tansy J, Newbold CI, Marsh K (1989) Intercellular adhesion molecule-1 is an endothelial cell adhesion receptor for Plasmodium falciparum. Nature 341:57–59.

41. Greve JM, Davies G, Meyer AM, Forte CP, Yost SC, Marlow CW, Kamarck ME, McClelland A (1989) A major human rhinovirus receptor is ICAM-1. Cell 56:839–847.

42. Tomassini JE, Graham D, DeWitt CM, Lineberger DW, Rodkey JA, Colonno RJ (1989) cDNA cloning reveals that the major group rhinovirus receptor on HeLa cells is intercellular adhesion molecule-1. Proc Natl Acad Sci USA 86:4907–4911.

43. Miller J, Knorr R, Ferrone M, Houdei R, Garron S, Dustin ML (1995) Intercellular adhesion molecule-1 dimerisation and its consequences for adhesion mediated by lymphocyte function associated-1. J Exp Med 182:1231–1241

44. Pober JS, Gimbrone MA Jr, Lapierre LA, Mendrick DL, Fiers W, Rothlein R, Springer TA (1986) Overlapping patterns of activation by human endothelial cells by interleukin-1, tumor necrosis factor and immune interferon. J Immunol 137:1893–1896.

45. Staunton DE, Dustin ML, Springer TA (1989) Functional cloning of ICAM-2, a cell adhesion ligand for LFA-1 homologous to ICAM-1. Nature 339:61–64

46. de Fougerolles AR, Stacker SA, Schwarting R, Springer TA (1991) Characterisation of ICAM-2 and evidence for a third counter-receptor for LFA-1. J Exp Med 174:253–267.

47. de Fougerolles AR, Springer TA (1992) Intercellular adhesion molecule 3, a third adhesion counter receptor for lymphocyte function-associated molecule-1 on resting lymphocytes. J Exp Med 175:185–190.

48. Thornhill MH, Wellicome SM, Mahiouz DL, Lanchbury JS, Kyan-Aung U, Haskard DO (1991) Tumor necrosis factor combines with IL-4 or IFN-α to selectively enhance endothelial cell adhesiveness for T-cells. J Immunol 146:592.

49. Bochner BS, Klunk DA, Sterbinsky SA, Coffman RL, Schleimer RP (1995) IL-13 selectively induces vascular cell adhesion molecule-1 expression in human endothelial cells. J Immunol 154:799–803.

50. Schwartz BR, Wayner EA, Carlos TM, Ochs HD, Harlan JM (1990) Identification of surface proteins mediating adherence of CD11/18-deficient lymphoblastoid cells to cultured endothelium. J Clin Invest 85:2019–2022.

51. Walsh GM, Hartnell A, Mermod JJ, Kay AB, Wardlaw AJ (1991) Human eosinophil, but not neutrophil adherence to IL-1 stimulated HUVEC is a4b1 (VLA-4) dependent. J Immunol 146:3419–3423.

52. Bochner BS, Lusckinskas FW, Gimbrone MA, Newman W, Sterbinsky A, Derse-Anthony CP, Klunk D, Schleimer RP (1991) Adhesion of human basophils and eosinophils to IL-1 activated human vascular endothelial cells: contribution of endothelial cell adhesion molecules. J Exp Med 173:1552.

53. Dobrina A, Menegazzi R, Carlos TM, Nardon E, Cramer R, Zacchi T, Harlan JM, Patriarca P (1991) Mechanisms of eosinophil adherence to cultured vascular endothelial cells: eosinophils bind to the cytokine induced endothelial ligand vascular cell adhesion molecule-1 via the very late antigen-4 receptor. J Clin Invest 88:20.

54. Weller PF, Rand TH, Golez SE, Chi-Rosso G, Lobb RR (1991) Human eosinophil adherence to vascular endothelium mediated by binding to vascular cell adhesion molecule-1 and endothelial leukocyte adhesion molecule-1. Proc Natl Acad Sci USA 88:7430.

55. Campanero MR, Puliod R, Ursa MA, Rodriguez-Moya M, de Landazuri MO, Sanchez-Madrid F (1990) An alternative leukocyte adhesion mechanism, LFA-1/ICAM-1 independent, triggered through the human VLA-4 integrin. J Cell Biol 110:2157–2165.

56. Hemler ME (1988) Adhesive protein receptors on haemopoietic cells. Immunol Today 9:109–113.

57. Shyjan AM, Bertagnolli M, Kenney CJ, Briskin MJ (1996) Human mucosal addressin cell adhesion molecule-1 (MAdCAM-1) demonstrates structural and functional similarities to the $\alpha4\beta7$-integrin binding domains of murine MAdCAM-1, but extreme divergence of mucin-like sequences. J Immunol 156:2851–2857

58. Berlin C, Berg EL, Briskin MJ, Andrew DP, Kilshaw PJ, Holzman B, Weissman IL, Hamann A, Butcher EC (1993) $\alpha4\beta7$ integrin mediates lymphocyte binding to the mucosal vascular addressin MAdCAM-1. Cell 74:185–195.

59. Newman PJ, Berndt MC, Gorski J, White GC, Lyman S, Paddock C, Muller WA (1990) PECAM-1 (CD31) cloning and relation to adhesion molecules of the immunoglobulin gene superfamily. Science 247:1219–1222

60. Muller WA, Ratti CM, McDonnell SL, Cohn ZA (1989) A human endothelial cell-restricted, externally disposed plasmalemmal protein enriched in intercellular junctions. J Exp Med 170:399–414.

61. Liao F, Huynh HK, Eiroa A, Greene T, Polizzi E, Muller WA (1995) Migration of monocytes across endothelium and passage through extracellular matrix involve separate molecular domains of PECAM-1. J Exp Med 182:1337–1343.

62. Kyan-Aung U, Haskard DO, Poston RN, Thornhill MH, Lee TH (1991) Endothelial leukocyte adhesion molecule-1 and intercellular adhesion molecule-1 mediated the adhesion of eosinophils to endothelial cells in vitro and are expressed by endothelium in allergic cutaneous inflammation in vivo. J Immunol 146:521–528.

63. Leung YM, Pober JS, Cotran RS (1991) Expression of endothelial-leukocyte adhesion molecule-1 in elicited late phase allergic reactions. J Clin Invest 87:1805–1809.

64. Bentley AM, Durham SR, Robinson DS, Menz G, Storz C, Cromwell O, Kay AB, Wardlaw AJ (1993) Expression of endothelial and leukocyte adhesion molecules, intercellular adhesion molecule-1, E-selectin and vascular cell adhesion molecule-1 in the bronchial mucosa in steady state and allergen induced asthma. J Allergy Clin Immunol 92:857–868.

65. Montefort S, Gratziou C, Goulding D, Polosa R, Haskard DO, Howart PH, Holgate ST, Caroll M (1993) Upregulation of leukocyte-endothelial cell adhesion molecules 6 hours after local allergen challenge of sensitized asthmatic airways. J Clin Invest 93:1411–1421.

66. Murphy G, Leventhal L, Zweiman B (1994) Endothelial CD62 and E-selectin expression in developing late-phase IgE mediated skin reactions. J Allergy Clin Immunol 93:183 (abstract).

67. Lee B-J, Nacleiro RM, Bochner BS, Taylor RM, Lim MC, Baroody FM (1994) Nasal challenge with allergen upregulates the local expression of vascular endothelial adhesion molecules. J Allergy Clin Immunol 94:1006–1016.

68. Montefort S, Roche WR, Howarth PH, Djukanovic R, Gratziou C, Carroll M, Smith L, Britten KM, Haskard D, Lee TH, et al. (1992) Intercellular adhesion molecule-1 (ICAM-1) and endothelial leucocyte adhesion molecule-1 (ELAM-1) expression in the bronchial mucosa of normals and asthmatic subjects. Eur Respir J 5:815–823.

69. Ohkawara Y, Yamauchi K, Maruyama N, Hoshi H, Ohno I, Honma M, Tanno Y, Tamura G, Shirato K, Ohtani H (1995) In situ expression of the cell adhesion molecules in bronchial tissues from asthmatics with air flow limitation: in vivo evidence of VCAM-1/VLA-4 interaction in selective eosinophil infiltration. Am J Respir Cell Mol Biol 12:4–12.

70. Gosset P, Tillie-Leblond I, Janin A, Marquette CH, Copin MC, Wallaert B, Tonnel AB (1995) Expression of E-selectin, ICAM-1 and VCAM-1 on bronchial biopsies from allergic and non-allergic asthmatic patients. Int Arch Allergy Immunol 106:69–77.

71. Fukuda T, Fukushima Y, Numao T, Ando N, Arima M, Nakajima H, Sagara H, Adachi T, Motojima S, Makino S (1996) Role of interleukin-4 and vascular cell adhesion molecule-1 in selective eosinophil migration into the airways in allergic asthma. Am J Respir Cell Mol Biol 14:84–94.

72. Montefort S, Feather IH, Wilson SJ (1992) The expression of leukocyte endothelial adhesion molecules is increased in perennial allergic rhinitis. Am J Respir Cell Mol Biol 7:393–398.

73. Symon FA, Walsh GM, Watson SR, Wardlaw AJ (1994) Eosinophil adhesion to nasal polyp endothelium is P-selectin dependent. J Exp Med 180:371–376.

74. Jahnsen FL, Haraldsen G, Aanesen JP, Haye R, Brandtzeg P (1995) Eosinophil infiltration is related to increased expression of vascular cell adhesion molecule-1 in nasal polyps. Am J Respir Cell Mol Biol 12:624–632.

75. Wakita H, Sakamoto T, Tokura Y, Takigawa W (1994) E-selectin and vascular cell adhesion molecule 1 as critical adhesion molecules for infiltration of T lymphocytes and eosinophils in atopic dermatitis. J Cutan Pathol 21:33–99.

76. Maestrelli P, diStefano A, Occari P, Turato G, Milani G, Pivirotto F, Mapp CE, Fabbri LM, Saetta M (1995) Cytokines in the airway mucosa of subjects with asthma induced by toluene diisocyanate. Am J Respir Crit Care Med 151:607–612.

77. Smith CH, Barker JNWN, Morris RW, MacDonald DM, Lee TH (1993) Neuropeptides induce rapid expression of endothelial cell adhesion molecules and elicit granulocytic infiltration in human skin. J Immunol 151:3274–82.

78. Vignola AM, Campbell AM, Chanez P, Lacoste P, Michel FB, Godard P, Bousquet J (1993) HLA-DR and ICAM-1 expression on bronchial epithelial cells in asthma and chronic bronchitis. Am Rev Respir Dis 147:529–534.

79. Manolitsas ND, Trigg CJ, McAulay AE, Wang JH, Jordan SE, D'Ardenne AJ, Davies RJ (1994) The expression of intercellular adhesion molecule-1 and the β1-integrins in asthma. Eur Respir J 7:1439–1444.

80. Ciprandi G, Pronzato C, Ricca V, Passalacqua G, Bagnasco M, Canonica GW (1994) Allergen specific challenge induces intercellular adhesion molecule-1 (ICAM-1/CD54) expression on nasal epithelial cells in allergic subjects. Relationship with early and late inflammatory phenomena. Am J Respir Crit Care Med 150:1653–1659.

81. Ciprandi G, Buscaglia S, Pesce GP, Villaggio B, Bagnesco M, Canonica GW (1993) Allergic subjects express intracellular adhesion molecule 1 (ICAM-1 or CD54) on epithelial cells of conjunctiva after allergen challenge. J Allergy Clin Immunol 91:783–792

82. Gearing AJ, Newman W (1993) Circulating adhesion molecules in disease. Immunol Today 14:506–512

83. Montefort S, Lai CKW, Kapahi P, Leung J, Lai KN, Chan HS, Haskard DO, Howarth PH, Holgate ST (1994) Circulating adhesion molecules in asthma. Am J Respir Crit Care Med 149:1149–1152.

84. Kobayashi T, Hashimoto S, Imai K, Amemiya E, Yamaguchi M, Yachi A, Horie T (1994) Elevation of serum soluble intercellular adhesion molecule-1 (sICAM-1) and sE-selectin levels in bronchial asthma. Clin Exp Immunol 96:110–115.

85. Koizumi A, Hashimoto S, Kobayashi T, Imai K, Yachi A, Horie T (1995) Elevation of serum soluble vascular cell adhesion molecule-1 (sVCAM-1) levels in bronchial asthma. Clin Exp Immunol 101:468–473.

86. Kowalzick L, Kleinheinz A, Neuber K, Weichenthal M, Kohler I, Ring J (1995) Elevated serum levels of soluble adhesion molecules ICAM-1 and ELAM-1 in patients with severe atopic eczema and influence of UVA-1 treatment. Dermatology 190:14–18.

87. Georas SN, Liu MC, Newman W, Beall LD, Stealey BA, Bochner BS (1992) Altered adhesion molecule expression and endothelial cell activation accompany the recruitment of human granulocytes to the lung after segmental antigen challenge. Am J Respir Cell Mol Biol 7:261–269.

88. Takahashi N, Liu MC, Proud D, Yu, X-Y, Hasegawa S, Spannhake EW (1994) Soluble intercellular adhesion molecule-1 in bronchoalveolar lavage fluid of allergic subjects following segmental antigen challenge. Am J Respir Crit Care Med 150:704–709.

89. Zangrilli JG, Shaver JR, Cirelli RA, Cho SK, Garlisi CG, Falcone A, Cuss FM, Fish JE, Peters SP (1995) sVCAM-1 levels after segmental allergen challenge correlates with eosinophil influx, IL-4 and IL-5 production and the late pahse response. Am J Respir Crit Care Med 151:1346–1353.

90. Wardlaw AJ, Walsh GM, Symon FA (1994) Mechanisms of eosinophil and basophil migration. Allergy 49:797–807.

91. Bochner BS, Schleimer RP (1994) The role of adhesion molecules in human eosinophil and basophil recruitment. J Allergy Clin Immunol 94:427–438.

92. Knol EF, Kansas GS, Tedder TF, Schleimer RP, Bochner BS (1993) Human eosinophils use L-selectin to bind to endothelial cells under non static conditions. J Allergy Clin Immunol 91:334.

93. Smith JB, Kunjummen RD, Kishimoto TK, Anderson DC (1992) Expression and regulation of L-selectin on eosinophils from human adults and neonates. Pediatr Res 32:465–471.

94. Georas SN, Liu MC, Newman W, Beall LD, Stealey BA, Bochner BS (1992) Altered adhesion molecule expression and endothelial cell activation accompany the recruitment of human granulocytes to the lung after segmental antigen challenge. Am J Respir Cell Mol Biol 7:261–269.

95. Wein M, Sterbinsky SA, Bickel CA, Schleimer RP, Bochner BS (1995) Comparison of human eosinophil and neutrophil ligands for P-selectin: Ligands for P-selectin differ from those for E-selectin. Am J Respir Cell Mol Biol 12:315–319.

96. Bochner BS, Sterbinsky SA, Bickel CA, Werfel S, Wein M, Newman W (1994) Differences between human eosinophils and neutrophils in the function and expression of sialic acid containing counter-ligands for E-selectin. J Immunol 152:774–782.

97. Symon FA, Lawrence MB, Williamson M, Walsh GM, Watson SR, Wardlaw AJ (1996) Characterisation of the eosinophil P-selectin ligand. J Immunol 157:1711–1719.

98. Kimani G, Tonnensen MG, Henson PM (1988) Stimulation of eosinophil adherence to human vascular endothelial cell in vitro by platelet activating factor. J Immunol 140:3161.

99. Lamas AMC, Mulroney CM, Schleimer RP (1988) Studies of the adhesive interaction between purified human eosinophils and cultured vascular endothelial cells. J Immunol 140:1500.

100. Walsh GM, Hartnell A, Wardlaw AJ, Kurihara K, Sanderson CJ, Kay AB (1990) Il-5 enhances the in vitro adhesion of human eosinophils, but not neutrophils in a leucocyte integrin (CD11/18) dependent manner. Immunology 71:258–265.

101. Moser R, Fehr J, Olgati L, Bruijnzeel PLB (1992) Migration of primed human eosinophils across cytokine activated endothelial cell monolayers. Blood 79:2937–2945.

102. Ebisawa M, Bochner BS, Georas SN, Schleimer RP (1992) Eosinophil transendothelial migration induced by cytokines. Role of the endothelial and eosinophil adhesion molecules in IL-1b induced transendothelial migration. J Immunol 149:4021–4028.

103. Schleimer RP, Sterbinsky SA, Kaiser J, Bickel CA, Klunk DA, Tomioka K, Newman W, Luscinskas FW, Gimbrone MA, McIntyre BW, Bochner B (1992) IL-4 induces adherence of human eosinophils and basophils, but not neutrophils to endothelium. Association with expression of VCAM-1. J Immunol 148:1086–1092.

104. Hartnell A, Robinson DS, Kay AB, Wardlaw AJ (1993) CD69 is expressed by human eosinophils activated in vivo in asthma and in vitro by cytokines. Immunology 80:281–286.

105. Desreumaux P, Janin A, Colomble JF (1992) Interleukin 5 messenger RNA expression by eosinophils in the intestinal mucosa of patients with coeliac disease. J Exp Med 175:293–296.

106. Azzawi M, Bradley B, Jeffery PK, Frew A, Wardlaw AJ, Knowles G, Assoufi B, Collins JV, Durham S, Kay AB (1990) Identification of activated T lymphocytes and eosinophils in bronchial biopsies in stable atopic asthma. Am Rev Respir Dis 142:1407–1413.

107. Kroegel C, Liu MC, Hubbard WC, Lichenstein LM, Bochner BS (1994) Blood and bronchoalveolar eosinophils in allergic subjects after segmental antigen challenge: surface phenotype, density heterogeneity and prostanoid production J Allergy Clin Immunol 93:725–734.

108. Mengelers HJJ, Kaikoe T, Hooibrink B, et al. (1993) Down modulation of L-selectin expression on

eosinophils recovered from bronchoalveolar lavage fluid after allergen provocation. Clin Exp Allergy 23:196–204.

109. Dri P, Cramer R, Spessotto P, Romano M, Patriarca P (1991) Eosinophil activation on biologic surfaces. J Immunol. 147:613–620.

110. Anwar ARE, Cromwell O, Walsh GW, Kay AB, Wardlaw AJ (1994) Adhesion to fibronectin primes eosinophils via a4/b1. Immunology 82:222–228.

111. Neeley SP, Hamann KJ, Dowling T, McAllister KT, White SR, Leff AR (1994) Augmentation of stimulated eosinophil degranulation by VLA-4 (CD49d)-mediated adhesion to fibronectin. Am J Respir Cell Mol Biol 11:206–213.

112. Kita H, Horie S, Gleich GJ (1996) Extracellular matrix proteins attenuate activation and degranulation of stimulated eosinophils. J Immunol 156:1174–1181.

113. Anwar ARE, Cromwell O, Walsh GM, Kay AB, Wardlaw AJ (1993) Adhesion to fibronectin prolongs eosinophil survival. J Exp Med 177:839–843.

114. Walsh GM, Symon FA, Wardlaw AJ (1995) Human eosinophils preferentially survive on tissue fibronectin compared with plasma fibronectin. Clin Exp Allergy 25:1128–1136.

115. Mould AP, Wheldon A, Komoriya EA, Wayner EA, Yamada KM, Humphries MJ (1990) Affinity chromatic isolation of the melanoma adhesion receptor for the IIICS region of fibronectin and its identification as the integrin α4β1. J Biol Chem 265:4020.

116. Walsh GM, Symon FA, Lazarovits AI, Wardlaw AJ (1996) Integrin α4β7 mediates human eosinophil interaction with MAdCAM-1, vascular cell adhesion molecules-1 and fibronectin. Immunology 89:112–119.

117. Georas SN, McIntyre WB, Ebisawa M, Bednarczyk JL, Sterbinsky SA, Schlemier RP, Bochner BS (1993) Expression of a functional laminin receptor α6β1 (very late activation antigen-6) on human eosinophils. Blood 82:2872–2879.

118. Tourkin A, Anderson T, Carwile, Le-Roy E, Hoffman S (1993) Eosinophil adhesion and maturation is modulated by laminin. Cell Adhesion Commun 1:161.

119. Walsh GM, Wardlaw AJ (1997) Matrix protein induced eosinophil survival is inhibited by dexamethasone. J Allergy Clin Immunol 100:208–215.

120. Jalkanen S, Bargatze RF, de los Toyos JM, Butcher EC (1987) Lymphocyte recognition of high endothelium: antibodies to distinct epitopes of an 85–95 kd glycoprotein antigen differentially inhibit binding to lymph node, mucosal or synovial endothelial cells. J Cell Biol 105:983–990.

121. Picker LJ, Kishimoto TK, Smith CW, Warnock RA, Butcher EC (1991) ELAM-1 is an adhesion molecule for skin-homing T cells. Nature 349;796.

122. Picker LJ, Martin RJ, Trumble AE, et al. (1994) Control of lymphocyte re-circulation in man: differential expression of homing associated adhesion molecules by memory/effector T cells in pulonary versus cutaneous effector sites. Eur J Immunol 24:1269–1277.

123. Abernathy-Carver KJ, Sampson HA, Picker LJ, Leung DYM (1995) Milk-induced eczema is associated with the expansion of T cells expressing cutaneous lymphocyte antigen. J Clin Invest 95:913–918.

124. Babi LFS, Picker LJ, Soler MTP (1995) Circulating allergen reactive T cells from patients with atopic dermatitis and allergic contact dermatitis express the skin-selective homing receptor the cutaneous lymphocyte associated antigen (CLA). J Exp Med 181:747–753.

125. Corrigan CJ, Kay AB (1992) In: Barnes PJ, Rodger IW, Thomson NC, eds. T Lymphocytes Ch. 9. In Asthma: Basic Mechanisms and Clinical Management. Academic Press, U.K. London, pp. 125–142.

126. Kennedy JD, Hatfield CA, Fidler SF, Winterrowd GE, Haas JV, Chin JE, Richards IM (1995) Phenotypic characterisation of T lymphocytes emigrating into lung tissue and the airway lumen after antigen inhalation in sensitised mice. Am J Respir Cell Mol Biol 12:613–623.

127. Columbo M, Bochner BS, Marone G (1995) Human skin mast cells express functional β1 integrins that mediate adhesion to extracellular matrix proteins. J Immunol 154:6058–6064.

128. Sperr WR, Agis H, Czerwenka K, Klepetko K, Kubista E, Boltz-Nitulescu G, Lechner K, Valent P (1992) Differential expression of cell surface integrins on human mast cells and human basophils. Ann Hematol 65:10.

129. Lavens SE, Goldring K, Thomas LH, Warner JA (1996) Effects of integrin clustering on human lung mast cells and basophils. Am J Respir Cell Mol Biol 14:95–103.

130. Sriramarao P, von Adrian UH, Butcher EC, Bourdon MA, Broide DH (1994) L-selectin and very late antigen-4 integrin promote eosinophil rolling at physiological sheer street rate in vivo. J Immunol 153:4238–4246.

131. Gundel RH, Wegner CD, Torcellini CA, Clarke CC, Haynes N, Rothlein R, Smith CW, Letts LG (1991) ELAM-1 mediates antigen-induced acute airway inflammation and late phase obstruction in monkeys. J Clin Invest 88:1407–1411.

132. Wegner CD, Grundel RH, Reilly P, Haynes N, Letts GL, Rothlein R (1990) ICAM-1 in the pathogenesis of asthma. Science 247:416–418.

133. Wegner CD, Gundel RH, Churchill L, Letts LG (1993) Adhesion glycoproteins as regulators of airway inflammation; emphasis on the role of ICAM-1. In: Holgate ST, Austen KF, Lichtenstein LF, Kay AB, eds. Asthma: Physiology Pharmacology and Treatment. Academic, London, pp. 227–242.

134. Abraham WM, Sielczak MW, Ahmed A, et al. (1993) α4 integrins mediate antigen-induced late bronchial responses and prolonged airway hyperresponsiveness in sheep. J Clin Invest 776–87.

135. Rabb HA, Olivenstein R, Issekutz TB, Renzl PM, Martin JG (1994) The role of the leucocyte adhesion molecules VLA-4, LFA-1 and Mac-1 in allergic airway in rat. Am J Respir Crit Care Med 149: 1186–1191.

136. Weg VB, Williams TJ, Lobb PR, Nourshargh S (1993) A monoclonal antibody recognizing the very late activation antigen-4 inhibits eosinophil accumulation in vivo. J Exp Med 177:561–566.

137. Pretolani MC, Ruffie C, de Silva L, Joseph D, Lobb R, Vargaftig B (1994) Antibody to very late activation antigen 4 presents antigen-induced bronchial hyperreactivity and cellular infiltration in the guinea pig airways. J Exp Med 180:795–805.

138. Nakajima H, Sano H, Nishimura T, Yoshida S, Iwanoto I (1994) Role of vascular cell adhesion molecule 1/very late antigen 4 and intercellular adhesion molecule 1 interactions in antigen-induced eosinophil and T cell recruitment into the tissue. J Exp Med 179:1145–1154.

139. Metzger WJ, Ridgr V, Tollefson V, Arrheius T, Gaeta FCA, Elices M (1994) Anti-VLA-1 antibody and CS1 peptide inhibitor modify airway inflammation and bronchial airway hyperresponsiveness (BHR) in the allergic rabbit. J Allergy Clin Immunol 93:183 (abstract).

19 Cell/Cytokine Interactions

David H. Broide, MBChB

CONTENTS

INTRODUCTION

Cytokines provide an important local mechanism for inflammatory cells at sites of allergic inflammation to communicate with each other in orchestrating the inflammatory response. Cytokines regulate a number of cellular functions important to allergic inflammation, including the regulation of immunoglobulin E (IgE) synthesis, the regulation of the expression of adhesion molecules by endothelium, and the regulation of inflammatory cell function (1). Our understanding of the relative importance of individual cytokines to allergic inflammation has been advanced by the cloning of cytokines and cytokine receptors, the elucidation of the crystal structure of cytokines suggesting important ligand binding sites, and in vitro functional studies using recombinant cytokines and individual cell types important to allergic function (i.e., mast cells, eosinophils, T-cells, B-cells, endothelium, epithelium). We will review cell/cytokine interactions in the context of these studies, focusing particularly on cytokine interactions with eosinophils, as well as review important advances in understanding the in vivo role of individual cytokines in studies using cytokine transgenic mice (mice overexpressing a particular cytokine) (2) or cytokine knockout mice (mice deficient in a particular cytokine) (3) (Table 1).

MECHANISM OF CELL/CYTOKINE INTERACTIONS: CYTOKINE RECEPTORS

Cytokines released at sites of allergic inflammation induce their biologic effect by binding to cytokine cell surface receptors. At least five cytokine receptor families have been identified and characterized based on a shared family structure (4) (Table 2). Class I cytokine

From: *Allergy and Allergic Diseases: The New Mechanisms and Therapeutics*
Edited by: J. A. Denburg © Humana Press Inc., Totowa, NJ

Table 1
Cytokine Knockout and Transgenic Mice

Cytokine	Knockout mice	Transgenic mice
IL-4	Th2-dependent immune responses impaired	Inflammatory lesion of external eye
	Decreased IgE response	Increased IgE
	Attenuation of eosinophilic inflammation and IL-5 secretion following aerosol antigen inhalation	
IL-5	No eosinophilia following aerosol inhalation antigen challenge	Peripheral-blood eosinophilia
	Airway hyperreactivity abolished in antigen-challenged mice (C57BL/6 strain)	Tissue eosinophilia
GM-CSF	No major perturbation of hematopoesis	Ocular, skeletal-muscle, and peritoneal lesions characterized by an accumulation of macrophages
	Characteristic pulmonary pathology resembling alveolar proteinosis	Increased numbers of activated pleural and peritoneal macrophages

Table 2
Cytokine Receptor Families

1. Class I (hematopoetic receptors)
   Common β-chain (IL-3, IL-5, GM-CSF)
   Common γ-chain (IL-2, IL-4, IL-13)
   Common chain (IL-6, IL-11)

2. Class II
   Interferon receptors

3. Immunoglobin superfamily
   IL-1, CSF-1

4. TNF-like receptors
   TNF, nerve growth factor

5. G-protein-coupled receptors
   Chemokines

receptors (hematopoietic receptors) and G-protein-coupled receptors (chemokine receptors) are particularly important to eosinophils. For example, members of the class I hematopoietic receptor family (interleukin [IL]-5, granulocyte-macrocyte colony-stimulating factor [GM-CSF], and IL-3 receptors) all express a common β-chain *(5)*. The demonstration that the IL-5, GM-CSF, and IL-3 receptors all share a common β-chain responsible for signal transduction explains many of the overlapping biologic properties of IL-5, GM-CSF, and IL-3 in terms of their ability to maintain eosinophil proliferation, viability, and effector function. Each of these three cytokines binds to a unique α-chain but shares a common β-signal transduction chain *(5)*.

Eosinophil chemotaxis into tissues is likely to be regulated in part by chemokines such as eotaxin and RANTES members of the C-C subclass of chemokines *(6)*. Chemokines exert their biologic effect by coupling to a family of seven transmembrane-spanning G-protein-coupled receptors *(6)*. Thus, class I receptors and the family of G-protein-coupled chemokine receptors are likely to play an important role in eosinophilic inflammation.

Cytokines such as IL-1 and tumor necrosis factor (TNF) induce endothelial cells to express adhesion molecules such as intercellular adhesion molecule (ICAM), vascular cell adhesion molecule (VCAM), and E-selectin and are therefore likely to play an important role in the interaction of circulating inflammatory cells and endothelium. These cytokines exert their effect through individual receptors belonging to specific families. For example, the IL-1 receptor belongs to the immunoglobulin supergene family of receptors, whereas the TNF 55 receptor present on the endothelial cell belongs to the TNF-like receptor family whose members include receptors for TNF and nerve growth factor *(4)*. In addition to IL-1 and TNF, IL-4 and IL-13 are cytokines that induce adhesion molecule expression (i.e., VCAM) by endothelial cells *(7)*. In contrast to the IL-1 receptor and TNF receptor, the IL-4 and IL-13 receptors belong to the class I family of hematopoietic receptors *(4)*. As the IL-4 and IL-13 receptors signal endothelial cells to express VCAM (but not ICAM or E-selectin) whereas the IL-1 and TNF receptors signal endothelial cells to express VCAM as well as ICAM and E-selectin, these postreceptor signal transduction pathways in endothelial cells are likely to differ depending on the receptor family initiating the signaling *(5)*.

IMPORTANCE OF CELL/CYTOKINE INTERACTIONS TO ALLERGIC INFLAMMATION: INSIGHTS FROM CYTOKINE TRANSGENIC AND CYTOKINE KNOCKOUT MICE

IL-4 Transgenic Mice

In vitro IL-4 exerts important functional effects relevant to allergic inflammation, including regulating IgE synthesis and inducing endothelial cell adhesion molecule expression. IL-4 transgenic mice display an "allergic" phenotypic abnormality in that all the mice display inflammatory lesions of the external eye characterized by marked swelling and erythema of the eyelid *(8)*. Histologic analysis of the ocular lesion demonstrates a dense inflammatory cell infiltrate composed of mononuclear cells, eosinophils, and mast cells *(8)*. The development of IL-4 transgenic mice has demonstrated the importance of IL-4 to IgE synthesis in vivo, as these mice express markedly increased IgE levels in vivo *(9)*. In addition, B-cells from these IL-4 transgenic mice synthesize increased amounts of IgE when stimulated in vitro with lipopolysaccharide *(9)*. The increased production of antigen-specific IgE in IL-4 transgenic mice occurs in response to T-cell-dependent but not to T-cell-independent antigens *(9)*.

IL-5 Transgenic Mice

IL-5 transgenic mice are phenotypically normal except for mild splenomegaly *(10,11)*. Bone marrow from IL-5 transgenic mice have increased numbers of IL-5-dependent eosinophil precursors. IL-5 transgenic mice have markedly increased numbers of eosinophils in peripheral blood (~40% of peripheral-blood leukocytes), demonstrating the importance of IL-5 in lineage-specific eosinophil proliferation *(10)*. In addition to the increased number of blood eosinophils, a variety of tissues (bone marrow, spleen, lungs, Peyers patches, mesenteric lymph nodes, and gut lamina propria) exhibit eosinophilia.

GM-CSF Transgenic Mice

GM-CSF, like IL-5, is able to influence eosinophil proliferation, viability, and effector function in vitro. Whereas GM-CSF transgenic mice exhibit eosinophilia in vivo, the level of eosinophilia is mild compared to that noted with IL-5 transgenic mice *(12)*. The functional effect of GM-CSF in these transgenic mice appears to be particularly targeted to marcrophages, which are present in increased numbers in peritoneal and pleural cavities. These macrophages appear to be activated, as assessed by increased expression of macrophage activation markers (MAC2 and MAC3) as well as elevated basal and stimulated superoxide production. Phenotypically, GM-CSF transgenic mice develop characteristic ocular, skeletal-muscle, and peritoneal lesions characterized by an accumulation of macrophages *(12)*.

GM-CSF Knockout Mice

Although GM-CSF is a hematopoetic growth factor, GM-CSF knockout mice do not exhibit any significant perturbation of hematopoesis *(13)*. However, GM-CSF knockout mice develop a characteristic pulmonary pathology resembling human alveolar proteinosis. As alveolar macrophage function is regulated by GM-CSF, the accumulation of lipoproteinacious material in the alveoli of GM-CSF knockout mice is most likely due to impaired macrophage function in these mice.

Interferon-γ Knockout Mice

The interferon-γ (IFNγ) knockout mice have normal development and are healthy in the absence of pathogenic infection *(14–16*. They have no alterations in splenic and thymic cell populations or peripheral blood cells. However, in response to infection with *Mycobacterium bovis*, IFNγ knockout mice have impaired production of nitric oxide and superoxide anion, as well as reduced expression of major histocompatibility complex (MHC) class II on macrophages. The IFNγ knockout mice exhibit significantly increased mortality in response to sublethal infection with *M. bovis*.

IL-4 Knockout Mice

IL-4 knockout mice exhibit a number of functional deficiencies important to allergic inflammation. For example, IL-4-deficient mice have significantly reduced levels of IgE and do not develop an IgE response to a nematode parasitic infection *(17,18)*. Although there is normal T- and B-cell development in these mice, T helper 2 (Th2)-dependent immune responses are impaired in that CD-4$^+$ T-cells from naive IL-4 knockout mice do not produce Th2 cytokines. In addition, CD-4$^+$ T-cells derived from *Nippostrongylus brasiliensis*-infected IL-4 knockout mice generate markedly reduced amounts of Th2-type cytokines, which correlates with a reduced helminth-induced eosinophilia.

IL-4 Knockout Mice: Inhalation Antigen Challenge

Aerosol antigen challenge of ovalbumin-sensitized wild-type mice induces an eosinophilic airway inflammatory response that is dependent on IL-5 and CD-4$^+$ T-lymphocytes *(19)*. In contrast, antigen challenge of IL-4 knockout mice results in a marked attenuation of eosinophilic inflammation and IL-5 secretion *(19)*. In vitro stimulation of T-lymphocytes derived from the lungs of IL-4 knockout mice fail to induce secretion of IL-4 as well as IL-5 after crosslinking of the CD-3/T-cell receptor complex.

Studies using a neutralizing monoclonal antibody to IL-4 (11B11), as opposed to studies using IL-4 knockout mice, demonstrated that when 11B11 was injected during the 3-wk allergen sensitization procedure (i.e., before the second injection of ovalbumin on d 14 of the

21-d sensitization protocol) there was greater than 90% inhibition of eosinophil recruitment into the lung *(20)*. In contrast, when an anti-IL-4 antibody was administered on d 21, 4 h before the final aerosol antigen challenge, there was no significant inhibition of eosinophil recruitment into the lung *(20)*. In contrast to these findings, studies using a polyclonal antibody to IL-4, administered immediately before antigen challenge, inhibited the recruitment of eosinophils into the lungs *(21)*. Whether the differences in these results with neutralizing antibodies to IL-4 are a result of differences in monoclonal (MAb) vs polyclonal anti-IL-4 antibodies used or other methodologic differences is not clear at present.

IL-5 Knockout Mice

IL-5 deficient mice are phenotypically normal and do not respond with eosinophilia following aerosol inhalation antigen challenge *(22)*. Lung histology and eosinophil numbers in bronchoalveolar lavage fluid and blood taken from IL-5 knockout mice resemble those of mice that are not actively sensitized with allergen *(22)*. In contrast, lymphocyte numbers in bronchoalveolar lavage fluid are significantly elevated after allergen challenge of IL-5 knockout mice, although increases in lymphocyte number are less marked than in wild-type mice challenged with allergen *(22)*. Following ovalbumin sensitization, ovalbumin-specific IgE is detected at similar levels in sera from IL-5 knockout and wild-type mice after aerosol allergen challenge. Airway hyperreactivity to methacholine is also abolished in aerosol antigen-challenged IL-5 knockout mice. The central role of IL-5 in aerosol allergen-induced eosinophilic recruitment into the airway was further suggested from studies reconstituting IL-5 production in the lungs of IL-5 knockout mice by using a recombinant vaccinia virus expressing IL-5. The lungs of allergen-sensitized IL-5 knockout mice exposed via the airway to the control virus (not expressing IL-5) showed highly localized pockets of airway inflammation that were not characterized by eosinophilic infiltration and that correlated with the sites of virus infection *(22)*. Exposure of these mice to aerosolized ovalbumin did not induce further airway inflammation or lung damage. In contrast, when IL-5 knockout mice had IL-5 restored in the airway by intranasal inoculation of recombinant vaccinia virus-IL-5 and were then challenged with ovalbumin, they developed significant peripheral-blood eosinophilia, severe pulmonary eosinophilic inflammation, and airway hyperreactivity *(22)*. Lungs of IL-5 knockout mice given recombinant vaccinia virus-IL-5 in the absence of ovalbumin sensitization and aerosolization showed some evidence of eosinophil migration, which was primarily localized to the sites of recombinant vaccinia virus-IL-5 infection but was not accompanied by dense cellular infiltration or changes in lung morphology. These studies suggest that IL-5 is essential for mounting aerosol allergen-induced pulmonary and blood eosinophilia as well as the subsequent onset of airway hyperreactivity and lung damage in vivo.

In contrast to this study using IL-5-deficient mice *(22)*, a study using neutralizing antibodies to IL-5 did not demonstrate an important role for IL-5 *(23)* and eosinophils in the development of bronchial hyperreactivity. In these studies mice were given a combination of two neutralizing anti-IL-5 MAbs (TRFK-4 and TRFK-5, a rat IgG_{2a} and IgG_1 MAb, respectively) intraperitoneally weekly throughout the experimental period. In these experiments the percentage of eosinophils following anti-IL-5 treatment could be reduced from ~44% to ~2% without changes in airway pressure from baseline. In contrast to mice treated with anti-IL-5 antibodies, mice treated with neutralizing anti-IL-4 monoclonal antibodies throughout the period of immunization had substantial blockade of airway hyperreactivity that was not associated with a significant effect on levels of eosinophils in the lung, suggesting that the effects of IL-4 were independent of effects on eosinophil recruitment into the lung *(23)*. Although at present it is not clear why studies with neutralizing antibodies to IL-5 as compared to IL-5 knockout mice have produced divergent results, a few potential explanations are possible *(24)*.

These include genetic differences in the strains of mice used in the two studies (C57BL/6 mice in IL-5 knockout studies and balb/c mice in studies using neutralizing antibodies to IL-5), potential methodologic concerns when using either knockout mice or MAb treatments, and finally the reproducibility and accuracy of physiologic measurements of airway hyperreactivity in small animals such as mice. In terms of the C57BL/6 mice, studies have revealed that this mouse strain is deficient in the low-molecular-weight secretory phospholipase A_2, an enzyme that has been implicated in facilitating exocytosis in mast cells by generating lysophospholipids for fusion of the perigranular and plasma membranes, and in providing some of the arachidonic acid used for eicosanoid biosynthesis *(24)*. In addition, C57BL/6 mice have a point mutation that prevents the C57BL/6 mouse from producing one of seven mast cell proteases, namely, mast cell protease seven *(24)*. It is speculated that because of these and perhaps other genetic deficiencies, the C57BL/6 mouse is resistant to the induction of mast cell-dependent airway hyperresponsiveness. These studies suggest that there may be eosinophil-dependent (C57BL/6 mice; IL-5 knockout studies) and eosinophil-independent (balb/c mice; anti-IL-4 antibody studies) pathways to generate the clinical phenotype of airway hyperresponsiveness. This may be relevant and applicable to human asthma, in which it is likely that multiple cellular pathways may lead to the expression of airway hyperresponsiveness, depending on the genetic background of the host. In addition to genetic differences in mouse strains used in the above studies, there are also technical concerns about using either knockout mice or neutralizing antibodies. Whereas the strength of using knockout mice in studies of allergic inflammation is that a particular single gene is deficient in the knockout mouse, the confounding potential for a counterregulatory cytokine gene to be expressed in response to the mutation must always be considered. Studies using neutralizing antibodies to cytokines also have the potential for producing false negative results (depending on dose, route, and timing of administration of antibody, affinity of antibody) or false positive results (nonspecific binding of antibody to Fc receptors on inflammatory cells and not to the cytokine being studied). It should also be noted that measurements of airway hyperresponsiveness in mice are technically demanding and the accuracy and reproducibility of such measurements require considerable expertise. Advances in knockout mice technology permitting the generation of tissue-specific and time-inducible gene knockouts as well as the use of $F_{(ab)}$ fragments in neutralizing antibody studies will enhance the interpretation of studies using cytokine knockout mice or neutralizing antibodies to cytokines.

IL-12 AND MURINE MODELS OF ASTHMA

IL-12, a cytokine produced by monocytes and macrophages in response to infections, induces cell-mediated immune functions, upregulates Th1 cytokines, especially IFNγ, and inhibits or downregulates Th2 cytokines. In in vivo murine models of parasitic infection, administration of IL-12 suppresses the expression of Th2 cytokines and the associated responses, including eosinophilia, serum IgE, and mucosal mast cell proliferation *(25)*. In an in vivo murine model of asthma, IL-12 was also able to abrogate antigen-induced airway hyperresponsiveness and pulmonary eosinophilia concomitant with suppression of Th2 cytokine expression *(26)*. The effect of IL-12 in this murine model of airway inflammation is partially dependent on IFNγ, as IL-12-treated mice treated concurrently with an anti-IFNγ antibody had an approx 50% inhibition in eosinophil recruitment as compared to isotype control antibody-treated IL-12-challenged mice. The anti-IFNγ MAb therefore partially reversed the IL-12-induced inhibition of airway hyperresponsiveness in IL-12-challenged mice. These studies suggest that the beneficial effect of IL-12 is partially mediated through IFN-γ in inhibiting Th2 cytokine production. In addition, IL-12 may directly suppress airway hyperresponsiveness or eosinophil production or stimulate production of mediators other than IFN-γ

Table 3
Cytokine Regulation of Eosinophil Adhesion to Endothelium

Cytokinea	Adhesion molecule
	Endothelial adhesion-molecule expression
IL-1, TNF	(a) ICAM, VCAM, E-selectin
IL-4, IL-13	(b) VCAM (but not ICAM or E-selectin)
	Eosinophil adhesion molecule
GM-CSF, IL-5	(a) Regulates number of receptors
	β2-integrin upregulation
	L-selectin shedding
GM-CSF	(b) Regulates function of receptor VLA-4

[a]Examples of cytokines that regulate the expression or function of endothelial- or eosinophil-expressed adhesion molecules.

that could have these effects. Alternatively, the lack of complete IFNγ dependency of IL-12 effects on allergic responses may be caused by incomplete neutralization of IL-12 by the anti-IFNγ antibody used *(26)*.

CYTOKINE REGULATION OF EOSINOPHIL ADHESION

Cytokines are likely to play an important role in eosinophil adhesion to endothelium, both at the level of inducing endothelial cells to express adhesion molecules as well as at the level of regulating the expression of adhesion receptors by eosinophils (Table 3). In vivo studies using intravital video microscopy have demonstrated that IL-1 can induce eosinophil rolling and firm adhesion to endothelium under conditions of blood flow in vivo *(27)*. In these experiments the rabbit mesentery microcirculation was stimulated with IL-1 to induce adhesion molecule expression in the microvascular endothelium. Human peripheral-blood eosinophils were purified and fluorescently labeled and injected into the mesenteric circulation. In contrast to unstimulated endothelium, IL-1-stimulated endothelium induced significant rolling and adhesion of eosinophils in the microcirculation. The rolling of eosinophils in the microcirculation could be inhibited with neutralizing antibodies to either L-selectin or very late activation antigen (VLA)-4 integrin expressed on the eosinophil cell surface, whereas only antibodies to L-selectin were required to inhibit neutrophil rolling along endothelium. These studies demonstrate that eosinophils and neutrophils use different receptors for the initial rolling along vascular endothelium, with both cell types using L-selectin, whereas eosinophils utilize VLA-4 in addition to L-selectin to roll along IL-1-stimulated vascular endothelium.

These and other studies have demonstrated that the paradigm of selectin-mediated leukocyte rolling mediated solely by selectins and firm adhesion mediated by integrins does not hold for all leukocytes in vivo. Whereas the recognition of selectins as leukocyte rolling receptors has been extensively documented, the ability of integrins such as VLA-4 to function as rolling receptors has only recently been demonstrated in eosinophils and lymphocytes. The ability of integrins such as VLA-4 to subserve both a leukocyte rolling function as well as a firm adhesion function is suggested from in vitro studies in which the functional state of VLA-4 can be regulated from a low-affinity to a high-affinity state by cellular agonists. Using a single-cell micropipet adhesion assay, we have demonstrated that a cytokine such as GM-CSF can increase the affinity of eosinophil-expressed VLA-4 binding to its counter-receptors VCAM and CS-1 and that this increase in binding affinity is not associated with alterations in VLA-4 receptor number (assessed by FACS analysis) or VLA-4 receptor distri-bution (assessed by confocal microscopy) *(28)*. GM-CSF is also able to upregulate the number of β2-integrin receptors expressed by eosinophils and induce the shedding of L-selectin from the eosinophil cell surface, although this is less efficiently performed than GM-CSF-induced shedding of L-selectin by neutrophils *(29)*. Overall, these studies suggest that cytokines such as GM-CSF can have important effects on adhesion receptors expressed by eosinophils, both in terms of the number of receptors expressed (increased number of β2-integrin receptors and decreased number of L-selectin cell surface receptors) *(29)* as well as induce changes in the functional nature of the VLA-4 receptor from a low-avidity to a high-avidity state without affecting VLA-4 receptor number or distribution. These cytokine-induced changes in the num-ber and function of eosinophil adhesion receptors may alter the eosinophil from a cell express-ing rolling receptors prior to GM-CSF stimulation (eosinophils express L-selectin, low-avidity VLA-4, and low levels of β2-integrins pre GM-CSF exposure) to an eosinophil expressing firm adhesion receptors post GM-CSF exposure (eosinophil express increased β2-integrins and high-avidity VLA-4 and shed L-selectin).

The importance of cytokine-induced endothelial adhesion molecules to eosinophil recruit-ment is also suggested from in vivo studies with P-selectin- and ICAM-deficient mice *(30)*. Eosinophil recruitment in ragweed-challenged P-selectin-deficient mice (approx 75% inhi-bition of eosinophil recruitment) and ICAM-1-deficient mice (approx 67% inhibition of eosinophil recruitment) was significantly reduced compared to wild-type mice. In contrast to studies evaluating neutrophil recruitment in P-selectin/ICAM double mutant mice (neutrophil recruitment is inhibited ~100% following peritoneal *Streptococcus* pneumonia infection) *(31)*, eosinophil recruitment was not completely inhibited in P-selectin/ICAM-1 double mutant mice (eosinophil recruitment inhibited ~62%). Studies using intravital microscopy demon-strate that eosinophil rolling and firm adhesion are significantly reduced in P-selectin-deficient mice and that P-selectin and ICAM-1 are both important to eosinophil peritoneal recruitment following ragweed challenge. However, P-selectin/ICAM-1-independent eosinophil recruit-ment pathways, most likely utilizing VLA-4/VCAM (contributing ~25–38% to eosinophil recruitment), are also evident following allergen challenge.

Eosinophils and neutrophils share the ability to roll on endothelial-expressed P-selectin and firmly adhere to endothelial-expressed ICAM. In contrast, endothelial-expressed E-selectin preferentially supports neutrophil but not eosinophil rolling in vivo *(32)*. In addition, as eosinophils but not neutrophils express the integrin VLA-4, only eosinophils are able to roll on and adhere to endothelium expressing the VLA-4 ligand VCAM.

SUMMARY

Cytokine are likely to play an important role in the pathogenesis of allergic inflammation by modulating IgE synthesis and adhesion-molecule expression by endothelial cells and by regulating inflammatory cell function. Studies with individual cytokines have revealed that several cytokines share overlapping functions, rendering the neutralization of a single cytokine potentially ineffective as a mode of therapy. However, it is also likely that there is a hierarchy in terms of the importance of individual cytokines to allergic inflammation, with some cytokines being more important than others. For example, IL-5 appears very important to eosinophilic inflammation, and IL-4 to IgE synthesis. Studies using either neutralizing antibodies to cytokines or cytokine knockout mice will provide important insights into the hierarchy of importance of individual cytokines to allergic inflammation in murine models. The translation of these insights into advances in the treatment of human allergic inflammation is eagerly awaited.

REFERENCES

1. Broide DH (1995) Cytokines and adhesion molecules in asthma. Curr Allergy Clin Immunol 8:19–22.
2. Hanahan D (1989) Transgenic mice as probes into complex systems. Science 246:1265–1275.
3. Lewis J, Yang B, Detloff P, Smithies O (1996) Gene modification via "plug and socket" gene targeting. J Clin Invest 97:3–5.
4. Nicola NA (1995) Structural aspects of cytokine/receptor interactions. Ann NY Acad Sci 766:253.
5. Ihle JN (1995) Cytokine receptor signalling. Nature 377:591.
6. Schall TJ, Bacon KB (1994) Chemokines, leukocyte trafficking, and inflammation. Curr Opin Immunol 6:8651–873.
7. Bochner BS, Klunk DA, Sterbinsky SA, Coffman RL, Schleimer RP (1995) Interleukin-13 selectively induces vascular cell adhesion molecule-1 (VCAM-1) expression in human endothelial cells. J Immunol 154:799–803.
8. Tepper RI, Levinson DA, Stanger BZ, et al. (1990) IL-4 induces allergic-like inflammatory disease and alters T cell development in transgenic mice. Cell 62:457–467.
9. Burstein HJ, Tepper RI, Leder P, Abbas AK (1991) Humoral immune functions in IL-4 transgenic mice. J Immunol 147:2950–2956.
10. Dent LA, Strath M, Mellor AL, Sanderson CJ (1990) Eosinophil in transgenic mice expressing interleukin 5. J Exp Med 172:1425–1431.
11. Tominaga A, Takaki S, Koyama N, et al. (1991) Transgenic mice expressing a B cell growth and differentiation factor gene (Interleukin 5) develop eosinophilia and autoantibody production. J Exp Med 173:429–437.
12. Elliott MJ, Strasser A, Metcalf D (1991) Selective up-regulation of macrophage function in granulocyte-macrophage colony-stimulating factor transgenic mice. J Immunol 147:2957–2963.
13. Stanley E, Lieschke GJ, Grail D, et al. (1994) Granulocyte/macrophage colony-stimulating factor-deficient mice show no major perturbation of hematopoiesis but develop a characteristic pulmonary pathology. Proc Natl Acad Sci USA 90:770–774.
14. Huang S, Hendriks W, Althage A, et al. (1993) Immune response in mice that lack the interferon-γ receptor. Science 250:1742–1745.
15. Dalton DK, Pitts-Meek S, Keshav S, et al. (1993) Multiple defects of immune cell function in mice with disrupted interferon-γ genes. Science 259:1739–1742.
16. Amiri P, Haak-Frendscho M, Robbins K, et al. (1994) Anti-immunoglobulin E treatment decreases worm burden and egg production in *Schistosoma mansoni*-infected norma and interferon-γ knockout mice. J Exp Med 180:43–51.
17. Kuhn R, Rajewsky K, Muller W (1991) Generation and analysis of interleukin-4 deficient mice. Science 254:707–710.
18. Kopf M, LeGros G, Bachmann, et al. (1993) Disruption of the murine IL-4 gene blocks Th2 cytokine responses. Nature 362:245–248.
19. Brusselle G, Kips J, Joos G, et al. (1995) Allergen-induced airway inflammation and bronchial responsiveness in wild-type and interleukin-4-deficient mice. Am J Respir Cell Mol Biol 12:254–259.
20. Coyle AJ, Le Gros G, Bertrand C, et al. (1995) Interleukin-4 required for the induction of lung Th2 mucosal immunity. Am J Respir Cell Mol Biol 13:54–59.
21. Lukacs MW, Strieter RM, Chensue SW, and Kunkel SL (1994) IL-4 dependent eosinophil infiltration in a murine mouse model of asthma. Am J Respir Cell Mol Biol 10:526–533.
22. Foster PS, Hogan SP, Ramsay AJ, et al. (1996) Interleukin 5 deficiency abolishes eosinophilia, airways hyperreactivity and lung damage in a mouse asthma model. J Exp Med 183:195–201.
23. Corry DB, Folkesson HG, Warnock ML, et al. (1996) Interleukin 4, but not interleukin 5 or eosinophils, is required in a murine model of acute airway hyperreactivity. J Exp Med 183: 109–117.
24. Drazen JM, Arm JP, Austen KF (1996) Sorting out the cytokines of asthma. J Exp Med 183:1–5.
25. Finkelman FD, Madden KB, Cheever AW, et al. (1994) Effects of interleukin-12 on immune responses and host protection in mice infected with intestinal nematode parasites. J Exp Med 179:1563–1572.
26. Gavett SH, O'Hearn DJ, Li X, et al. (1995) Interleukin 12 inhibits antigen-induced airway hyper-responsiveness, inflammation, and Th2 cytokine expression in mice. J Exp Med 182:1527–1536.
27. Sriramarao P, Von Andrian UH, Butcher EC, et al. (1994) $\alpha_4\beta_1$, integrin and L-selectin mediate eosinophil rolling at physiological shear rates in vivo. J Immunol 153:4238–4246.
28. Sung KLP, Yang L, Elices M, et al. (1996) GM-CSF regulates the functional adhesive state of VLA-4 expressed by eosinophils. J Immunol 158:919–927.

29. Sriramarao P, Broide DH (1996) Differential regulation of eosinophil adhesion under conditions of flow *in vivo*. Ann NY Acad Sci 796:218–225.
30. Broide DH, Humber D, Sullivan S, et al. (1996) Inhibition of eosinophil rolling and recruitment in P-selectin and ICAM deficient mice. Blood. In Press.
31. Bullard DC, Qin L, Lorenzo I, et al. (1995) P-selectin/ICAM-1 double mutant mice: acute emigration of neutrophils into the peritoneum is completely absent but is normal into pulmonary alveoli. J Clin Invest 95:1782
32. Sriramarao P, CR, Norton P, Borgstrom R, DiScipio BA, Wolitzky DH, Broide (1996) E-selectin preferentially supports neutrophil but not eosinophil rolling under conditions of flow in vitro and in vivo. J Immunol 157:4672–4680.

IV SIGNALING IN ALLERGIC REACTIONS

20

Signaling in Mast Cells

Anthony P. Sampson, MA, PhD
and Martin K. Church, M.Pharm, PhD, DSc

CONTENTS

INTRODUCTION

Mast cells release preformed granule-associated mediators (histamine, tryptase, and cytokines) and *de novo*-synthesized mediators (eicosanoids) when antigen crosslinks immunoglobulin E (IgE) bound to its high-affinity receptor (FcεRI). These mediators play central roles in the immediate reactions to allergen exposure in rhinitis and asthma and may also initiate and perpetuate chronic inflammation. The biochemical mechanisms that transduce and amplify the antigen-binding signal into a cellular response are not fully understood even in animal cell lines *(1)* and are complicated by crosstalk between different signaling pathways. This complexity may arise from the need for a mast cell to remain quiescent when IgE binds to its high-affinity receptor but to release mediators explosively when IgE receptors are crosslinked by multivalent antigen. Understanding this unique complexity may help in the development of novel pharmacological agents for antiallergy therapy. This chapter will outline the emerging consensus on the most prominent signal transduction pathways in mast cells.

MORPHOLOGY OF MAST CELL DEGRANULATION

The mast cell triggering signal requires bridging of two or more IgE molecules, as shown by studies with bivalent haptens of defined length and with chemically linked IgE dimers *(2,3)*. Only about 1% of the IgE molecules on the mast-cell surface need to be bridged to completely activate histamine release. Crosslinking of diffusely distributed FcεRI molecules causes interaction with the cytoskeleton to form aggregated patches and eventual capping at one pole

From: *Allergy and Allergic Diseases: The New Mechanisms and Therapeutics*
Edited by: J. A. Denburg © Humana Press Inc., Totowa, NJ

of the cell *(4)*. These aggregated receptors may then be internalized. Within minutes, distinct morphological changes occur that characterize compound exocytosis and that are visible by light and transmission electron microscopy *(5)*. Cells extend pseudopodia, taking on a "ruffled" appearance. Individual granules swell and the electron-dense granule contents fuse to form an interconnected network with alterations of the granule matrix. Formation of pores between the granular membrane and the plasma membrane is associated with the appearance of distinct cytoskeletal filaments followed by extrusion of granule contents into the extra-cellular medium.

ACTIVATION OF TYROSINE KINASES

Phosphorylation of tyrosine residues on a number of intracellular proteins has been increasingly recognized as an early event in signal transduction in many cells. Tyrosine kinase (TK) activity was initially characterized as an intrinsic property of some growth factor receptors, such as epidermal growth factor *(6)*. The c-*kit* receptor for stem cell factor (SCF) also has intrinsic TK activity *(7)*. These receptor tyrosine kinases dimerize upon ligand binding and are activated by autophosphorylation *(8)*, allowing high-affinity binding of a number of proteins involved in subsequent signal transduction steps, including phospholipases and enzymes involved in the phosphoinositide cycle. These proteins generally contain specific *src* homology 2 (SH2) domains *(9)*, which interact with an SH2-containing adaptor protein (Shc) to activate transcription factors, including c-*myc*, c-*fos*, and c-*jun*.

In contrast, the FcεRI lacks intrinsic tyrosine kinase activity *(10)*. However, at least 10 families of nonreceptor or cytoplasmic tyrosine kinases have been described, including the Abl, Brk, Csk, Src, Syk/Zap-70, and Tec families, and these may associate with surface receptors that lack intrinsic tyrosine kinase activity to allow signal transduction to proceed. FcεRI is a tetrameric complex of an IgE-binding α subunit, a β subunit, and a disulfide-linked homo-dimer of γ subunits. Like the T-cell receptor and the B-cell antigen receptor, the α subunit of FcεRI belongs to the immunoglobulin superfamily. The cytoplasmic domains of the β and γ subunits share a tyrosine-containing motif (D/E-X_7, D/E-X_2-Y-X_2-L/I-X_7-Y-X_2-L/I) thought to be essential for cell activation and known variously as the antigen receptor activation motif (ARAM), the tyrosine activation motif (TAM), or antigen receptor homology 1 (ARH1) *(11)*. In rodents, IgE crosslinking leads within 5–15 sec to association of FcεRI with members of the *src* family of nonreceptor TKs, particularly *lyn* and c-*yes* *(12–14)*. These TKs may phosphorylate the ARAMs in the FcεRI β- and γ-subunits *(12,15,16)*. Other studies demonstrate in addition serine and threonine phosphorylation of the β and γ subunits, respectively *(17)*, possibly by the action of a protein kinase C (PKC-δ). Together, these may cause conformational changes that allow binding of further TKs of the *syk* family and their tyrosine phosphorylation, either directly by *lyn* *(18)* or by autophosphorylation by the two phosphorylated tyrosine residues of the ARAM on FcεRI (Fig. 1).

Receptor crosslinking in rodent mast cells and rat basophil leukemia cells also causes tyrosine phosphorylation of the protein tyrosine kinase. PTK72, a nonreceptor tyrosine kinase that does not belong to the *src* family *(14,19,20)*. PTK72 may be identical to the p72[syk] previously identified associating with the B-cell antigen receptor and that has been shown to be expressed in human lung mast cells *(21)*. Tyrosine phosphorylation of PTK72 does not occur after calcium ionophore stimulation or after phorbol ester stimulation, showing that it is specific for the pathway induced by FcεRI aggregation. However, in rat basophil leukemia cells it does not seem to be a prerequisite for activation of the phosphatidylinositol cycle or histamine secretion, suggesting the presence of other independent signal transduction pathways *(22)*.

A number of other proteins, most containing SH2 and/or SH3 domains, are tyrosine-phosphorylated after FcεRI activation in mast cells, including the 47-kDa Nck, which contains

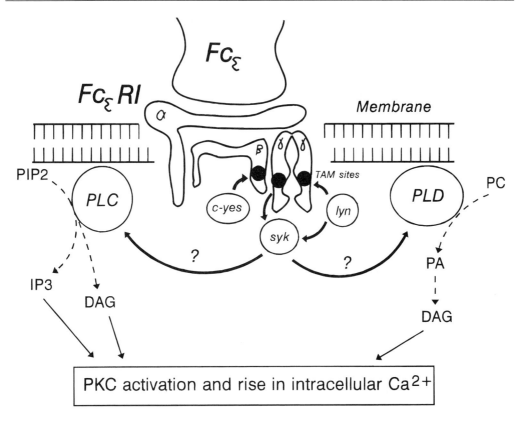

Fig. 1. IgE crosslinking leads to conformational changes in the cytoplasmic domains of the β- and γ-chains of FcεRI allowing phosphorylation of the TAMs by *src* family TKs, including *lyn* and c-*yes*. Further phosphorylation steps involving *syk* family TKs lead to activation of PLC and PLD.

almost exclusively three SH3 domains and one SH2 domain. Nck is also phosphorylated by growth factors and may act in a number of cells as an adaptor molecule to transmit a range of stimuli to downstream effector pathways regulating cell proliferation *(23)*. Bruton's tyrosine kinase (BTK) is activated after FcεRI crosslinking, but it does not appear to interact directly with FcεRI in mouse mast cells, and its function remains unclear. A central regulatory pathway of mast-cell activation and differentiation is mediated by tyrosine phosphorylation of Raf-1, which results in activation via MEK (MAP or ERK kinase) of mitogen-activated protein (MAP) kinases (or extracellular signal-regulated kinases [ERKs]). These integrate signals from surface receptors, including cytokine receptors and FcεRI, and transmit them by serine–threonine phosphorylation of proteins such as c-*jun* and c-*fos* to activate gene transcription and protein synthesis *(23)*.

The degree of activation of mast cells may depend on the balance between phosphorylation by tyrosine kinases and dephosphorylation by tyrosine phosphatases. One such phosphatase is leukocyte common antigen (CD45), which plays a role in T-cell signaling, probably by dephosphorylating the *src* family kinase p56^{lck} associated with CD4 and CD8 molecules *(24)*. In human basophils, monoclonal antibodies to CD45 specifically inhibit IgE-dependent histamine release *(25)*, possibly the result of a conformational change that enhances dephosphorylation of activated proteins in the FcεRI signaling cascade. Preincubation of human lung mast cells with okadaic acid and other inhibitors of serine–threonine phosphatases reduces IgE-stimulated histamine release and leukotriene C$_4$ (LTC$_4$) synthesis *(26)*. Constitutive activity of such phosphatases may restore the capacity of mast cells to respond to stimuli by returning previously phosphorylated signaling proteins to the dephosphorylated state.

PHOSPHOINOSITIDE HYDROLYSIS
AND CHANGES IN INTRACELLULAR CALCIUM

An important link between FcεRI activation and subsequent events is the tyrosine phosphorylation of phospholipases, particularly phospholipase C (PLC). The activity of PLC is critical in initiating phosphoinositide turnover. Phosphatidylinositol (PI), phosphatidylinositol-4-phosphate (PIP), and phosphoinositol-4,5-bisphosphate (PIP$_2$) are broken down after FcεRI crosslinking and produce water-soluble inositol phosphates (IPs) (especially IP$_3$), which release Ca^{2+} from intracellular stores, and diacylglycerol (DAG), which together with Ca^{2+} activates PKC. PLC also generates large quantities of DAG from phosphatidylcholine (PC) *(27)*, and DAG may furthermore be generated by an indirect pathway utilizing phospholipase D (PLD). Like PLC, PLD is activated by phosphorylation.

There are a number of PLC isozymes *(28)*, some of which are activated by tyrosine phosphorylation (PLC-γ1) *(29)* and others of which require a G protein. Classical G proteins are high-molecular-weight heterotrimeric guanosine triphosphate (GTP)-binding proteins that transduce signals from surface receptors to intracellular effectors *(30)*. A second group of G proteins are low-molecular-weight monomers such as the proto-oncogene product *ras*. Injection of *ras* into rat mast cells induces exocytosis *(31)*, but little is known about these G-proteins in human mast cells. Although the subunits of FcεRI (α, β, and two γ) together have seven transmembrane regions, the FcεRI does not have sequence homology with other classical G-protein-linked seven-transmembrane-region receptors (such as muscarinic and adrenergic receptors). Studies in rodent mast cells and basophil lines with GTP-γ-S, a stable GTP analog, and with GTP-β-S, a G-protein inhibitor, have nevertheless confirmed that a G protein is involved in PIP$_2$ hydrolysis, the rise in [Ca^{2+}]$_i$, and subsequent histamine release *(32–34)*. Pertussis toxin inactivation of G$_i$ does not block IgE-dependent responses in most mast cell and basophil lines but may block responses to other stimuli such as compound 48/80, showing that a multiplicity of G proteins may be involved *(35,36)*.

Cytosolic calcium ion concentrations ([Ca^{2+}]$_i$) rise markedly after IgE crosslinking on mast cells. Experiments with calcium ionophores, fusion with Ca^{2+}-containing liposomes, and direct microinjection have shown a rise in [Ca^{2+}]$_i$ to be an essential activator of histamine release and lipid mediator synthesis *(37,38)*, although other signals are also required. Many of the actions of Ca^{2+} are mediated by binding to the 17-kDa protein calmodulin. In rat basophilic leukemia (RBL)-2H3 cells, only a transient increase in [Ca^{2+}]$_i$ is seen in the absence of extracellular Ca^{2+}; the physiological source of the rise in [Ca^{2+}]$_i$ is therefore thought to be a release from intracellular stores, caused by inositol phosphates, preceding an influx of extracellular Ca^{2+}, at least partly triggered by DAG–PKC interaction *(39–43)*. Similar Ca^{2+} fluxes occur in human lung mast cells *(44)*, although the relative importance of the intracellular and extracellular fluxes may vary between cell types and between species. The mechanism by which extracellular Ca^{2+} enters the cell is at present unclear, as FcεRI-linked calcium channels have not been described.

PROTEIN KINASE C

PKC is not a single enzyme but a family of serine–threonine kinases that are activated by Ca^{2+} and by phospholipids, particularly DAG released during PI turnover, an action that is mimicked by phorbol esters. FcεRI activation may cause an early translocation of PKC from the cytoplasm to the plasma membrane *(45)*, and phorbol esters enhance secretion of histamine

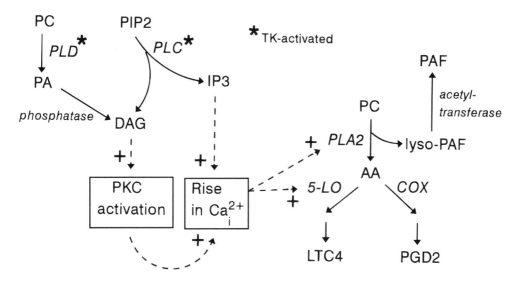

Fig. 2. IgE-dependent triggering of lipid mediator synthetic pathways. TK activation of PLC and PLD leads to a rise in intracellular Ca^{2+} via release of DAG and IP_3 from PIP_2 and PC. Ca^{2+}-activated PLA_2 acts on PC to liberate arachidonic acid (AA), the substrate for the formation of LTs and prostanoids (PGs) and lyso-PAF, the precursor of PAF.

from mast cells and basophils *(46,47)*. However, complete depletion of PKC activity by long-term incubation with phorbol esters reduces but does not abolish histamine release. It is likely that protein phosphorylation by PKC modulates histamine release in rat mast cells by priming them for responses to other Ca^{2+}-dependent stimuli but that PKC in itself is not an essential link in mast-cell signal transduction *(48,49)*.

Mast cells have been shown to synthesize, store, and release a number of cytokines implicated in asthma and allergy. Human lung mast cells constitutively express messenger ribonucleic acid (mRNA) for interleukin (IL)-5, IL-6, IL-8, IL-10, granulocyte-macrophage colony-stimulating factor (GM-CSF), and tumor necrosis factor (TNF)α *(50)*. IgE-dependent activation upregulates message transcription for IL-5, IL-8, and IL-13 and initiates message expression for IL-3 and IL-4. Little is known about the signals that transduce FcεRI crosslinking into cytokine expression, but cytokine production may be strictly regulated by PKC activity *(1)*.

FORMATION OF EICOSANOIDS

Human lung mast cells are sources of potent bronchoconstrictor and vasoactive eicosanoids, including cysteinyl-LTs and prostaglandin D_2 (PGD_2) (Fig. 2). Arachidonate is found at the *sn*-2 position of phospholipids, including PC, phosphatidylserine (PS), and PI, and the source of arachidonate for eicosanoid synthesis may depend on the stimulus. Activation of PLC by G-protein- or tyrosine kinase-dependent mechanisms after FcεRI activation causes phosphoinositide turnover and a rise in $[Ca^{2+}]_i$ and [DAG]. DAG may also be provided by the sequential action of PLD, producing phosphatidic acid, and a phosphatase. Arachidonate may be formed by cleavage from DAG by DAG lipase. However, a rise in Ca^{2+} activates cytosolic phospholipase A_2 ($cPLA_2$), which directly liberates arachidonate from PC, PS, or PI and also activates 5-lipoxygenase, (5-LO) the initial enzyme of the leukotriene synthetic pathway. The activity of $cPLA_2$ is increased many-fold in vitro by phosphorylation by MAP kinase *(51,52)*, and this may be one pathway by which cytokines prime mast cells and basophils for enhanced eicosanoid synthesis in response to a second stimulus. Release of arachidonate from PC also produces 1-alkyl-2-lyso-PC, the unacetylated precursor of platelet-activating factor (PAF) *(53)*. Both the PLC and PLA_2 pathways are induced by GTP-γ-S, showing involvement of a G protein *(54)*. Further metabolism of arachidonate occurs predominantly by the sequential action of 5-LO, five-lipoxygenase activating protein (FLAP), and LTC_4 synthase to the first of the cysteinyl-LTs, LTC_4, and by the action of cyclooxygenase (COX) and PGD_2 synthase to PGD_2, the principal mast-cell prostanoid *(55)*. Smaller amounts of thromboxane A_2 and PGE_2 may also be formed. Both 5-LO and LTC_4 synthase have phosphorylation sites for PKC, and phorbol esters reduce LTC_4 synthesis in eosinophil-like cell lines *(56)*.

ACTIVATION OF ADENYLATE CYCLASE AFTER IgE-DEPENDENT ACTIVATION

A rise in intracellular cyclic adenosine monophosphate (cAMP) occurs after crosslinkage of FcεRI on human mast cells *(57,58)*, and as this seems to precede Ca^{2+} influx and not to be dependent on extracellular Ca^{2+}, it has been proposed as a central pathway of mast-cell signaling. However, it does not occur in the rat basophil line RBL-2H3 *(59)*, and it is more likely that it represents a normal inhibitory mechanism in mast cells to damp down mediator release. A rise in intracellular cAMP also occurs after activation of adenylate cyclase by pharmacological agents, including PGs, $β_2$-agonists, and histamine (H_2), acting at G-protein-linked receptors, and after phosphodiesterase inhibition by theophylline. Raised cAMP activates cAMP-dependent protein serine kinases (PKA), which inhibit histamine and other mediator release.

FUTURE DIRECTIONS

Despite rapid advances in recent years, particularly in the tyrosine kinase area, many of the signaling events following allergenic stimulation of mast cells remain to be elucidated, and a coherent overall picture has yet to emerge. Research on mast cells is hampered by the difficulty of purifying sufficient cells from human tissues, and as a consequence much of our knowledge is based on work with rat peritoneal mast cells, a rat basophil leukemia cell line, and bone-marrow-derived murine mast cells cultured in the presence of IL-3. Heterogeneity in mast-cell and basophil signal transduction pathways may prevent conclusions based on this work from being valid in human mast cells.

The central role played by the mast cell in allergic disease, both as a precipitator of the early-phase response and as a producer of proinflammatory cytokines, nevertheless makes it a prime target for development of drug therapy. Although the development of anti-IgE antibodies to prevent allergic activation of mast cells will represent a major advance, this is a long-term therapy that may turn out to be contraindicated in areas in which parasitic infections are common. Thus, a drug that would "disable" the mast cell in a temporary and reversible manner by uncoupling the activation–secretion pathway would be a great benefit to our therapeutic armory.

ACKNOWLEDGMENTS

The authors thank Jane Warner and Sandra Lavens-Phillips (Department of Physiology and Pharmacology, University of Southampton) for helpful discussions and for access to unpublished data. The first author is supported by the Frances and Augustus Newman Foundation and the Royal College of Surgeons of England.

REFERENCES

1. Razin E, Pecht I, Rivera J (1995) Signal transduction in the activation of mast cells and basophils. Immunol Today 16:370–373.
2. Siraganian RP, Hook WA, Levine BB (1975) Specific *in vitro* histamine release from basophils by bivalent haptens: evidence of activation by simple bridging of membrane bound antibody. Immunochemistry 12:149–156.
3. Segal DM, Taurog JD, Metzger H (1977) Dimeric immunoglobulin E serves as a unit signal for mast cell degranulation. Proc Natl Acad Sci USA 74:2993–2997.
4. Robertson D, Holowka D, Baird B (1986) Cross-linking of immunoglobulin E-receptor complexes induces their interaction with the cytoskeleton of rat basophilic leukemia cells. J Immunol 136:4565–4572.
5. Caulfield JP, El Lati S, Thomas G, Church MK (1990) Dissociated human foreskin mast cells degranulate in response to anti-IgE and substance P. Lab Invest 63:502–510.
6. Ullrich A, Schlessinger J (1990) Signal transduction by receptors with tyrosine kinase activity. Cell 61:203–205.
7. Schrader JW, Welham MJ, Leslie KB, Duronio V (1995) Cytokine-mediated signal transduction in mast cells. In: Kitamura Y, Yamamura S, Galli SJ, Greaves MW, eds. Biological and Molecular Aspects of Mast Cell and Basophil Differentiation and Function. Raven, New York, pp. 65–77.
8. Bertics PJ, Gill GN (1985) Self-autophosphorylation enhances the protein tyrosine kinase activity of the epidermal growth factor receptor. J Biol Chem 260:14,642–14,647.
9. Koch CA, Anderson D, Moran MF, Ellis C, Pawson T (1991) SH2 and SH3 domains: elements that control interactions of cytoplasmic signalling proteins. Science 252:668–674.
10. Benhamou M, Gutking JS, Robbins KC, Siraganian RP (1990) Tyrosine phosphorylation coupled to IgE receptor mediated signal transduction and histamine release. Proc Natl Acad Sci USA 87:5327–5332.
11. Gauen LK, Zhu Y, Letourneur F, Hu Q, Bolen JB, Matis LA, Klausner RD, Shaw A (1994) Interactions of p59(fyn) and Zap-70 with T-cell receptor activation motifs: defining the nature of a signalling motif. Mol Cell Biol 14:3729–3741.
12. Eiseman E, Bolen JB (1992) Engagement of the high affinity IgE receptor activates src protein related tyrosine kinases. Nature 355:78–80.
13. Jouvin MH, Adamczewski M, Numerof R, Letourneur O, Valle A, Kinet JP (1994) Differential control of the tyrosine kinases *lyn* and *syk* by the two signalling chains of the high affinity immunoglobulin E receptor. J Biol Chem 269:5918–5925.
14. Penhallow RC, Class K, Sonoda H, Bolen JB, Rowley RB (1995) Temporal activation of nontransmembrane protein tyrosine kinases following mast cell FcεRI engagement. J Biol Chem 270:23, 362–23,365.
15. Oliver JM, Burg DL, Deanin GG, Mclaughlin JL, Geahlen RL (1994) Role of the protein tyrosine kinase, *syk*, in signal transduction in mast cells: inhibition of FcεRI-mediated signalling by the *syk*-selective inhibitor, piceatannol. J Biol Chem 269:29,697–29,703.
16. Wilson BS, Kapp N, Lee RJ, Pfeiffer JR, Martinez AM, Platt Y, Letourneur F, Oliver JM (1995) Distinct functions of the FcεRI γ and β subunits in the control of FcεRI-mediated tyrosine kinase activation and signalling responses in RBL-2H3 mast cells. J Biol Chem 270:4013–4022.
17. Paolini R, Jouvin MH, Kinet JP (1991) Phosphorylation and dephosphorylation of the high-affinity receptor for immunoglobulin E immediately after receptor engagement and disengagement. Nature 353:855–858.
18. Kinet JP (1992) The gamma-zeta dimers of Fc receptors as connectors to signal transduction. Curr Opin Immunol 4:43–48.
19. Hutchcroft JE, Geahlen RL, Deanin GG, Oliver JM (1992) FcεRI-mediated tyrosine phosphorylation and activation of the 72kDa protein tyrosine kinase, PTK72, in RBL-2H3 rat tumor mast cells. Proc Natl Acad Sci USA 89:9107–9111.
20. Minoguchi K, Benhamou M, Swaim WD, Kawakami Y, Kawakami T, Siraganian RP (1994) Activation of the protein tyrosine kinase p72[syk] by FcεRI aggregation in rat basophilic leukemia cells. J Biol Chem 269:16,902–16,908.
21. Lavens SE, Peachell PT, Warner JA (1992) Role of tyrosine kinases in IgE-mediated signal transduction in human lung mast cells and basophils. Am J Respir Cell Mol Biol 7:637–644.

22. Stephan V, Benhamou M, Gutkind JS, Robbins KC, Siraganian RP (1992) FcεRI-induced protein-tyrosine phosphorylation of pp72 in rat basophilic leukemia cells (RBL-2H3): evidence for a novel signal transduction pathway unrelated to G protein activation and phophatydylinositol hydrolysis. J Biol Chem 267:5434–5441.

23. Kawakami T, Kawakami Y, Yao L, Fukamachi H, Matsuoka S, Miura T (1995) Tyrosine kinases and their substrates in the FcεRI signaling pathway. In: Kitamura Y, Yamamura S, Galli SJ, Greaves MW, eds. Biological and Molecular Aspects of Mast Cell and Basophil Differentiation and Function. Raven, New York, pp. 249–261.

24. Turner JM, Brodsky MH, Irving BA, Levin SD, Perlmutter RM, Littman DR (1990) Interaction of the unique N-terminal region of tyrosine kinase p56[lck] with cytoplasmic domains of CD4 and CD8 is mediated by cysteine motifs. Cell 60:755–765.

25. Hook WA, Berenstein EH, Zinsser FU, Fischler C, Siraganian RP (1991) Monoclonal antibodies to the leukocyte common antigen (CD45) inhibit IgE-mediated histamine release from human basophils. J Immunol 147:2670–2676.

26. Peachell PT, Munday MR (1993) Regulation of human lung mast cell function by phosphatase inhibitors. J Immunol 151:3808–3816.

27. Kennerly DA (1990) Phosphatidylcholine is a quantitatively more important source of increased 1, 2-diacylglycerol than is phosphatidylinositol in mast cells. J Immunol 144:3912–3919.

28. Rhee SG, Suh PG, Ryu SH, Lee SY (1989) Studies of inositol phospholipid-specific phospholipase C. Science 244:546–550.

29. Nishibe S, Wahl MI, Hernandez-Sotomayor SM, Tonks NK, Rhee SG, Carpenter G (1990) Increase of the catalytic activity of phospholipase C-gamma 1 by tyrosine phosphorylation. Science 250:1253–1256.

30. Stryer L, Bourne HR (1986) G proteins: a family of signal transducers. Annu Rev Cell Biol 2:391–419.

31. Bar-Sagi D, Gomperts BD (1988) Stimulation of exocytotic degranulation by microinjection of the *ras* oncogene protein in rat mast cells. Oncogene 3:463–468.

32. Cunha-Melo JR, Gonzago HM, Ali H, Huang FL, Huang KP, Beaven MA (1989) Studies of protein kinase C in the rat basophilic leukemia (RBL-2H3) cell reveal that antigen-induced signals are not mimicked by the actions of phorbol myristate acetate and Ca^{2+} ionophore. J Immunol 143:2617–2625.

33. Ali H, Collado-Escobar DM, Beaven MA (1989) The rise in concentration of free Ca^{2+} and of pH provides sequential, synergistic signals for secretion in antigen-stimulated rat basophilic leukemia (RBL-2H3) cells. J Immunol 143:2626–2633.

34. Von zur Mühlen F, Eckstein F, Penner R (1991) Guanosine 5'-[beta-thio]triphosphate selectively activates calcium signalling in mast cells. Proc Natl Acad Sci USA 88:926–930.

35. Nakamura T, Ui M (1983) Suppression of passive cutaneous anaphylaxis by pertussis toxin, an islet-activating protein, as a result of inhibition of histamine release by mast cells. Biochem Pharmacol 32:3435–3441.

36. Saito H, Okajima F, Molski TF, Sha'afi RI, Ui M, Ishizaka T (1988) Effect of cholera toxin on histamine release from bone marrow-derived mouse mast cells. Proc Natl Acad Sci USA 85:2504–2508.

37. Bennett JP, Cockcroft S, Gomperts BD (1981) Rat mast cells permeabilized with ATP secrete histamine in response to calcium ions buffered in the micromolar range. J Physiol (Lond) 317:335–345.

38. Theoharides TC, Douglas WW (1978) Secretion in mast cells induced by calcium entrapped within phospholipid vesicles. Science 201:1143–1145.

39. Takaishi T, Siraganian RP (1985) Changes in $^{45}Ca^{2+}$ flux following the activation of rat basophilic leukemia cells for histamine release. Ann Allergy 55:353 (abstract).

40. Stump RF, Oliver JM, Cragoe EJ, Deanin GG (1987) The control of mediator release from RBL-2H3 cells: roles for Ca^{2+}, Na^+, and protein kinase C1. J Immunol 139:881–886.

41. Mohr FC, Fewtrell C (1987) The relative contributions of extracellular and intracellular calcium to secretion from tumor mast cells: multiple effects of the proton ionophore carbonyl cyanide m-chlorophenylhydrazone. J Biol Chem 262:10,638–10,643.

42. Matthews G, Neher E, Penner R (1989) Second messenger-activated calcium influx in rat peritoneal mast cells. J Physiol (Lond) 418:105–130.

43. Penner R, Matthews G, Neher E (1988) Regulation of calcium influx by second messengers in rat mast cells. Nature 334:499–501.

44. MacGlashan DW (1989) Single cell analysis of Ca^{2+} changes in human lung mast cells: graded vs. all-or-nothing elevations after IgE-mediated stimulation. J Cell Biol 109:123–134.

45. White JR, Pluznik DH, Ishizaka K, Ishizaka T (1985) Antigen-induced increase in protein kinase C activity in plasma membrane of mast cells. Proc Natl Acad Sci USA 82:8193–8197.

46. Sagi-Eisenberg R, Pecht I (1984) Protein kinase C, a coupling element between stimulus and secretion of basophils. Immunol Lett 8:237–241.

47. Sagi-Eisenberg R, Lieman H, Pecht I (1985) Protein kinase C regulation of the receptor-coupled calcium signal in histamine-secreting rat basophilic leukaemia cells. Nature 313:59–60.

48. Howell TW, Kramer IM, Gomperts BD (1989) Protein phosphorylation and the dependence on Ca^{2+} and GTP-γ-S for exocytosis from permeabilised mast cells. Cell Signal 1:157–163.

49. Koopmann WR, Jackson RC (1990) Calcium- and guanine-nucleotide-dependent exocytosis in permeabilized mast cells: modulation by protein kinase C. Biochem J 265:365–373.

50. Okayama Y, Semper A, Holgate ST, Church MK (1995) Multiple cytokine mRNA expression in human mast cells stimulated via FcεRI. Int Arch Allergy Immunol 107:158–159.

51. Lin L-L, Lin AY, Knopf JL (1992) Cytosolic phospholipase A_2 is coupled to hormonally-regulated release of arachidonic acid. Proc Natl Acad Sci USA 89:6147–6151.

52. Lin L-L, Wartmann M, Lin AY, Knopf JL, Seth A, Davis RJ (1993) cPLA$_2$ is phosphorylated and activated by MAP kinase. Cell 72:269–278.

53. Snyder F (1985) Chemical and biochemical aspects of platelet activating factor: a novel class of acetylated ether-linked choline phospholipids. Med Res Rev 5:107–140.

54. Narasimhan V, Holowka D, Baird B (1990) A guanine nucleotide binding protein participates in IgE receptor-mediated activation of endogenous and reconstituted phopholipase A_2 in a permeabilized cell system. J Biol Chem 265:1459–1464.

55. Murakami M, Austen KF, Arm JP (1995) Cytokine regulation of arachidonic acid metabolism in mast cells. In: Kitamura Y, Yamamura S, Galli SJ, Greaves MW eds. Biological and Molecular Aspects of Mast Cell and Basophil Differentiation and Function. Raven, New York, pp. 25–37.

56. Ali A, Ford-Hutchinson AW, Nicholson DW (1994) Activation of protein kinase C down-regulates leukotriene C_4 synthase activity and attenuates cysteinyl leukotriene production in an eosinophilic substrain of HL-60 cells. J Immunol 153:776–788.

57. MacGlashan DW, Schleimer RP, Peters SP, Schulman ES, Adams GK, Kagey-Sobotka A, Newball HH, Lichtenstein LM (1983) Comparative studies of human basophils and mast cells. Fed Proc 42:2504–2509.

58. Peachell PT, MacGlashan DW, Lichtenstein LM, Schleimer RP (1988) Regulation of human basophil and lung mast cell function by cyclic adenosine monophosphate. J Immunol 140:571–579.

59. Morita Y, Siraganian RP (1981) Inhibition of IgE-mediated histamine release from rat basophilic leukemia cells and rat mast cells by inhibitors of transmethylation. J Immunol 127:1339–1344.

21 Signaling in Human Basophils

Donald MacGlashan, Jr., MD, PHD

CONTENTS

INTRODUCTION

Allergic diseases occur when immunoglobulin E (IgE) antibodies, bound to specific high-affinity receptors on mast cells and basophils, are aggregated by specific antigens to induce the release of mediators, such as histamine, from these two cell types. In a search for new therapies to inhibit this allergic response, it is reasonable to explore the possibility of shutting off mediator release with an agent that interferes with the biochemical reactions that occur in these cells after aggregation occurs. Signal transduction is a general descriptive term for these biochemical events and refers to the fact that the extracellular signal, antigen binding to cell surface IgE in this case, is transduced into a cascade of biochemical changes that ultimately cause the cell to secrete preformed granules and synthesize new lipids or proteins. The motivation for such an approach comes from spectacular past successes, although these past successes, such as glucocorticosteroids, were only appreciated as signal transduction regulators long after they had become important clinical therapies. It is expected that if the signal transduction process can be understood well enough, specific therapies that only modify mast cell or basophil behavior could be developed.

The field of signal transduction has exploded in recent years, driven quite effectively by the ability to modify specific components of the biochemical pathways with genetic techniques. Many of these techniques apply only to cells that proliferate in culture, and often these are cell lines of either human or animal origin. To understand mast cell or basophil signal transduction biology, investigators first began with studies of rat peritoneal mast cells but moved on to study several types of cell lines, most notably the rat basophilic leukemia cell (RBL-2H3 cells, the 2H3 designation referring to a variant that degranulates in response to IgE-mediated signals). Much of our understanding of IgE-mediated signal transduction comes from studies of RBL cells, but there have been many advances in the understanding of human mast cell and basophil biology as well. These human cells are difficult to obtain in purity and quantity sufficient for signal transduction studies, but new technologies have begun to open these cells for study. Signal transduction issues, as they relate to RBL cells or murine mast

From: *Allergy and Allergic Diseases: The New Mechanisms and Therapeutics*
Edited by: J. A. Denburg © Humana Press Inc., Totowa, NJ

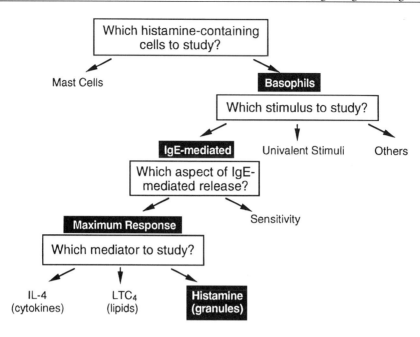

Fig. 1. Possible areas of study related to the problem of releasability.

cells, are well discussed in several other current reviews (e.g. *[1]*), so this will not be the explicit topic of this chapter. Instead, some interesting issues of human basophil and mast cell biology will be discussed in the context of signal transduction, drawing information from studies of both human cells and RBL cells. One of the advantages to studying human cells, besides the more immediate relationship to the human condition, derives from the availability of patients with different clinical histories. There are so many potential points of regulation in the IgE-mediated signal transduction cascade that identifying points for intervention is not easy. However, if one can identify how natural control is exerted, through the ability to study specific patients, specific targets may be more readily identified. More importantly, once these points of control are identified, the biological pathways that lead to their modulation in certain patients can also be identified, offering another therapeutic route. Glucocorticosteroids represent this kind of possibility, although once again, this is a retrospective conclusion. Indeed, the exact modification in the IgE-mediated signal transduction pathway in human basophils that results from treatment with steroids remains unknown. It is instead the fact that an exogenous modulator can operate to shut down this specific pathway that is interesting *(2)*.

As noted above, there are now a vast array of topics that fall under the purview of signal transduction. This chapter will cover basophil or mast cell biology as it relates to the clinical behavior of a patient. These topics will revolve around the issue of releasability. This catch-all term generally refers to the ability of the cell itself to respond to stimulation. It is a very broad subject and to keep the issue of signal transduction in focus, the chapter will narrow the subject in the manner shown in Fig. 1. Starting at the top of the figure and working down, I shall discuss some of the branch points in some detail but finally focus on the last branch point in order to discuss issues relating to signal transduction.

Table 1
Some General Methods of Assessing Basophil Responsiveness

Spontaneous histamine release ± enhancing agents (e.g., D_2O)
Response to non-IgE-dependent stimuli (e.g., C5a, chemokines)
Maximum response to polyclonal anti-IgE antibody
Cell surface density of antigen-specific IgE to obtain:
   half-maximal release
   fixed amount of histamine release (e.g., 25%)
Response to IgE-dependent histamine releasing factors
Response to cytokines

RELEASABILITY

Mast Cells or Basophils?

The study of FcεRI-bearing/histamine-containing cells in vitro leads to the first decision at the top of Fig. 1. Mast cells have relevance to the immediate hypersensitivity reaction, as they are the cells present in the tissues of anatomical structures that interface with the environment (airways, gut, skin). Despite advances in the preparation of these cells to obtain cells that are of sufficient purity for biochemical study *(3,4)*, they remain difficult and expensive to study. Furthermore, it is nearly impossible to obtain cells from chosen donors; tissues are always obtained as a byproduct of surgical procedures for other reasons. Consequently, comparative studies are extremely difficult with the current technologies used to study signal transduction. Basophils, on the other hand, can be obtained from whole blood *(5–7)* and are more available for comparative studies. Previous reviews have presented the evidence that the allergic reaction is composed of at least two phases *(8–10)*. The so-called late-phase reaction results from the migration of circulating leukocytes, specifically basophils, eosinophils, and lymphocytes *(11–13)*. There is good evidence that the basophil plays a role in the late-phase reaction in the airway *(11,14)* and is therefore not only a surrogate for mast-cell studies but useful to examine in its own right. There are some very interesting differences between mast cells and basophils, at the level of signal transduction, so some of these issues will be discussed below. However, most of the studies that can be discussed relate to human basophils.

Releasability and the Class of Stimulus

As noted above, releasability is a catch-all term for a number of observations made over the last 30 yr. It is appealing to imagine that some of the differences between atopics and nonatopics or between atopic patients with different sensitivities to allergens result from differences in the intrinsic sensitivity of their basophils (or mast cells) to stimulation. Although it seems clear that antigens drive a classical immediate hypersensitivity reaction, presumably through the IgE receptor (FcεRI), it is not necessarily clear that all of the allergic or asthmatic pathology is a result of this kind of activation. Human basophils respond to quite a few stimuli. Examples include formyl-met-leu-phe (FMLP; a bacterial N-terminal blocked tripeptide) *(15)*, anaphylatoxins C5a and C3a *(16)*, platelet activating factor *(17,18)*, chemokines such as monocyte chemotactic protein (MCP)-1 *(19)*, IgE-dependent histamine releasing factor (HRF) *(20,21)*, major basic protein *(22)*, polyamines *(23)*, and some cytokines (in a donor-specific manner) *(24)*. Differences between atopics and nonatopics, or differences within the atopic group of subjects themselves, might involve these alternate ways of activating the cells. Table 1 includes some ways that basophil responsiveness has been examined.

Stimulation through receptors other than FcεRI appears to involve a different set of signal transduction steps *(25–32)*. This may ultimately be useful in the design of a therapeutic strategy that specifically alters IgE-mediated secretion, but it also useful to delineate what steps need to be in operation in order for secretion to occur. Although mediator secretion will be discussed at greater length below, it should be noted that to date, secretagogues are generally defined by their ability to induce histamine release. It is not a given that other mediators will be secreted. One of the first clear examples of differential release was the observation that C5a did not induce leukotriene C_4 (LTC_4) release *(25)*. This occurs despite a very brisk histamine release response. FMLP and C5a are two stimuli that induce a fast histamine release response that is inhibited by pertussis toxin *(28)*. The implication is that they both utilize a pertussis toxin-sensitive guanosine triphosphate (GTP) binding protein to mediate the earliest signal transduction steps. This is a well characterized type of signal transduction that includes a ligand-induced change in the receptor such that it becomes capable of binding a GTP protein (Gs, for example), which in turn is capable of activating phospholipase Cβ. This phospholipase C (PLC) can generate second messengers that lead to a nearly universal appearance of an elevation in cytosolic free Ca^{2+} ($[Ca^{2+}]_i$) and the activation of protein kinase C (PKC). However, although both FMLP and C5a induce a brisk degranulation, only FMLP is able to induce a strong LTC_4 secretion. The basis for the distinction is not yet in hand; however, its resolution might shed some light on the requirements for LTC_4 release that would also apply to IgE-mediated release.

Although the study of non-IgE-dependent secretagogues helps us to understand secretion in general (and is more useful because purified basophils generally respond better to FMLP or C5a than to IgE-mediated stimuli), it is not yet clear what role they play in allergic reactions (with the possible exception of chemokines, although signal-transduction issues haven't been well studied for these stimuli). IgE-mediated secretion, on the other hand, has a clear role. Consequently, the releasability issue is often examined in the context of IgE-mediated secretion.

Maximal Histamine Release or Cellular Sensitivity

The parameter most often examined for IgE-mediated secretion is the maximum histamine release that can be obtained with a stimulus that operates through the cell-bound IgE and its high-affinity receptor. The stimuli used most often are either antigens to which the donor's basophils are sensitive or a less specific stimulus like polyclonal anti-IgE antibody. Histamine release is generally expressed as a percentage of the total cellular histamine, since this mediator is preformed and no one has yet found a clear instance of histamine being synthesized during secretion (or even following secretion). It is convenient to normalize the release in this manner, allowing a sense that the relative levels of stimulation among donors can be better appreciated. However, the downside is that the relationship between the amount of signal transduction (e.g., the magnitude of the $[Ca^{2+}]_i$ response) and histamine release is not necessarily linear across the entire range of 0–100% histamine release. This is particularly true because it is often the case that the best combination of IgE-mediated stimuli can only induce a partial release of the cell's histamine *(33)*. We have found no evidence that partial histamine release represents only a fraction of the cells releasing their entire complement of histamine *(27,34–36)*, although this conclusion remains somewhat controversial *(37–39)*.

So if there are no clear subpopulations, then additional factors must modulate the extent to which the cells release. Several years ago, we considered the possibility that basophils from different donors had a very broad range of sensitivity to IgE-mediated stimulation. It was known that the endogenous IgE density (IgE molecules per basophil) varied remarkably among donors *(40,41)*. We hypothesized that the sensitivity also varied considerably and explained the maximal release variability. For example, suppose that two basophil preparations had cell

Table 2
Factors Regulating the Response of a Donor's Basophils to Stimulation
with a Specific Antigen: Determinants of the Antigen Dose Response Curve

Number of FcεRI per basophil—correlated to the serum IgE antibody titer
Fraction of the total IgE specific for the antigen under study—this must factor in the
    donor's IgE-specific response to the antigen's specific epitopes
Nature of the antigen, number of epitopes, and their affinity for the donor's IgE antibodies
Maximal mediator release
Absolute sensitivity of the basophils under study—number of IgE molecules required for
    50% of the maximal response, a result of both intrinsic and extrinsic factors impinging
    on basophil function

surface IgE densities of 200,000. However, for one donor 400,000 IgE aggregates were required for 50% histamine release, whereas only 10,000 were required in the second donor. Clearly, the maximum release that could be obtained in the less sensitive donor would be less than 50%, whereas for the more sensitive donor we would expect nearly 100% histamine release for a general crosslinking agent like anti-IgE antibody. In this model, no special conditions need to be invoked to explain the limited histamine release in some donors except for a difference in sensitivity. This hypothesis was tested and found incorrect *(33)*. There are two parameters to IgE-mediated histamine release that appear to be regulated independently. Maximal histamine release and the sensitivity of the cell to IgE-mediated stimulation do not correlate. Therefore, maximal histamine release and basophil sensitivity are independent parameters regulated by unknown mechanisms within the cell. This would suggest that both parameters need to be evaluated in the context of signal transduction biochemistry. However, determining sensitivity is not technically straightforward and would be difficult to execute routinely. So most studies focus on maximum release. The magnitude of basophil histamine release is an interesting topic when considered in the context of the patient's sensitivity to antigen exposure. One would assume that aspects of what is known about basophils would apply to mast cells as well. When planning studies of basophil response, there are several other known factors that must be considered. These are summarized in Table 2.

Which Mediator to Examine?

The framework for releasability studies and signal transduction is therefore to study IgE-mediated histamine release from basophils and to generally examine the relationship of signal transduction events to maximum histamine release among donors. The final branch point in the flow diagram in Fig. 1 is "which mediator to study?" This may be a relevant question because as we shall see, the signal transduction events differ for each of the mediators. However, if the cause of variability among donors results from modulation of very early events, this may not be as relevant a question.

Human basophils are now known to secrete three classes of mediators. Historically, histamine release was first studied, although it required 10 yr (from 1960–1970) to determine that leukocyte histamine release really meant basophil histamine release. This mediator is preformed and stored in basophil granules. Thus, the act of degranulation allows histamine to be secreted. There are a host of other granule contents that accompany histamine; a reasonably complete list has only recently been compiled but not yet published *(42)*. The typical image of basophil degranulation includes the fusion of granules to the plasma membrane prior to exposure of the contents to the extracellular medium. This form of degranulation has been termed

AND (anaphylactic degranulation) (for review *see* ref. *43*). It is generally common to all stimuli studied, but it is not the sole means of getting histamine out of the cell. Many years ago, studies of tissue sections containing basophils revealed another form of degranulation. This is termed PMD (piecemeal degranulation) *(43)*. In essence, the basophil uses small vesicles to transport the contents of the large granules to the plasma membrane for expulsion. Stimulation increases the rate of vesicular traffic with the effect of slowly transferring the granule's contents to the outside of the cell without explicit fusion of the granules to the plasma membrane *(44)*. It is not yet clear whether all of a granule's contents are transferred this way, but it appears that histamine is transferred. The image that comes to mind is of synaptic vesicles being secreted in nerve cell terminals.

This is quite a different picture of degranulation than has been traditionally envisioned. What makes this particularly intriguing is that the relative contribution of PMD and AND to the degranulation process appears to depend on the stimulus and also the point in time following stimulation. PMD is a strong characteristic of basophils stimulated with phorbol esters *(45)*. This nonphysiologic stimulus appears to define one end of a continuum. At the other end of the continuum is AND, which is the predominant mode of degranulation for IgE-mediated release *(39)*. A stimulus like FMLP appears to induce both forms of degranulation, with PMD predominating early in the reaction and AND becoming apparent later *(46)*. Furthermore, FMLP induces enormous enlargement of the granules, forming what have been called degranulation sacs *(46)*. These sacs are often large enough, under conditions of strong stimulation, that the cell looks like a thin torus when viewed by light microscopy. It is interesting that histamine release following stimulation with FMLP is essentially complete within 15–30 sec, the time when PMD predominates. If most of the histamine is released by this mechanism, then it is not clear why the cell continues on to AND. It is possible that not all granule contents are released by PMD and the AND mechanism allows these to be released on a slightly different time scale. There are some indications that the nature of the secretion may also change according to whether the cell is in suspension or attached to a surface *(35,43,47)*. The relevance of these observations to the biology of secretion is not yet clear, except that they indicate that the signal transduction pathways may be distinctive for the different types of degranulation.

Historically, the next class of mediators to be associated with IgE-mediated secretion from human basophils (and mast cells) are the newly synthesized lipids, leukotrienes for basophils *(48)* and leukotrienes and prostaglandins for lung mast cells *(49,50)* (the relative amounts of these lipoxygenase and cyclooxygenase metabolites vary among mast cells from different tissues *[51]*). The inability of basophils to secrete any cyclooxygenase products is interesting, but there is little developmental biology available to provide an explanation for the absence of this enzyme(s). Lipid metabolism that involves arachidonic acid has at various times been implicated in the control of degranulation, but no current studies clearly define a direct role for arachidonic acid (AA) in degranulation. However, there is an interesting development from studies on the mechanisms of AA generation following stimulation that may impinge on the control of histamine release. First, some studies in rat mast cells indicated that secretory type II phospholipase A_2 ($sPLA_2$) was involved in histamine release *(52)*. It may not be the generated arachidonic acid that is relevant in this observation but the generation of deacylated phospholipids that influences granule fusion. In human basophils, this kind of result is not obtained *(53)*.

In recent years, the study of leukotriene and prostaglandin synthesis in stimulated cells has taken an interesting turn. One strongly held paradigm that is quite recent in origin is that leukotriene release takes place on the nuclear membrane rather than the plasma membrane. The enzymes responsible for its synthesis translocate to, or are present in, the nuclear membrane, and the synthesized LTC_4 is actively transported out of the cell from this location

(54,55). It is felt by many that a cystolic PLA_2 ($cPLA_2$) (85 kDa) is responsible for the initial step, and this enzyme appears to be somewhat selective for phospholipids containing sn-2 AA *(56)*. This enzyme can also be found to translocate to the nuclear membrane *(56)*. In contrast, the $sPLA_2$ (14 kDa) is found to either operate in the extracellular environment or be partially accessible to reagents in the extracellular environment. Consequently, this enzyme is not thought to contribute free AA for LTC_4 synthesis.

The current twist to this picture of events is that the source of AA for LT synthesis versus prostaglandin synthesis is not always the same. Furthermore, it appears that AA derived from $sPLA_2$ can be the sole source for leukotriene synthesis. A recent study using human monocytes has shown that prostaglandin synthesis uses AA derived from $cPLA_2$ *(57)*, whereas LT synthesis uses AA derived from $sPLA_2$. If antisense oligonucleotides are used to downregulate $cPLA_2$ in these cells, the cells lose the ability to secrete prostaglandins, although LT synthesis remains intact *(58)*. This seems to be a common theme for human leukocytes *(59)*. Our recent studies of basophils indicate that an $sPLA_2$ generates the AA used for LTC_4 synthesis *(53)*. Interestingly, this AA is typically not observable, with the implication that its generation is tightly coupled to 5-lipoxygenase (5-LO). This AA can be made observable if a 5-LO inhibitor is used. There is another source of AA in stimulated basophils that is unaffected by $sPLA_2$ inhibitors, and it appears that it may be derived from a $cPLA_2$ that is present in reasonable abundance in basophils. One model that fits the data thus far is that $sPLA_2$ is embedded in the plasma membrane, accessible to extracellular antibodies but with an active site inside the cell. For example, extracellularly applied $sPLA_2$ generates remarkable amounts of AA but this AA has no effect on the amount of LTC_4 synthesis *(53)*. A transition-state analog inhibitor of $sPLA_2$ that cannot penetrate the plasma membrane effectively inhibits this extracellularly applied $sPLA_2$ but has no effect on the endogenous $sPLA_2$ *(53)*. However, a monoclonal antibody to $sPLA_2$ inhibits its activity in intact cells (*see* below for a similar situation for anti-CD45 monoclonal antibodies [MAb]). Our speculation is that this $sPLA_2$ acts on inner leaflet phospholipids to generate an AA that is transferred to a closely approximated 5-LO so that no free AA "leaks." Although it is not known whether 5-LO translocates or resides on the nuclear membrane in basophils, this model can accommodate such a possibility by simply postulating that the topologies of the nuclear and plasma membranes are such that 5-LO on the nuclear membrane could be brought into apposition with the plasma-membrane $sPLA_2$.

LTC_4 is synthesized after histamine release in human basophils *(25)*. For FMLP, its synthesis begins after histamine release is complete, whereas for anti-IgE antibody, its synthesis lags behind histamine release but is complete at about the same time *(25)*. The generation of AA also lags behind histamine release, both the $sPLA_2$- and $cPLA_2$-derived AA (assuming that the normally observable AA is derived from the action of $cPLA_2$) *(60)*. These data indicate that the signals for LT synthesis differ from those for histamine release and may even suggest that degranulation must occur for AA to occur. However, this latter point cannot be stretched too far since the correlation between LTC_4 release and histamine release is only weak ($Rs = 32$), suggesting that there are other factors that contribute to the secretion of LTs. A final point is that not all stimuli induce the secretion of LTC_4. Of the physiological stimuli, IgE- and FMLP-mediated stimulation cause LTC_4 release, whereas C5a generally causes no LTC_4 release in most donors *(25,27)*. Of the nonphysiologic stimuli, ionomycin induces significant LTC_4 release, whereas phorbol esters like PMA induce none *(25)*. It is likely that the magnitude of the $[Ca^{2+}]_i$ response is a necessary moderator for LTC_4 secretion (but not a sufficient condition, since maitotoxin, a flagellate toxin, causes marked increases in $[Ca^{2+}]_i$ with no subsequent LTC_4 release *[61]*). Phorbol myristic acid (PMA) induces no $[Ca^{2+}]_i$ response *(26)*, and C5a induces only a transient $[Ca^{2+}]_i$ response *(27,60)*. Since AA generation occurs only 1–2 min after stimulation with FMLP (after the initial transient Ca has passed and during the second elevation, which depends on extracellular Ca^{2+}), we might surmise that in the absence of a second $[Ca^{2+}]_i$ phase, little AA, and therefore little or no LTC_4, is generated.

The final category of secreted mediators is the cytokines, which may be representative of other transcriptionally regulated mediators yet to be identified. Basophils appear to secrete several cytokines, with interleukin (IL)-4 being the first one demonstrated *(7,62)*. Recent reports indicate that IL-13 and MIP1-α are also synthesized *de novo* and secreted during IgE-mediated stimulation *(63,64)*. As with LTC_4, there is only a weak correlation between histamine release and IL-4 secretion among different donors *(62,65)*. Extensive studies of IL-4 secretion seem to demonstrate that the contaminating cells do not contribute to its production during IgE-mediated secretion *(62,65)*. Indeed, even using an optimal stimulus like A23187 and PMA, we find that a general population of lymphocytes (for example, those that contaminate basophil preparations at lower purities) secretes only one-tenth the IL-4 generated by basophils (on a per cell basis). Consequently, it now seems feasible to use highly sensitive IL-4 enzyme-linked immunosorbent assay (ELISA) kits to perform IL-4 studies on rather impure basophils (2–5%) *(65)*. As noted above, an optimal stimulus for lymphocytes is a combination of a calcium ionophore like ionomycin and a phorbol ester like PMA. Ionomycin alone is a weak stimulus for lymphocytes, and PMA induces little or no IL-4 release. In contrast, basophils are optimally stimulated with ionomycin, and much better release follows ionomycin than even a strong IgE-mediated response. PMA also induces little or no IL-4 release but inhibits ionomycin-induced release *(66)*. This is distinct from the behavior of lymphocytes *(66)*, RBL cells *(67)*, and possibly human lung mast cells *(68)*. Preliminary evidence from some studies in Jurkat cells (that paradoxically behave like basophils rather than T-cells in this context) suggests that this occurs at the level of transcription regulation; a recent study of the IL-4 promoter demonstrates that there is an NF-kB-sensitive element in competition with an NF-AT element *(69)*. In other words, if both transcriptional factors are present, they compete to occupy a nearly common promoter sequence. Since NF-kB activity is increased by PKC activation, this may provide an explanation for the effect of PMA on ionomycin-induced IL-4 release in basophils. PMA effectively suppresses the $[Ca^{2+}]_i$ signal that follows IgE-mediated stimulation (it has no effect on the ionomycin-induced change in $[Ca^{2+}]_i$), which makes it difficult to perform a test of its effects on this stimulus (if $[Ca^{2+}]_i$ elevations are required for NF-AT activity, then the application of PMA would not test the same mechanism as it does with ionomycin-induced IL-4 release). However, we have found that the relatively specific second-generation PKC inhibitor BIS-2 (bis-indoylmaleimide II) enhances IgE-mediated IL-4 secretion, supporting the concept that PKC activation during IgE-mediated stimulation could be a downregulatory element for this mediator.

IL-4 secretion is a rather slow process, on average requiring ≈2 h for half-maximal release and ranging from 0.5 to 4 h, which is in keeping with it being synthesized *de novo* during IgE-mediated stimulation. The process is sensitive to cycloheximide *(62)*, which suggests that protein synthesis is required, although it might only indicate that some other signal transduction factor (indirectly involved in IL-4 secretion) requires protein synthesis. With the advent of extremely sensitive IL-4 ELISA kits, lysates of resting cells are sometimes found to contain very low levels of IL-4, and the first 30 min of histamine secretion releases this IL-4. This fraction may be 1–5% of the total IL-4 ultimately secreted. This might explain reports that some IL-4 can be found in resting cells using immunocytochemical techniques. The significance of a small amount of IL-4 in resting cells is not clear; possibly it indicates a previous state of activation or a low level of activation in vivo. Stimulation results in the upregulation of messenger ribonucleic acid (mRNA) for IL-4, with message being apparent after 30 min of activation. If the cells are stimulated with a multivalent antigen like penicillin-HSA (BPO-HSA) and the reaction is stopped by adding univalent hapten (BPO-lysine) at a time point in the early phase of secretion, 30–60 min, no further release occurs. The implication is that secretion is dependent on the maintenance of crosslinks, although the mRNA may be present. Studies in RBL cells support the view that secretion itself is dependent on the maintenance of crosslinks; intracellular tumor necrosis factor (TNF) synthesized in the first hour was not secreted when cross links were disrupted with monovalent hapten and gradually disappeared from the intracellular compartment *(67)*.

THE ROLE OF DESENSITIZATION

One aspect of mediator release not yet discussed is desensitization. It is noteworthy that most often basophils or mast cells do not release all of their available mediators. For histamine secretion, this means that not all of a preformed mediator is secreted, but for newly formed mediators like LTC_4 or IL-4, this statement needs to be restated: IgE-mediated release does not often lead to secretion as great as can be obtained with other powerful stimuli like ionomycin. Indeed, the IgE-mediated process generally falls far short of what is possible. One way to interpret these observations is that there is an intrinsic mechanism to limit secretion. IgE-mediated release (for any mediator) requires extracellular calcium, so it is possible to reconfigure the experimental protocol and stimulate the cells under suboptimal conditions—the absence of extracellular calcium *(70)*. When this is done, crosslinks are established, and it appears that some aspects of activation are engaged but no secretion occurs until calcium is added to the extracellular medium. The longer one waits before adding the calcium back, the poorer the subsequent release. Thus, IgE-mediated histamine release decays with a half-life of ≈15 min under this experimental protocol *(70,71)*. There are many experiments that indicate that this approach to studying autoregulation provides some insights into the downregulatory mechanisms inherent in these activation reactions *(72,73)*. With the recognition that IL-4 secretion occurs, and it occurs long after histamine release is complete, our hypothesis that downregulation events shut off early signal transduction events needed modification. Clearly, if some process is operating to shut off histamine release, it must not have an effect on IL-4 secretion. This suggests that there are different signal transduction pathways for histamine and IL-4 secretion. Furthermore, desensitization mechanisms that operate on histamine release must not operate on the very earliest stages of signal transduction, since these would be required to maintain the signals for IL-4 secretion (*see* the above comments about dissociating cross links). Therefore, our current belief is that there are somewhat independent mechanisms for the downregulation of each of the mediators.

SIGNAL TRANSDUCTION: GENERAL CONSIDERATIONS

IgE-mediated secretion (Fig. 2) is dependent on the aggregation of the high-affinity receptor FcεRI. Today, it is possible to speculate on the reason for the requirement for aggregation, although at this time nearly all this speculation must be based on studies performed in RBL cells. The notion of aggregation by its very nature suggests the assemblage of several components, and this in fact is what appears to occur. FcεRI, which is composed of four subunits, α, β, and disulfide-linked γ2, has no apparent intrinsic enzymatic activity *(74)*. Instead, the β and γ subunits act to focus the activity of associated tyrosine kinases *(75–80)*. Although the precise picture is not yet clear, it seems that the Src-family protein (a family of membrane-associated tyrosine kinases) *lyn* is associated with FcεRI *(81–84)*. When aggregation occurs, *lyn* may crossphosphorylate the β-chain of the crosslinked FcεRI on a site referred to as an immunoreceptor tyrosine-based activation motif (ITAM) *(79,84,85)*. There is one site each for the β- and γ-chains. *lyn* may then bind to this β-chain ITAM through its SH2 domain (src-homology 2 domain) to be further activated so that it then phosphorylates the γ-chain

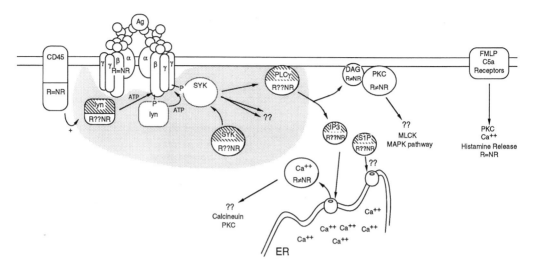

Fig. 2. Partial schematic of the signal transduction pathways involved in IgE-mediated stimulation. For each of the steps in the cascade, there is an indication of whether the component has been studied using human basophils. If the component is shaded in the upper half, it has not been adequately studied. In the lower half of each of the components depicted, there is an indication of whether releasing (R) and non-releasing (NR) basophils show similar levels of response or expression of the particular component. R??NR means that the comparison has not been made, R = NR means the expression or response is similar, and R ≠ NR usually means that releasing basophils express or show a response for the component whereas nonreleasing basophils do not. The shaded region around FcεRI indicates that these early components have not generally been studied in human basophils or studies are underway. Note that for non-IgE mediated stimulation (far right of the figure), basophils that don't respond to IgE-mediated stimulation do respond to FMLP or C5a to a degree that is indistinguishable from basophils that do respond to IgE-mediated stimulation. For the abbreviations *see* the text.

ITAM *(79)*. The SH2 domain of another tyrosine kinase, *syk*, can recognize this particular phosphorylated ITAM, which therefore causes *syk* to be recruited to the membrane FcεRI *(75–77,81,84,86–88)*. *syk* appears to phosphorylate several proteins, although the precise details of the cascade are not as clear beyond this point. Indeed, the above scenario is still tentative, since it is also clear that there are other associated kinases and phosphatases that regulate the initial events during receptor aggregation. *syk* can probably phosphorylate phospholipase Cγ (PLC-γ) *(87)*, which enables the next well-studied cascades of PKC activation and Ca^{2+} mobilization. PLC-γ does this by metabolizing phosphatidyl inositol into its two active components, diacylglycerol (DAG) and inositol triphosphate (IP3). DAG can promote the activation of PKC, whereas IP_3 induces the IP_3 receptor on the cell's endoplasmic reticulum (ER) or calcisomes to release stored Ca^{2+}.

There are further details for downstream signal transduction events. For example, $[Ca^{2+}]_i$ probably regulates calcineurin (a Ca^{2+}/calmodulin-dependent phosphatase), which in turn regulates the phosphorylation state of transcriptional factors and thus may be critical for the cytokine secretion now understood to be a part of the late secretory reaction. A second well-studied pathway, the mitogen-activated protein (MAP) kinase (MAPK) pathway *(89)*, may depend on both $[Ca^{2+}]_i$ and PKC activation, and MAPK, in coordination with $[Ca^{2+}]_i$, activates $cPLA_2$ *(90)*. PKC may also regulate the activity of myosin light chain kinase (MLCK) *(91,92)*, which participates in the regulation of the cytoskeleton *(93)*. Beyond these few pathways, the steps leading to secretion of each of the three types of mediators remain ill-defined.

SIGNAL TRANSDUCTION EVENTS IN HUMAN BASOPHILS

How might these observations be applied to the study of human basophil releasability? First, it is necessary to review what events have been studied in human basophils. The early events that describe the ability of FcεRI to initiate a phosphorylation reaction are essentially unstudied. It is quite likely that the general scheme being discovered in RBL cells will be operative, but the particular details may differ, and it may be these details that are relevant to understanding the control of mediator release. As will become clear below, it will probably be necessary to examine these early events in order to understand releasability.

Intermediate Events

Given the number of early events now being found to precede an elevation in $[Ca^{2+}]_i$, one might consider $[Ca^{2+}]_i$ changes as an intermediate event (although the full length of the cascade is unknown). The average net $[Ca^{2+}]_i$ signal is well correlated with histamine release. The Spearman rank correlation coefficient for these two parameters is 0.78 ($n = 44$) *(26)*. The initial changes in cytosolic $[Ca^{2+}]_i$ significantly precede histamine release (and LTC_4 and IL-4 release as well), so there may be a causal relationship *(26)*. It has been difficult to dissociate the change in $[Ca^{2+}]_i$ from histamine release, although some unusual experimental designs can approach this condition (these will not be discussed). A close inspection of the $[Ca^{2+}]_i$/histamine-release correlation reveals a reasonably large amount of variability in the $[Ca^{2+}]_i$ response (for a given amount of histamine release), especially in the lower regions of the response range. Moreover, an elevation in $[Ca^{2+}]_i$ alone is clearly not sufficient to initiate secretion. These observations suggest that additional factors contribute to the response. This is not a new perspective, and numerous studies of secretory cells have suggested that PKC is a participant (this will be discussed below, e.g., *[94]*). Ionomycin is a strong stimulus for the release of all mediators, but in terms of the magnitude of the induced $[Ca^{2+}]_i$ response, this is actually a poor stimulus for histamine release when compared to anti-IgE antibody. The half maximal response (EC_{50}) for anti-IgE antibody is approximately 100 nM (net elevation for the period of histamine release, ≈15 min), whereas for ionomycin, the EC_{50} is ≈700 nM. This is not true for LTC_4 and IL-4 release, however. It appears that for LTC_4 release, a similar elevation in $[Ca^{2+}]_i$ for anti-IgE and ionomycin results in similar levels of LTC_4 release. Ionomycin appears to induce the release of 2–3-fold more IL-4 than anti-IgE antibody when the $[Ca^{2+}]_i$ elevations are similar. The reasons for this are not entirely clear but may relate to the fact that ionomycin induces a sustained $[Ca^{2+}]_i$ response whereas the $[Ca^{2+}]_i$ response following anti-IgE does eventually decay. This decay following anti-IgE antibody appears quite slow, and it is certainly sustained far longer than histamine release occurs. But, it does decay with a half-life of approx 30–60 min, whereas the $[Ca^{2+}]_i$ response following ionomycin is generally constant. Extensive correlations between the $[Ca^{2+}]_i$ response and LTC_4 or IL-4 release have not been performed, but the fact that all experimental maneuvers that eliminate the $[Ca^{2+}]_i$ response (or more precisely, suppressing the second phase of the $[Ca^{2+}]_i$ response) stop these reactions, even for stimuli for which such maneuvers do not stop histamine release, suggests that they would be highly correlated. The end result of the studies of $[Ca^{2+}]_i$ elevations and mediator release indicates that $[Ca^{2+}]_i$ is probably a critical second messenger. Indeed, in nonreleasers, in which IgE-mediated release is near zero, the second phase of the $[Ca^{2+}]_i$ response is also near zero, and the initial phase is weak. Therefore, it is likely that control of secretion is exerted at an earlier level than the elevation in $[Ca^{2+}]_i$. Substances that mediate cytosolic Ca^{2+} changes, such as IP_3 or sphingosine-1-phosphate (S1P) *(95)*, or the enzymes that produce them during IgE-mediated release have not been measured in human basophils.

The activation of PKC is also an event downstream of the early tyrosine kinase activation events described above, but probably not too many steps downstream. Like the $[Ca^{2+}]_i$ signal, PKC activation precedes histamine release by a substantial margin of time (6). Also, like the $[Ca^{2+}]_i$ response, it appears that PKC activation is reasonably correlated with histamine release (6). Indeed, PKC activity rises and falls on a time scale that might explain the cessation of histamine release. However, these studies of PKC activation must be interpreted cautiously. The studies are dependent on measuring the activity of an enzyme capable of phosphorylating a foreign substrate, histone III. This substrate is certainly not relevant to IgE-mediated signal transduction, so the evidence rests with the observation that this *ex situ* kinase activity is Ca^{2+}- and phosphatidylserine-dependent, a hallmark of PKC-like activity used in the 1980s. Until more relevant substrates have been examined either *in situ* or *ex situ*, the data remains preliminary. A further confounding problem is that PKC is a family of enzymes that appear to have conflicting activities. In RBL cells, PKC-α and -ε appear to be inhibitory, whereas PKC-β and -δ are activators of degranulation (96,97). Therefore, the measurement of a generalized PKC activity is difficult to properly interpret.

In the last few years there has been a reinspection of the role of PKC in various secretory reactions because the causal evidence has generally depended on pharmacological agents that were thought to be specific for PKC. All of the original class of PKC inhibitors have been found to be nonselective, which shouldn't be all that surprising since many of these inhibitors were adenosine triphosphate (ATP) analogs. Recent studies using overexpression or dominant-negative expression techniques haven't exactly clarified the issue (for a brief review *see [98]*). Recently, several new inhibitors have been developed that appear to have better selectivity, although time will probably alter this perspective. Indeed, one new inhibitor, Go-6976, was actually thought to be specific for PKC-α and -β but now appears to inhibit some tyrosine kinases. Thus far, the bis-indoylmaleimide derivatives appear to be selective in a number of systems, or at least don't inhibit early signal transduction kinases. Surprisingly, while the indoylmaleimide class of inhibitors are very effective inhibitors of PMA-induced histamine release from human basophils, they have no effect on (or slight enhancement of) IgE-mediated histamine release. This is a rather surprising result, especially for human basophils. Of the histamine-containing cells activated through IgE (human or rodent), the human basophil is unique for its ability to degranulate in response to the sole application of PMA (99). Since phorbol esters are still thought to be specific activators of PKC isozymes, these observations have certainly indicated that the basophil degranulation apparatus was uniquely capable of responding to PKC activation, i.e., PKC activity alone is sufficient. Indeed, PMA can induce this response even in buffers devoid of meaningful Ca^{2+} concentrations (high-EGTA buffers) as well as basophils heavily loaded with a cell-permeant calcium buffer like BAPTA (which completely suppresses the $[Ca^{2+}]_i$ response to any physiological stimulus and allows only weak elevations of $[Ca^{2+}]_i$ even with ionomycin). However, if cells are treated with very low levels of PMA such that secretion occurs at a very slow rate, and a small amount of ionomycin is added, the basophil degranulates within a minute. Clearly the synergy of the two agents is a strong activator of the downstream events leading to degranulation. These results pave the way for a model that places PKC in a central role for the degranulation process. Thus, this absence of an effect on IgE-mediated responses by clearly effective PKC inhibitors is surprising and intriguing. One caveat to these observations is the result of studies with calphostin C. This is a unique class of PKC inhibitors that effectively inhibits PKC through its regulatory domain rather than the catalytic domain (100). It inhibits PMA, anti-IgE antibody, and FMLP-induced histamine release and does not inhibit the $[Ca^{2+}]_i$ signal following anti-IgE antibody. However, calphostin C is also found to inhibit ionomycin-induced release at similar concentrations. No other PKC inhibitor does this, and this result raises the possibility that it affects other signal transduction events not yet measured.

While exploring the role of PKC in the IgE-mediated activation of human basophils we have stumbled upon an intriguing observation that may partially explain the effects of PMA on basophil secretion. An initial survey of the PKC isozymes present in basophils turned up two notable absences. Lymphocytes and monocytes express moderate amounts of PKC-α, βI, βII, δ, ϵ, and η (all class I and class II PKC isozymes with the exception of PKC-γ, which is only found in brain tissue). RBL cells also show a similar profile *(96)*. However, basophils lack both PKC-α and -η (using basophils purified to nearly 100%). The surprise is the absence of PKC-α, which is generally a ubiquitous isozyme. Results in the literature might have predicted this situation, however. Both neutrophils and eosinophils appear to lack PKC-α *(101–103)*. In addition, the expression of PKC-δ is substantially greater than found in lymphocytes or monocytes, 4–5-fold greater (PKC-βI, βII, and -ϵ are similar to lymphocytes and monocytes). Preliminary studies of human lung mast cells, on the other hand, indicate levels of PKC-α expression similar to lymphocytes or monocytes but PKC-δ is expressed only weakly. If the functional results from RBL cells can be applied to basophils, then the absence of PKC-α might mean that an important negative regulator of secretion is missing and the strong presence of an important activator, PKC-δ, allows PMA to induce histamine release in basophils, although it has no direct effects on mast cells. It remains to be seen if this is true and it also remains to be seen if these observations have relevance to histamine release. As with the $[Ca^{2+}]_i$ correlation, the bottom line of the PKC studies is that PKC activity appears to correlate with histamine release, and this suggests that regulation of releasability is exerted prior to this signal transduction event.

Early Signal Transduction Events

Events earlier than these processes are not well studied in human basophils or mast cells. There are pharmacological agents that are thought to inhibit tyrosine kinases, and some do inhibit histamine release, but these results should be viewed cautiously *(104)*. Preliminary studies indicate the presence of both *lyn* and SYK in human basophils *(105)* and mast cells, but no functional correlates of their behavior have been examined. CD45 is a tyrosine phosphatase that is expressed at high levels on all leukocytes and is considered critical to the functioning of *lyn*. Phosphorylation of *lyn* at one of its tyrosines results in inhibition of its catalytic activity (presumably folding the phosphorylated tyrosine and the surrounding peptide into its own catalytic site). CD45 removes this phosphate and maintains the activity of *lyn (106)*. We have examined two classes of donors for CD45 expression, those that don't secrete mediators in response to IgE-mediated stimulation and those that show marked secretion. Both groups expressed similar levels of CD45 using a monoclonal antibody previously found to inhibit IgE-mediated release through CD45 *(107)*. This is a crude measure and ignores the possibility that the activity of CD45 differs between the two groups. However, such studies are not yet feasible in human basophils. In a similar context, we have examined another tyrosine phosphatase, PTP1c, which appears to regulate the sensitivity of B-cells to stimulation *(108)*. Basophils express high levels of PTP1c, but these levels are essentially equivalent in all basophils, releasers, poor releasers, or nonreleasers. Again, it may be more relevant to examine PTP1c activity, but the tools don't yet exist for the small numbers of cells available.

MODULATION OF RELEASABILITY

Table 3 presents some of the broad categories that could or should be investigated to address the issue of releasability in basophils and its relationship to signal transduction. The possibilities revolve around intrinsic factors, either activators or inhibitors, and extrinsic factors that modulate the intrinsic factors, either positively or negatively. In the context of intrinsic mechanisms,

Table 3
Some Possible Causes for the "Releasability" Variable

Intrinsic
  Control is exerted through a missing or inactive component of the IgE-mediated signal
    transduction pathway
  Control is exerted through the activity of a down-regulatory pathway, e.g.,
    desensitization

Extrinsic
  Variations in release result from regulation by an extrinsic promoter of basophil
    function, specifically for the IgE-mediated signal transduction pathway
  Variations in release result from inhibitory regulation by extrinsic factors

it is useful to note that there is good correlation between the rate at which a basophil desensitizes
(as measured by the technique described above) and the maximum histamine release. In other
words, if a basophil has an active desensitization pathway, one might expect that the maximum
response would be blunted. This viewpoint makes sense in light of the observation that the sensitivity of the basophil to crosslinks and the maximal release are independent parameters.
Desensitization events presumably require early signals, although not necessarily the same pathways used for activation, so the desensitization pathway must be able to sense crosslinks in a
manner similar to activation. Thus both activation and desensitization are started on an equal
footing with regard to the initial crosslinking, but if the desensitization process is overly active,
the maximal response is suppressed. It is clear that desensitization exerts effects on early signal
transduction events and therefore provides an intrinsic process to regulate secretion and
potentially explain the releasability question.

Most notable among the explanations that involve extrinsic factors is the possibility that
cytokines are critical. There are several cytokines that markedly affect basophil function, but
the most efficacious and possibly most potent is IL-3. IL-3 can induce marked changes in the
responsiveness of basophils, affecting all stimuli and the release of all mediators. It certainly
has marked effects on basophils that release poorly to IgE-mediated stimulation, but until
recently, it had no apparent effect on the IgE-mediated response of the so-called nonreleasers
(*see* above). Thus, it was difficult to explain the continuum of releasability by differences in
IL-3 control. However, in a recently published paper, it was found that long-term culture (4–7 d)
of nonreleasing basophils with IL-3 appears to convert them to releasing basophils. We have
verified this observation, and it suggests that the entire continuum of releasability could
be explained by an extrinsic factor like IL-3. The data suggest that either donors express variable amounts of circulating IL-3 or the basophils express variable levels of the IL-3 receptor.
Since basophils from any class of donor seem to respond well to even short treatments with
IL-3 (even nonreleasers in which IL-3 doesn't alter the IgE-mediated response but does
enhance stimuli like FMLP or C5a), it appears that the problem is not clearly with the expression of IL-3 receptor. This suggests that circulating IL-3 levels may play a role.

These observations also direct studies to determining how IL-3 exerts its effects on
basophils. This problem is multifaceted. IL-3 appears to have three effects that occur in three
time domains. A short treatment of the cells with IL-3 (5–15 min) markedly upregulates histamine and LTC_4 secretion and has variable enhancing effects on IL-4 release. However,
with one possible exception, we have yet to find an early signal transduction event that is
upregulated on this time scale (the exception is that free AA levels are increased following
C5a stimulation, and as noted above *(60)*, this may indicate the activity of a $cPLA_2$ whose

role in basophil secretion is uncertain). Surprisingly, this early enhancement is not inhibited by several effective tyrosine inhibitors (the IL-3 receptor appears to signal through some tyrosine kinases like JAK-family kinases). On the other hand, 24 h with IL-3 renders a basophil even more responsive. Histamine release is not enhanced too much further, but LTC_4 and IL-4 release are enhanced 10-fold. $[Ca^{2+}]_i$ signals are also increased markedly, 3–4-fold *(60)*. At the 24-h time point, nonreleasing basophils are not yet affected by IL-3 treatment *(109)*. The third phase of the IL-3 effect may take place on the time scale of days, and it is during this period that nonreleasing basophils convert *(110)*. No signal transduction studies have been conducted at this stage of its effects. It appears that a phenotypic change may occur during these long incubations, which implies that a marked number of changes probably occur. Thus, it may be difficult to pin the effects on releasability on a change in any one signal transduction event, but such a study will probably yield some valuable insights into how releasability in regulated.

To summarize, releasability, measured as the maximum histamine release to polyclonal anti-IgE antibody, appears to be regulated at a point preceding the elevation in $[Ca^{2+}]_i$ and PKC activity. Intrinsic control may be exerted through a desensitization process, and extrinsic control through the activity of IL-3.

REFERENCES

1. Scharenbery AM, Kinet JP (1995) Early events in mast cell signal transduction. Chem Immunol 61:72.
2. Schleimer RP, MacGlashan DW Jr, Gillespie E, Lichtenstein LM (1982) Inhibition of basophil histamine release by anti-inflammatory steroids. II. Studies on the mechanism of action. J Immunol 129:1632.
3. Schulman ES, MacGlashan DW Jr, Peters SP, Schleimer RP, Newball HH, Lichtenstein LM (1982) Human lung mast cells: purification and characterization. J Immunol 129:2662.
4. Glaum MC, Jaffe JS, Gillespie DH, Raible DG, Post TJ, Wang Y, Dimitry E, Schulman ES (1995) IgE-dependent expression of interleukin-5 mRNA and protein in human lung: modulation by dexamethasone. Clin Immunol Immunopathol 75:171.
5. MacGlashan DW Jr, Lichtenstein LM (1980) The purification of human basophils. J Immunol 124:2519.
6. Warner JA, MacGlashan DW Jr (1989) Protein kinase C (PKC) changes in human basophils. IgE-mediated activation is accompanied by an increase in total PKC activity. J Immunol 142:1669.
7. Brunner T, Heusser CH, Dahinden CA (1993) Human peripheral blood basophils primed by interleukin-3 (IL-3) produce IL-4 in response to immunoglobulin E receptor stimulation. J Exp Med 177:605.
8. Naclerio RM, Kagey SA, Lichtenstein LM, Togias AG, Iliopoulos O, Pipkorn U, Bascom R, Norman PS, Proud D (1987) Observations on nasal late phase reactions. Immunol Invest 16:649.
9. Charlesworth EN, Hood AF, Soter NA, Kagey SA, Norman PS, Lichtenstein LM (1989) Cutaneous late-phase response to allergen: Mediator release and inflammatory cell infiltration. J Clin Invest 83:1519.
10. Olson R, Karpink MH, Shelanski S, Atkins PC, Zweiman B (1990) Skin reactivity to codeine and histamine during prolonged corticosteroid therapy. J Allergy Clin Immunol 86:153.
11. Liu MC, Hubbard WC, Proud D, Stealey BA, Galli SJ, Kagey SA, Bleecker ER, Lichtenstein LM (1991) Immediate and late inflammatory responses to ragweed antigen challenge of the peripheral airways in allergic asthmatics. Cellular, mediator, and permeability changes. Am Rev Respir Dis 144:51.
12. Wardlaw AJ, Dunette S, Gleich GJ, Collins JV, Kay AB (1988) Eosinophils and mast cells in broncho-alveolar lavage in mild asthma: relationship to bronchial hyperreactivity. Am Rev Resp Dis 137:62.
13. Azzawi M, Bradley B, Jeffery PK, Frew AJ, Wardlaw AJ, Knowles G, Assoufi B, Collins JV, Durham S, Kay AB (1990) Identification of activated T-lymphocytes and eosinophils in bronchial biopsies in stable atopic asthmatics. Am Rev Resp Dis 142:1407.
14. Iliopoulos O, Baroody F, Naclerio RM, Bochner BS, Kagey-Sobotka A, Lichtenstein LM (1992) Histamine containing cells obtained from the nose hours after antigen challenge have functions and phenotypic characteristics of basophils. J Immunol 148:2223.
15. Siraganian RP, Hook WA (1977) Mechanism of histamine release by formyl methionine-containing peptides. J Immunol 119:2078.
16. Siraganian RP, Hook WA (1976) Complement-induced histamine release from human basophils. II. Mechanism of the histamine release reaction. J Immunol 116:639.

17. Brunner T, de Weck AL, Dahinden CA (1991) Platelet-activating factor induces mediator release by human basophils primed with IL-3, granulocyte-macrophage colony-stimulating factor, or IL-5. J Immunol 147:237.

18. Columbo M, Casolaro V, Warner JA, MacGlashan DW Jr, Kagey-Sobotka A, Lichtenstein LM (1990) The mechanism of mediator release from human basophils induced by platelet-activating factor. J Immunol 145:3855.

19. Bischoff SC, Krieger M, Brunner, T, Dahinden CA (1992) Monocyte chemotactic protein 1 is a potent activator of human basophils. J Exp Med 175:1271.

20. MacDonald SM, Lichtenstein LM, Proud D, Plaut M, Naclerio RM, MacGlashan DW, Kagey SA (1987) Studies of IgE-dependent histamine releasing factors: heterogeneity of IgE. J Immunol 139:506.

21. MacDonald S, Lichtenstein LM (1995) Cloning and expression of histamine releasing factor. Science 269:688.

22. O'Donnell MC, Ackerman SJ, Gleich GJ, Thomas LL (1983) Activation of basophil and mast cell histamine release by eosinophil granule major basic protein. J Exp Med 157:1981.

23. Foreman JC, Lichtenstein LM (1980) Induction of histamine secretion by polycations. Biochim Biophys Acta 629:587.

24. MacDonald SM, Schleimer RP, Kagey SA, Gillis S, Lichtenstein LM (1989) Recombinant IL-3 induces histamine release from human basophils. J Immunol 142:3527.

25. Warner JA, Peters SP, Lichtenstein LM, Hubbard W, Yancey KB, Stevenson HC, Miller PJ, MacGlashan DW Jr (1989) Differential release of mediators from human basophils: differences in arachidonic acid metabolism following activation by unrelated stimuli. J Leukocyte Biol 45:558.

26. Warner JA, MacGlashan DW Jr (1990) Signal transduction events in human basophils—a comparative study of the role of protein kinase-C in basophils activated by anti-IgE antibody and formyl-methionyl-leucyl-phenylalanine. J Immunol 145:1897.

27. MacGlashan DW Jr, Warner JA (1991) Stimulus-dependent leukotriene release from human basophils: a comparative study of C5a and Fmet-leu-phe. J Leukocyte Biol 49:29.

28. Warner JA, Yancey KB, MacGlashan DW Jr (1987) The effect of pertussis toxin on mediator release from human basophils. J Immunol 139:161.

29. Botana LM, MacGlashan DW Jr (1991) Differential effects of cAMP on mediator release in human basophils. FASEB J 5:A1007.

30. Ali H, Cunha MJR, Saul WF, Beaven MA (1990) Activation of phospholipase C via adenosine receptors provides synergistic signals for secretion in antigen-stimulated RBL-2H3 cells: evidence for a novel adenosine receptor. J Biol Chem 265:745.

31. Collado ED, Cunha MJR, Beaven MA (1990) Treatment with dexamethasone down-regulates IgE-receptor-mediated signals and up-regulates adenosine-receptor-mediated signals in a rat mast cell (RBL-2H3) line. J Immunol 144:244.

32. Collado EH, Ali H, Beaven MA (1990) On the mechanism of action of dexamethasone in a rat mast cell line (RBL-2H3 cells). Evidence for altered coupling of receptors and G-proteins. J Immunol 144:3449.

33. MacGlashan DW Jr (1993) Releasability of human basophils: Cellular sensitivity and maximal histamine release are independent variables. J Allergy Clin Immunol 91:605.

34. MacGlashan DW Jr, Botana L (1993) Biphasic Ca^{++} responses in human basophils: evidence that the initial transient elevation associated with mobilization of intracellular calcium is an insufficient signal for degranulation. J Immunol 150:980.

35. MacGlashan DW Jr, Bochner B, Warner JA (1994) Graded changes in the response of individual human basophils to stimulation: Distributional behavior of early activation events. J Leukocyte Biol 55:13.

36. MacGlashan DW Jr (1995) Graded changes in the response of individual human basophils to stimulation: distributional behavior of events temporally coincident with degranulation. J Leukocyte Biol 58:177.

37. Knol EF, Mul FPJ, Jansen H, Calafat J, Roos D (1991) Monitoring human basophil activation via CD63 monoclonal antibody 435. J Allergy Clin Immunol 88:328.

38. Pruzansky JJ, Zeiss CR, Patterson R (1980) A linear correlation between histamine release and degranulation of human basophils by specific antigen or the ionophore A23187. Immunology 40:411.

39. Dvorak AM, Newball HH, Dvorak HF, Lichtenstein LM (1980) Antigen-induced IgE-mediated degranulation of human basophils. Lab Invest 43:126.

40. Conroy MC, Adkinson NFJ, Lichtenstein LM (1977) Measurement of IgE on human basophils: relation to serum IgE and anti-IgE-induced histamine release. J Immunol 118:1317.

41. Malveaux FJ, Conroy MC, Adkinson NFJ, Lichtenstein LM (1978) IgE receptors on human basophils. Relationship to serum IgE concentration. J Clin Invest 62:176.

42. Wilde C (1994) Cabo San Lucas Meeting: The Role of Basophils and Eosinophils in Human Disease.

43. Dvorak AM (1992) Basophils and mast cells: Piecemeal degranulation in situ and ex vivo: A possible mechanism for cytokine-induced function in disease. In: Coffey RG, ed. Granulocyte Responses to Cytokines, Marcel Dekker, New York, p. 169.

44. Dvorak AM, Morgan ES, Lichtenstein LM, MacGlashan DW Jr (1994) Activated human basophils contain histamine in cytoplasmic vesicles. Int Arch Allergy Immunol 105:8.

45. Dvorak AM, Warner JA, Morgan E, Kissell-Rainville S, Lichtenstein LM, MacGlashan DW Jr (1992) An ultrastructural analysis of tumor-promoting phorbol diester-induced degranulation in human basophils. Am J Pathol 141:1309.

46. Dvorak AM, Warner JA, Kissell S, Lichtenstein LM, MacGlashan DW Jr (1991) F-met peptide-induced degranulation of human basophils. Lab Invest 64:234.

47. Warner JA, Bochner BS, MacGlashan DW Jr (1990) Cytoskeletal rearrangement and shape change in human basophils. J Allergy Clin Immunol 146:1a.

48. MacGlashan DW Jr, Peters SP, Warner J, Lichtenstein LM (1986) Characteristics of human basophil sulfidopeptide leukotriene release: releasability defined as the ability of the basophil to respond to dimeric cross-links. J Immunol 136:2231.

49. MacGlashan DW Jr, Schleimer RP, Peters SP, Schulman ES, Adams GK, Newball HH, Lichtenstein LM (1982) Generation of leukotrienes by purified human lung mast cells. J Clin Invest 70:747.

50. Lewis RA, Soter NA, Diamond PT, Austen KF, Oates JA, Roberts LJ (1982) Prostaglandin D2 generation after activation of rat and human mast cells with anti-IgE. J Immunol 129:1627.

51. Lawrence ID, Warner JA, Cohan VL, Hubbard WC, Kagey SA, Lichtenstein LM (1987) Purification and characterization of human skin mast cells. Evidence for human mast cell heterogeneity. J Immunol 139:3062.

52. Murakami M, Kudo I, Suwa Y, Inoue K (1992) Release of 14-kDa group II phospholipase A2 from activated mast cells and its possible involvement in the regulation of the degranulation process. Eur J Biochem 209:257.

53. Hundley TR, Marshall L, Hubbard WC, MacGlashan DW Jr (1998) Arachidonic acid release for leukotriene C4 synthesis in human basophils is mediated by a secretory phospholipase A2, J Pharmacol Exp Ther.

54. Schievella AR, Regier MK, Smith WL, Lin LL (1995) Calcium-mediated translocation of cytosolic phospholipase A2 to the nuclear envelope and endoplasmic reticulum. J Biol Chem 270:30,749.

55. Woods JW, Evans JF, Ethier D, Scott S, Vickers PJ, Hearn L, Heibein JA, Charleson S, Singer II (1993) 5-lipoxygenase and 5-lipoxygenase-activating protein are localized in the nuclear envelope of activated human leukocytes. J Exp Med 178:1935.

56. Clark JD, Lin LL, Kriz RW, Ramesha CS, Sultzman LA, Lin AY, Milona N, Knoph JL (1991) A novel arachidonic acid-selective cytosolic PLA2 contains a Ca^{2+}-dependent translocation domain with homology to PKC and GAP. Cell 65:1043.

57. Roshak A, Sathe G, Marshall LA (1994) Supression of monocyte 85-kDa phospholipase A2 by antisense and effects on endotoxin-induced prostaglandin biosynthesis. J Biol Chem 269:25,999.

58. Marshall LA, Bolognese B, Roshak A (1997) Distinct phospholipase A2 enzymes differentially mediate human monocyte eicosanoid formation. J Biol Chem 272:759.

59. Marshall LA, Hall RH, Winkler JD, Bolognese B, Roshak A, Flamburg PL, Sung SM, Chabot-Fletcher M, Adams JL, Mayer RJ (1995) SB 203347, an inhibitor of 14 kDa phospholipase A2, alters neutrophil arachidonic acid release and metabolism and prolongs survival in murine edndtoxin shock. J Pharmacol Exp Therap 274:1254.

60. MacGlashan DW Jr, Hubbard WC (1993) Interleukin-3 alters free arachidonic acid generation in C5a-stimulated human basophils. J Immunol 151:6358.

61. Columbo M, Taglialalatela M, Warner JA, MacGlashan DW Jr, Yasumoto T, Annunziato L, Marone G (1992) Maitotoxin, a novel activator of mediator release from human basophils, induces large increases in cytosolic calcium resulting in histamine, but not leukotriene C4 release. J Pharmacol Exp Therap 263:979.

62. MacGlashan DW Jr, White JM, Huang SK, Ono SJ, Schroeder J, Lichtenstein LM (1994) Secretion of interleukin-4 from human basophils: The relationship between IL-4 mRNA and protein in resting and stimulated basophils. J Immunol 152:3006.

63. Sim TC, Li H, Reece LM, Alam R (1996) Interleukin-13 production by human basophils. J Allergy Clin Immunol 97:358a.

64. Li H, Sin TC, Grant JA, Alam R (1996) The production of MIP-1a by basophils and its comparison to the production by other leukocytes. J Allergy Clin Immunol 97:267a.

65. Schroeder JT, MacGlashan DW Jr, Kagey-Sobotka A, White JM, Lichtenstein LM (1994) The IgE-dependent IL-4 secretion by human basophils: The relationship between cytokine production and histamine release in mixed leukocyte cultures. J Immunol 153:1808.

66. Schroeder JT, Lichtenstein LM, Kagey-Sobotka A, MacGlashan DW Jr (1996) IL-4 secretion by human basophils and lymphocytes is differentially regulated by protein kinase C activation, submitted.

67. Baumgartner RA, Yamada K, Deramo VA, Beaven MA (1994) Secretion of TNF from a rat mast cell line is a brefeldin A-sensitive and calcium/protein kinase C-regulated process. J Immunol 153:2609.

68. Jaffe JS, Glaum MC, Raible DG, Post TJ, Dimitry E, Govindarao D, Wang Y, Schulman ES (1995) Human lung mast cell IL-5 gene and protein expression: temporal analysis of upregulation following IgE-mediated activation. Am J Respir Cell Mol Biol 13:665.

69. Casolaro V, Georas S, Song Z, Zubkoff ID, Abdulkadir SA, Thanos D, Ono SJ (1995) Inhibition of NFATp-dependent transcription by NFkB. Implications for differential gene expression in T cell subsets. Proc Natl Acad Sci USA 92:11,623.

70. Lichtenstein LM, De Bernardo R (1971) IgE mediated histamine release: in vitro separation into two phases. Int Arch Allergy Appl Immunol 41:56.

71. Sobotka AK, Dembo M, Goldstein B, Lichtenstein LM (1979) Antigen-specific desensitization of human basophils. J Immunol 122:511.

72. Dembo M, Goldstein B (1980) A model of cell activation and desensitization by surface immunoglobin: the case of histamine release from human basophils. Cell 22:59.

73. Kazimierczak W, Mier HL, MacGlashan DW Jr, Lichtenstein LM (1984) An antigen-activated DFP-inhibitable enzyme controls basophil desensitization. J Immunol 132:399.

74. Blank U, Ra C, Miller L, White K, Metzger H, Kinet JP (1989) Complete structure and expression in transfected cells of high affinity IgE receptor. Nature 337:187.

75. Benhamou M, Gutkind JS, Robbins KC, Siraganian RP (1990) Tyrosine phosphorylation coupled to IgE receptor-mediated signal transduction and histamine release. Proc Natl Acad Sci USA 87:5327.

76. Benhamou M, Stephan V, Gutkind SJ, Robbins KC, Siraganian RP (1991) Protein tyrosine phosphorylation in the degranulation step of RBL-2H3 cells. FASEB J 5:A1007.

77. Stephan V, Benhamou M, Gutkind JS, Robbins KC, Siraganian RP (1992) Fc epsilon RI-induced protein tyrosine phosphorylation of pp72 in rat basophilic leukemia cells (RBL-2H3). Evidence for a novel signal transduction pathway unrelated to G protein activation and phosphatidylinositol hydrolysis. J Biol Chem 267:5434.

78. Paolini R, Jouvin MH, Kinet JP (1991) Phosphorylation and dephosphorylation of the high affinity receptor for immunoglobulin E immediately after receptor engagement and disengagement. Nature 353:855.

79. Yamashita T, Mao SY, Metzger H (1994) Aggregation of the high-affinity IgE receptor and enhanced activity of p53/56lyn protein-tyrosine kinase. Proc Natl Acad Sci USA 91:11,251.

80. Eiseman E, Bolen JB (1992) Signal transduction by the cytoplasmic domains of Fc epsilon RI-gamma and TCR-zeta in rat basophilic leukemia cells. J Biol Chem 267:21,027.

81. Jouvin MH, Adamczewski M, Numerof R, Letourneur O, Valle A, Kinet JP (1994) Differential control of the tyrosine kinase lyn and syk by the two signaling chains of the high affinity immunoglobulin E receptor. J Biol Chem 269:5918.

82. Eiseman E, Bolen JB (1992) Engagement of the high-affinity IgE receptor activates src protein-related tyrosine kinases. Nature 355:78.

83. Kihara H, Siraganian RP (1994) Src homology 2 domains of Syk and Lyn bind to tyrosine-phosphorylated subunits of the high affinity IgE receptor. J Biol Chem 269:22,427.

84. Scharenberg AM, Lin S, Cuenod B, Yamamura H, Kinet JP (1995) Reconstitution of interactions between tyrosine kinases and the high affinity IgE receptor which are controlled by receptor clustering. EMBO J 14:3385.

85. Cambier JC (1995) Antigen and Fc receptor signaling. The awesome power of the immunoreceptor tyrosine-based activation motif (ITAM) (review). J Immunol 155:3281.

86. Hutchcroft JE, Geahlen RL, Deanin GG, Oliver JM (1992) Fc epsilon RI-mediated tyrosine phosphorylation and activation of the 72-kDa protein-tyrosine kinase, PTK72, in RBL-2H3 rat tumor mast cells. Proc Natl Acad Sci USA 89:9107.

87. Li W, Deanin GG, Margolis B, Schlessinger J, Oliver JM (1992) FceRI-mediated tyrosine phosphorylation of multiple proteins including phospholipase C gamma 1 and the receptor beta/gamma2 complex in RBL-2H3 cells. Mol Cell Biol 12:3176.

88. Shiue L, Zoller MJ, Brugge JS (1995) Syk is activated by phosphotyrosine-containing peptides representing the tyrosine-based activation motifs of the high affinity receptor for IgE. J Biol Chem 270:10,498.

89. Hirasawa N, Scharenberg A, Yamamura H, Beaven MA, Kinet JP (1995) A requirement for Syk in the activation of the microtubule-associated protein kinase/phospholipase A2 pathway by Fc epsilon R1 is not shared by a G protein-coupled receptor. J Biol Chem 270:10,960.

90. Lin LL, Wartmann M, Lin A, Knoph JL, Seth A, Davis RJ (1993) cPLA2 is phosphorylated and activated by MAP kinase. Cell 72:269.

91. Ludowyke RI, Peleg I, Beaven MA, Adelstein RS (1989) Antigen-induced secretion of histamine and the phosphorylation of myosin by protein kinase C in RBL cells. J Biol Chem 264:12,492.

92. Choi OH, Adelstein RS, Beaven MA (1994) Secretion from RBL-2H3 cells is associated with phosphorylation of myosin light chains by myosin light chain kinase as well as phosphorylation by protein kinase C. J Biol Chem 269:536.

93. Hamawy MM, Mergenhagen SE, Siraganian RP (1993) Tyrosine phosphorylation of pp125FAK by the aggregation of high affinity immunoglobulin E receptor requires adherence. J Biol Chem 268:6851.

94. Beaven MA, Guthrie DF, Moore JP, Smith GA, Hesketh TR, Metcalfe JC (1987) Synergistic signals in the mechanism of antigen-induced exocytosis in 2H3 cells: evidence for an unidentified signal required for histamine release. J Cell Biol 105:1129.

95. Choi OH, Kim JH, Kinet JP (1996) Calcium mobilization via sphingosine kinase in signaling by the FceRI antigen receptor. Nature 380:634.

96. Ozawa K, Szallasi Z, Kanzanietz MG, Blumberg PM, Mischak H, Mushinski JF, Beaven MA (1993) Ca^{2+}-dependent and Ca^{2+}-independent isozymes of protein kinase C mediate exocytosis in antigen-stimulated rat basophilic RBL-2H3 cells: reconstitution of secretory responses with Ca^{2+} and purified isozymes in washed permeabilized cells. J Biol Chem 268:1749.

97. Ozawa K, Yamada K, Kanzanietz MG, Blumberg PM, Beaven MA (1993) Different isozymes of protein kinase C mediate feedback inhibition of phospholipase C and stimulatory signals for exocytosis in rat RBL-2H3 cells. J Biol Chem 268:2280.

98. Dekker LV, Parker PJ (1994) Protein kinase C: a question of specificity. Trends Biochem Sci 19:73.

99. Schleimer RP, Gillespie E, Lichtenstein LM (1981) Release of histamine from human leukocytes stimulated with the tumor promoting phorbol esters. I. Characterization of the response. J Immunol 126:570.

100. Tamaoki T, Takahashi I, Kobayashi E, Nakano H, Akinaga S, Suzuki K (1990) Calphostin (UCN1028) and calphostin related compounds, a new class of specific and potent inhibitors of protein kinase C. Adv Second Messenger Phosphoprotein Res 24:497.

101. Devalia V, Thomas SB, Roberts PJ, Jones M, Linch (1992) Down-regulation of human protein kinase C alpha is associated with terminal neutrophil differentiation. Blood 80:68.

102. Dang PM, Rais S, Hakim J, Perianin A (1995) Redistribution of protein kinase C isoforms in human neutrophils stimulated by formyl peptides and phorbol myristate acetate. Biochem Biophys Res Comm 212:664.

103. Bates ME, Bertics PJ, Calhoun WJ, Busse WW (1993) Increased protein kinase C activity in low density eosinophils. J Immunol 150:4486.

104. Lavens SE, Peachell PT, Warner JA (1992) Role of tyrosine kinases in IgE-mediated signal transduction in human lung mast cells and basophils. Am J Respir Cell Mol Biol 7:637.

105. Lavens SE, Warner JA (1995) The role of the tyrosine kinase, SYK, in IgE-mediated signal transduction in human lung mast cells and basophils. FASEB J 9:A781.

106. Berger SA, Mak TW, Paige CJ (1994) Leukocyte common antigen (CD45) is required for immunoglobulin E-mediated degranulation of mast cells. J Exp Med 180:471.

107. Hook WA, Berenstein EH, Zinsser FU, Fishler C, Siraganian RP (1991) Monoclonal antibodies to the leukocyte common antigen (CD45) inhibit IgE-mediated histamine release from human basophils. J Immunol 147:2670.

108. Pani G, Kozlowski M, Cambier JC, Mills GB, Siminovitch KA (1995) Identification of the tyrosine phosphatase PTP1C as a B cell antigen receptor-associated protein involved in the regulation of B cell signaling. J Exp Med 181:2077.

109. Nguyen KL, Gillis S, MacGlashan DW Jr (1990) A comparative study of releasing and nonreleasing human basophils: nonreleasing basophils lack an early component of the signal transduction pathway that follows IgE cross-linking. J Allergy Clin Immunol 85:1020.

110. Yamaguchi M, Hirai K, Ohta K, Suzuki K, Kitani S, Takaishi T, Ito K, Ra C, Morita Y (1996) Culturing in the presence of IL-3 converts anti-IgE nonresponding basophils into responding basophils. J Allergy Clin Immunol 97:1279.

22

Eosinophil Signal Transduction

Hirohito Kita, MD

CONTENTS

INTRODUCTION

Eosinophils are important effector cells in host defense against parasites, in allergic diseases such as bronchial asthma and atopic dermatitis, and in diseases associated with eosinophilia (1,2). The eosinophil is an important source of cytotoxic proteins, lipid mediators, and oxygen metabolites, which have the potential to induce pathology in disease. However, little is known about the mechanisms coupling receptors and effector functions of eosinophils. Studies in eosinophils have been hampered because eosinophils represent only a small fraction of peripheral white blood cells, and the isolation of large numbers of cells for biochemical studies has been difficult. However, recent advances in procedures have enabled us to isolate eosinophils from normal individuals with high purity and reasonable recovery. Furthermore, techniques have become available to analyze intracellular events at a single-cell level. This chapter will review recent advances in the studies of eosinophil signal transduction, in the hope of finding ways to modulate eosinophil activation therapeutically in patients with eosinophil-associated diseases.

EOSINOPHIL RECEPTOR FUNCTIONAL RELATIONSHIPS

As shown in Table 1, eosinophils generate an array of inflammatory mediators, including granule proteins, lipid mediators, and oxygen metabolites, in response to a number of agonists. Eosinophils are also potential sources of cytokines and growth factors. Although various functions of eosinophils and stimuli are described in detail in another chapter of this book, two important points need to made. First, single functions of eosinophils can be induced by a number of physiologic stimuli activating on their receptors. For instance, eosinophil degranulation

From: *Allergy and Allergic Diseases: The New Mechanisms and Therapeutics*
Edited by: J. A. Denburg © Humana Press Inc., Totowa, NJ

Table 1
Activators and Regulators of Eosinophil Functions[a]

Activators and regulators	Degranulation	Production of lipid mediators	Superoxide production	Cytotoxicity against Ab-coated targets	Priming[b]	Chemotaxis/ chemokinesis	Adhesion	Survival	Cytokine production
Immunoglobulins									
IgG	↑	↑	↑	↑			↑		↑
IgE	↑	↑		↑					↑
IgA	↑								↑
Secretory IgA	↑								↑
Complements									
C3a	↑		↑			↑			↑[c]
C5a	↑		↑			↑			
Zymosan	↑	↑	↑						
Lipid mediators and small molecules									
PAF	↑	↑	↑	↑	↑	↑	↑		↑[d]
LTB4			↑			↑			
Cytokines									
IL-1	↑↓		↑↓						
IL-3	↑	↑	↑	↑	↑	↑	↑		
IL-4	↑→			↑→					
IL-5	↑	↑	↑	↑	↑	↑	↑	↑	↑
GM-CSF	↑	↑	↑	↑	↑	↑	↑	↑	↑
TNFα				↑				↑	
IFNγ	↑↓						↑→	↑	↑
TGFβ	↑↓								
Chemokines									
IL-8						↑[d]			
RANTES	↑[e]					↑			↑[d]
MCP3	↑[e]					↑			
MCP4						↑			
MIP-1α	↑[e]					↑			

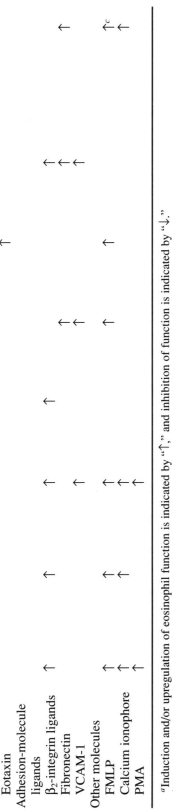

Eotaxin
Adhesion-molecule ligands
β_2-integrin ligands
Fibronectin
VCAM-1
Other molecules
FMLP
Calcium ionophore
PMA

[a]Induction and/or upregulation of eosinophil function is indicated by "↑," and inhibition of function is indicated by "↓."
[b]"Priming" means enhancement of eosinophil function (e.g., superoxide production, chemotaxis) induced by other agonists.
[c]In the presence of cytochalasine B.
[d]In the presence of priming factors.
[e]At high concentrations.

is induced by immunoglobulins (Ig) such as IgG and IgA *(3–5)*, serum-opsonized zymosan *(6)*, complement fragment C5a *(7,8)*, platelet-activating factor (PAF) *(9)*, and cytokines such as interleukin (IL)-5, granulocyte-macrophage colony-stimulating factor (GM-CSF), regulated upon activation in normal T cells expressed and secreted (RANTES), and macrophage inflammatory protein (MIP)-1α *(10–13)*. Eosinophil oxidative metabolism is also stimulated by a variety of stimuli, including PAF *(14)*, leukotriene (LT) B_4 *(15)*, C3a *(16)*, zymosan *(17)*, IgG-coated surface *(18)*, and immobilized vascular cell adhesion molecule (VCAM)-1 *(19)*. These observations suggest a redundancy in the signaling mechanisms leading to effector function of eosinophils and indicate the presence of common pathway(s) through which signals generated by various receptors merge. Second, engagement and perturbation of a single receptor provokes a wide variety of cellular functions. For example, IL-5 promotes proliferation and differentiation of eosinophil progenitors *(20,21)*, as well as stimulating a number of mature-eosinophil functions, including survival *(22)*, degranulation, LTC_4 and superoxide production, helminthotoxic activity, and IL-8 production *(22–24)*. IL-5 also has a chemokinetic activity for eosinophils *(25)* and induces the integrin-dependent adhesion of eosinophils to plasma-coated glass and endothelial cells *(26)*. Thus, stimulation of a given eosinophil receptor will likely lead to a variety of intracellular and extracellular events, including gene transcription, translocation of enzymes for lipid metabolism and oxidative burst, and activation of the exocytotic machinery and integrin molecules. Therefore, questions remain regarding divergent signaling mechanism(s) that couple a single receptor to multiple cellular functions. Although it is almost impossible to explore intracellular mechanisms for all the functions and receptors of eosinophils, recent studies on two major areas of eosinophil signal transduction, including the intracellular mechanisms leading to eosinophil effector functions and cytokine-induced signal transduction, provide useful insights. An overview of these two mechanisms may help us to understand the complex world of eosinophil signal transduction.

SIGNAL TRANSDUCTION
FOR EOSINOPHIL EFFECTOR FUNCTIONS (FIG. 1)

Role of Calcium in Eosinophil Activation

Recently, several studies have investigated exocytotic mechanisms in eosinophils. The experimental approach is to permeabilize the eosinophils in order to manipulate the composition of the cytosol. This can be done through the use of the patch-clamp technique in a single cell or by the treatment of cells with the bacterial cytolysin Streptolysin-*O*. The patch-clamp technique is a very sensitive way to measure membrane currents, which can then be used to measure membrane capacitance at high resolution (index of membrane area) *(27)*; furthermore, the intracellular space can be dialyzed with an appropriate solution *(28)*. At a Ca^{2+} concentration buffered at 1 μM, the introduction of the nonhydrolyzable guanosine-5′-*O*-(3-thiotriphosphate) (GTP) analog GTP-γS into a single guinea pig eosinophil elicited a two- to threefold increase in membrane capacitance, which suggested an exocytotic degranulation of the cell *(29)*. Comparable results are obtained with human eosinophils, in which the intracellular application of Ca^{2+}, 10 μM, and GTP-γS, 100 μM, induces fusion of eosinophil peroxidase (EPO)-containing granules with the cell surface membrane; this fusion is associated with a marked increase in membrane capacitance *(30)*. Ca^{2+} alone causes granule fusion and GTP-γS alone causes a gradual degranulation; together, both of them synergistically induce a marked degranulation. These results provide evidence that Ca^{2+}-dependent factors and GTP-binding proteins (G proteins), presumably small G protein as described below, act cooperatively in granule release from eosinophils.

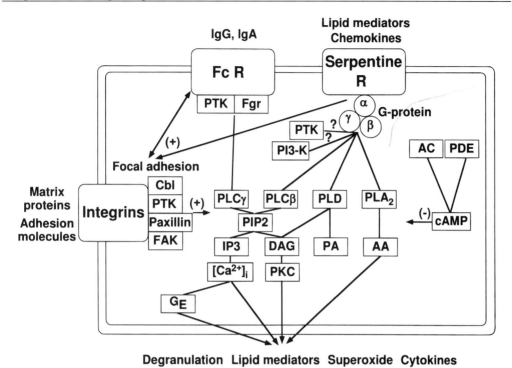

Fig. 1. Signal transduction for eosinophil effector functions. Information described in the text is summarized. The abbreviations are explained in the text.

Other evidence to suggest that a rise in $[Ca^{2+}]_i$ is one of the prerequisite signals for eosinophil activation is that the calcium ionophore A23187 induces degranulation and respiratory burst in eosinophils *(14,31)* and the production of LTC_4 by eosinophils *(32)*. Furthermore, eosinophil degranulation induced by secretory IgA (sIgA)- or IgG-coated Sepharose 4B beads is completely abrogated by chelating extracellular Ca^{2+} by ethylene glycol-bis (B-amino-ethyl ether) N,N,N',N'-tetraacetic acid (EGTA) (H. Kita, unpublished observations, 1990). More recently, a study of movement in eosinophils suggests the importance of $[Ca^{2+}]_i$ gradient: $[Ca^{2+}]_i$ gradients in eosinophils moving persistently in one direction are highest at the rear of the cell and lowest at the front of the cell *(33)*. When eosinophils reverse their direction, the region of the cell that becomes the new leading edge has the lowest $[Ca^{2+}]_i$. These results suggest that the rise in $[Ca^{2+}]_i$, as well as the gradient of $[Ca^{2+}]_i$, are both important in degranulation and movement of eosinophils.

Although Ca^{2+} is likely required for the full function of eosinophils, calcium dependency seems to vary among the various functions of eosinophils. As described above, elevation of $[Ca^{2+}]_i$ is absolutely required for degranulation and exocytosis. In contrast, the shape change of eosinophils stimulated by PAF and C5a is independent of the extracellular Ca^{2+} *(8)*. The respiratory burst of eosinophils can also occur without involvement of calcium. For example, SK&F 96365, a receptor-operated, calcium-channel inhibitor, inhibits the $[Ca^{2+}]_i$ rise in LTB_4 stimulated guinea pig eosinophils, but has no effect on the respiratory burst *(34)*. PAF-induced degranulation and elevation of $[Ca^{2+}]_i$ is dependent on extracellular Ca^{2+}, whereas PAF-stimulated superoxide generation is dependent on the presence of extracellular Mg^{2+} *(35)*. Furthermore, phorbol 12-myristate 13-acetate (PMA) induces a faster and larger respiratory burst from human eosinophils than does calcium ionophore A23187, whereas A23187 induces larger amounts of degranulation than PMA *(36)*. In the future, it will be important to characterize and differentiate the signaling involved in these different functions of eosinophils.

Mechanisms of Calcium Mobilization

AGONISTS THAT INDUCE CALCIUM MOBILIZATION INTO EOSINOPHILS

Several agonists can induce an elevation of $[Ca^{2+}]_i$ in eosinophils from various species. In guinea pig peritoneal eosinophils, the resting $[Ca^{2+}]_i$ is 120 nM and $[Ca^{2+}]_i$ increases rapidly following stimulation of the cells by PAF *(37)*. This effect of PAF is transient, peaking after 10–15-sec exposure and returning to resting levels within 60 s *(37)*; it is concentration-dependent (half maximal response $[EC_{50}]$ ~15 nM), and inhibited by a PAF receptor antagonist, apafant *(37)*. Similar results have been obtained in human eosinophils *(37)*. The response to PAF is dependent on external Ca^{2+}, since it is inhibited by EGTA and Ni^{2+}, but not by the dihydropyridine antagonist nifedipine, suggesting that Ca^{2+} entry stimulated by PAF involves receptor-operated calcium channels *(37)*. Pharmacologic examination suggests the presence of two distinct PAF receptors on human eosinophils *(39)*. In addition to PAF, LTB_4, complement fragment C5a, and *N*-formyl-methionyl-leucyl-phenylalanine (FMLP) also induce elevations in $[Ca^{2+}]_i$ in both guinea pig and human eosinophils *(8,38)*, as do the C-C chemokines, RANTES *(40,41)*, MIP-1α *(40,41)*, monocyte chemotactic protein (MCP)2 *(42)* and MCP3 *(43)* also elicit a rise in $[Ca^{2+}]_i$ in human eosinophils. The common denominator of these agonists is the structure of the corresponding receptors, which all contain seven transmembrane domains *(44)*, the so-called "serpentine" receptor family.

PRODUCTION OF INOSITOL PHOSPHATES AND CALCIUM MOBILIZATION

What is the mechanism that induces the rise in $[Ca^{2+}]_i$? In general, intracellular Ca^{2+} can be released from the endoplasmic reticulum and mobilized from the extracellular milieu into the cells by inositol-1,4,5-triphosphate (IP_3) *(45)*. IP_3, together with diacylglycerol (DAG), is generated by hydrolysis of a membrane phospholipid, phosphatidylinositol 4,5-bisphosphate (PIP_2). These mechanisms may also operate in eosinophils, because PAF elicits a rapid and transient increase in IP_3 mass in guinea pig eosinophils, as described above *(47)*. PAF also stimulates GTP hydrolysis in guinea pig eosinophil membranes *(47)*. The rise in $[Ca^{2+}]_i$ induced by PAF is preceded by the increase in IP_3, consistent with a causal relationship between these two events *(48)*. Other agonists, including LTB_4 and C5a, also promote the accumulation of IP_3 in guinea pig eosinophils *(48)*. In murine eosinophils, IgG stimulates phosphoinositide hydrolysis, which is considered to be an important step in the activation of 5'-lipoxygenase *(49)*. In human eosinophils, sIgA and IgG immobilized to Sepharose 4B beads cause a rapid hydrolysis of PIP_2 as detected by the production of $[^3H]$inositol phosphates $([^3H]IP)$ *(36)*. Eosinophil degranulation occurs after IP_3 production and calcium influx *(36,48)*, suggesting that the IP_3 induced elevation in $[Ca^{2+}]_i$ is an early step in the eosinophil degranulation response. Thus, the hydrolysis of PIP_2 and the production of IP_3 following receptor–ligand interaction seem to be important steps in the elevation of $[Ca^{2+}]_i$ and activation of eosinophils.

ACTIVATION OF PHOSPHOLIPASE C (PLC)

In numerous receptor systems, ligand binding triggers a rapid increase in phosphoinositide hydrolysis induced by PLC activation *(50)*. PLC-mediated hydrolysis of PIP_2 generates at least two second messengers, IP_3 and DAG, which, in turn, trigger intracellular calcium mobilization and protein kinase C (PKC) activation, as described above *(51)*. PLC consists of several isoforms divided into three classes termed β, γ, δ (52). The mechanism leading to PLC activation is variable depending on the isoform of the enzyme. Direct coupling between the PLC-β1 isoform and a pertussis toxin (PTX)-insensitive G protein, G_q, has been shown and PLC-β2 is likely regulated by a PTX-sensitive G protein, such as G_{i2} $(53,54)$. PLC-β3 could underlie both PTX-sensitive and PTX-insensitive receptor-linked phosphoinositide hydrolysis. In contrast, the PLC-γ isoforms appear to be regulated by tyrosine kinases and not by G proteins (55). Activation of PLC-δ has not yet been reported, and it has been speculated that this class may be the target for PTX-sensitive G proteins (55). The PLC isoforms present in eosinophils are unknown. Our preliminary results suggest that human eosinophils possess PLC-γ2 and PLC-β2, but not PLC-γ1 or PLC-β1 (56).

Several lines of evidence suggest that PLC is activated after receptor ligation of eosinophils. Several agonists, including PAF, LTB_4, and C5a, elicit a rapid and transient increase in IP_3 mass in guinea pig eosinophils $(46,48)$. In [^{3}H]inositol-labeled murine eosinophils, crosslinking of Fcγ receptor (FcγR) by anti-IgG $F(ab')_2$ fragments [$F(ab')_2$] stimulates phosphoinositide hydrolysis and production of IP_3 within 15 min (49). The response is inhibited by a PLC-inhibitor, neomycin. In human eosinophils, secretory IgA and IgG immobilized to Sepharose 4B beads and FMLP cause a rapid hydrolysis of PIP_2 as detected by the production of [^{3}H]IP within 30 min (36). The PLC in human eosinophils is likely coupled to a PTX-sensitive G protein, as described in detail later in this chapter.

PLC likely plays an important role in the activation of eosinophils. For example, inhibition of PLC activity by neomycin results in both inhibition of IP_3 production and LTC_4 production in murine eosinophils (49). Similarly, human eosinophil degranulation, stimulated by sIgA- and IgG-coated Sepharose beads and detected by the release of eosinophil-derived neurotoxin (EDN), is inhibited by PTX. The similarity in the kinetic effects of PTX on IP production and EDN release suggests a causal relationship between PLC activation and degranulation of eosinophils (10). Furthermore, as mentioned above, human eosinophils possess PLC-γ2, and it is tyrosine phosphorylated when cells are treated with a tyrosine phosphatase inhibitor, pervanadate. Pervanadate treatment of eosinophils results in IP production and subsequent degranulation of eosinophils (see Role of PTX Sensitive Heterotrimeric G Protein in Eosinophil Activation). Although these observations provide indirect evidence, there is no reason to doubt that PLC is activated after the ligation of various receptors and that the enzyme is important for the activation of eosinophils. In the future, it will be important to further characterize the PLC isoforms present in eosinophils and to dissect the mechanisms involved in PLC activation by various ligands.

Role of PTX-Sensitive Heterotrimeric G Protein in Eosinophil Activation

Recent studies have defined transmembrane receptors that regulate various second messenger-generating enzymes through intermediate G proteins (57). In contrast to intracellular small G proteins, the G proteins implicated in receptor-mediated signaling are membrane-bound αβγ-heterotrimers. Upon receptor activation, the α subunit of G protein (Gα subunit) dissociates from the Gβγ subunits and liberated Gα and Gβγ subunits activate various effector molecules, such as PLC-β isoforms, phospholipase A_2 (PLA_2), adenylate cyclase (AC), guanylate cyclase, and several ion channels $(58,59)$.

PTX is an useful pharmacologic tool to study the role of G proteins in receptor-mediated cell signaling. Certain α subunits of heterotrimeric G proteins serve as specific substrates for adenosine 5′-diphosphate (ADP) ribosylation by PTX (60). ADP ribosylation of the α subunit of G proteins disrupts G-protein-effector coupling. For example, PTX pretreatment of neutrophils inhibits the coupling of the FMLP receptor to PLC activity in these cells (61). The major substrate for ADP ribosylation by PTX in neutrophil membranes is a 41-kDa protein, G_{i2} αsubunit *(62)*.

There are several lines of evidence to indicate that the eosinophil response to FMLP is mediated by a heterotrimeric G protein. First, PTX pretreatment of eosinophils for 2 h markedly reduced the degranulation response of human eosinophils to FMLP in a concentration-dependent manner. The relatively long preincubation period required for the PTX effects is consistent with cumulative modification and inactivation of a critical intermediate G protein by the ADP biosyltransferase activity of PTX catalytic subunits *(63)*. In contrast, degranulation induced by PMA, which directly activates PKC independent of cell surface stimulation, is unaffected by pretreatment of eosinophils with PTX. Second, as described above, the activation of the cAMP pathway inhibits the stimulus-dependent degranulation response by human eosinophils *(64)*. However, treatment of eosinophils with PTX for 2 h fails to increase cyclic adenosine monophosphate (cAMP) levels, indicating that the suppressive effect of PTX on stimulus-induced eosinophil degranulation is not explained by a cAMP-dependent negative regulatory mechanism. Third, eosinophil lysates incubated with activated PTX in the presence of [^{32}P] nicotinamide-adenine dinucleotide (NAD) result in the transfer of [^{32}P]NAD-ribose to a prominent 41-kDa protein substrate *(65)*. The ADP ribosylation of this protein is absolutely dependent on the presence of PTX in the in vitro reaction mixture. Furthermore, pretreatment of intact eosinophils with PTX for 2 h before ADP ribosylation of cellular proteins in vitro leads to inhibition of radiolabeling of the 41-kDa protein. Collectively, these data are most consistent with the possibility that ADP ribosylation by PTX functionally inactivates the G protein responsible for the coupling of FMLP receptors to the exocytotic mechanism of eosinophils.

The modification of these G proteins renders them incapable of coupling cell surface receptor ligation to the activation of intracellular effector enzymes, including PLC-β. As described earlier, stimulation of myo[^{3}H]inositol-labeled eosinophils with FMLP for 30 min induces marked increases in total IP accumulation, suggesting that this stimulus transduces signals, at least in part, through membrane receptors coupled to phosphoinositide-specific PLC activity. Pretreatment of eosinophils with PTX virtually abolishes the production of IP induced by FMLP *(63)*. Recent evidence indicates that the neutrophil FMLP receptor is coupled to intracellular PLC through a PTX-sensitive G_i-like protein. The major substrate in neutrophil membranes is a 41-kDa membrane protein identified as the α-subunit of the G_{i2} heterotrimer *(62)*. Likewise, we have observed that the predominant substrate for PTX in eosinophils is also a 41-kDa membrane protein. The PTX-dependent ADP ribosylation of the 41-kDa protein paralleled the inhibitory action of PTX on the functional responsiveness of eosinophils to FMLP. In another study, a 40-kDa protein, reactive with anti-G_i-α antibody, was detected in eosinophil membrane preparation by immunoblot analysis *(66)*. Taking these data together, the 41-kDa PTX substrate may represent a G-protein αsubunit (possibly G_{i2}-α) involved in the transduction of activation signals, such as IP, from FMLP receptors on eosinophils.

We have also found that the eosinophil degranulation response induced by sIgA and IgG immobilized to Sepharose 4B beads is also inhibited by exposure of eosinophils to PTX for 2 h. Furthermore, increases in phosphoinositide hydrolysis in eosinophils stimulated by immobilized sIgA and IgG is inhibited by PTX, suggesting that eosinophil receptors to sIgA and IgG are also coupled to a PTX-sensitive G protein. These findings contrast with those found in neutrophils, in which functions induced by FcγR-mediated stimuli are largely insensitive to PTX. Several other receptor functions of eosinophils are sensitive to PTX. For example, PTX inhibits the specific binding of [^{3}H]PAF to human eosinophils *(47)*. In addition, pretreatment of eosinophils with PTX attenuates [Ca^{2+}]$_i$ changes and EPO release induced by C5a and PAF *(8)*. The production of reactive oxygen species from eosinophils stimulated by

RANTES, C3a, and C5a is also completely inhibited by PTX *(16,67)*. Thus, eosinophil receptors for PAF, C3a, C5a, and RANTES are likely coupled to PTX-sensitive G proteins, consistent with the current knowledge regarding coupling of "serpentine" receptors with PTX-sensitive G proteins. In contrast, the IgG receptor for eosinophils is FcγRII (CD32), which is a single polypeptide chain with only one transmembrane domain. The reason why eosinophil signaling mediated by this receptor is sensitive to G protein is still unclear. Perhaps, other signaling molecules, such as tyrosine kinases, intervene between Ig receptors and G proteins. Alternatively, eosinophil activation induced by IgG or sIgA may be mediated by an autocrine production of chemotactic factors, such as PAF, which activates eosinophils through PTX-sensitive G proteins.

Roles of Small GTP-Binding Proteins in Eosinophil Degranulation

As described earlier, exocytosis from streptolysin *O*-permeabilized guinea pig eosinophils is dependent on Ca^{2+} and GTP-γS *(68)*. In addition, adenosine triphosphate (ATP) augments exocytosis in permeabilized cells by increasing the affinities of both Ca^{2+} and GTP-γS for their respective binding proteins *(68)*. In cells treated with 2-dideoxyglucose and antimycin-A to suppress the endogenous level of ATP, neither Ca^{2+} nor GTP-γS is alone able to induce eosinophil exocytosis. In contrast, when GTP-γS and Ca^{2+} are used together, they promote the marked release of β-hexosaminidase even in the absence of ATP. Because GTP-γS is a non-hydrolyzable analog of GTP that cannot function as a phosphoryl donor, the exocytosis of permeabilized eosinophils must occur independent of protein phosphorylation. ATP is thought to be required to maintain the concentration of PIP_2 and to provide sufficient GTP for G protein activation. Therefore, the ability of GTP-γS together with Ca^{2+} to elicit exocytosis, even in the absence of ATP, dissociates PIP_2 and its products from the exocytotic mechanism of eosinophils. These findings suggest that a novel G protein, G_E, which is distinctive from the heterotrimeric membrane-bound G proteins coupled to PLC activity, may directly mediate a distal process of exocytosis in eosinophils *(69)*.

The nature of this G_E protein in eosinophils is not clear yet; however, it is reported that small G proteins are implicated in the regulation of the secretory process of mammalian cells *(70)*. Furthermore, messenger ribonucleic acid (mRNA) for one of the small G proteins, rab1, which is homologous to a protooncogene *ras* p21, is expressed in human eosinophils *(30)*. Another small G protein, Ras, is also found in eosinophils *(28)*. Therefore, small G proteins, such as those in the Ras superfamily, may be candidates for G_E protein for eosinophils.

If G_E can directly mediate exocytosis in eosinophils, then how does ATP increase the Ca^{2+}/GTP-γS-mediated exocytosis of eosinophils? This may be due to the activation of PKC through diglycerides cleaved from membrane phospholipids by PLC or phospholipase D (PLD) and the subsequent phosphorylation of Ca^{2+}-binding protein and G_E. In fact, GTP-γS-induced β-hexosaminidase release from eosinophils can be inhibited by an inhibitor of PKC *(68)*. From these data, we can speculate about the important roles for Ca^{2+}-binding protein, G_E, and PKC in the exocytotic processes of eosinophils.

Roles of PLA$_2$ and PLD in Eosinophil Activation

As described above, second messengers such as IP_3 and DAG are generated as a consequence of the activation of PLC. Other phospholipases that are involved in the generation of second messengers include: PLA_2, which hydrolyses phosphatidylcholine (PC) and/or phosphatidylethanolamine (PE) to produce arachidonic acid (AA) and lyso-PC and/or lyso-PE; and PLD, which hydrolyses PC to produce phosphatidic acid (PA) and choline *(71)*. There are several lines of evidence to suggest that these phospholipases also participate in eosinophil activation.

PHOSPHOLIPASE A$_2$

PLA$_2$ can mediate a variety of actions within cells, either directly or via subsequent transformation of its products, one of which, AA, is metabolized into prostaglandins, leukotrienes, thromboxanes, and lipoxins. Another product, lyso-PC, is acetylated to form PAF *(72)*. As described above, eosinophils can synthesize LTC$_4$, LTD$_4$, and PAF. Guinea pig eosinophils release thromboxane B$_2$, LTB$_4$, and 5-hydroxy eicosatetraenoic acid (5-HETE) following calcium ionophore *(73)*. Indeed, as suspected, the activity of PLA$_2$ has been documented in guinea pig eosinophils. The activity of PLA$_2$ was first confirmed in guinea pig eosinophils *(74)*. Stimulation of [^{3}H]AA-labeled guinea pig eosinophils with calcium ionophore A23187 results in the release of AA in parallel to the hydrolysis of endogenous PC. This ionophore-induced AA release is inhibited by the chelation of intracellular calcium, but not by extracellular calcium, suggesting that PLA$_2$ activity is dependent on the mobilization of intracellular calcium. In contrast to findings in other cell types such as macrophages, IL-1β inhibits PLA$_2$ activity and subsequent release of AA by guinea pig eosinophils.

The role of PLA$_2$ in eosinophil function can be examined by using agonists and antagonists. The respiratory burst of membrane-permeabilized bovine eosinophils induced by G-protein-dependent stimuli, such as the nonhydrolyzable GTP analog GTP-γS and the aluminum tetrafluoro complex AlF$_4^-$ is enhanced by 0.1–1 μM of AA and inhibited by the PLA$_2$ inhibitor 4-bromophenacylbromide *(75)*. The PLA$_2$ activator adriamycin enhances this response. Similarly, 4-bromophenacylbromide and another class of PLA$_2$ inhibitor, mepacrine, inhibit degranulation, LTC$_4$ production, and the respiratory burst in human eosinophils stimulated by FMLP plus cytochalasin B *(76)*. The effects of mepacrine can be reversed by the addition of AA. At least two mechanisms may involve the action of PLA$_2$ on eosinophil function. First, the respiratory burst of eosinophils by opsonized zymosan, is prevented by preincubation of cells with a PAF inhibitor, WEB 2086, suggesting a role for PAF synthesis and PAF release in the activation of the respiratory burst by opsonized zymosan *(77)*. Indeed, PAF is detected in the supernatant of opsonized zymosan-stimulated eosinophils. Furthermore, addition of AA itself (50 μM) to purified human eosinophils leads to the formation of LTC$_4$ and 15-leukotrienes *(78)*. Second, exogenously added porcine PLA$_2$ induces noncytotoxic eosinophil degranulation, and this effect is blocked by 4-bromophenacylbromide *(79)*. These findings suggest that PLA$_2$ activates the eosinophil secretory process either by directly acting on eosinophils or by inducing the generation of bioactive AA and phospholipid metabolites.

PHOSPHOLIPASE D

It is well known that PLD is activated in neutrophils by chemoattractants, such as FMLP *(80)*. The activation of PLD generates PA and choline from cellular PC, and the resultant PA is then dephosphorylated by PA phosphohydrolase to form DAG. Information available now suggests that PLD in eosinophils can also be activated following receptor ligation. Human eosinophils labeled in alkyl-PC with ^{32}P produce alkyl-[^{32}P]PA and alkyl-[^{32}P]phosphatidylethanol (alkyl-[^{32}P]PEt) when stimulated by C5a, A23187, or PMA in the presence of ethanol *(81)*. Because cellular ATP does not contain ^{32}P, alkyl-[^{32}P]PA cannot be formed by the combined actions of PLC and DAG kinase, suggesting that hydrolytic action of PLD is involved alkyl-[^{32}P]PA production. Alkyl-[^{32}P]PEt formation also parallels that of alkyl-[^{32}P]PA, suggesting that a PLD-catalyzed transphosphatidylation reaction occurs between alkyl-PC and ethanol. Thus, PLD is likely activated in eosinophils following receptor- and nonreceptor-mediated activation.

What is the role for PLD activation in eosinophil function? In neutrophils, PLD-mediated hydrolysis of PC leads to large and sustained increases in DAG *(82)*. This increased DAG may prolong PKC activation and cause sustained cellular responses. A similar mechanism may be occur in eosinophils. Koenderman et al. reported that opsonized zymosan-induced respiratory burst in human eosinophils can be divided arbitrarily into two components, initiation and maintenance, and that the maintained component of the respiratory burst is inhibited by staurosporine, suggesting that it is reliant on PKC-dependent phosphorylation reactions *(83)*. The maintenance component of the respiratory burst is accompanied by a delayed accumulation of diglycerides, and not by an increase in $[Ca^{2+}]_i$. This observation suggests that the parent phospholipid from which diglyceride is derived is not PIP_2. Therefore, it is tempting to speculate that in opsonized zymosan-treated eosinophils PC may provide the primary source of diglycerides required for maintenance of the respiratory burst. Further studies are required to examine the potential role for PLD in eosinophil activation and to compare its function with other phospholipases such as PLC.

Roles of Protein Phosphorylation in Activation of Eosinophils

Leukocytes contain a variety of serine/threonine kinases and tyrosine kinases *(83)*. Many of these are targets for specific second messengers and are likely to be important mediators for transducing signals generated by receptor/ligand complexes. The physical presence of these kinases in eosinophils is not well known, probably because of the difficulties in obtaining large numbers of cells for the necessary biochemical studies. However, several lines of evidence suggest that eosinophils possess some kinases and that they play important roles in eosinophil function.

PROTEIN PHOSPHORYLATION

Protein phosphorylation is one of the mechanisms cells use to respond to extracellular signals. As a result of a receptor ligation, protein kinases are activated and catalyze the transfer of a phosphate group from a nucleotide triphosphate to a serine, threonine, or tyrosine residue of a substrate protein. This covalent modification alters the structure and function of the substrate protein and, consequently, the function of the cells. A number of eosinophil intracellular proteins are phosphorylated following receptor-mediated or nonreceptor-mediated stimulation of eosinophils *(82)*. For example, opsonized zymosan induces the phosphorylation of 30-, 34-, 59-, 67-, and 93-kDa proteins in human eosinophils. Different stimuli, such as calcium ionophore A23187 and PMA, phosphorylate distinctive, but not exclusive, sets of protein. The phosphorylation of resting eosinophils seems to be different and depends on the activation stage of the cells. As described above, eosinophils are divided into two groups: high-density eosinophils and low-density eosinophils. It is generally accepted that low-density eosinophils result from in vivo and/or in vitro activation, rendering them more active than high-density eosinophils in a variety of functional tests *(85,86)*. Indeed, the incorporation of ^{32}P into the protein bands of low-density eosinophils is more intense than that of high-density eosinophils from the same subjects *(87)*. Thus, various intracellular proteins are phosphorylated in eosinophils following activation; the degree of protein phosphorylation may provide a clue regarding functional heterogeneity of activated and nonactivated eosinophils.

ACTIVATION AND ROLES OF TYROSINE KINASES

Engagement of cell surface receptors initiates a cascade of biochemical events, one of which is an increase in the phosphorylation of proteins on tyrosine residues *(88,89)*. Tyrosine phosphorylation initiated by protein tyrosine kinase (PTK) is recognized as a critical event in a variety of cellular signaling pathways. Protein tyrosine phosphorylation also seems to be an early event in the activation of eosinophils induced by various stimuli. Stimulation of eosinophils with sIgA or IgG immobilized to Sepharose beads rapidly induces the tyrosine phosphorylation of a number of eosinophil proteins with molecular masses of 50–56, 73, 78, 100, 105, and 120 kDa within 10 min after stimulation *(65)*.

The activation of tyrosine kinases and tyrosine phosphorylation of proteins are likely important for eosinophil effector function. When tyrosine phosphorylation is blocked by PTK inhibitors, such as genistein and herbimycin A, the ability of eosinophils to degranulate in response to immobilized sIgA and IgG is abolished *(65)*. Conversely, when tyrosine phosphorylation of eosinophil proteins is enhanced by the tyrosine phosphatase inhibitor pervanadate, the eosinophil degranulation response is enhanced *(65)*. Furthermore, the activity of PLC can be inhibited by genistein and enhanced by pervanadate, suggesting that tyrosine kinases are involved in early signal transduction of eosinophils, at least in part *(65)*. These observations suggest that PTK is activated when eosinophils are stimulated with immobilized Ig or growth factors and that protein tyrosine phosphorylation likely plays a critical role in eosinophil functions, such as degranulation. Characterization of PTK showed that an src family PTK, Fgr, is activated in eosinophils stimulated by IgG *(65)*. Phosphatidylinositol 3-kinase (PI3-K) may be also activated by FcγRII in eosinophils because IgG-induced superoxide production is inhibited by wortmannin, a specific PI3-K inhibitor *(90)*. Interestingly, PI3-K is implicated in the rearrangement of actin filament, suggesting a potential role of this molecule in eosinophil effector function *(91)*. More studies are needed to identify the specific PTK coupled to the specific receptor and function of eosinophils.

ACTIVATION AND ROLES OF PKC

PKC is a serine/threonine kinase and a target for most of the known second messengers generated in leukocytes (e.g., Ca^{2+}, DAG, PA, AA). The PKC is activated intracellularly by these phospholipids and, in some instances, by calcium; the affinity of PKC for these activators is increased by the transient second messenger DAG *(92)*, which is the product of activated PLC and/or PLD.

The activation of PKC leads to the phosphorylation of the target proteins and the propagation of signals needed for the functional response of the cells. PKC is a family of eight isoforms that can be divided into two groups: Ca^{2+}-dependent, dependent, consisting of α, $β_I$, $β_{II}$, and γ; and Ca^{2+}-independent, consisting of δ, ε, ζ, and η *(93)*. Neutrophils contain predominantly $β_{II}$, δ, and ζ isoforms, with lower amounts of α and $β_I$ *(94–96)*. Only one study has examined the presence of PKC in eosinophils. The β isoform of PKC, but not α or γ, was detected in eosinophils by Western blotting with isoform-specific monoclonal antibodies *(97)*. In addition, the enzymatic activity of PKC was confirmed by the phosphatidyl serine-dependent transfer of ^{32}P from γ-$[^{32}P]$ATP to a protein substrate, histone. While the PKC activity of resting eosinophils is similar to that of neutrophils, low-density eosinophils have greater PKC activity than do high-density eosinophils *(97)*.

There are several lines of indirect evidence suggesting that PKC is important for eosinophil activation. For example, the PKC activator PMA induces a variety of eosinophil functions, such as adhesion *(98)*, respiratory burst *(99)*, and degranulation *(36,100)*. Another class of PKC agonist, 4-β-phorbol dibutyrate, also induces the production of hydrogen peroxide from guinea pig eosinophils *(101)*. In addition, the eosinophil degranulation induced by PMA is insensitive to a G-protein modulator, PTX *(36)*, or to a tyrosine kinase inhibitor, genistein *(65)*, suggesting that PKC is involved either directly in the exocytosis machinery or in the distal part of eosinophil signal transduction. Conversely, a PKC inhibitor, staurosporine, inhibits the respiratory burst of eosinophils stimulated by opsonized zymosan *(17)*. Staurosporine also inhibits the eosinophil degranulation induced by sIgA- or IgG-coated Sepharose beads with an IC_{50} of 30 nM *(102)*. Furthermore, the concentration-response curve of hydrogen peroxide production stimulated by LTB_4 is shifted fourfold to the right by the competitive PKC inhibitor 1-O-hexadecyl-2-O-methylglycerol *(101)*. Taken together, these findings suggest that various receptor agonists of eosinophils induce the respiratory burst and exocytosis in eosinophils via a mechanism involving PKC.

REGULATORY ROLES OF THE AC SYSTEM IN EOSINOPHIL ACTIVATION

The activation of AC, generation of cAMP, and subsequent activation of protein kinase A (PKA) are known to regulate the function of various types of cells. Although PKA and its substrate are still not identified in eosinophils, pharmacological evidence suggests that cAMP is playing an important regulatory role in eosinophil function.

Human eosinophils possess a homogeneous population of β2-adrenoreceptors with very high affinity (dissociation constant $[K_d]$ ~26 pM, 4300 sites/cell) *(103)*. These data are compatible with finding the β-adrenoreceptor agonist coupled to adenylyl cyclase, because isoproterenol induces the elevation of intracellular cAMP in guinea pig eosinophils and activates cAMP-dependent protein kinase *(104)*. Similar data are available for the selective β-adrenoreceptor agonist salbutamol with human eosinophils *(64,103)*. Functionally, β-adrenoreceptor agonists can suppress eosinophil function, although the time of preincubation is important because of the tachyphylaxis of the receptor *(64,105)*. β-adrenoreceptor agonists, such as isoproterenol and salbutamol, inhibit sIgA- and IgG-mediated degranulation of eosinophils *(64)*. The finding that β-adrenoreceptor agonists are potentiated by the phosphodiesterase (PDE) inhibitor isobutyl-methylxanthine (IBMX) further supports the possibility that these compounds are both acting on the AC system. Isoproterenol also inhibits LTC_4 production of human eosinophils induced by FMLP plus cytochalasin B *(106)*.

Cyclic nucleotide-PDE hydrolyses the 3'-ribose phosphate bond of 3', 5'-cyclic monophosphate to form the biologically inert 5'-nucleoside monophosphates. To date, five isoenzymes of PDE have been identified according to criteria that include substrate specificity, inhibitor sensitivity, allosteric modulation, and Ca^{2+} and calmodulin dependence *(107)*. Guinea pig eosinophils express predominantly a high-affinity, membrane-bound cAMP PDE with the characteristics of a PDE IV *(104)*. There is no enzymological evidence of PDE I, II, III, and V. Drugs that have been categorized as PDE IV antagonists (i.e., rolipram, denbufylline) potently increase the intracellular cAMP concentration, activate cAMP-dependent protein kinase, and abrogate both respiratory burst and PAF-induced Ca^{2+} mobilization in guinea pig eosinophils *(105,107)*. In contrast, the selective inhibitors of PDE III (SK&F 94120) and PDE I (zaprinast) are inactive.

The nonselective PDE inhibitors also show inhibitory effects on eosinophil function. In both guinea pig and human eosinophils, theophylline attenuates respiratory burst induced by opsonized zymosan at a relatively high concentration (~100 µM) *(109)*. The structural analog of theophylline, 8-phenyltheophylline, which is not a PDE inhibitor, is inactive even at higher concentrations; this supports the belief that the suppressive effect of theophylline is a result of PDE inhibition. Theophylline also inhibits sIgA- and IgG-induced degranulation of human eosinophils *(64)*. Furthermore, a potent PDE-inhibitor, IBMX, also inhibits sIgA- and IgG-induced eosinophil degranulation *(64)*. The supposition that this is mediated via a cAMP/AC-dependent mechanism is provided by the observation that IBMX potentiates the inhibitory effects of the β2-adrenoreceptor agonists isoproterenol and salbutamol. Thus, PDE inhibitors, especially PDE IV inhibitors, downregulate the various effector functions of eosinophils.

The inhibitory effects of the AC system on eosinophil function are further supported by two different groups of pharmacological agents. First, the degranulation of human eosinophils induced by immunoglobulins is inhibited by lipophilic cAMP analogs such as dibutyryl cAMP, 8-bromo cAMP, and N^6-benzoyl cAMP *(64)*. Second, cholera toxin treatment increases intracellular cAMP levels through the ADP ribosylation of the α-subunit of the stimulatory guanine nucleotide binding protein (G protein) for adenylyl cyclase, resulting in persistent stimulation of this enzyme activity *(110)*. Eosinophils treated with cholera toxin for 2 h exhibit fourfold increases in cAMP *(64)*. The degranulation responses of eosinophils to sIgA- and IgG-coated Sepharose 4B are progressively impaired by cholera toxin treatment. The latency period of 1 h to inhibit the degranulation by cholera toxin is consistent with the time lag required for catalytic modification of G protein by this toxin. Thus, these observations strongly suggest that the AC system inhibits the function and, probably, the receptor/ligand-mediated activation signal of eosinophils.

Among the various stimulators of the AC system, the PDE inhibitors are the most intriguing. With the advent of molecular biology, evidence now available suggests the presence of 20–30 different mammalian PDE isoenzymes. Although the precise significance and tissue/cell localization of these isoenzymes are still unknown, this diversity provides a unique therapeutic opportunity for the highly selective PDE inhibitors and the inhibition of specific types of cells such as eosinophils.

CYTOKINE-INDUCED SIGNAL TRANSDUCTION OF EOSINOPHILS

IL-3/IL-5/GM-CSF Receptors on Eosinophils

IL-3, IL-5, and GM-CSF, besides being a growth maturation factor for eosinophils, also stimulate a number of mature human eosinophil functions: It has been shown that eosinophils possess receptors for IL-3, IL-5, and GM-CSF (approx 1000 receptors/cell) *(111–112)*. The receptors for these cytokines consist of two noncovalently associated two chains, namely a ligand-specific α-chain (60–80 kDa), which binds the cognate ligand with low affinity (K_d of 10 n*M*) *(113–116)*, and a 120-kDa common β-chain ($β_c$), which confers high-affinity binding to the ligand and signal transduction *(117)*. The affinity of the complete GM-CSF receptor (K_d of 44 p*M*) *(112)* on human eosinophils is approx 10 times higher than for IL-3 ($K_d = 470$ p*M*) *(112)* and IL-5 ($K_d = 518$ p*M*) *(111)*. The sharing of $β_c$ among the receptors for GM-CSF, IL-3, and IL-5 may explain the crosscompetition between these cytokines; this competition may be viewed as the "sequestering" of the common β-chain by excess heterologous competitor *(118)*. It is likely that $β_c$ is present in numbers similar to each of the α-chains, but less than the three α-chains combined. In addition, membrane proximal cytoplasmic regions of α-chains of GM-CSF and/or IL-5 receptors that are critical for regulation of cell growth have been identified, indicating that α-chains are also important for signal transduction *(119–121)*.

Regulation of the Expression of the IL-5 Receptor

Characterization of the promoter of the IL-5 receptor α-chain (IL-5Rα) has led to the identification of a 34-bp functional region that lacks consensus sequences for known transcription factors *(122)*. This 34-bp sequence is important for maximal expression of the IL-5Rα gene and binds nuclear factor(s) from myeloid and eosinophilic cell lines. Restricted expression of this nuclear factor(s) and the 34-bp target promoter sequence may account for selective expression of the IL-5Rα gene in basophil and eosinophil lineages. A similar mechanism may be involved in the transcription of the Charcot-Leyden crystal (CLC) protein gene. Characterization of the CLC protein gene promoter suggests the presence of a regulatory element that positively regulates transcription in the eosinophilic HL-60 cell line, but has a neg-

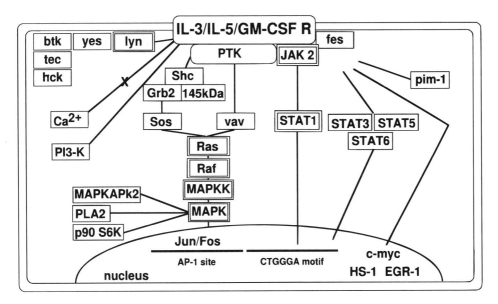

Fig. 2. Signal transduction from IL-3/IL-5/GM-CSF receptors. Information described in the text is summarized. Double rectangles denote the molecules confirmed in IL-5 signaling of human eosinophils.

ative regulatory function in other myeloid and nonmyeloid cells *(123)*. In addition, the CLC protein gene and the IL-5Rα gene promoters contain putative binding sites for GATA proteins, a family of hematopoietic zinc-finger transcription factors *(122,123)*. mRNA for GATA-1, GATA-2, and GATA-3 is expressed in human eosinophils and basophils, and expression of GATA-1 mRNA is upregulated in an eosinophilic HL-60 cell line in response to IL-5 *(124)*. Therefore, GATA proteins may regulate transcription of eosinophil/basophil characteristic genes such as CLC protein and IL-5Rα. In addition, putative PU.1-binding sites are present in CLC protein promoter, whereas consensus binding sequences for AP-1 are found in IL-5Rα promoter *(122,123)*. Up to now, no definite eosinophil-specific regulatory deoxyribonucleic acid (DNA) element(s) or transcription factor(s) have been identified.

Signal Transduction from IL-3/IL-5/GM-CSF Receptors (Fig. 2)

ACTIVATION OF TYROSINE KINASES

It is unlikely that ligation of IL-3/IL-5/GM-CSF receptors directly stimulates the elevation of $[Ca^{2+}]_i$ and activates PKC. Alternatively, GM-CSF, IL-3, and IL-5 clearly induce tyrosine phosphorylation of a number of intracellular proteins, including those belonging to the Ras pathway and the Janus kinase (JAK)/signal transducers and activators of transcription (STAT) pathway *(125–128)*. Experiments using various hematopoietic cell lines expressing GM-CSF, IL-3, or IL-5 receptor suggests that multiple tyrosine kinases are activated by these cytokines, including *lyn (129,130)*, *hck (131)*, *yes (130)*, *btk (132)*, *tec (133)*, c-*fes (134)*, and Janus kinase JAK2 *(see* below for details) *(132,135,136)*. Furthermore, IL-5 induces tyrosine phosphorylation of P13-K in a murine IL-5-dependent cell line, Y16 *(132)*. JAK2 and c-*fes* associate directly with β_c of the IL-3/Il-5/GM-CSF receptors *(134,136)*, suggesting that activation of these kinases indicates early events in cytokine signaling.

Because IL-3, IL-5, and GM-CSF share β_c, which is important for signal transduction, it was considered that these cytokines use the same signaling pathways. In fact, a common set of proteins was phosphorylated on tyrosine in eosinophils stimulated by IL-3, IL-5, or GM-CSF

(137). On the other hand, in a human erythroleukemia cell line, TF-1, cell proliferation in response to IL-3 or GM-CSF was inhibited by tyrosine kinase inhibitors, whereas that in response to IL-5 was enhanced by these drugs *(138)*. Furthermore, inhibitors of PKC inhibited IL-3- but not IL-5-induced proliferation. These observations suggest that the signal transduction pathways and the role of tyrosine kinase in cell proliferation differ among these three cytokines at least in the TF-1 cell line, but this hypothesis remains to be tested in eosinophils. Activation of tyrosine kinases also appears to be cell type-specific. For example, *hck* is activated by GM-CSF in dimethyl sulfoxide (DMSO)-differentiated HL-60 cells *(131)*, but not in human neutrophils or the TF-1 cell line *(130)*. The human nuclear tyrosine kinase c-*fes* is activated in TF-1 cell line in response to GM-CSF or IL-3 *(134)*, whereas c-*fes* is not activated in MO7e cells stimulated by GM-CSF *(139)*.

In human eosinophils, *lyn (140)* and JAK2 *(141–142)* have recently been identified as tyrosine kinase involved in IL-5 signaling. Tyrosine phosphorylation and activation of these kinases were inhibited by treatment of eosinophils by transforming growth factor (TGF)-β, suggesting a mechanism for the inhibitory activity of TGF-β on eosinophils *(143)*. Although physiologic meanings of the activation of *lyn* and JAK2 in eosinophil function are unknown, a study reported that GM-CSF-induced survival of eosinophils was inhibited by a tyrosine kinase inhibitor, genistein *(144)*. Conversely, a tyrosine phosphatase inhibitor enhanced the survival of eosinophils *(144)*. Furthermore, IL-5-induced chemokinesis is also dependent on tyrosine kinase(s) *(145)*. Thus, the tyrosine kinase activated by IL-5 likely plays an important role in the functions of eosinophils. Whether additional tyrosine kinases are activated by IL-5 in eosinophils and whether they are involved in eosinophils function need further investigation.

ACTIVATION OF THE RAS PATHWAY

The Ras pathway is activated by various cytokines *(146)*. IL-3, IL-5, and GM-CSF also activate several components of the Ras signaling cascade. For example, Ras is activated by IL-3, IL-5, and GM-CSF *(147)*. When stimulated by IL-3 and GM-CSF, the 52-kDa adapter protein Shc is phosphorylated on tyrosine and becomes associated with another adapter protein, Grb2 *(148,149)*. IL-3 and GM-CSF also induce the tyrosine phosphorylation of an unknown 145-kDa protein that binds to the Grb2-binding site of Shc *(150,151)*. Others reported the association of an unknown 140-kDa protein with Grb2 *(152)*. Thus, these 140- and 145-kDa proteins may be potential regulators of Ras activity. It is also possible that activation of Ras stimulated by IL-3, IL-5, and GM-CSF is mediated by a guanine nucleotide exchange factor, Vav *(153)*, because IL-5 induces tyrosine phosphorylation of this protein *(132)*. The downstream molecules of the Ras pathway, including Raf-1 *(154)*, two distinct forms of mitogen-activated protein kinase kinase (MAPKK) *(155)*, and mitogen-activated protein kinase (MAPK) (p42 and p44) *(156)*, as well as the potential targets of MAPK, such as mitogen-activated protein kinase activated protein (MAPKAP) kinase 2 and p90 S6 kinase *(157,158)*, are activated by IL-3 and GM-CSF. GM-CSF-induced activation of MAPKK and MAPK is slower and more persistent compared to that induced by FMLP *(155)*. In human eosinophils, IL-5 induces activation of Ras, Raf, MAPKK (p41 and p45), and MAPK (p44) *(140)*. In this study, only the p44 form of MAPK, but not the p42 form, was detected by eosinophils, although further studies are needed to fully characterize the MAPKK and MAPK involved in eosinophil signal transduction.

ACTIVATION OF TRANSCRIPTION FACTORS

Recently, a number of studies have shown that receptors for various cytokines associate with and activate members of the JAK family of cytoplasmic protein tyrosine kinases *(159)*. JAK physically associates with the membrane-proximal region of the ligand-bound receptor, leading to tyrosine phosphorylation and activation of JAK. The activated JAK phosphorylates the receptors as well as cytoplasmic proteins belonging to a family of transcription factors, called STAT. On activation (i.e., phosphorylation), STAT proteins form homo- or heterodimers, translate to nucleus, bind to defined DNA sequences, and regulate transcription *(159)*. At least seven members (Stat1α, Stat1β, Stat2, Stat3, Stat4, Stat5, and Stat6) belong to the STAT family *(160)*.

In human monocytes, U937 cells, and BaF3/ER cells, IL-3 and GM-CSF induce a single DNA binding complex containing an 80-kDa tyrosine phosphorylated protein (p80) that can be distinguished from the Stat1α homodimer induced by inteferon (IFN)γ *(161,162)*. Likewise, IL-5 induces an uncharacterized DNA binding complex in human basophils *(161)*. Recently, it was demonstrated that IL-3 and GM-CSF induce activation of Stat5 homologs in various myeloid cells *(163–165)*. Moreover, IL-3 induces tyrosine phosphorylation of Stat6 *(166)*. Stat3 is induced by IL-5 in BaF3 cells stably transfected with human IL-5R *(167)*. Another study reported weak tyrosine phosphorylation of Stat1α in BaF3 cells in response to IL-3 *(168)*.

In human eosinophils, IL-5 as well as IL-3 and GM-CSF induce two DNA binding complexes when the IFNγ/IL-6 response element of the intercellular adhesion molecule (ICAM)-1 promoter is used as a probe *(141)*. One of these DNA binding complexes contains Stat1α as a homodimer. Similarly, when stimulated by IL-5, JAK2 is rapidly tyrosine-phosphorylated, and Stat1 is identified in the nuclear extract using DNA sequence from the ly6 promoter *(142)*.

IL-3, IL-5, and GM-CSF induce many other nuclear proteins. Long-term stimulation with IL-3, IL-5, and GM-CSF leads to the induction of the transcription factor c-myc *(120,158,169)*. A hematopoietic serine/threonine kinase, *pim*-1, is induced by GM-CSF *(158,170)*. mRNA for the transcription factors c-*fos (120,158,169)* and c-*jun (120,158)* are induced by IL-3, IL-5, and GM-CSF. A putative transcription factor that is specifically expressed in hematopoietic cells, HS-1, is also tyrosine-phosphorylated upon stimulation with IL-5 *(132,171)*. IL-3 and GM-CSF induces transcription of the early growth response gene 1 (EGR-1), mediated by a cAMP responsive element (CRE), suggesting that a CREB-family member can be activated by these cytokines as well *(172)*. Studies need to be done to examine the presence and activation of these transcription factors in eosinophils. Furthermore, the roles of transcription factors in proliferation and differentiation of eosinophil precursors and in *de novo* synthesis of various genes in mature eosinophils remain to be resolved.

GENERATION AND MODULATION
OF CELL ACTIVATION SIGNAL BY INTEGRINS

Integrins and Signaling

Integrins are heterodimer molecules expressed on many types of cells and play important roles in cell adhesion, spreading, migration, and activation. Recent studies suggest that integrins play a pivotal role in the formation of focal adhesion, which is essential for cellular function. Focal adhesion sites are composed of actin filaments, cytoskeletal proteins structurally associated with actin filaments, such as talin, vinculin, paxillin, filamin, and tensin, and several signal transduction molecules. These proteins include focal adhesion kinase (FAK), P13-K, Grb2, Soc, and Crk *(173)*. The cytoskeletal proteins may coordinate the assembly of a focal adhesion site and link integrins to microfilaments *(173)*. Furthermore, crosslinking of a β$_2$-integrin, α$_M$β$_2$, leads to cocapping of this integrin with other cell surface molecules, such as α$_L$β$_2$, FcγRIII, and the FMLP receptor *(174,175)*. Thus, several receptors and signaling molecules are highly concentrated at the focal adhesion sites, making efficient intracellular signaling possible.

Activation of Tyrosine Kinases by Integrins

Crosslinking of β_1-integrins results in activation and tyrosine phosphorylation of a 125-kDa protein, FAK *(173)*. Activated FAK is associated with other signaling molecules, such as Src, Grb2, and Sos *(176)*. FAK also associates and phosphorylates the p85 subunit of PI3-K *(177)*. Because Grb2 and PI3-K are implicated in the Ras signaling pathway and mitogenic signaling, respectively, the activation of FAK is potentially involved in various effector functions and gene induction of adherent cells. Ligation of a β_2-integrin, $\alpha_L\beta_2$, in lymphocytes induces tyrosine phosphorylation of p130^{cas} and its association with an adapter protein, Crk *(178)*. Furthermore, in neutrophils stimulated with tumor necrosis factor (TNF) α, an *src* family tyrosine kinase, Fgr, and paxillin were phosphorylated on tyrosine *(179)*.

Tyrosine kinases are also likely involved in eosinophil activation mediated by integrins. Nagata et al. *(19)* showed that genistein, a tyrosine kinase inhibitor, did not affect eosinophil adhesion to VCAM-1 immobilized onto tissue culture plates through a β_1-integrin, $\alpha_4\beta_1$. In contrast, this genistein did inhibit superoxide production by eosinophils adherent to VCAM-1, suggesting that PTK is involved in intracellular signaling generated by eosinophils adherent to VCAM-1 but that PTK is not involved in adhesion of eosinophils to VCAM-1. In fact, they could identify increased tyrosine phosphorylation of several 30- and 40-kDa proteins in eosinophils adherent to VCAM-1. We also found that eosinophils stimulated by anti-CD11b monoclonal antibody (MAb) (antibody against $\alpha_M\beta_2$) coupled to polystyrene microbeads showed tyrosine phosphorylation of intracellular proteins, including paxillin and several proteins with molecular-weight ranges of 115–125 kDa *(180)*. Eosinophils stimulated by IL-5 and adherent to protein-coated surfaces in an $\alpha_M\beta_2$-dependent manner showed tyrosine phosphorylation of a number of intracellular proteins; tyrosine phosphorylation of 115-kDa protein was specifically inhibited when anti-CD18 MAb prevented eosinophil adhesion. Preliminary studies suggest that FAK is constitutively tyrosine-phosphorylated in resting eosinophils, and one of the proteins with 115–125-kDa molecular-weight range is in fact a multifunctional adapter protein, Cbl *(181)*. Thus, the activation of tyrosine kinases and the tyrosine phosphorylation of cellular proteins are likely involved in transmembrane signaling mediated by integrin adhesion molecules in eosinophils. Further studies are required to characterize individual proteins and to analyze the functional significance of the proteins.

Activation of PLC by Integrins

As described above, ligand binding to various receptors triggers a rapid increase in phosphoinositide hydrolysis induced by PLC activation. Crosslinking of a β_2-integrin, $\alpha_L\beta_2$, also results in tyrosine phosphorylation of PLC-γ in lymphocytes *(182)*. β_2-integrins also mediate IP$_3$ accumulation, an increase in [Ca^{2+}]$_i$, activation of PLD, and actin polymerization in neutrophils *(183–185)*.

In human eosinophils, we showed that, when eosinophils are incubated in plates coated with human serum albumin (HSA) and stimulated by PAF, they adhere to HSA-coated wells through β_2-integrin and show a sixfold increase in PLC activity *(186)*. In contrast, when plates are coated with laminin, a ligand for $\alpha_6\beta_1$, PAF-stimulated increase in PLC activity is markedly decreased. This lower PLC activity is also associated with a decreased degranulation response by the cells. Similarly, activation of PLC in eosinophils stimulated by IL-5 and adherent to HSA-coated plates is inhibited when adhesion is prevented by pretreatment of the cells with anti-CD18 MAb *(180)*. Conversely, engagement of the $\alpha_M\beta_2$ on eosinophils by anti-CD11b MAb coupled to polystyrene beads results in increased PLC activity in eosinophils. Thus, cellular adhesion through β_2-integrins is likely playing an important role in the activation of PLC in eosinophils, culminating in a generation of second messengers and the induction of effector functions.

CONCLUSIONS

Eosinophils are important effector cells in the host defense against parasites, allergic diseases, and diseases associated with eosinophilia. An increasing number of studies on the biochemistry and pharmacology of eosinophils have been done recently to delineate the intracellular mechanisms of the cells. It seems clear that eosinophil functions are regulated by a number of intracellular molecules, including phospholipases, secondary and tertiary messengers, G proteins, and protein phosphorylation. The information available also suggests that eosinophils share common signaling pathways with other types of leukocytes. In the future, it will be interesting to test whether there are any differences at the levels of signal transduction between eosinophils and other cell types. Further studies of eosinophil immunology, biochemistry, and pharmacology may lead us to identify critical molecule(s) that play a pivotal role in eosinophil effector functions, and may result in the development of new classes of drugs/modulators for the treatment of eosinophil-associated inflammatory disorders.

ACKNOWLEDGMENTS

The author's studies have been supported in part by grants (AI 34577, AI 34486) from the National Institute of Health and from the Mayo Foundation.

REFERENCES

1. Gleich GJ, Adolphson CR (1986) The eosinophilic leukocyte: structure and function. Adv Immunol 39:177.
2. Butterfield JH, Leiferman KM, Gleich GJ (1995) Eosinophil-associated diseases. In: Frank MM, Austen KF, Claman HN, Unanue ER, eds. Samter's Immunological Diseases, Fifth edition. Little, Brown, Boston, p. 501.
3. Abu-Ghazaleh RI, Fujisawa T, Mestecky J, Kyle RA, Gleich GJ (1989) IgA-induced eosinophil degranulation. J Immunol 142:2393.
4. Capron MC, Tomassin M, Voist EVD, Kuznierz J-P, Papin J-P, Capron A (1988) Existence and function of receptor for immunoglobulin A on human eosinophils. C R Acad Sci Paris 307:397.
5. Fujisawa T, Abu-Ghazaleh RI, Kita H, Sanderson CJ, Gleich GJ (1990) Regulatory effect of cytokines on eosinophil degranulation. J Immunol 144:642.
6. Winqvist I, Olofsson T, Olsson I (1984) Mechanisms for eosinophil degranulation: release of eosinophil cationic protein. Immunology 51:1.
7. Takafuji S, Tadokoro K, Ito K, Dahinden CA (1994) Degranulation of eosinophils stimulated with C3a and C5a. Int Arch Allergy Appl Immunol 104:27.
8. Kernen P, Wymann MP, Von Tscharner V, Deranleau DA, Tai PC, Spry CJ, Dahinden CA, Baggiolini M (1991) Shape changes, exocytosis, and cytosolic free calcium changes in stimulated human eosinophils. J Clin Invest 87:2012.
9. Kroegel C, Yukawa T, Dent G, Venge P, Chung KF, Barnes PJ (1989) Stimulation of degranulation from human eosinophils by platelet activating factor. J Immunol 142:3518.
10. Kita H, Weiler DA, Abu-Ghazaleh R, Sanderson CJ, Gleich GJ (1992) Release of granule proteins from eosinophils cultured with IL-5. J Immunol 149:629.
11. Horie S, Kita H (1994) CD11b/CD18 (Mac-1) is required for degranulation of human eosinophils induced by human recombinant granulocyte-macrophage colony-stimulating factor and platelet-activating factor. J Immunol 152:5457.
12. Alam R, Stafford S, Forsythe P, Harrison R, Faubion D, Lett-Brown MA, Grant JA (1993) RANTES is a chemotactic and activating factor for human eosinophils. J Immunol 150:3442.
13. Rot A, Krieger M, Brunner T, Bischoff SC, Schall TJ, Dahinden CA (1992) RANTES and macrophage inflammatory protein 1 alpha induce the migration and activation of normal human eosinophil granulocytes. J Exp Med 176:1489.
14. Sedgwick JB, Vrtis RF, Gourley MF, Busse WW (1988) Stimulant-dependent differences in superoxide anion generation by normal human eosinophils and neutrophils. J Allergy Clin Immunol 81:876.

15. Palmblad J, Gyllenhammar H, Lindgren JA, Malmstern CL (1984) Effects of leukotrienes and f-Met-Leu-Phe on oxidative metabolism of neutrophils and eosinophils. J Immunol 132:3041.

16. Elsner J, Oppermann M, Czech W, Dobos G, Schopf E, Norgauer J, Kapp A (1994) C3a activates reactive oxygen radical species production and intracellular calcium transients in human eosinophils. Eur J Immunol 24:518.

17. Koenderman L, Tool ATJ, Roos D, Verhoeven AJ (1990) Priming of the respiratory burst in human eosinophils is accompanied by changes in signal transduction. J Immunol 145:3883.

18. Bach MK, Brashler JR, Petzold EN, Sanders ME (1992) Superoxide production by human eosinophils can be inhibited in an agonist-selective manner. Agents Actions 35:1.

19. Nagata M, Sedgwick JB, Bates ME, Kita H, Busse WW (1995) Eosinophil adhesion to vascular cell adhesion molecule-1 activates superoxide anion generation. J Immunol 155:2194.

20. Saito H et al. (1988) Selective differentiation and proliferation of hematopoietic cells induced by recombinant human interleukins. Proc Natl Acad Sci USA 85:2288.

21. Sanderson CJ, Warren DJ, Strath M (1985) Identification of a lymphokine that stimulates eosinophil differentiation in vitro: its relationship to interleukin 3, and functional properties of eosinophils produced in cultures. J Exp Med 162:60.

22. Rothenberg ME et al. (1989) IL-5-dependent conversion of normodense human eosinophils to the hypodense phenotype uses 3T3 fibroblasts for enhanced viability, accelerated hypodensity, and sustained antibody-dependent cytotoxicity. J Immunol 143:2311.

23. Lopez AF et al. (1988) Recombinant human interleukin 5 is a selective activator of human eosinophil function. J Exp Med 167:219.

24. Nakajima H, Gleich GJ, Kita H (1996) Constitutive production of IL-4 and IL-10 and stimulated production of IL-8 by normal peripheral blood eosinophils. J Immunol 156:4859.

25. Walsh GM et al. (1990) Il-5 enhances the in vitro adhesion of human eosinophils, but not neutrophils, in a leucocyte integrin (CD11/18)-dependent manner. Immunology 71:258.

26. Wang JM et al. (1989) Recombinant human interleukin 5 is a selective activator of human eosinophil function. Eur J Immunol 19:701–705.

27. Neher E, Marty A (1982) Discrete changes of cell membrane capacitance observed under condition of enhanced secretion in bovine adrenal chromaffin cells. Proc Natl Acad Sci USA 79:6712.

28. Fernandez JM, Neher E, Gomperts BD (1984) Capacitance measurements reveal stepwise fusion events in degranulating mast cells. Nature 312:453.

29. Nusse O, Lindau M, Cromwell O, Kay AB, Gomperts BD (1990) Intracellular application of guanosine-5′-O-(3-thiotriphosphate) induces exocytotic granule fusion in guinea-pig eosinophils. J Exp Med 171:775.

30. Aizawa T, Kakuta Y, Yamauchi K, Ohkawara Y, Maruyama N, Nitta Y, Tamura G, Sasaki H, Takishima T (1992) Induction of granule release by intracellular application of calcium and guanosine-5′-O-(3-thiotriphosphate) in human eosinophils. J Allergy Clin Immunol 90:789.

31. Fukuda T, Ackerman SJ, Reed CE, Peters MS, Dunnette SL, Gleich GJ (1985) Calcium ionophore A23187 calcium-dependent cytolytic degranulation in human eosinophils. J Immunol 135:1349.

32. Owen WF Jr, Soberman RJ, Yoshimoto T, Schaller AL, Lewis RA, Austen KF (1987) Synthesis and release of leukotriene C_4 by human eosinophils. J Immunol 138:532.

33. Brundage RA, Fogarty KE, Tuft RA, Fay FS (1991) Calcium gradients underlying polarization and chemotaxis of eosinophils. Science 254:703.

34. Subramanian N et al. (1992) Leukotriene B_4 induced steady state calcium rise and superoxide anion generation in guinea pig eosinophils are not related events. Biochem Biophys Res Commun 187:670.

35. Kroegel C, Yukawa T, Westwick J, Barnes PJ (1989) Evidence for two platelet activating receptors on eosinophils: dissociation between PAF-induced intracellular Ca^{2+}-mobilization, degranulation and superoxide anion generation in eosinophils. Biochem Biophys Res Commun 162:571.

36. Kita H, Abu-Ghazaleh RI, Gleich GJ, Abraham RT (1991) Role of pertussis toxin-sensitive G proteins in stimulus dependent human eosinophil degranulation. J Immunol 147:3466.

37. Kroegel C, Pleass R, Yukawa T, Chung KF, Westwick J, Barnes PJ (1989) Characterization of platelet activating factor-induced elevation of cytosolic free calcium concentration in eosinophils. FEBS Lett 243:41.

38. Kroegel C, Giembycz MA, Barnes PJ (1990) Characterization of eosinophil activation by peptides: differential effects of substance P, melittin, and fMet-Leu-Phe. J Immunol 145:2581.

39. Hwang SB (1990) Specific receptors of platelet-activating factor, receptor heterogeneity, and signal transduction mechanisms. J Lipid Med 2:123.

40. Rot A, Krieger M, Brunner T, et al. (1992) RANTES and macrophage inflammatory protein 1 alpha induce the migration and activation of normal human eosinophil granulocytes. J Exp Med 176:1489.

41. Schweizer RC, Welmers BAC, Raaijmakers JAM, et al. (1994) RANTES and interleukin-8-induced responses in normal human eosinophils: effects of priming with interleukin-5. Blood 83:3697.

42. Weber M, Uguccioni M, Ochensberger B, et al. (1995) Monocyte chemotactic protein MCP-2 activated human basophil and eosinophil leukocytes similar to MCP-3. J Immunol 154:4166.

43. Dahinden CA, Geiser T, Brunner T, et al. (1994) Monocyte chemotactic protein 3 is a most effective basophil- and eosinophil-activating chemokine. J Exp Med 179:751.

44. Murphy PM (1994) The molecular biology of leukocyte chemoattractant receptors. Annu Rev Immunol 12:593.

45. Berridge MJ (1987) Inositol triphosphate and diacylglycerol: two interacting second messengers. Annu Rev Biochem 56:159.

46. Kroegel C, Chilvers ER, Barnes PJ (1990) Platelet activating factor (PAF) stimulates phosphoinositide (PI) metabolism in guinea-pig eosinophils. Clin Sci 76:54P.

47. Dent G, Barnes PJ (1991) Platelet activating factor simulates a pertussis toxin-sensitive GTPase activity in guinea-pig eosinophil membrane. Br J Pharmacol 104:86P.

48. Kroegel C, Chilvers ER, Giembycz MA, Challiss RAJ, Barnes PJ (1991) Platelet activating factor stimulates a rapid accumulation of inositol (1,4,5)triphosphate in guinea-pig eosinophils: relationship to calcium mobilization and degranulation. J Allergy Clin Immunol 88:114.

49. De Andres B, Del Pozo V, Cardaba B, Martin E, Tramon P, Lopez-Rivasa A, Palonino P, Lahoz C (1991) Phosphoinositide breakdown is associated with Fc-γRII mediated activation of 5'-lipoxygenase in murine eosinophils. J Immunol 146:1566.

50. Cockcroft S (1992) G-protein-regulated phospholipase C, D and A_2-mediated signalling in neutrophils. Biochim Biophys Acta 1113:135.

51. Abdel-Latif AA (1986) Calcium-mobilizing receptors, polyphosphoinositides, and the generation of second messengers. Pharmacol Rev 38:227.

52. Berridege MJ (1993) Inositol triphosphate and calcium signaling. Nature 361:315.

53. Taylor SJ, Chae HZ, Rhee SG, Exton JH (1991) Activation of the β1 isozyme of phospholipase C by α subunit of the G_q class of G proteins. Nature 350:516.

54. Katz A, Wu D, Simon MI (1992) Subunits beta gamma of heterotrimeric G protein activate beta 2 isoform of phospholipase C. Nature 360:686.

55. Rhee SG (1991) Inositol phospholipid-specific phospholipase C: interaction of γ1 isoform with tyrosine kinase. Trends Biochem Sci 16:297.

56. Kato M, Kita H, manuscript in preparation.

57. Gilman AG (1987) G proteins: transducers of receptor-generated signals. Annu Rev Biochem 56:615.

58. Neer EJ (1995) Heterotrimeric G proteins: organizers of transmembrane signals. Cell 80:249.

59. Clapham DE, Neer EJ (1993) New roles of G-protein $\beta\gamma$ dimers in transmembrane signaling. Nature 365:403.

60. Bokoch GM, Katada T, Northup JK, Newlett EL, Gilman AG (1983) Identification of the predominant substrate for ADP-ribosylation by islet activating protein. J Biol Chem 258:2072.

61. Okajima F, Katada T, Ui M (1985) Coupling of the guanine nucleotide regulatory protein chemotactic peptide receptors in neutrophil membrane and its uncoupling by islet-activating protein, pertussis toxin: A possible role of the toxin substrate in Ca^{2+}-mobilizing receptor-mediated signal transduction. J Biol Chem 260:6761.

62. Snyderman R, Perianin A, Evans T, Polakis P, Didsbury J (1990) G proteins and neutrophil function. In: Moss J, Vaughan M, eds. ADP-Ribosylating Toxin and G Proteins. American Society for Microbiology, Washington, p. 295.

63. Ui M (1990) Pertussis toxin as valuable probe for G-protein involvement in signal transduction. In: Moss J, Vaughan M, eds. ADP-Ribosylating Toxins and G Proteins. American Society for Microbiology, Washington, p. 45.

64. Kita H, Abu-Ghazaleh RI, Gleich GJ, Abraham RT (1991) Regulation of Ig-induced eosinophil degranulation by adenosine-3',5'-cyclic monophosphate. J Immunol 146:2712.

65. Kato M, Abraham RT, Kita H (1995) Tyrosine phosphorylation is required for eosinophil degranulation induced by immobilized immunoglobulin. J Immunol 155:357.

66. Agrawal DK, Ali N, Numao T (1992) PAF receptors and G-proteins in human blood eosinophils. J Lipid Med 5:101.

67. Kapp A, Zeck-Kapp G, Czech W, Schopf E (1994) The chemokine RANTES is more than a chemoattractant: characterization of its effect on human eosinophil oxidative metabolism and morphology in comparison with IL-5 and GM-CSF. J Invest Dermatol 102:906.

68. Cromwell O, Bennett JP, Hide I, Kay AB, Comperts BD (1991) Mechanisms of granule enzyme secretion from permeabilized guinea-pig eosinophils. Dependence on Ca^{2+} and guanine nucleotide. J Immunol 147:1905.

69. Gomperts BD (1990) G_E: a GTP-binding protein mediating exocytosis. Annu Rev Physiol 52:591.

70. Barbacid M (1987) *ras* genes. Annu Rev Biochem 56:779.

71. McPhil LC, Strum SL, Leone PA, Sozzani S (1992) The neutrophil respiratory burst mechanism. In: Coffey R, ed. Granulocyte Responses to Cytokines: Basic and Clinical Research. Marcel Dekker, New York, p. 47.

72. Dennis EA, Rhee SG, Billah MM, Hannun YA (1991) Role of phospholipases in generating lipid second messengers in signal transduction. FASEB J 5:2068.

73. Sun FF, Czuk CI, Taylor BM (1989) Arachidonic acid metabolism in guinea pig eosinophils: synthesis of thromboxane B2 and leukotriene B4 in response to soluble or particulate activators. J Leukocyte Biol 46:152.

74. Debbaghi A, Hidi R, Vargaftig BB, Touqui L (1992) Inhibition of phospholipase A2 activity in guinea pig eosinophils by human recombinant IL-1 beta. J Immunol 149:1374.

75. Aebischer CP, Pasche I, Jorg A (1993) Nanomolar arachidonic acid influences the respiratory burst in eosinophils and neutrophils induced by GTP-binding protein. A comparative study of the respiratory burst in bovine eosinophils and neutrophils. Eur J Biochem 218:669.

76. White SR, Strek ME, Kulp GV, Spaethe SM, Burch RA, Neeley SP, Leff AR (1993) Regulation of human eosinophil degranulation and activation by endogenous phospholipase A2. J Clin Invest 91:2118.

77. Tool AT, Koenderman L, Kok PT, Blom M, Roos D, Verhoeven AJ (1992) Release of platelet-activating factor is important for the respiratory burst induced in human eosinophils by opsonized particles. Blood 79:2729.

78. Kok PT, Hamelink ML, Kijne GM, Verhagen J, Koenderman L, Veldink GA, Bruynzeel PL (1989) Leukotriene C4 formation by purified human eosinophils can be induced by arachidonic acid in the absence of calcium-ionophore A23187. Agents Actions 26:96.

79. Henderson WR, Chi EY, Jorg A, Klebanoff SJ (1983) Horse eosinophil degranulation induced by the ionophore A23187. Ultrastructure and role of phospholipase A2. Am J Pathol 111:341.

80. Korchak HM, Vosshall LB, Haines KA, Wilkenfeld C, Lundquist KF, Weissmann G (1988) Activation of the human neutrophil by calcium-mobilization ligands. II. Correlation of calcium, diacylglycerol, and phosphatidic acid generation with superoxide anion generation. J Biol Chem 263:11098.

81. Minnicozzi M, Anthes JC, Siegel MI, Billah M, Egan RW (1990) Activation of phospholipase D in normodense human eosinophils. Biochem Biophys Res Commun 170:540.

82. Billah MM, Anthes JC (1990) The regulation of cellular functions of phosphatidylcholine hydrolysis (review). Biochem J 269:281.

83. Huang, C-K (1989) Protein kinases in neutrophils: a review. Membr Biochem 8:61.

84. Ramesh KS, Rocklin RE, Pincus SH (1987) Phosphorylation and dephosphorylation of soluble proteins in human eosinophils. J Cell Biochem 34:203.

85. Pincus SH, Schooley WR, DiNapoli AM, Broder S (1981) Metabolic heterogeneity of eosinophils from normal and hypereosinophilic patients. Blood 58:1175.

86. Kajita T, Yui Y, Mita H, Taniguchi N, Saito H, Mishima T, Shida T (1985) Release of leukotriene C_4 from human eosinophils and its relation to cell density. Int Arch Allergy Appl Immunol 78:406.

87. Kurosawa M, Shimizu Y, Tsukagoshi H (1992) Human peripheral blood hypodense eosinophil proteins are more labeled with ^{32}P than the normodense eosinophil proteins. Int Arch Allergy Immunol 97:283.

88. Perlmutter RM, Levin SD, Appleby MW, Anderson SJ, Alberola-Iia J (1993) Regulation of lymphocyte function by protein phosphorylation. Annu Rev Immunol 11:451.

89. Chan AC, Desai DM, Weiss A (1994) The role of protein tyrosine kinases and protein tyrosine phosphatases in T cell antigen receptor signal transduction. Annu Rev Immunol 12:555.

90. Bach MK, Brashler JR, Petzold EN, Sanders ME (1992) Superoxide production by human eosinophils can be inhibited in an agonist-selective manner. Agents Actions 35:1.

91. Kapeller R, Cantley LC (1994) Phosphatidylinositol 3-kinase. BioEssays 16:565.

92. Nishizuka Y (1988) The molecular heterogeneity of protein kinase C and its implications for cellular regulation. Nature 334:661.

93. Bell RM, Burns, DJ (1991) Lipid activation of protein kinase C. J Biol Chem 266:4641.

94. Pontremoli S, Melloni E, Sparatore B, Michetti M, Salamino F and Horecker BL, (1990) Isozymes of protein kinase C in human neutrophils and their modification by two endogenous proteinases. J Biol Chem 265:706.

95. Stasia MJ, Strulovici B, Daniel-Issakani S, Pilosin JM, Dianoux AC, Chambaz E, Vignais PV (1990) Immunocharacterization of β- and ζ-subspecies of protein kinase C in bovine neutrophils. FEBS Lett 274:61.

96. Smallwood JI, Malawista SE (1992) Protein kinase C isoforms in human neutrophil cytoplasts. J Leukocyte Biol 51:84.

97. Bates ME, Bertics PJ, Calhoun WJ, Busse WW (1993) Increased protein kinase C activity in low density eosinophils. J Immunol 150:4486.

98. Dobrina A, Menegazzi R, Carlos TM, Narden E, Cramer R, Zacchi T, Harlan JM, Patricia P (1991) Mechanisms of eosinophil adherence to cultured vascular endothelial cells. J Clin Invest 88:20.

99. Sedgwick JB, Geiger KM, Busse WW (1990) Superoxide generation by hypodense eosinophils from patients with asthma. Am Rev Respir Dis 142:120.

100. Egesten A, Gullberg U, Olsson I, Richter J (1993) Phorbol ester-induced degranulation in adherent human eosinophil granulocytes is dependent on CD11/CD18 leukocyte integrins. J Leukocyte Biol 53:287.

101. Rabe KF, Giembycz MA, Dent G, Barnes PJ (1992) Activation of guinea pig eosinophil respiratory burst by leukotriene B4; role of protein kinase C. Fund Clin Pharmacol 6:353.

102. Kita H, Horie S, Okubo Y, Weiler D, Gleich GJ (1993) Pharmacologic modulation of eosinophil degranulation. J Allergy Clin Immunol 91:332.

103. Yukawa T, Ukena D, Kroegel C, Chanez P, Dent G, Chung KF, Branes PJ (1990) Beta$_2$-adrenergic receptors on eosinophils. Binding and functional studies. Am Rev Respir Dis 141:1446.

104. Souness JE, Carter CM, Diocee BK, Hassall GA, Wood LJ, Turner NC (1991) Characterization of guinea-pig eosinophil phosphodiesterase activity. Assessment of its involvement in regulating superoxide generation. Biochem Pharmacol 42:937.

105. Rabe KF, Giembycz MA, Dent G, Evans PM, Barnes PJ (1991) β$_2$-adrenoceptor agonists and respiratory burst activity in guinea-pig and human eosinophils. Fund Clin Pharmacol 5:402.

106. Munoz NM, Vita AJ, Neeley SP, McAllister K, Spaethe SM, White SR, Leff AR (1994) Beta adrenergic modulation of formyl-methionyl-leucyl-phenylalanine-stimulated secretion of eosinophil peroxidase and leukotriene C4. J Pharmacol Exp Ther 268:139.

107. Nicholson CD, Challiss RAJ, Shahid M (1991) Differential modulation of tissue function and therapeutic potentials of selective inhibitors of cyclic nucleotide phosphodiesterase isoenzymes. Trends Pharmacol Sci 12:19.

108. Dent G, Giembycz MA, Rabe KF, Barnes PJ (1991) Inhibition of eosinophil cyclic nucleotide PDE activity and opsonized zymosan-stimulated respiratory burst by "type IV"-selective PDE inhibitor. Br J Pharmacol 103:1339.

109. Yukawa T, Kroegel C, Dent G, Chanez P, Ukena D, Barnes PJ (1989) Effect of theophylline and adenosine on eosinophil function. Am Rev Respir Dis 140:327.

110. Cassel D, Selinger Z (1997) Mechanism of adenylate cylase activation by cholera toxin: inhibition of GTP hydrolysis at the regulatory site. Proc Natl Acad Sci USA 74:3307.

111. Chihara J, et al. (1990) Characterization of a receptor for interleukin 5 on human eosinophils: Variable expression and induction by granulocyte-macrophage colony-stimulating factor. J Exp Med 172:1347.

112. Lopez AF, Eglinton JM, Gillis D, et al. (1989) Reciprocal inhibition of binding between interleukin 3 and granulocyte-macrophage colony-stimulating factor to human eosinophils. Proc Natl Acad Sci USA 86:7022.

113. Gearing DP, et al. (1989) Expression cloning of a receptor for human granulocyte-macrophage colony-stimulating factor. EMBO J 8:3667.

114. Kitamura T, et al. (1991) Expression cloning of the human IL-3 receptor cDNA reveals a shared β subunit for the human IL-3 and GM-CSF receptors. Cell 66:1165.

115. Murata Y, et al. (1992) Molecular cloning and expression of the human interleukin 5 receptor. J Exp Med 175:341.

116. Tavernier J, et al. (1991) A human high affinity interleukin-5 receptor, IL5R, is composed of an IL5-specific alpha chain and a beta chain shared with the receptor for GM-CSF. Cell 66:1175.

117. Hayashida K, Kitamura T, Gorman DM, et al. (1990) Molecular cloning of a second subunit of the

receptor for human granulocyte-macrophage colony-stimulating factor (GM-CSF): reconstitution of a high-affinity GM-CSF receptor. Proc Natl Acad Sci USA 87:9655.

118. Lopez AF, et al. (1992) GM-CSF, IL-3 and IL-5: cross-competition on human haemopoietic cells. Immunol Today 13:495.

119. Weiss M, Yokoyama C, Shikama Y, Naugle C, Druker B, Sieff CA (1993) Human granulocyte-macrophage colony-stimulating factor receptor signal transduction requires the proximal cytoplasmic domains of the alpha and beta subunit. Blood 82:3298.

120. Takaki S, Kanazawa H, Shiiba M, Takatsu K (1994) A critical cytoplasmic domain of the interleukin-5 (IL-5) receptor α chain and its function in IL-5 mediated growth signal transduction. Mol Cell Biol 14:7404.

121. Polotskaya A, Zhao Y, Lilly MB, Kraft AS (1994) Mapping the intracytoplasmic regions of the alpha granulocyte-macrophage colony-stimulating factor receptor necessary for cell growth regulation. J Biol Chem 269:14,607.

122. Sun Z, Yergeau DA, Tuypens T, Tavernier J, Paul CC, Baumann MA, Tenen DG, Ackerman SJ (1995) Identification and characterization of a functional promotor region in the human eosinophil IL-5 receptor α subunit gene. J Biol Chem 270:1462.

123. Gomolin HI, Yamaguchi Y, Paulpillai AV, Dvorak LA, Ackerman SJ, Tenen DG (1983) Human eosinophil Charcot-Leyden crystal protein: cloning and characterization of a lysophospholipase gene promoter. Blood 82:1868.

124. Zon LI, Yamaguchi Y, Yee K, Albee EA, Kimura A, Bennett JC, Orkin SH, Ackerman SJ (1993) Expression of mRNA for the GATA-binding proteins in human eosinophils and basophils: potential role in gene transcription. Blood 81:3234.

125. Gomez Cambronero J, Yamazaki M, Metwally F, Molski TF, Bonak VA, Huang CK, Becker EL, Sha'afi RI (1989) Granulocyte-macrophage colony-stimulating factor and human neutrophils: role of guanine nucleotide regulatory proteins. Proc Natl Acad Sci USA 86:3569.

126. Koyasu S, Tojo A, Miyajima A, Akiyama T, Kasuga M, Urabe A, Schreur J, Arai KI, Takaku F, Yahana I (1987) Interleukin 3-specific tyrosine phosphorylation of a membrane glycoprotein of M_r 150,000 in multi-factor-dependent myeloid cell line. EMBO J 6:3979.

127. Sorensen PHB, Mui ALF, Murthy SC, Krystal G (1989) Interleukin-3, GM-CSF and TPA induce distinct phosphorylation events in an interleukin 3-dependent multipotential cell line. Blood 73:406.

128. Murata Y, Yamaguchi N, Hitoshi Y, Tominaga A, Takatsu K (1990) Interleukin 5 and interleukin 3 induce serine and tyrosine phosphorylation of several cellular proteins in an interleukin 5-dependent cell line. Biochem Biophys Res Commun 173:1102.

129. Torigoe T, O'Connor R, Santoli D, Reed JC (1992) Interleukin-3 regulates the activity of the LYN protein-tyrosine kinase in myeloid-committed leukemic cell lines. Blood 80:617.

130. Corey S, Eguinoa A, Puyana-Theall K, Bolen JB, Cantley L, Mollinedo F, Jackson TR, Hawkins PT, Stephens LR (1993) Granulocyte macrophage-colony stimulating factor stimulates both association and activation of phosphoinositide 3OH-kinase and src-related tyrosine kinase(s) in human myeloid derived cells. EMBO J 12:2681.

131. Linnekin D, Howard OMZ, Park L, Farrar W, Ferris D, Longo DL (1994) Hck expression correlates with granulocyte-macrophage colony-stimulating factor induced proliferation in HL-60 cells. Blood 84:94.

132. Sato S, Katagiri T, Takaki S, Kikuchi Y, Hitoshi Y, Yonehara S, Tsukada S, Kitamura D, Watanabe T, Witte O, Takatsu K (1994) IL-5 receptor-mediated tyrosine phosphorylation of SH2/SH3-containing proteins and activation of Bruton's tyrosine kinase and Janus 2 kinases. J Exp Med 180:2101.

133. Mano H, Yamashita Y, Sato K, Yazaki Y, Hirai H (1995) Tec protein-tyrosine kinase is involved in interleukin-3 signaling pathway. Blood 85:343.

134. Hanazono Y, Chiba S, Sasaki K, Mano H, Miyajima A, Arai KI, Yazaki Y, Hirai H (1993) c-fps/fes protein-tyrosine kinase is implicated in a signaling pathway triggered by granulocyte-macrophage colony-stimulating factor and interleukin-3. EMBO J 12:1641.

135. Silvennoninen O, Witthuhn BA, Quelle FW, Cleveland JL, Yi T, Ihle JN (1993) Structure of the murine JAK2 protein tyrosine kinase and its role in interleukin 3 signal transduction. Proc Natl Acad Sci USA 90:8429.

136. Quelle FW, Sato N, Witthuhn BA, Inhorn RC, Eder M, Miyajima A, Griffin JD, Ihle JN (1994) JAK2 associates with the beta c chain of the receptor for granulocyte-macrophage colony-stimulating factor, and its activation requires the membrane-proximal region. Mol Cell Biol 14:4335.

137. van der Bruggen T, Kok PTM, Raaijmakers JAM, Verhoeven AJ, Kessels RGC, Lammers JWJ,

Koenderman L (1993) Cytokine priming of the respiratory burst in human eosinophils is Ca^{2+} independent and accompanied by induction of tyrosine kinase activity. J Leukocyte Biol 53:347.

138. Mire-Sluis A, Page LA, Wadhwa M, Thorpe R (1995) Evidence for a signaling role for the α chains of granulocyte-macrophage colony-stimulating factor (GM-CSF), interleukin-3 (IL-3), and IL-5 receptor: divergent signaling pathways between GM-CSF/IL-3 and IL-5. Blood 86:2679.

139. Linnekin D, Mou SM, Greer P, Longo DL, Ferris DK (1995) Phosphorylation of a fes-related protein in response to granulocyte-macrophage colony-stimulating factor. J Biol Chem 270:4950.

140. Pazdrak K, Schreiber D, Forsythe P, Justement L, Alam R (1995) The intracellular signal transduction mechanisms of interleukin 5 in eosinophils: the involvement of lyn tyrosine kinase and the ras-raf-MEK-microtubulus-associated protein kinase pathway. J Exp Med 181:1827.

141. van der Bruggen T, Caldenhoven E, Kanters D, Coffer P, Raaijmakers JAM, Lammers JWJ, Koenderman L (1995) IL-5 signaling in human eosinophils involves JAK2 tyrosine kinase and Stat1α. Blood 85:1442.

142. Pazdrak K, Stafford S, Alam R (1995) The activation of the JAK-Stat1 signaling pathway by IL-5 in eosinophils. J Immunol 155:397.

143. Pazdrak K, Justment L, Alam R (1995) Mechanism of inhibition of eosinophil activation by transforming growth factor-β: Inhibition of Lyn, MAP, Jak2 Kinase and STAT1 nuclear factor. J Immunol 155:4454.

144. Yousefi S, Green DR, Blaser K, Simon HU (1994) Protein tyrosine phosphorylation regulates apoptosis in human eosinophils and neutrophils. Proc Natl Acad Sci USA 91:10,868.

145. Schweizer RC, Kessel-Welmers BAC, Warringa RAJ, Maikoe T, Raaijmakers JAM, Lammers JWJ, Koenderman L (1996) Mechanisms involved in eosinophil migration. Platelet-activating factor-induced chemotaxis and interleukin 5-induced chemokinesis are mediated by different signals. J Leukocyte Biol 59:347.

146. Satoh T, Nakafuku M, Kaziro Y (1992) Function of ras as a molecular switch in signal transduction. J Biol Chem 267:24149.

147. Satoh T, Nakafuku M, Miyajima A, Kaziro Y (1993) Involvement of ras p21 protein in signal-transduction pathways from interleukin 2, interleukin 3, and granulocyte/macrophage colony stimulating factor, but not from interleukin 4. Proc Natl Acad Sci USA 88:3314.

148. Cutler RL, Liu L, Damen JE, Krystal G (1993) Multiple cytokines induce the tyrosine phosphorylation of Shc and its association with Grb2 in hemopoietic cells. J Biol Chem 268:21463.

149. Welhaum MJ, Duronio V, Lislie KB, Bowtell D, Schrader JW (1994) Multiple hemopoietins, with the exception of interleukin-4, induce modification of Shc and mSos1, but not their translocation. J Biol Chem 269:21,165.

150. Matsuguchi T, Salgia R, Hallek M, Eder M, Druker B, Ernst TJ, Griffin JD (1994) Shc phosphorylation in myeloid cells is regulated by granulocyte macrophage colony-stimulating factor, interleukin-3, and steel factor and is constitutively increased by p210 BCR/ABL. J Biol Chem 269:5016.

151. Liu L, Damen JE, Cutler RL, Krystal G (1994) Multiple cytokines stimulate the binding of a common 145-kilodalton protein to Shc at the Grb2 recognition site of Shc. Mol Cell Biol 14:6926.

152. Lanfrancone L, Pelicci G, Brizzi MF, Arouica MG, Carciani C, Giuli S, Pegoraro L, Pawson T, Pelicci PG (1995) Overexpression of shc proteins potentiates the proliferative response to the granulocyte-macrophage colony-stimulating factor and recruitment of Grb2/Sos and Grb2/p140 complexes to the β receptor subunit. Oncogene 10:907.

153. Gulbins E, Coggeshall KM, Baier G, Katzav S, Burn P, Atlman A (1993) Tyrosine kinase-stimulated guanine nucleotide exchange activity of Vav in T cell activation. Science 260:822.

154. Carroll MP, Clark Lewis I, Rapp UR, May WS (1990) Interleukin-3 and granulocyte-macrophage colony-stimulating factor mediate rapid phosphorylation and activation of cytosolic c-raf. J Biol Chem 265:19,812.

155. Thompson HL, Marshall CJ, Saklatvala J (1994) Characterization of two different forms of mitogen-activated protein kinase induced in polymorphonuclear leukocytes following stimulation by N-formyl-methionyl-leucyl-phenylalaine or granulocyte-macrophage colony-stimulating factor. J Biol Chem 269:9486.

156. Welham MJ, Duronio V, Sanghera JS, Peleshi SL, MA Shrader (1992) Multiple hemopoietic growth factors stimulate activation of mitogen-activated protein kinase family members. J Immunol 149:1683.

157. Ahlers A, Engel K, Scott C, Gaestel M, Herrmann F, Brach MA (1994) Interleukin-3 and granulocyte-macrophage colony-stimulating factor induce activation of the MAPKAP kinase 2 resulting in in vitro serine phosphorylation of the small heat shock protein (Hsap 27). Blood 83:1791.

158. Satoh N, Sakamaki K, Terada N, Arai K, Miyajima A (1993) Signal transduction by the high-affinity GM-CSF receptor: two distinct cytoplasmic regions of the common beta subunit responsible for different signaling. EMBO J 12:4181.

159. Darnell JE Jr, Kerr IM, Stark GR (1994) Jak-stat pathways and transcriptional activation in response to IFNs and other extracellular signaling proteins. Science 264:1415.

160. Ihle JN, Kerr IM (1995) JAKs and Stats in signaling by the cytokine receptor superfamily. Trends Genetics 11:69.

161. Larner AC, David M, Feldman GM, Igarashi K, Hackett RH, Webb DSA, Sweitzer SM, Petricoin EF III, Finbloom DS (1993) Tyrosine phosphorylation of DNA binding proteins by multiple cytokines. Science 261:1730.

162. Lamb P, Kessler LV, Suto C, Levy DE, Seidel HM, Stein RB, Rosen J (1994) Rapid activation of proteins that interact with the interferon-γ activation site in response to multiple cytokines. Blood 83:2063.

163. Mui ALF, Wakao H, O'Farrell AM, Hanada N, Miyajima A (1995) Interleukin-3, granulocyte-macrophage colony stimulating factor and interleukin-5 transduce signals through two STAT5 homologs. EMBO J 14:1166.

164. Azam M, Erdjument-Bromage H, Kreider BL, Xia M, Quelle F, Basu R, Saris C, Tempst P, Ihle JN, Schindler C (1995) Interleukin-3 signals through multiple isoforms of Stat5. EMBO J 14:1402.

165. Gouilleux F, Pallard C, Dusanter-Fourt I, Wakao H, Haldosen LA, Norstedt G, Levy D, Groner B (1995) Prolactin, growth hormone, erythropoietin and granulocyte-macrophage colony stimulating factor induce MGF-Stat5 DNA binding activity. EMBO J 14:2005.

166. Quelle FW, Shimoda K, Thierfelder W, Fisher C, Kim A, Rubin SM, Cleveland JL, Pierce JH, Keegan AD, Nelms K, Paul WE, Ihle JN (1995) Cloning of murine Stat6 and human Stat6, Stat proteins that are tyrosine phosphorylated in response to IL-4 and IL-13 but are not required for mitogenesis. Mol Cell Biol 15:3336.

167. Caldenhoven E, van Dijk T, Raaijmakers JAM, Lammers JWJ, Koenderman L, de Groot RP (1995) Activation of the Stat3/APRF transcription factor by interleukin-5. J Biol Chem 270:25,778.

168. Matsuda T, Hirano T (1994) Association of p72 tyrosine kinase with Stat factors and its activation by interleukin-3, interleukin-6, and granulocyte colony-stimulating factor. Blood 83:3457.

169. Conscience JF, Verrier B, Martin G (1994) Interleukin-3-dependent expression of the c-myc and c-fos proto-oncogene in hemopoietic cell lines. EMBO J 5:317.

170. Lilly M, Le T, Holland P, Hendrickson SL (1992) Sustained expression of the pim-1 kinase is specifically induced in myeloid cells by cytokines whose receptors are structurally related. Oncogene 7:727.

171. Kitamura D, Kaneko H, Miyagoe Y, Ariyasu T, Watanabe T (1989) Isolation and characterization of a novel human gene expressed specifically in the cells of hematopoietic lineage. Nucleic Acid Res 17:9367.

172. Sakamoto KM, Fraser JK, Lee HJ, Lehman E, Gasson JC (1994) Granulocyte-macrophage colony-stimulating factor and interleukin-3 signaling pathways converge on the CREB-binding site in the human egr-1 promoter. Mol Cell Biol 14:5975.

173. Clark EA, Grugge JS (1995) Integrins and signal transduction pathways: the road taken. Science 268:233.

174. Zhou MJ, Todd RF, van der Winkel JGJ, Petty HR (1993) Cocapping of the leukoadhesion molecules complement receptor type 3 and lymphocyte function-associated antigen-1 with Fcγ receptor III on human neutrophils. J Immunol 150:3030.

175. Petty HR, Todd RF III (1993) Receptor-receptor interactions of complement receptor type 3 in neutrophil membranes. J Leukocyte Biol 54:492.

176. Schlaepfer DD, Hanks SK, Hunter T, van der Geer P (1994) Integrin-mediated signal transduction linked to ras pathway by grb2 binding to focal adhesion kinase. Nature 372:786.

177. Chen HC, Guan JL (1994) Association of focal adhesion kinase with its potential substrate phosphatidylinositol 3-kinase. Proc Natl Acad Sci USA 91:10,148.

178. Petruzzelli L, Takami M, Herrera R (1996) Adhesion through the interaction of lymphocyte function-associated antigen-1 with intracellular adhesion molecule-1 induces tyrosine phosphorylation of p130^{cas} ant its association with c-CrkII. J Biol Chem 271:7796.

179. Berton G, Fumagalli L, Laudanna C, Sorio C (1993) β$_2$ integrin-dependent protein tyrosine phosphorylation and activation of the FGR protein tyrosine kinase in human neutrophils. J Cell Biol 126:1111.

180. Kato M, Abraham RT, Gleich GJ, Kita H (1996) Cross-linking and clustering of Mac-1 ($\alpha_M\beta_2$) molecules induces activation and degranulation of human eosinophils. Am J Respir Crit Care Med 153:A58.

181. Kato M, Abraham RT, Okada S, Kita H (1998) Ligation of the β_2 integrin triggers activation and degranulation of human eosinophils. Am J Respir Cell Mol Biol. In press.

182. Kanner SB, Grosmaire LS, Ledbetter JA, Damale NK (1993) $\beta2$-integrin LFA-1 signaling through phospholipase C-γ1 activation. Proc Natl Acad Sci USA 90:7099.

183. Fällman M, Andersson R, Andersson T (1993) Signaling properties of CR3 (CD11b/CD18) and CR1 (CD35) in relation to phagocytosis of complement-opsonized particles. J Immunol 151:330.

184. Jaconi MEE, Theler JM, Schlegel W, Appel RD, Wright SD, Lew PD (1991) Multiple elevations of cytosolic-free Ca^{2+} in human neutrophils: initiation by adherence receptors of the integrin family. J Cell Biol 112:1249.

185. Walzog B, Seifert R, Zakrzewicz A, Gaehtgens P, Ley K (1994) Cross-linking of CD18 in human neutrophils induces an increase of intracellular free Ca^{2+} exocytosis of azurophilic granules, qualitative up-regulation of CD18, shedding of L-selectin, and actin polymerization. J Leukocyte Biol 56:625.

186. Kita H, Horie S, Gleich GJ (1996) Extracellular matrix proteins attenuate activation and degranulation of stimulated eosinophils. J Immunol 156:1174.

V PATHOGENESIS

23

Pathogenesis of Allergic Rhinitis

Niels Mygind, MD and Ronald Dahl, MD

CONTENTS

INTRODUCTION

Allergic rhinitis is a well-defined disease. Especially seasonal allergic rhinitis is well suited for studies of pathogenesis and pathophysiology, as there are plenty of patients and as allergen challenge, outside the pollen season, can produce an experimental disease state with inflammation in the nasal mucous membrane. In addition, the nose is easily accessible for direct inspection, sampling of secretions and lavage fluids, and brush and mucosal biopsies. In recent years many researchers have taken advantages of these possibilities, and as a consequense, our knowledge of the pathogenesis and pathophysiology of allergic rhinitis has increased considerably (1–3).

This paper will discuss the pathogenesis and pathophysiology of allergic rhinitis, and emphasis will be on the description of structures and tissues believed to be responsible for the nasal symptoms. T-lymphocytes, cytokines, and adhesion molecules, important for the regulation of the immunoinflammatory reaction, are only mentioned briefly, as they are described in detail in other chapters.

NASAL PHYSIOLOGY AND ALLERGEN DEPOSITION

The specialized structure of the nose is important for its functions (Figs. 1 and 2): heating, humidification, and filtration of inhaled air. The nose protects the lower airways by act-

From: *Allergy and Allergic Diseases: The New Mechanisms and Therapeutics*
Edited by: J. A. Denburg © Humana Press Inc., Totowa, NJ

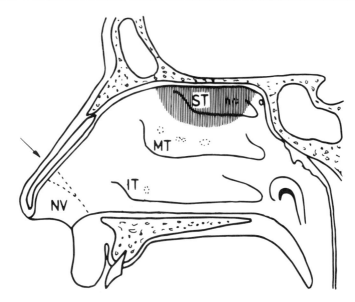

Fig. 1. Lateral wall of the nasal cavity. NV is the nasal vestibule, and the hatched area is the olfactory region. The openings from the nasolacrimal duct and paranasal sinuses are under the inferior (IT), middle (MT), and superior (ST) turbinates. The arrow points to the internal osteum, which is the narrowest part of the airway.

ing as a filter for inhaled particles. They impinge against the nasal mucosa because of the high linear velocity of inhaled air in the nose, the turbulence behind the narrow entrance to the nasal cavity (the internal ostium), and the bent route they travel through the nose. Filtration is very effective for large particles (>10 μm), and only a few pollen grains will reach the lower airways *(5)*.

Owing to its filter function, the nose receives an allergen burden, which per square centimeter must be considerably higher than in the lower airways. A prevalence of allergic rhinitis as high as 15–20% *(6)* seems to be the price to be paid for this protection of the bronchi.

As the outpost of the airways, the nose must be capable of expelling damaging inhaled substances as quickly as possible, and it is therefore understandable that neural reflexes play an important role in the nose, in which sneezing and reflex-mediated hypersecretion can quickly expel harmful substances.

Another function of the nose is provision, to the lower airways, of heating and humidification of the inhaled air. Of importance for this function is the close contact between inhaled air and the mucous membrane in the slit-like nasal cavity and the abundant vasculature in the nose *(7)*. Consequently, the nose can quickly and considerably change its baseline for airflow resistance, and it can become blocked in response to irritative stimuli and allergic inflammation.

It is a striking physiologic phenomenon, seen in a computerized tomography (CT)-scan examination, that the mucous membrane of the nasal lateral wall, at any time, is dynamically sculptured to form a template of the septal wall, maintaining the narrow slit-like cavity, of importance for normal nasal function. Contact between mucous membranes ("kissing mucous membranes") causes symptomatology (a feeling of stuffiness, hypersecretion) and perhaps also pathology owing to release of cytokines from perturbed epithelial cells.

The mechanism behind the maintenance of the slit-like cavity is unknown, but it is probably of neural origin and associated with the "nasal cycle" of alternating congestion of the two nasal cavities.

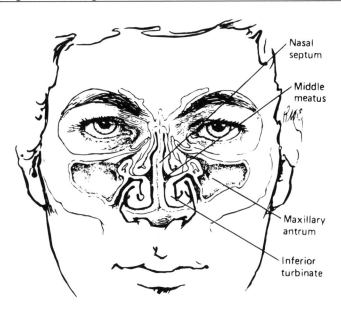

Nasal septum

Middle meatus

Maxillary antrum

Inferior turbinate

Fig. 2. Cross-section through the nasal cavities, showing turbinates and the slit-like passages. Reproduced from ref. *4* with permission.

ALLERGEN PENETRATION

The fate of inhaled allergen that becomes trapped in the nasal filter is largely unknown. Mucociliary transport carries it with a speed of 8 mm/min toward the nasopharynx, and it is swallowed and eliminated within 30 min. However, mucociliary transport also delivers a part of the trapped allergen to the adenoids, where it gets in close contact with the specialized immune system of the adenoids.

Obviously, the adenoids guard the upper airways, just as the tonsils guard the entrance to the gastrointestinal tract. However, the immunological role of the adenoids for nasal allergy has been completely neglected. Otolaryngologists just remove the tissue.

When an airborne pollen grain comes in contact with surface fluid on the nasal mucosa, allergenic molecules are eluted within seconds, and symptoms can be initiated within 30 sec *(7)*.

Probably only a small fraction of the allergen molecules will penetrate the epithelial lining, since proteins of this size (molecular weight of 10–20 kDa) are not easily absorbed from the nasal mucosa *(9)*. Little is known about allergen penetration into the human nasal mucosa, but in contrast to earlier belief, there is no evidence in support of the statement that allergen penetration is facilitated by allergic inflammation *(10)*.

The closer the immunoglobulin E (IgE)-bearing mast cells are to the airway lumen, the higher the allergen concentration to which they are exposed. Histological studies have shown that mast-cell degranulation predominantly takes place close to the epithelial surface and in the deeper parts of lamina propria, only following vigorous allergen challenge *(11,12)*.

ALLERGEN–IgE INTERACTION

In the mucous membrane, probably close to the epithelial surface, the allergen initiates an allergic reaction when it interacts with cell-attached IgE molecules. As described elsewhere in this volume, our knowledge about regulation of the IgE response has increased considerably in recent years. The high-affinity receptor (FcεRI) on mast cells and basophils (and probably on Langerhans cells) is now biochemically characterized, and low-affinity receptors (FcεRII) have been identified on T-lymphocytes, eosinophils, and other cell types. The role of FcεRII in the allergic reaction, however, remains to be defined.

ANTIGEN-PRESENTING CELLS

For allergen activation of T-lymphocytes there has to be an interaction with antigen-presenting cells. Within the airways the antigen-presenting cell appears to be the dendritic or Langerhans cell. These cells form a dendritic network within the mucosa, and studies by Fokkens and colleagues *(13)* have demonstrated a naturally occurring increase in Langerhans cells in seasonal allergic rhinitis that can be mimicked by repeated allergen challenge. Epithelial Langerhans cells are IgE bearing and may be able to react directly with allergen very close to the luminal surface of the mucous membrane. According to Fokkens et al. *(13)*, it is likely that aeroallergens cause a simultaneous stimulation of mast cells, as described in mast cells and basophils, and epithelial Langerhans cells, which by T-cell-dependent mechanisms are involved in the late phase response to allergen challenge and in the maintenance of chronic allergic rhinitis.

MAST CELLS AND BASOPHILS

These cells have a unique role to play in the pathogenesis of allergic rhinitis, since they express high-affinity receptors for IgE (FcεRI) and are the only cells that synthesize and release histamine.

The literature on the relative occurrence and importance of mast-cell subsets and basophils in the nose is somewhat confusing, and the results apparently conflicting, as different morphological *(14,15)* and immunohistochemical methods *(1,16,17)* have been used to identify the cells. However, taken together, the results give support to the statement that the mast cell is the predominant cell in the mucous membrane, whereas the basophil leucocyte, in the airway lumen, may be equal in number to the mast cell *(17)* or may even outnumber it *(1)*. Mast cells of the MC_T type are the most prevalent subset in the surface epithelium *(18)* and mast cells of the MC_{TC} type in the lamina propria *(16)*. Thus, it is clear that there are marked differences between the relative occurrence of these cell types in different compartments of the nasal mucosa.

During the early-phase response to allergen challenge there are morphological *(15)* and biochemical *(1)* signs of mast-cell degranulation. During the late-phase response there in an influx of basophils *(1)* and mast cells (MC_T) *(17)* to the surface epithelium, and the number of intraepithelial cells is increased in symptomatic allergic rhinitis, whereas the number of cells in lamina propria is unchanged *(16)*. The increased number of surface mediator cells may explain the priming phenomenon, which consists of an increasing nasal sensitivity to subsequent allergen provocations *(19)*.

Thus, it is well established that mast cells, by release of histamine and lipid mediators, elicit the symptoms of the early-phase response to allergen in the nose. More recently it has been shown that the mast cell also, by the synthesis and release of cytokines *(20)*, has the potential of contributing to the late-phase inflammatory response.

The intraepithelial cells are probably the most important mast cells, since they come in contact with allergen quickly and in large amounts. In addition, histamine release from these cells results in more symptomatology than release from submucosal cells. This can be illustrated by a simple experiment performed by M. Okuda. When histamine is dropped onto the mucous membrane it causes itching, sneezing, rhinorrhea, and blockage, whereas submucosal injection of the same amount of histamine only results in slight blockage.

It is sometimes difficult to reconcile the hypothesis of a central role played by intraepithelial mast cells with the fact that a pollen challenge readily induces symptoms outside the season, when the number of intraepithelial mast cells is close to zero *(16)*.

EOSINOPHILS

The simple counting of eosinophils in nasal secretion/smear, already introduced in 1922, is still the best parameter of allergic inflammation in the nose *(21)*. The role of the eosinophil in the pathogenesis of allergic rhinitis, however, is less clear.

It is obvious that the number of eosinophils increases in the epithelium and lamina propria during the late-phase response to allergen challenge in the nose and that these cells immunochemically show signs of activation, paralled by increased levels of eosinophil proteins (eosinophil cationic protein [ECP], major basic protein [MBP]) in nasal lavage fluid *(1,22)*. Similar findings, at lower quantitative levels, are seen in symptomatic allergic rhinitis *(16,23)*.

Eosinophil accumulation and activation, during the late-phase response, is paralleled in time by an increase in nonspecific nasal responsiveness. Knowing the cytotoxic potential of eosinophil proteins for airway epithelial cells, it is natural to postulate a causal relationship between eosinophil activation and the development of hyperresponsiveness. In favor of this hypothesis is that topical corticosteroids markedly reduce in parallel the clinical late-phase symptoms *(22)*, eosinophil accumulation and activation *(24)*, and the increase in responsiveness *(25)*. The correlation between late-phase eosinophilia and increased responsiveness has been investigated by two groups, with different results.

The late Ulf Pipkorn's group in Lund, Sweden *(25)*, did not find a positive correlation between eosinophil influx and increased responsiveness, measured by a nasal methacholine test, and they questioned the importance of eosinophils for the development of hyperresponsiveness. Konno's group, in Japan *(2)*, on the other hand, not only found a positive correlation between the two parameters, but also between the degree of steroid-induced improvement of nasal reactivity to histamine and the degree of decrease of ECP in nasal lavage fluid.

Although the problem has not been resolved, it seems fair to conclude that, at present, the release of eosinophil proteins seems to be the best candidate for the explanation of nonspecific nasal reactivity in allergic rhinitis.

A similar hypothesis is now widely, almost generally, accepted for the lower airways and asthma. It is claimed that the eosinophil-induced increased airway responsiveness is associated with gross damage to the epithelium and shedding of epithelial cells in the bronchi. However, in the nose the epithelial layer is intact in spite of local eosinophilia and hyperresponsiveness *(26)*. Perhaps the pronounced bronchial changes are a result of the combined effects of eosinophil proteins and mechanical pressure from mucus plugs and bronchoconstriction.

In spite of the morphologically intact nasal epithelium, it is still a tenable hypothesis that eosinophil proteins have a negative influence on epithelial cell function and perhaps impair cell attachment, rendering the epithelium more fragile. Many years ago we found more epithelial cells in smears from patients with allergic rhinitis than from normal controls *(27)*, and in a recent electron microscopic study Yang et al. *(28)* found an increased number of epithelial cells in suctioned secretions from allergic rhinitis patients.

The eosinophil may play another important role in the pathogenesis of allergic rhinitis. It is the quantitatively most important inflammatory cell in allergic inflammation and, as a rich source of leukotriene D_4 (LTD_4), it may contribute to nasal blockage during the late-phase response and in chronic allergic rhinitis. Terada et al. *(2)* found a good correlation between LTD_4 in nasal lavage fluid and nasal blockage. A significant pathogenic role of LTD_4 has

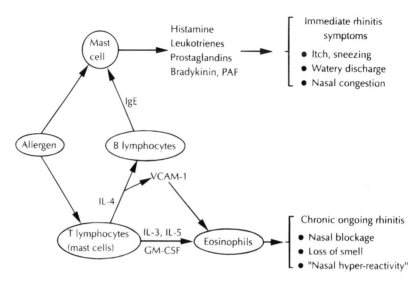

Fig. 3. Hypothesis on mechanisms of allergic rhinitis. From Stephen R. Durham, National Heart and Lung Institute, London.

recently been indicated by controlled studies, which showed effect on nasal blockage of a LTD_4-receptor antagonist *(29)* and a 5-lipoxygenase inhibitor *(30)*.

T-LYMPHOCYTES AND CYTOKINES

The interplay between T cells, cytokines, and adhesion molecules in the regulation of the immunoinflammatory reaction is described in other chapters, and we will confine our contribution to a brief description of the quantitative findings in studies of the human nasal mucosa. A simplified presentation is given in Fig. 3.

Normal Numbers of Total T-Cells

The number of $CD3^+$ total T-cells and $CD8^+$ cytotoxic T-cells in the nasal lamina propria is not increased following allergen challenge *(31)*, in seasonal *(16)* or perennial allergic rhinitis *(32)*. It is uncertain whether there are changes in the number of intraepithelial cells.

Increased Numbers of Activated and Memory T-Helper Cells

The number of $CD4^+$ T helper cells is increased following allergen challenge *(31)* and in perennial allergic rhinitis *(32,33)*, whereas the results in seasonal allergic rhinitis vary *(16,33)*. There is also an increase in the number of $CD25^+$ activated T-cells following allergen challenge *(31)* and exposure *(33)* and of $CD45RO^+$ memory T-cells in perennial allergic rhinitis *(32)*.

Increased T Helper 2 Cytokine Profile

In their classical *in situ* hybridization study, Durham et al. *(34)* showed increases in messenger ribonucleic acid positive ($mRNA^+$) cells for interleukin (IL)-3, IL-4, IL-5, and granulocyte-macrophage colony-stimulating factor (GM-CSF) following nasal allergen provocation and a positive correlation between IL-5 $mRNA^+$ cells and eosinophils.

Recently, two studies using reverse transcriptase polymerase chain reaction have been published. Karlsson et al. *(35)* found IL-4 mRNA almost exclusively in allergic patients following allergen challenge and exposure in the pollen season, whereas they did not find any difference with regard to IL-2 and IL-5. Studying epithelial scrapings and full nasal biopsies in patients with perennial allergic rhinitis, Pawankar et al. *(36)* found expression of IL-13 genes in intraepithelial T-lymphocytes and mast cells in 18 out of 19 patients and in none of five normal controls and six patients with chronic infective rhinitis. The level of IL-13 gene expression correlated strongly with the level of total serum IgE.

Other Sources of Cytokines

Studies of the nasal mucosa (in allergic rhinitis) have shown synthesis of IL-4, IL-5, and IL-6 in mast cells, IL-5 in eosinophils *(20)* and IL-1α, IL-6, and IL-8 in epithelial cells *(37)*.

ADHESION MOLECULES

Endothelial Cells

Lee et al. *(38)* found an upregulation of vasular cell adhesion molecule (VCAM)-1, but not intercellular adhesion molecule (ICAM)-1, on endothelial cells 24 h after allergen provocation. There was a weak positive correlation between VCAM-1 expression and the number of submucosal eosinophils.

Adhesion molecules are upregulated when stimulated by various substances, including inflammatory cytokines. Using the method of gene expression quantification, Terada et al. *(39)* showed that IL-5 can induce ICAM-1 gene expression in the nasal mucosa of patients with perennial allergic rhinitis, but not in patients with perennial nonallergic noneosinophilic rhinitis, suggesting that allergic reactions favor adhesion molecule induction by IL-5.

Epithelial Cells

Ciprandi et al. *(40)*, studying nasal epithelial cells, found expression of ICAM-1 (CD54) only during the pollen season in allergic subjects. They concluded that seasonal allergic rhinitis is characterized by an infiltration of inflammatory cells correlated with CD54 expression on nasal epithelial cells. These authors *(41)* considered CD54 to be an early and sensitive marker of an allergic reaction, since they found CD54 expression within 30 min of allergen provocation, lasting for at least 24 h, in patients but not in normal controls. It is thought-provoking that ICAM-1, so significantly upregulated by allergen exposure, is the human receptor for rhinovirus *(42)*.

EXPERIMENTAL ALLERGEN CHALLENGE AND NATURAL ALLERGEN EXPOSURE

A nasal allergen challenge is often used in the study of patogenesis and pathophysiology of allergic rhinitis. It is easy to perform, the nasal mucosa is accessible for examinations, there are many volunteers, and they can be studied outside and during the pollen season.

When the sensitized human nose is challenged with pollen outside the season, sneezing, watery rhinorrhea, and blockage follow within minutes. This early-phase response is caused by mediators predominantly released from mast cells, and histamine is by far the most important mediator.

The allergic response does not end with the early-phase symptoms within an hour. During the rest of the day many patients have occasional sneezing, nose blowings, and sustained nasal blockage. In contrast to the bronchial late-phase response, the one in the nose is considerably weaker than the early-phase response, and a biphasic pattern is not a typical feature *(22)*. The late-phase symptom response is associated with increased nasal responsiveness to allergen, histamine, and methacholine and an increased influx and activation of eosinophils, basophils, and mast cells (MC$_T$) to the epithelium, as described above.

Extravasation of albumin from postcapillary venules is used as a marker of inflammation *(10)*. However, the albumin content in nasal lavage fluid is considerably higher during the early-phase response than during the late-phase inflammatory response. In addition, glandular hypersecretion increases the albumin level on the epithelial surface *(43)*.

Although very useful for the study of basic mechanisms, a laboratory challenge is an artificial situation in which one single challenge is given with a hugh dose of allergen. Natural exposure to pollen in the season consists of 15,000 tiny challenges per day. Symptoms are caused by a mixture of early-phase and late-phase responses, hyperresponsiveness, reflex activity, and inflammation. The mutual relations between these pathophysiological factors may not be the same in artificial challenge and natural exposure. In nasal lavage fluid, Wang et al. *(44)* found a higher ratio between tryptase (marker of early phase) and ECP (marker of late phase) following artificial challenge than during natural exposure in the pollen season.

ITCHING AND SNEEZING: SENSORY NERVES

Itching in the nose, leading to sneezing attacks, is highly characteristic for allergic rhinitis. There are two lines of evidence indicating that histamine is the most important mediator of this symptom. First, intranasal spraying of histamine, but not leukotrienes, prostaglandins, and kinins, gives the same sensation of itch *(3)*. Second, an H_1 antihistamine can almost completely inhibit itching and sneezing in the early-phase nasal response and in seasonal allergic rhinitis as well *(45)*.

Histamine stimulates sensory nerve endings and induces neural reflexes, but H_1 receptors have not been identified on sensory nerve endings in the nose, so there is only indirect evidence for their existence.

Table 1 summarizes the association between putative mediators and nasal symptoms, and Fig. 4 gives a simplified presentation of the effects of histamine in the nose.

RHINORRHEA: SUBMUCOSAL GLANDS

In theory, nasal discharge can have a multitude of sources such as nasal glands, goblet cells, plasma exudation, secretions from paranasal sinuses, tears, and condensed expired water. There are about 100,000 submucosal glands in the human nose or $8/mm^2$, compared to $1/mm^2$ in the trachea *(46)*. The glands are mixed seromucous with 8 times as many serous as mucous acini (unpublished data). They are under the control of the parasympathetic nervous system, in contrast to the mucous goblet cells in the surface epithelium *(47)*. Whereas watery nasal secretion is predominantly derived from glands, mucous secretion from paranasal sinuses is mainly produced by goblet cells, as there are very few glands in the sinuses *(46)*.

The substance blown out of allergic noses has traditionally been called secretion. Recently, its origin from submucosal glands has been questioned, as plasma exudation is demonstrated as a consistent consequence of allergic airway inflammation *(48)*.

Although plasma products are found in nasal surface fluid and may contain molecules that contribute to nasal symptoms, a series of arguments speak against any significant contribution of plasma exudation to the volume and physical characteristics of nasal surface fluid:

1. The biophysical properties of nasal surface fluid, especially its high elasticity, convincingly show a contribution of glycoproteins from mucus-producing cells *(47)*.
2. Surface fluid collected during the early-phase response to allergen *(49)* and during natural pollen exposure *(50)* contains about 1 mg/mL of the plasma marker albumin, and this constitutes only 2–3% of normal plasma levels.

Table 1
Symptoms of Allergic Rhinitis and Putative Mediators

Symptom	Pathological features	Putative mediator
Itching	Sensory nerve stimulation	Histamine (H_1)
Sneezing	Sensory nerve stimulation, somatic reflex, and expiratory muscle contraction	Histamine (H_1)
Rhinorrhea	Sensory nerve stimulation and cholinergic glandular reflex	Histamine (H_1)
	Direct effect on glands	Histamine (H_2) Leukotrienes Other secretogoges
	Direct effect on goblet cells	Surface irritants
Nasal obstruction	Vasodilatation	Histamine (H_1) Histamine (H_2) Leukotrienes Prostaglandins? Vasoactive intestinal polypeptide (VIP)?
	Extravasation and edema formation	Histamine (H_1) Leukotrienes? Prostaglandins? Platelet-activating factor (PAF)? Substance P? Not histamine
Hyperirritability and hyper-responsiveness	Increased sensitivity of nerve endings	Eosinophil products? Not histamine
	Increased responsiveness of vasculature and glands	Eosinophil products?

3. The concentration of albumin in blown nasal secretions is similar following allergen challenge and glandular hypersecretion induced by a methacholine challenge *(49)*.
4. The formation of nasal fluids following an allergen challenge can be inhibited efficiently by pretreatment with atropine, which blocks the glandular cholinoceptors *(51)*.

These observations, in our opinion, give convincing evidence that nasal surface fluid in allergic rhinitis is mainly derived from submucosal glands.

BLOCKAGE: VASODILATATION AND EDEMA

The airway mucosa, including the nasal mucous membrane, contains postcapillary venules, which upon action from mediator substances, such as histamine, leak unfiltered plasma-proteins into the tissue with the subsequent formation of edema *(10)*. Most marked is the enormous tissue edema seen in nasal polyps, where gaps between endothelial cells are directly visible *(52)*.

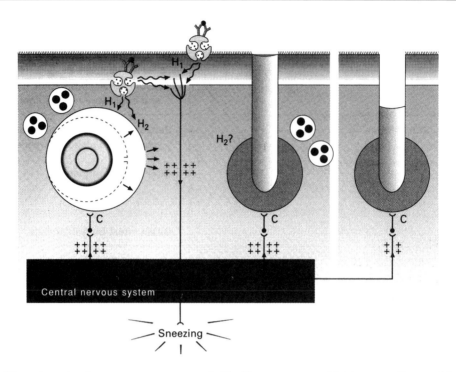

Fig. 4. Histamine stimulates sensory nerves, probably H_1 receptors, and initiates a reflex resulting in sneezing and a parasympathetic reflex that via cholinoceptors (C) results in bilateral hypersecretion and transient vasodilatation. Histamine causes vasodilatation by a direct effect on vascular H_1 and H_2 receptors and edema formation by an effect on vascular H_1 receptors. Glands possess H_2 receptors, but their significance in the airways is unknown.

The nose, in contrast to the remainder of the airway mucosa, has large venous sinusoids that can quickly change their volume and with that the degree of nasal congestion *(7)*.

We do not know precisely to what extent nasal blockage in rhinitis is caused by edema and vasodilatation, respectively. Pretreatment with a topical vasoconstrictor can inhibit the allergen-induced increase in nasal airway resistance during the early-phase response *(53)*, which points at vasodilatation as the most important factor for acute rhinitis. The contribution of edema formation probably increases in chronic disease.

PATHOPHYSIOLOGY AND PHARMACOTHERAPY

As mentioned earlier, H_1 antihistamines have a marked effect on itching and sneezing, a moderate effect on hypersecretion, and little or no effect on blockage *(45,54)*.

The effect on sneezing and rhinorrhea is mediated via nervous H_1 receptors and neural reflexes. The submucosal glands do not have H_1 receptors. They have H_2 receptors, but H_2 antihistamines are without any significant effect on nasal hypersecretion *(55)*. The lack of H_1 antihistamine effect on nasal blockage is surprising and difficult to explain, because antihistamines have proven antiexudation effects *(45)*, and the nasal vasculature possesses both H_1 and H_2 receptors *(55)*.

A part of the explanation is the contribution of other mediators to this symptom. As mentioned above, recent studies indicate that LTD_4 plays a role in mediating nasal blockage. For clinical use, it will be necessary to combine LTD_4 antagonists with H_1 antagonists in order to get an effect on all nasal symptoms. A series of nonsedating antihistamines have mast-cell-stabilizing or antiallergic effect in vitro *(45)*, but clinical trials have not shown superior efficacy of these compounds over the pure H_1 histamine receptor blockers. In general, the effect of so-called antiallergic compounds in the nose has been disappointing.

Prophylactic treatment with glucocorticoids has a more fundamental effect on mucosal inflammation. This effect is considered to be secondary to the regulatory effect on cytokine gene transcription, especially in T-lymphocytes *(35,56)*, which again is responsible for a reduction in the number of effector cells characteristic of allergic inflammation, i.e., mast cells and eosinophils *(57)*.

A glucocorticoid, preferably used topically, is the most effective therapy of rhinitis *(57)*. It is effective in all cases of allergic and in most cases of nonallergic rhinitis. Apparently, responsiveness to steroids is associated with T-cell-driven eosinophil-dominated inflammation, whereas neutrophil-dominated inflammation, for example in the common cold, responds poorly to corticosteroids. Reliable tests for the demonstration of nasal eosinophil inflammation may be helpful in the future for the identification of steroid responders among patients with perennial nonallergic rhinitis.

REFERENCES

1. Naclerio RM, Baroody FM, Kagey-Sobotka A, Lichtenstein LM (1994) Basophils and eosinophils in allergic rhinitis. J Allergy Clin Immunol 94:1303–1309.
2. Terada N, Konno A, Togawa K (1994) Biochemical proterties of eosinophils and their preferential accumulation mechanism in nasal allergy. J Allergy Clin Immunol 94:629–642.
3. Howarth PH (1995) The cellular basis for allergic rhinitis. Clin Exp Allergy 50 (Suppl 23):6–10.
4. Proctor DF (1989) The upper respiratory tract. In: Fishman AP, ed. Pulmonary Diseases and Disorders. McGraw-Hill, New York, pp. 209–223.
5. Andersen I, Proctor DF (1982) The fate and effects of inhaled materials. In: Proctor DF, Andersen I, eds. The Nose: Upper Airway Physiology and the Atmospheric Environment. Elsevier, Amsterdam, pp. 423–455.
6. Strachan DP (1995) Epidemiology of hay fever: towards a community diagnosis. Clin Exp Allergy 25:296–303.
7. Eccles R (1995) Nasal airways. In: Busse WW, Holgate ST, eds. Asthma and Rhinitis. Blackwell, Oxford, pp. 73–79.
8. Løwenstein H, Mygind N (1978) Extraction and degradation of timothy pollen allergen during simulated *in vivo* conditions. Allergy 33:238–240.
9. Chien YW, Su KSE, Chang S-F (1989) Nasal systemic drug delivery. Marcel Dekker, New York.
10. Persson CGA, Svensson C, Greif L, Andersson M, Wollmer P, Alkner U, Erjefält I (1992) The use of the nose to study the inflammatory response of the respiratory tract. Thorax 47:993–1000.
11. Viegas M, Gomez E, Brooks J, Davies RJ (1989) Changes in mast cell numbers in and out of the pollen season. Int Arch Allergy Appl Immunol 82:275–276.
12. Fokkens WJ, Godthelp T, Holm AF, Mulder PGH, Vroom TM, Rijntes E (1992) Dynamics of mast cells in the nasal mucosa of patients with allergic rhinitis and non-allergic controls. Clin Exp Allergy 22:701–710.
13. Fokkens WJ, Vroom TM, Rijntes E, Mulder PGH (1989) Fluctuation of the number of CD1a (T6)-positive dendritic cells, presumably Langerhans cells, in the nasal mucosa of patients with isolated grass-pollen allergy before, during and after the grass-pollen season. J Allergy Clin Immunol 84:39–43.
14. Okuda M, Sakaguchi Y, Suzuki F, Ohtsuka H, Kawabori S (1985) Ultrastructural heterogeneity of the basophilic cells in the allergic nasal mucosa. Ann Allergy 54:152–157.
15. Enerbäck L, Pipkorn U, Olafsson A (1986) Intraepithelial migration of mucosal mast cells in hay fever: ultrastructural observations. Int Arch Allergy Appl Immunol 81:289–297.
16. Bentley M, Jacobson MR, Cumberworth V, et al. (1992) Immunohistology of the nasal mucosa in seasonal allergic rhinitis: increases in activated eosinophils and epithelial mast cells. J Allergy Clin Immunol 89:877–883.
17. Juliusson S, Karlsson G, Bachert C, Enerbäck L (1994) Metachromatic, IgE-bearing and tryptase-containing cells on the nasal mucosal surface in provoked allergic rhinitis. Acta Pathologica Microbiologica et Immunologica Scandinavica 102:153–160.

18. Otsuka H, Inaba M, Fujikura T, Kunitomo M (1995) Histological and functional characteristics of metachromatic cells in the nasal epithelium in allergic rhinitis: studies of nasal scrapings and their disperse cells. J Allergy Clin Immunol 96:528–536.

19. Connell JT (1969) Quantitative intranasal pollen challenges. J Allergy Clin Immunol 43:33–44.

20. Bradding P, Feather IH, Wilson S, Bardin PG, Heusser CH, Holgate ST, Howarth PH (1993) Immunolocalization of cytokines in the nasal mucosa of normal and perennial rhinitis subjects. J Immunol 151:3853–3865.

21. Sulukvelidze I, Conway M, Evans S, Djuric V, Dolovich J (1995) Perennial allergic rhinitis: clinical and nasal irrigation fluid findings. J Allergy Clin Immunol 95:191 (abstract).

22. Grønborg H, Bisgaard H, Rømeling F, Mygind N (1993) Early and late nasal symptom response to allergen challenge. Allergy 48:87–93.

23. Wang D, Clement P, Smitz J, De Waele M, Derde M-P (1995) Correlations between complaints, inflammatory cells and mediator concentration in nasal secretions after nasal allergen challenge and during natural allergen exposure. Int Arch Allergy Immunol 106:278–285.

24. Bisgaard H, Grønborg H, Mygind N, Dahl R, Lindqvist N, Venge P (1990) Allergen-induced increase of eosinophil cationic protein in nasal lavage fluid: effect of the glucocorticoid budesonide. J Allergy Clin Immunol 85:891–895.

25. Klementsson H (1992) Eosinophils and the pathophysiology of allergic rhinitis. Clin Exp Allergy 22:1058–1064.

26. Lim MC, Taylor RM, Naclerio RM (1995) The histology of allergic rhinitis and its comparison to cellular changes in nasal lavage fluid. Am J Respir Crit Care Med 151:136–144.

27. Mygind N, Thomsen J (1973) Cytology of the nasal mucosa. Arch Klin Exp Ohr Nas Kehl Heilk 201:123–129.

28. Yang P-C, Okuda M, Pawankar R, Aihara K (1995) Electron microscopical studies of the cell population in nasal secretions. Rhinology 33:70–77.

29. Donelly AR, Glass M, Minkwitz C, Casale TB (1995) The leukotriene D_4-receptor antagonist, ICI 204,219, relieves symptoms of acute seasonal allergic rhinitis. Am J Respir Crit Care Med 151:1734–1739.

30. Howarth PH, Harrison K, Lau L (1995) The influence of a 5-lipoxygenase inhibitor in allergic rhinitis. Int Arch Allergy Immunol 107:423–424.

31. Varney VA, Jacobson MR, Sudderick RM, et al. (1992) Immunohistology of the nasal mucosa following allergen-induced rhinitis. Am Rev Respir Dis 146:170–176.

32. Pawankar RU, Okuda M, Okubo K, Ra S (1995) Lymphocyte subsets of the nasal mucosa in perennial allergic rhinitis. Am J Respir Crit Care Med 152:2049–2058.

33. Calderon MA, Lozewicz S, Prior A, Jordan S, Davies RJ (1994) Lymphocyte infiltration and thickness of the nasal mucous membrane in perennial and seasonal allergic rhinitis. J Allergy Clin Immunol 93:635–643.

34. Durham SR, Ying S, Varney V, et al. (1992) Cytokine messenger RNA expression for IL-3, IL-4, IL-5, and GM-CSF in the nasal mucosa after local allergen provoction: relationship to tissue eosinophilia. J Immunol 148:2390–2394.

35. Karlsson MG, Davidsson Å, Viale G, Grazziani D, Hellquist HB (1995) Nasal messenger RNA expression of interleukins 2, 4 and 5 in patients with allergic rhinitis. Diagn Mol Pathol 4:85–92.

36. Pawankar RU, Okuda M, Hasegawa S, et al. (1995) Interleukin-13 expression in the nasal mucosa of perennial allergic rhinitis. Am J Respir Crit Care Med 152:2059–2067.

37. Kenney JS, Baker C, Welch MR, Altman LC (1994) Synthesis of interleukin-1α, interleukin-6, and interleukin-8 by cultured human nasal epithelial cells. J Allergy Clin Immunol 93:1060–1067.

38. Lee B-J, Naclerio RM, Bochner BS, Taylor RM, Lim MC, Baroody FM (1994) Nasal challenge with allergen upregulates the local expression of vascular endothelial adhesion molecules. J Allergy Clin Immunol 94:1006–1016.

39. Terada N, Konno A, Fukasa S, et al. (1995) Interleukin-5 upregulates intercellular adhesion molecule-1 gene expression in the nasal mucosa in nasal allergy but not in nonallergic rhinitis. Int Arch Allergy Immunol 106:139–145.

40. Ciprandi G, Pronzato C, Ricca V, Bagnasco M, Canonica GW (1994) Evidence of intercellular adhesion molecule-1 expression on nasal epithelial cells in acute rhinoconjunctivitis caused by pollen exposure. J Allergy Clin Immunol 99:738–746.

41. Ciprandi G, Pronzato C, Ricca V, Passalacqua G, Bagnasco M, Canonica GW (1994) Allergen-specific challenge induces intercellular adhesion molecule 1 (ICAM-1 or CD54) on nasal epithelial cells in allergic subjects. Am J Respir Crit Care Med 1150:1653–1659.

42. Greve JM, Davis G, Meyer AM, et al. (1989) The major human rhinovirus receptor is ICAM-1. Cell 56:839–847.

43. Jacobi H, Stahl-Skov P, Bindslev-Jensen C, Prtorius C, Weeke B, Mygind N. Histamine and tryptase in nasal lavage fluid following challenge with allergen and methacholine. Clin Exp Allergy (in press).

44. Wang D, Clement P, Smitz J, Derde M-P (1994) Concentrations of chemical mediators in nasal secretions of patients with hay fever during natural allergen exposure. Acta Otolaryngol (Stockh) 114:552–555.

45. Simons FER (1993) Antihistamines. In: Mygind N, Naclerio RM, eds. Allergic and Non-allergic Rhinitis: Clinical Aspects. Munksgaard, Copenhagen, pp. 123–136.

46. Tos M (1982) Distribution of mucus producing elements in the respiratory tract. Eur J Respir Dis 64 (Suppl 128):269–279.

47. Mygind N (1993) Hypersecretion in the airways. In: Andrews P, Widdicombe J, eds. Pathophysiology of the Gut and Airways. Portland, London, pp. 47–57.

48. Persson CGA, Pipkorn U (1990) Pathogenesis and pharmacology of asthma and rhinitis. In: Mygind N, Pipkorn U, Dahl R, eds. Rhinitis and Asthma: Similarities and Differences. Munksgaard, Copenhagen, pp. 275–288.

49. Brofeldt S, Mygind N, Sørensen CH, Readman AS, Marriott C (1986) Biochemical analysis of nasal secretions induced by methacholine, histamine, and allergen provocation. Am Rev Respir Dis 133:1138–1142.

50. Mygind N, Weeke B, Ullman S (1974) Quantitative determination of immunoglobulins in nasal secretion. Int Arch Allergy Appl Immunol 49:99–107.

51. Konno A, Togawa K, Fujiwara T (1983) The mechanisms involved in onset of allergic manifestations in the nose. Eur J Respir Dis 64(128):155–166.

52. Cauna N, Hinderer KH, Manzetti GW, Swansson EW (1972) Fine structure of nasal polyps. Ann Otol Rhinol Laryngol 81:41–58.

53. Brooks CD, Karl KJ, Francom SF (1993) Effect of vasoconstrictor pre-treatment on obstruction, secretion and sneezing after nasal challenge with threshold and suprathreshold allergen doses. Rhinology 31:165–168.

54. Wihl J-Å, Petersen BN, Petersen BN, Gundersen G, Bresson K, Mygind N (1985) Effect of the non-sedative H_1-receptor antagonist astemizole in perennial allergic and nonallergic rhinitis. J Allergy Clin Immunol 75:720–772.

55. Secher C, Kirkegaard J, Borum P, Maansson A, Osterhammel P, Mygind N (1982) Significance of H_1 and H_2 receptors in the human nose. J Allergy Clin Immunol 70:211–218.

56. Rak S, Jacobson MR, Sudderick RM, et al. (1994) Influence of prolonged treatment with topical corticosteroid (fluticasone propionate) on early and late phase nasal responses and cellular infiltration in the nasal mucosa after allergen challenge. Clin Exp Allergy 24:930–939.

57. Mygrand N, Lund V (1996) Topical corticosteroid therapy of rhinitis. Clin Immunother 5:122–136.

24 Pathogenic Mechanisms of Urticaria

Allen P. Kaplan, MD

CONTENTS

INTRODUCTION

Urticaria and angioedema are common disorders affecting approx 20% of the population at some time during their lifetime. Urticaria (hives) is an intensely pruritic rash that consists of a centrally raised blanched wheal surrounded by an erythematous flare that is generally circular but can vary greatly in size and shape depending on the particular type. It is caused by inflammation that is localized to the venular plexuses of the superficial dermis. Angioedema (except hereditary and vibratory angioedema) has the same causes and pathogenic mechanisms as does urticaria, but the reaction occurs in the deep dermis and subcutaneous tissue and has swelling as the prominent manifestation with a normal external appearance of the skin.

Inflammatory mechanisms operative in urticaria can be divided into two general types, depending on the rate at which hive formation occurs and the length of time it is evident. One form of urticaria has lesions that last 1–2 h and results from degranulation of mast cells. The inciting stimulus is present only briefly, and there is no late component to the urticaria. Biopsy of such lesions reveals little or no cellular infiltrate. The second form has a prominent cellular infiltrate, and individual lesions can last from many hours to as long as 2 d. In this chapter I describe the various types of urticarias, ranging from those that are among the most fleeting (and simplest) to those of progressively longer duration. The focus will be on pathogenic mechanisms and the nature of the inflammatory reaction.

THE PHYSICAL URTICARIAS

Physically induced hives and/or swelling share the common property of being reproducibly induced by environmental factors such as a change in temperature or by direct stimulation of the skin by pressure, stroking, vibration, or light *(1)*. These disorders have been the subject of considerable investigation and serve as models *(2)* from which we have learned a great deal about pathogenic mechanisms leading to hive formation and swelling. A classification of these disorders is given in Table 1, which includes virtually all described types.

Cold-Dependent Disorders

Idiopathic cold urticaria is characterized by the rapid onset of pruritus, erythema, and swelling after exposure to a cold stimulus. The location of the swelling is confined to those

From: *Allergy and Allergic Diseases: The New Mechanisms and Therapeutics*
Edited by: J. A. Denburg © Humana Press Inc., Totowa, NJ

Table 1
Classification of Physically Induced Urticaria and/or Angioedema

1. Cold-dependent disorders
   a. Idiopathic cold urticaria
   b. Cold urticaria associated with abnormal serum proteins: cold agglutinins, cryo-globulin, cryofibrinogen, Donath-Landsteiner antibody
   c. Systemic cold urticaria
   d. Cold-induced cholinergic urticaria
   e. Cold-dependent dermatographism
   f. Delayed cold urticaria
2. Exercise-induced disorders
   a. Exercise-induced anaphylaxis: idiopathic or food-dependent
   b. Cholinergic urticaria (*see* item 1d for cold-dependent variant)
   c. Exercise-induced angioedema
3. Local heat urticaria
   a. Familial variant
4. Dermatographism
   a. Urticaria pigmentosa/systemic mastocytosis
   b. Cold-dependent variant (*see* item 1e)
   c. Delayed dermatographism
5. Pressure-induced urticaria/angioedema (delayed)
   a. Immediate-pressure urticaria
6. Solar urticaria
   a–f. Types I–VI
7. Aquagenic urticaria
8. Vibratory angioedema
   a. Familial
   b. Sporadic

parts of the body that have been exposed; in this sense it is a local, rather than a systemic, disorder. However, total body exposure such as occurs with swimming can cause massive release of vasoactive mediators, resulting in hypotension; if the subject "passes out," death by drowning can result. The disease can begin in any age group and has no obvious sex predilection. When suspected, an ice-cube test can be performed in which an ice cube is placed on the subject's forearm for 4–5 min. A positive reaction leads to formation of a hive the shape of the ice cube within 10 min *after* the stimulus is removed. The time course of this reaction, i.e., cold challenge followed by hive formation as the area returns to body temperature, demonstrates that a two-step reaction has occurred in which exposure to cold is a prerequisite but hive formation actually occurs as the temperature increases.

The term "idiopathic" was utilized to indicate that the cause of cold urticaria is unknown and is unassociated with abnormal circulating plasma proteins such as cryoglobulins or cold agglutinins. However, there is evidence that many of these are nevertheless caused by an immunologic reaction. Within this group, most have been shown to be immunoglobulin E (IgE)-dependent, based on passive-transfer studies *(3)*. Serum of the subject is injected intradermally into a normal recipient. After 48 h, the site is challenged with an ice cube. Although the incidence of positive transfer has varied in different studies, our experience suggests that about 10% clearly are positive. This is undoubtedly an underestimate, since the passive transfer is far less sensitive than doing an ice cube test in the propositus, and only those with sufficient pathogenic IgE in the circulation (rather than those bound to mast cells) are detected.

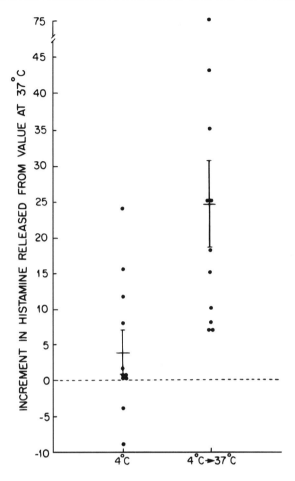

Fig. 1. In vitro histamine release upon challenge of skin biopsies by exposure to various temperatures. Using specimens maintained at 37°C as baseline, the increment in histamine release (ordinate) is compared to comparable samples from each subject that are either chilled to 4°C (left) or chilled for 10 min and then warmed to 37°C (right). The latter condition reproduces the ice cube test used to diagnose suspected patients and results in a prominent augmentation of histamine release.

In two cases, an IgM antibody was shown to mediate cold urticaria *(4)*. In these cases, passive transfer was positive after a short interval of 3–6 h but was negative at 48 h, in contrast to an IgE-mediated reaction, which remains positive at 48 h. We have also reported a similar passive transfer (i.e., positive only after short-term sensitization) that seemed to be caused by an IgG antibody *(5)*.

Studies of the pathogenesis of cold urticaria have demonstrated release of mediators into the circulation upon challenge of patients by placing one hand in ice water for 5 min and obtaining serial blood samples for 20 min thereafter. As with the ice-cube test, swelling is usually not evident while the hand is being chilled; instead, swelling appears between 4–8 min thereafter and is associated with marked pruritus. In this case, chilling occurs in the deep dermis and subcutaneous tissue in addition to more superficial skin layers; thus the entire hand swells and angioedema results. Studies have documented release of histamine *(6)*, eosinophilotactic peptides *(7)*, high-molecular-weight neutrophil chemotactic factor (NCF) *(8)*, platelet-activating factor *(9)*, and prostaglandin D_2 *(10,11)* into the circulation with a time course that parallels the

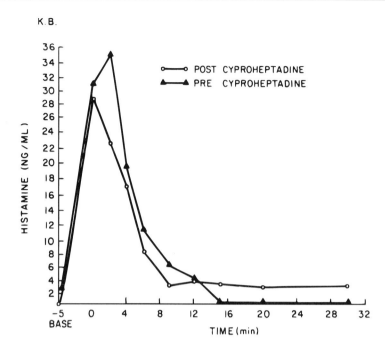

Fig. 2. Time course of histamine release on the challenge of a patient with cold urticaria by placing one hand in ice water and sampling venous blood draining that hand over time. The procedure was performed before and after treatment with cyproheptadine, demonstrating no change in histamine secretion, although no reaction was observed with treatment.

manifest swelling. It is proposed that chilling initiates a reaction mediated by IgE bound to mast cells and that, upon warming, mediators are released into the circulation.

When skin biopsy specimens were tested by chilling and warming, histamine release was also demonstrable *(6)* (Fig. 1); however, chilling and warming basophils of patients did not result in histamine release, even in those in whom IgE-mediated disease was documented. Thus, it appeared unlikely that the disorder was caused by a circulating IgE cryoglobulin (unless the patients' basophils are desensitized). Rather, the presence of skin and/or cutaneous mast cells seemed essential.

One proposal to explain such a result is that patients have an IgE autoantibody to a cold-induced skin antigen. Thus, sensitization might occur in the cold, and release of mediators proceeds as the cells warm. Studies to test this hypothesis have thus far been negative. We have also found high levels of IgM and IgG antibodies directed against the Fc portion of IgE in patients with cold urticaria *(5)* and, although the clinical significance of such autoantibodies is questionable *(12)*, one such serum was shown to cause release of histamine when incubated with normal basophils. However, this reaction was demonstrable at 37°C and did not require chilling followed by warming, so its relationship to the disease was not clear.

Cyproheptadine (Periactin) in divided doses is the drug of choice for cold urticaria. Histamine release, however, is unaffected by doses of cyproheptadine that completely control symptoms *(13)*; it appears, therefore, to act as a classical antihistamine, i.e., by blockade of H_1 receptors (Fig. 2). However, other antihistamines of comparable potency are less effective; the reason for this is uncertain. Although cyproheptadine has antiserotonin activity, serotonin does not appear to be released in cold urticaria. Some patients do not respond well to cyproheptadine, and it has been reported that symptoms do not always correlate well with histamine release *(14)*. Thus, other vasoactive factors may also make a significant contribution for some patients. Experimental cromolyn-like drugs, which inhibit mast-cell degranulation, are effective in controlling symptoms and suppressing the ice-cube test in patients who are poorly responsive to cyproheptadine *(15)*. Ketotifen, in particular, has been shown to inhibit histamine release and is effective in a variety of physically induced urticarias *(16)*.

Localized cold urticaria, in which only certain areas of the body urticate with cold contact, has been reported after predisposing conditions such as cold injury, or sites of intracutaneous allergen injections, ragweed immunotherapy, or insect bites. We have described a patient with cold urticaria confined to the head and face in whom there was no identifiable antecedent or associated event *(16)*. Such cases argue against the presence of a circulatory factor and speak in favor of a local abnormality of (possibly) mast cells.

Cold urticaria has also been described as being associated with the presence of cryoproteins such as cold agglutinins, cryoglobulins, cryofibrinogen, and the Donath-Landsteiner antibody seen in secondary syphilis (paroxysmal cold hemoglobinuria). The only reported studies that address mechanisms of hive formation are those performed in patients with associated cryoglobulins. The isolated proteins appear to transfer cold sensitivity and activate the complement cascade upon in vitro incubation with normal plasma *(17,18)*. Thus, it is possible that hive formation in these subjects is due to cold-dependent anaphylatoxin release.

It is clear that a disorder such as cryoglobulinemia can be associated with cutaneous vasculitis as well as cold urticaria, and other associations between these two entities have been reported. Eady and Greaves *(19)* reported that frequent and repeated cooling of the skin in patients with idiopathic cold urticaria can cause vasculitic lesions. In one case, immune reactants (IgM and C3) deposited in the vessels of such lesions *(20)*. In two other patients, leukocytoclastic vasculitis was seen in association with cold urticaria, and circulating immune complexes were clearly evident *(2,21)*. It appeared that the mediator release caused by cold challenge could localize immune complexes to cutaneous sites, where they then caused vasculitis *(2)*. Sites of typical urticarial vasculitis independent of temperature change were also evident *(21)*. Therapy in these cases is directed toward the underlying disease, leading to cryprotein production, plus antihistamines.

Other cold-dependent syndromes have been reported, but the incidence of such cases is unknown. A delayed form of cold urticaria was described *(22)* in which swelling appeared 9–18 h after cold exposure. Studies of mediator release were unrevealing, the cold sensitivity could not be passively transferred, and biopsy of a lesion revealed edema and a mononuclear cell infiltrate. Family studies suggested a dominant mode of inheritance. A series of four patients have been described in whom exercise in a cold environment induced hives similar to those seen with cholinergic urticaria; however, hive formation did not occur if exercise was performed in a heated environment. In this disorder the cold exposure is systemic rather than local, and it should be suspected in any patient whose symptoms are suggestive of either cold urticaria or cholinergic urticaria and in whom standard tests for each disorder are negative *(23)*. Exercise in a cold room or running on a winter's day will lead to generalized urticaria and confirm the diagnosis. Because of the visual resemblance of the lesions to those of typical cholinergic urticaria, the disorder has been called *cold-induced cholinergic urticaria*. A study of 13 patients with symptoms suggestive of cold urticaria and cholinergic urticaria revealed two who did not have both disorders but had the cold-induced cholinergic type hives *(24)*.

Another related disorder called *systemic cold urticaria* yields severe generalized hive formation upon systemic cold challenge occurring over covered or uncovered parts of the body. Symptoms are unrelated to exercise or other activities *(25)*, and the ice-cube test is negative. Histamine release upon cold challenge (with or without exercise) has been observed in cold-induced cholinergic urticaria as well as systemic cold urticaria. Treatment regimens of

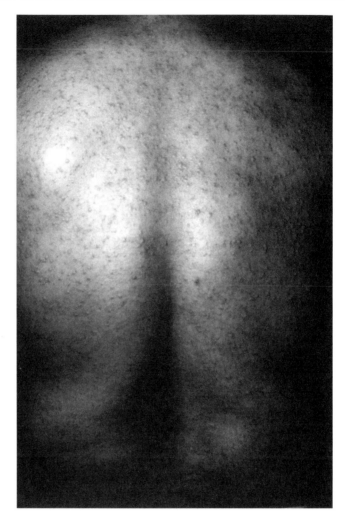

Fig. 3. Typical lesion of cholinergic urticaria (generalized heat urticaria) induced by exercise in place for 10 min.

hydroxyzine plus cyproheptadine in high dosage *(26)* or Doxepin *(27)* have been utilized successfully.

Another disorder called *cold-dependent dermatographism* has been reported in which prominent hive formation is seen if the skin is scratched and then chilled *(25)*. In this disorder the ice-cube test and systemic cold challenge yield no hives. Simply scratching the skin yields a weakly positive dermatographic response, but dramatic accentuation is seen when the scratched area is chilled. Treatment once again is high-dose antihistamines, e.g., 200 mg of diphenhydramine/d or a combination of hydroxyzine (100–200 mg/d) and cyproheptadine (8–16 mg/d).

Finally, a disorder called localized *cold reflex urticaria* has been reported in which the ice-cube test is positive, but hives form in the vicinity of the contact site, and not precisely where the cube is applied *(28,29)*. The appearance of the hives resembles the punctate lesions of cholinergic urticaria and there is no confluent hive where the ice cube is applied. A methacholine or acetylcholine skin test for cholinergic urticaria is negative, although the symptoms of one such patient resembled cold-induced cholinergic urticaria in that exercise-induced hives were seen in a cold environment *(28)*.

Exercise-Induced Disorders

Cholinergic or generalized heat urticaria is characterized by the onset of small punctate wheals surrounded by a prominent erythematous flare associated with exercise, hot showers, sweating, and anxiety *(30)*. Typically, lesions first appear about the neck and upper thorax; and when viewed from a distance, hives may not be perceived and the patient appears flushed (Fig. 3). However, pruritus is a prominent feature of the reaction; on close inspection, small punctate wheals can be discerned, sometimes as small as 1 mm in diameter, that are surrounded by a prominent flare. Gradually the lesions spread distally to involve the face, back, and extremities, and the wheals increase in size. In some patients the hives become confluent and resemble angioedema *(31)*. Also occasionally seen are symptoms of more generalized cholinergic stimulation such as lacrimation, salivation, and diarrhea. These various stimuli have the common feature of being mediated by cholinergic nerve fibers that innervate the musculature via parasympathetic neurons and innervate the sweat glands by cholinergic fibers that travel with the sympathetic nerves *(32)*.

The characteristic lesion of cholinergic urticaria can be reproduced by intradermal injection of 100 μg of methacholine (Mecholyl) in 0.1 mL saline. When positive, the resulting localized hive surrounded by satellite lesions is indistinguishable from spontaneous lesions, and confirms the diagnosis. However, we have found that only about one-third of patients give a clearly positive skin test; these are generally the most severe cases. Challenge by exercise (e.g., running in an 85°C warmed room or using a bicycle ergometer for 10–15 min) is a far more sensitive test. Thus, the skin test can be used to confirm the diagnosis but cannot be used as a diagnostic test *(33,34)*. Those patients who have a positive methacholine skin test demonstrate a "hypersensitivity" to cholinergic mediators, but they have no evidence of an immunoglobulin-mediated allergy to acetylcholine.

It is possible that the disorder is due to an intrinsic cellular abnormality that results in abnormal mediator release in the presence of cholinergic agents. One study addressing this issue demonstrated an increased number of muscarinic receptors at urticarial sites. These receptors were further augmented when exercise followed patch-testing to copper-containing materials *(35)*. This increased number of acetylcholine binding sites may be an important key to understanding the pathogenesis of cholinergic urticaria. The importance of copper is unclear, but it may affect ligand–receptor affinity.

There is evidence that a reflex consisting of afferent humoral and efferent neurogenic components is involved in this urticarial disorder. When one places a patient's hand in warm water with a tourniquet tied proximally, there is no urticaria until the tourniquet is released. A generalized eruption then ensues. Thus, a central perception of a temperature change transmitted via the circulation appears to be followed by an efferent reflex leading to urticaria. Such a reflex could also account for the association of hives with anxiety *(36)*, although it should be emphasized that in these instances the emotional reaction may be completely appropriate. Cholinergic urticaria is the only form of hives in which emotional stimuli can, in some patients, initiate an urticarial reaction.

Studies of mediator release during attacks of cholinergic urticaria have demonstrated that, in most cases, elevated plasma histamine levels parallel the onset of pruritus and urticaria *(34)*. Subsequent studies have confirmed the presence of histaminemia in association with cholinergic urticaria *(34,37)*, and the release of eosinophilotactic peptides and NCF *(38)*. When patients are challenged while wearing a plastic occlusive suit to produce maximal changes in cutaneous and core body temperature, significant falls in forced expired volume in 1 (FEV_1), maximal midexpiratory flow rate, and specific conductance are observed, associated with a rise in residual volume. Thus, under such conditions, an abnormality in pulmonary function can be detected, reflecting either primary pulmonary involvement or altered pulmonary mechanics secondary to circulating mediators. A clinically significant alteration in pulmonary function is unusual in cholinergic urticaria and has no clear association with exercise-induced asthma.

Kaplan et al. *(39)* also described two cases of typical cholinergic urticaria in whom lesions became confluent and were associated with prominent elevation of plasma histamine as well as recurrent episodes of hypotension. Thus, some extreme cases of cholinergic urticaria can resemble the exercise-induced anaphylactic syndrome. An important distinguishing feature is that an increase in core body temperature of greater than 0.7°C using hyperthermic blankets or submersion in warmed water causes hives, histamine release, and anaphylactic symptoms in cholinergic urticaria patients, but not in the exercise-induced anaphylactic syndrome *(40)* (*see* Exercise-Induced Anaphylaxis). One should also point out that combinations of "physical urticarias" can occur in the same patient, i.e., cold urticaria *(37)* or dermatographism *(38)* in association with cholinergic urticaria. Furthermore, combined cold and cholinergic urticaria, fulfilling separate criteria for each disorder *(24,37)*, is to be distinguished from cold-induced cholinergic urticaria *(23)*.

Treatment of cholinergic urticaria generally consists of hydroxyzine (100–200 mg/d) in divided doses *(36)*. Many, but certainly not all, patients respond to this regimen. Anticholinergic agents such as atropine or propantheline bromide (Pro-Banthine) have little effect, perhaps owing to an inability to attain sufficient systemic levels; however, injected atropine can reverse the methacholine skin test *(37)*.

Exercise-Induced Anaphylaxis

The syndrome of exercise-induced anaphylaxis was first described in a series of patients in whom combinations of pruritus, urticaria, angioedema, wheezing, and hypotension occurred as a result of exercise. Symptoms did not occur, however, with each exercise experience, and most described patients were accomplished athletes *(41)*. The disorder is distinguished from cholinergic urticaria by the following criteria: First, although exercise is the precipitating stimulus of each disorder, hot showers, sweating in the absence of exercise, and anxiety do not trigger attacks of exercise-induced anaphylaxis as they do in cholinergic urticaria *(30)*. Second, the hives seen with exercise-induced anaphylaxis are large (10–15 mm), in contrast to the punctate lesions characteristic of cholinergic urticaria. Finally, when patients with exercise-induced anaphylaxis are challenged in an occlusive suit, no change in pulmonary function is seen, although histamine release can be documented *(42)*. Optimal therapy for the exercise-induced anaphylactic syndrome is uncertain, and attempts at prophylaxis utilizing H_1 and H_2 antagonists have not generally been effective *(43)*. In contrast, classic cholinergic urticaria is usually responsive to prophylactic use of hydroxyzine.

Subtypes of exercise-induced anaphylaxis have also been described that are food-related. In one case, exercise-induced anaphylaxis occurred if the exercise took place 5–24 h after eating shellfish, whereas exercise alone or eating shellfish alone did not cause any symptoms *(44)*. In five other reported cases, two had symptoms only if exercise followed the ingestion of any food within 2 h *(44,45)*; in the remaining three cases, symptoms were precipitated by the specific ingestion of celery within 2 h of exercise *(46)*. The latter patients also had positive skin tests to celery. Thus, various forms of food-dependent, exercise-induced anaphylaxis are possible, and treatment requires the avoidance of specific foodstuffs prior to exercising or avoiding exercise within certain time intervals after eating. Kivity et al. *(47)* performed skin tests to compound 48/80 (a cutaneous mast cell degranulating agent) and histamine, demonstrating augmented wheal responses to 48/80 but not histamine in subjects with food-induced (skin test positive), exercise-induced anaphylaxis. Food or exercise alone did not affect the 48/80 response, suggesting increased mast cell releasability caused by the combination of food plus exercise. It is also of interest that one patient with cholinergic urticaria and associated anaphylaxis was successfully treated by vigorous daily exercise such that desensitization occurred within a week *(39)*. The number of patients with cholinergic urticaria or the exercise-induced anaphylactic syndrome that might respond to such treatment is unknown, although it is more likely to be effective in cholinergic urticaria with or without hypotension because symptoms occur reproducibly each time an exercise challenge is done.

Other Physically Induced Forms of Urticaria or Angioedema

The remaining forms of physically induced hives or swelling are, with the exception of dermatographism, relatively rare disorders. These include local heat urticaria, pressure-induced urticaria/angioedema, solar urticaria, aquagenic urticaria, and vibratory angioedema.

LOCALIZED HEAT URTICARIA

A local form of heat urticaria is a rare disorder in which urticaria develops within minutes after exposure to applied heat *(48)*. Sixteen cases have thus far been reported, most of which appear in females. When suspected, it can be tested by application of a test tube of warm water at 44°C to the arm for 4–5 min. If positive, a hive is seen a few minutes after the test tube is removed. Studies of mediator release in local heat urticaria resemble those reported in cold urticaria; plasma histamine levels peak 5–10 min after heat exposure *(49,50)*, although passive-transfer studies have been negative. NCF was also found to be released in one study *(50)*; thus, mast-cell degranulation in response to heat challenge seems likely. In one report, complement abnormalities were reported in the absence of histamine release *(51)*. Association with other forms of physical urticaria is also sometimes seen, e.g., combined cold urticaria and local heat urticaria *(52)*. Therapy has been problematic, since antihistamines such as hydroxyzine or cyproheptadine as well as oral disodium cromoglycate have been ineffective. One patient was successfully desensitized by repeated daily immersion in hot baths, but caution is in order as systemic reactions are possible *(51)*.

A variant of this disorder has been described that was familial and in which urticaria occurred 1.5–2 h after application of a warm stimulus *(53)* and persisted for 6–10 h. Sunbathing with pronounced heating of skin produced wheals as a result of the temperature effect, whereas sunlight itself could be tolerated. Desensitization of an area was achieved with repeated challenge every few days. Skin biopsy demonstrated a pronounced inflammatory cell infiltrate in the upper dermis and around hair follicles. The pathogenesis of this form of local heat urticaria is unknown. Partial control was achieved with oral antihistamines.

DERMATOGRAPHISM

The ability to write on skin, termed *dermatographism*, can occur as an isolated disorder that often presents as traumatically induced urticaria. It can be diagnosed by observing the skin after stroking it with a tongue depressor or fingernail. In such patients, a white line secondary to reflex vasoconstriction is followed by pruritus, erythema, and a linear wheal, as is seen in a classic wheal-and-flare reaction. It is said to be present in 2–5% of the population *(54,55)*; however, only a small fraction of these are of sufficient severity to warrant treatment. Biopsy of the skin reveals few changes, but most occur in the epidermis and consist of vacuolation of keratinocytes and basal epidermal-cell pseudopodia, as well as the appearance of typical mast-cell granules *(56)*. In approx 50% of cases, passive-transfer studies have demonstrated an IgE-dependent mechanism *(57,58)*. Thus, many patients have an abnormal circulating IgE that confers a particular form of pressure sensitivity to dermal mast cells. Such observations further suggest that histamine is one of the mediators of dermatographism, although demonstration of such release has been difficult because of the localized nature of the reaction. Early studies, however, did suggest that histamine is released into whole blood *(59)*, induced blisters over lesions contain elevated histamine levels *(60)*, 24-h urine histamine levels are elevated *(48)*, and histamine is increased in the perfusate, as shown by in vivo subcutaneous perfusion studies *(61)*. In a single, unusually severe case of IgE-mediated dermatographism, elevation of plasma histamine levels was documented within 1 min of stroking the skin, and the baseline histamine level was abnormal in multiple determinations, suggesting that "leakage" of histamine was ongoing *(62)*.

Although the evidence is often anecdotal, dermatographism appears to be a consequence of drug reactions *(63)*; in one case, dermatographism could be observed only upon challenge with the offending agent—in this instance, penicillin *(64)*. Therapy for dermatographism consists of antihistamines *(65,66)* for severe symptoms, and high doses may be needed. The initial objective of therapy is to decrease pruritus so that the stimulus for scratching is diminished; many patients complain of a sensation of itching or "skin crawling" that is readily relieved by antihistamines. At higher doses, one can show that the wheal-and-flare reaction to stroking is also markedly diminished.

Dermatographism also occurs in association with other disorders; for example, a mild form may be seen in some patients with chronic urticaria. Severe dermatographism is also associated with mast-cell proliferative disorders, in which a marked increase in dermal mast cells is seen, e.g., urticaria pigmentosa or systemic mastocytosis. Release of histamine in these disorders has been demonstrated *(48)*. It is also possible that other vasoactive agents released from cutaneous mast cells can be implicated in dermatographism and, in fact, in all forms of physically induced urticaria. An example is the elevation of prostaglandin D_2 (PGD_2) metabolites seen in the urine of patients with systemic mastocytosis, which may contribute to the hypotension associated with this disorder *(67)*.

PRESSURE-INDUCED URTICARIA/ANGIOEDEMA

Pressure-induced urticaria differs from most of the aforementioned types of hives or angioedema in that symptoms typically occur 4–6 h after pressure has been applied *(68)*. The disorder is clinically heterogeneous: for example, some patients may complain of swelling secondary to pressure with normal-appearing skin (i.e., no erythema or superficial infiltrating hive); the term *angioedema* is more appropriate in these cases. In other patients, the lesions are predominantly urticarial and may or may not be associated with significant swelling. When urticaria is present, an infiltrative lesion is seen, characterized by a perivascular mononuclear-cell infiltrate and dermal edema similar to that observed in chronic idiopathic urticaria *(69)*. Immediate dermatographism is not present, but delayed dermatographism is seen and may represent the same disorder *(26)*. Symptoms can be provoked by tight clothing, the hands may swell with activity such as hammering, foot swelling is common after walking, and buttock swelling may be prominent after sitting for a few hours. Testing can be performed using a sling (with a 5–15-lb weight attached) that is placed over the forearm or shoulder for 10–20 min. Gradual pressure applied by devices in g/mm^2 can also be used *(69)*. There are few available studies regarding pathogenesis; however, mediators that cause pain rather than pruritus (i.e., kinins) have been considered, because the lesions are typically described as burning or painful. Nevertheless, skin blisters induced over lesions reveal histamine release following the time course of hive formation *(60)*. Antihistamines, however, have little effect on the disorder, and patients with severe disease often have to be treated with corticosteroids.

Table 2
Solar Urticaria

Type	Wave length, nm	Passive transfer	Identified factor
1	280–320	+	IgE
2	320–400	–	—
3	400–500	–	—
4	400–500	+	IgE in some
5	280–500	–	—
6	400	–	Ferrochetalase deficiency

Although pressure urticaria/angioedema can occur as an isolated disorder, it is most often seen in association with chronic urticaria. Therapy is then usually directed toward the chronic urticaria. There are data to suggest an increased incidence of food allergy in those patients with chronic urticaria in whom pressure-induced symptoms are also prominent *(70)*.

Immediate-pressure urticaria has been described in patients with the hypereosinophilia syndrome characterized by an acute wheal-and-flare reaction within 1–2 min of applied pressure, i.e., pressing on the back with one's thumb. Those patients also are dermatographic, although patients with dermatographism alone typically do not have immediate-pressure urticaria and require a stroking motion to produce a hive *(71)*.

SOLAR URTICARIA

Solar urticaria is a rare disorder in which brief exposure to light causes the development of urticaria within 1–3 min. Typically, pruritus occurs first, in about 30 s, followed by edema confined to the light-exposed area and surrounded by a prominent erythematous zone caused by an axon reflex. The lesions then usually disappear within 1–3 h. When large areas of the body are exposed, systemic symptoms may occur, including hypotension and asthma. Although most reported patients have been in their third and fourth decades, the disorder can occur in any age group and has no association with other allergic disorders.

Solar urticaria has been classified into six types (Table 2), depending on the wavelength of light that induces lesions and the ability or inability to passively transfer the disorder with serum *(72–74)*. Types I and IV can be passively transferred and may therefore by immunologically (IgE?) mediated; they are associated with wavelengths of 280–320 n and 400–500 nm, respectively. The antigen has not been identified. Histamine release, mast-cell degranulation *(75)*, and formation of chemotactic factors for eosinophils and neutrophils *(76)* have been observed coincident with induction of lesions by ultraviolet light (type I).

Type VI solar urticaria, activated by light at 400 nm, is due to an inherited metabolic disorder in which protoporphyrin IX acts as a photosensitizer and is synonymous with erythropoietic protoporphyria. It is caused by ferrochetalase deficiency *(77,78)*. In contrast to other forms of porphyria, the urinary porphyrin excretion is normal; however, red-blood-cell protoporphyrin and fecal protoporphyrin and coproporphyrin levels are elevated. Irradiation of serum samples of such patients results in activation of the classic complement pathway and generation of C5a chemotactic activity *(79)*; this activity is proportional to the serum level of protoporphyrin *(80)*. Irradiation of the forearms of two such patients resulted in in vivo complement activation as assessed by a diminution of titers of C3 and C5 and generation of C5a *(81)*. Consistent with these observations is that deposition of C3 and accumulation of neutrophils is seen in the dermis *(82,83)*, and complement fragments can be detected in the serum and suction blister fluid of irradiated skin *(82)*. This condition responds to oral β-carotene, which absorbs light at the same wavelengths as protoporphyrin IX *(84)*.

The mechanism by which urticaria is produced in types II, III, and V is unknown, but these are induced by inciting wavelengths of 320–400, 400–500 and 280–500 nm, respectively. As a simple screen, fluorescent tubes that emit a broad, continuous spectrum can be used to test the patient, and filters can then be used to define the specific wavelengths that cause urticaria. Therapy of this disease requires avoidance of sunlight, protective garments to cover the skin, and use of topical preparations to absorb or reflect light. A 5% solution of paraaminobenzoic acid in ethanol, as in sunscreen lotions, can be helpful in the 280–320-nm range; however, it is more difficult to screen out the visible spectrum. The most effective agents for this purpose contain titanium oxide and/or zinc oxide. The efficacy of antihistaminics, antimalarials, and corticosteroids in these disorders is not clear and needs to be evaluated.

Aquagenic Urticaria

Thirteen cases have been reported of patients who developed small wheals after contact with water, regardless of its temperature, and who were distinguishable from patients with cold urticaria or cholinergic urticaria. This disorder has been termed *aquagenic urticaria (85)*. Direct application of a compress of tap water or distilled water to the skin is used to test for its presence. The diagnosis should be reserved for those rare cases that test positively for water but negatively for all other forms of physical urticaria. Combined cholinergic and aquagenic urticaria has been reported, and histamine release into the circulation has been documented upon challenge with water *(86)*.

Hereditary Vibratory Angioedema

Hereditary vibratory angioedema has been described in a single family in whom it was inherited in an autosomal dominant pattern. It is properly viewed as a physically induced angioedema, since patients complain of intense pruritus and swelling within minutes after vibratory stimuli *(87)*. The patients are not dermatographic and do not have pressure-induced urticaria. Lesions can be reproduced by gently stimulating the patient's forearm with a laboratory vortex for 4 min. Rapid swelling of the entire forearm and a portion of the upper arm ensues, and histamine has been shown to be released secondary to such a vibratory stimulus *(88)*. With care, patients can avoid vibratory stimuli, and their symptoms can otherwise be partially relieved with diphenhydramine. Nonfamilial, sporadic cases have also been described.

ACUTE NONPHYSICALLY INDUCED URTICARIA

Acute urticaria is a commonly encountered disorder that can be caused by a wide variety of agents. Most prominent are drug reactions, allergy to foods, and urticaria in association with infection or other systemic diseases. Episodes of acute urticaria usually last from a few days to 2–3 wk. When the urticarial episode exceeds 6 wk, it is arbitrarily designated "chronic."

The hive due to a food or drug reaction differs from that seen with the various physical urticarias in that individual lesions can remain prominent from many hours to 1–2 d. In this respect, the lesions more closely resemble chronic urticaria rather than the physical urticarias *(89)*. An allergic mechanism, in the strictest sense, requires an interaction of IgE antibody with the allergen (i.e., food or drug) followed by degranulation of cutaneous mast cells. However, it has been observed that when an allergic person is skin-tested (e.g., intracutaneous administration of ragweed antigen to a person with ragweed-induced rhinitis), the immediate wheal-and-flare reaction lasts a few minutes and disappears; it may then be followed by a swelling, 4–6 h later, which is called a *late-phase reaction (90)*. It has been shown that late-phase reactions are dependent on the prior IgE reaction *(91)*. They consist of a mixed cellular infiltrate containing mononuclear cells, neutrophils, eosinophils, and basophils *(92,93)* and are associated with a second wave of secretion of histamine *(94)* and other vasoactive substances. Cutaneous injection of 48/80, a polypeptide that causes mast-cell degranulation, can also lead to late-phase reactions *(95)*. It appears that the late-phase reaction in the skin requires something besides a single burst of mast-cell degranulation, but no data are available regarding this issue. We can theorize that mast-cell degranulation that persists over time and/or persistence of antigenic stimulation over time is the critical difference. This would be absent in virtually all the physical urticarias except delayed pressure urticaria. Perhaps the persistence of the hive in food or drug reactions is related to this phenomenon.

Urticaria has also been well documented during viral infections such as hepatitis *(96)* or infectious mononucleosis *(97)*, and a large number of helminthic parasites are associated with hives. Serum sickness reactions (including the prodrome of hepatitis-B infection) can be seen as a manifestation of drug reactions, and on biopsy one observes evidence of a small-vessel cutaneous vasculitis *(98)*. Urticaria in association with systemic lupus erythematosus *(99,100)* or other vasculitides appears similar: there is necrosis of the vessel wall (most prominent in small venules), infiltration with neutrophils, and deposition of immunoglobulins and complement. It is thought that these disorders are caused by immune complex deposition in the dermal vasculature and release of histamine (and other mediators) from perivenular mast cells caused by local formation of the anaphylatoxins C3a, C5a, and C4a *(101)*. IgE antibody to the initiating antigen may also be contributory.

CHRONIC IDIOPATHIC URTICARIA AND IDIOPATHIC ANGIOEDEMA

Reports of the frequency of identification of the etiologic agent in chronic urticaria and angioedema vary from 10 to 80%. However, the rate of successful diagnosis in most studies is probably not greater than 20%, and is likely much less. Different populations of patients or referral patterns may in part account for the wide variance reported. One may also confuse chronic urticaria with recurrent urticaria due to a repeatedly encountered allergen. We have studied over 700 patients with chronic urticaria for whom no etiologic agent could be identified after evaluation by primary care and consultant physicians in the community, with a success rate for identification of a causal factor of less than 5%. Most patients appear to have an idiopathic disorder. As a group they are not atopic, i.e., there is no increased incidence of eczema, allergic rhinitis, or asthma compared with the general population; IgE levels as a group are within normal limits. Some patients are dermatographic, although this is usually of milder degree than is seen with the IgE-dependent dermatographism described earlier, and curiously the dermographism may wax and wane just as the urticaria may vary from severe to mild or may intermittently subside. Some have symptoms consistent with pressure urticaria, i.e., areas subject to pressure are particularly likely to erupt with hives, but most hives are unassociated with pressure. These patients have a normal white blood count and sedimentation rate and have no evidence of systemic disease.

Pathogenesis

The lesion seen in chronic urticaria is different from that seen in most of the physically induced urticarial disorders. Biopsy of lesions of patients with cold urticaria or dermatographism reveals evidence of increased vascular permeability and edematous tissue, but no cellular infiltrate. The lesions appear quickly, usually disappear in less than 2 h, and do *not* have a late-phase component. Thus a single burst of mast-cell degranulation may be insufficient to cause a late-phase reaction *(102)*. Reactions to foods or drugs may be similar; how-

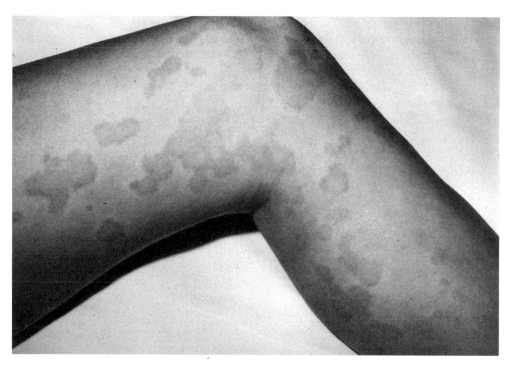

Fig. 4. Lesions of chronic "idiopathic" urticaria demonstrating elevated erythematous lesions that vary in shape and size, although most are annular.

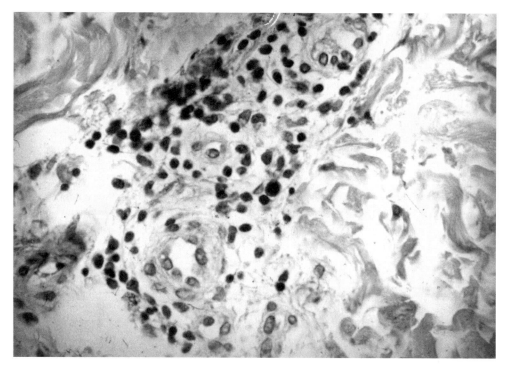

Fig. 5. Skin biopsy of chronic urticaria demonstrating a nonnecrotizing perivascular infiltration with mononuclear cells.

Table 3
Infiltrating Cells in Skin Biopsy Specimens from Patients
with Chronic Urticaria and Normal Controls

	Number of cells, mean (range)[a]	
Cell Type	Patients[a]	Control[b]
Eosinophils	1.2 (0–12)	0
Basophils	0.35 (0–2)	0
Neutrophils	3.0 (0–50)	0.14 (0–10)
Mononuclear cells	52.4 (16–247)	13.4 (3–25)
Mast cells	7.6 (0–19)	0.71 (0–3)

[a]N = 43.
[b]N = 7.

ever, there can be a late-phase component with a cellular infiltrate, so such lesions may resemble that seen in chronic urticaria. Of the physically induced disorders discussed herein, only skin biopsy specimens of patients with delayed pressure urticaria reveal pathology that is virtually indistinguishable from that seen in chronic urticaria.

External examination of patients with chronic urticaria reveals infiltrative hives with palpably elevated borders, sometimes varying greatly in size and/or shape but generally being rounded (Fig. 4). The typical lesion consists of a nonnecrotizing perivascular mononuclear cell infiltrate (Fig. 5). However, many types of histopathologic processes can occur in the skin and manifest as hives. For example, patients with hypocomplementemia and cutaneous vasculitis can have urticaria (angioedema), and biopsies of patients with urticaria, arthralgias, myalgias, and elevated erythrocyte sedimentation rate (ESR) as a manifestation of necrotizing venulitis revealed fibroid necrosis with a predominant neutrophilic infiltrate *(103,104)*. These latter urticarial lesions may be indistinguishable from those seen in the more typical, nonvasculitic cases. Hydroxychloroquine (Plaquanil) 200–400 mg/d can control symptoms in this unusual subpopulation of chronic urticaria patients.

Other studies *(105–108)* have examined the incidence of vasculitis in patients with urticaria, with a wide variety of results. Mathison and colleagues *(105)* found that 10 of 78 patients had hypocomplementemia, many with evidence of activation of the classic complement pathway; six of the 10 had elevated levels of circulating immune complexes. If hypocomplementemia and vasculitis are equated, the incidence of presumed vasculitis was 14%. Monroe and coworkers *(106)* found neutrophilic leukocytoclastic angiitis in 20% of patients; the other 80% had a perivascular infiltrate (not true vasculitis) of mononuclear cells that was classed as dense or sparse. Interestingly, the "vasculitic," "dense infiltrate," and "sparse infiltrate" groups had circulating immune complex levels of 33, 29, and 13%, respectively, as measured by multiple assays. Phanuphak and colleagues *(108)* used the criterion of significant cellular infiltrate within vessel walls to define vasculitis rather than that of endothelial damage, nuclear dust, fibrin deposition, or red-cell extravasation. They found a 52% incidence of vasculitis with various types of predominant cells and a 48% incidence of perivascular mononuclear-cell infiltrate. Deposition of immune complexes in the skin was seen in 18% of the vasculitis group—almost exclusively in those with an abundance of neutrophils.

We have reported results of a histopathologic study of chronic idiopathic urticaria in 43 consecutive patients *(107)*. All but one of the group had a nonnecrotizing perivascular infiltrate consisting primarily of lymphocytes. We therefore found vasculitis to be rare in urticaria; our patient group is probably comparable to the group without vasculitis in the study of Mathison and colleagues (105), the "sparse" and/or "dense" infiltrate groups of Monroe and coworkers (106), and the "perivasculitis group" of Phanuphak and colleagues (108).

We also noted a tenfold increase in number of mast cells and a fourfold increase in number of mononuclear cells in skin biopsy specimens from the patients with chronic urticaria compared with those from normal controls (Table 3). No increase in basophil number was seen, although basophils of patients with chronic urticaria are reported to be less responsive to anti-IgE than those of normal control subjects, suggesting in vivo desensitization (109). Thus, the increase in mast cells observed may be reflected in the increased amount of histamine found in blister fluid suctioned from patients with chronic urticaria compared with normal control subjects (60), and in the increased level of total skin histamine content reportedly present in such patients (110). A more recent study (111) did not confirm an increased number of mast cells based on tryptase staining and speculated that basophils or an increased amount of histamine per cell might account for the aforementioned observations. Differences in sampling and level of mast-cell degranulation are other variables to consider.

More recent studies have attempted to subtype the mononuclear-cell infiltrate using monoclonal antibodies (MAbs). A predominance of T-helper lymphocytes has been reported (112). We have found 50% T-lymphocytes, no B-cells, 20% monocytes, and 10% mast cells (113); however, T-cell subtyping fails to reveal a predominant pattern. Although eosinophils were not often seen in the skin biopsies of our patients, when considered as a group, an occasional patient had a prominent eosinophil accumulation. Deposition of eosinophil major basic protein in skin specimens of 50% of patients with chronic urticaria has been demonstrated, although only a fraction of the patients had obvious eosinophil infiltration (114). It is possible that degranulated eosinophils are present and more common than previously appreciated.

The 20% unidentified mononuclear cells might represent $\gamma\delta$ T-lymphocytes, and this will require reassessment with additional antisera. Because lymphocytes, monocytes, and mast cells all accumulate, it is hypothesized that a lymphokine or monokine may be released that causes mast-cell proliferation (or accumulation) and degranulation. Histamine-releasing factors (HRFs) that can cause cutaneous mast cell degranulation are being sought as a potential cause of histamine release in this disorder. Evidence for HRF release in patients with chronic urticaria has, in fact, been reported (115); however, the specific factor was not identified.

Chronic urticaria is most frequently characterized by a nonnecrotizing perivascular lymphocyte infiltrate with an accumulation of histamine-containing cells and augmented releasability. Patients with vasculitis and urticaria probably represent a separate subpopulation in whom the pathogenesis of hive formation likely involves immune complexes, complement activation, anaphylatoxin formation, histamine release, and neutrophil accumulation, activation, and degranulation.

Recently, there is considerable renewed interest in the possibility that chronic urticaria may be an autoimmune disorder. Perhaps the first suggestion for this arose from data that demonstrated an association of chronic urticaria with autoimmune hypothyroidism (Hashimoto's thyroiditis) and, more specifically, with the presence of antibodies to peroxidase or thyroglobulin. The incidence was 12–14% in two studies of chronic urticaria patients (116,117). However, it was noted that thyroid status did not relate to the occurrence of urticaria and that typically, hives did not remit when a euthyroid status was achieved. However, thyroid autoantibodies in these patients typically persist as well.

Gruber et al. (118) reported the presence of circulating IgG or IgM anti-IgE antibodies in chronic urticaria subjects. The incidence was approx 10% and was not seen in normal con-

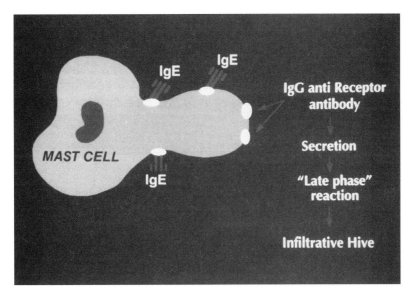

Fig. 6. Proposed mechanism of hive formation in chronic urticaria demonstrating that an IgG antibody directed against the α-subunit of the IgE receptor can cause mast-cell secretion and, as a consequence, a perivascular infiltrate and hives.

trols or patients with other types of urticaria, except cold urticaria. The underlying hypothesis was that such an antibody could degranulate cutaneous mast cells in vivo and lead to acute hives or even a late-phase reaction and its concomitant cellular infiltrate. Most recently, Hide et al. *(119)* reported the presence of anti-IgE receptor antibodies in 30–40% of chronic urticaria patients and an additional 10% with anti-IgE antibodies. These studies demonstrated autoreactivity to autologous serum in such subjects, i.e., injections of serum into the patient induced a wheal and flare reaction *(119)*. These sera could degranulate basophils to release histamine, and those reactive with cells stripped of their IgE were presumed reactive with the IgE receptor. The sera were inhibitable with either the α-subunit of their IgE receptor or with IgE itself, confirming the functional reactivity. Our preliminary data confirm the presence of reactivity with the α-subunit of the IgE receptor in about one-third of patients, using activated rat basophil leukemia cells transfected with the α-subunit of the IgE receptor *(120)*. If anti-IgE pathogenicity can be proven, then an autoimmune etiology can be inferred in 40–50% of patients. The cause in the others remains uncertain.

The above data suggest that the perivascular infiltrate seen in patients with chronic urticaria is a late-phase reaction or at least a variant thereof. However, there are some discrepancies between the histologic description of late-phase reactions and the lesions described in chronic urticaria. For example, basophils are prominent in the late-phase reaction in the nose, lung, or skin *(121,122)*, but no increase in basophils has yet been demonstrated in chronic urticaria *(113)*. Eosinophils are very prominent in asthma or nasal polyps and in induced or naturally occurring late-phase reactions in the lung and nose. They are somewhat less prominent in the skin; however, the lesions of chronic urticaria vary from eosinophils being very prominent to not being seen at all; the latter is the more common scenario. Since eosinophil cationic protein can be demonstrated in about two-thirds of biopsies of chronic-urticaria subjects, eosinophils may be present transiently or not identifiable for unknown technical reasons. Monocytes are minimally elevated in late-phase reactions of the lung, nose, and skin but can comprise 20%

of the cells of chronic urticaria; this is a prominent difference. Lymphocytes are also more prominent in chronic urticaria; subpopulations of such cells are known to "home" to the skin. Much more information is needed to relate the lesions observed to the putative consequences of an autoimmune reaction involving cutaneous mast cells. Further, some explanation is needed to understand the localization of such reactions to the skin, since mast cells in the nose or lung should be responsive to the same circulating autoantibody. A theoretical diagram depicting this mechanism for hive induction in chronic urticaria is shown in Fig. 6. Therapy consists of antihistamines in high dosage and alternate-day corticosteroids as outlined previously *(123)*. Experimental protocols based on a presumed autoimmune basis are being explored, including use of methotrexate, cyclosporine, plasmapheresis, and intravenous gamma globulin, particularly in steroid-resistant groups.

REFERENCES

1. Gorevic P, Kaplan AP (1980) The physical urticarias. Int J Dermatol 19:417.
2. Soter NA, Mihm MC, Jr, Dvorak HF, et al. (1978) Cutaneous necrotizing venulitis: a sequential analysis of the morphological alterations occurring after mast cell degranulation in a patient with a unique syndrome. Clin Exp Immunol 32:46.
3. Houser DD, Arbesman CE, Ito K, et al. (1970) Cold urticaria: immunologic studies, Am J Med 49:23.
4. Wanderer AP, Maselli R, Ellis EF, et al. (1971) Immunologic characterization of serum factors responsible for cold urticaria, J Allergy Clin Immunol 48:13.
5. Gruber BL, Marchese M, Ballan D, et al. (1986) Anti IgG autoantibodies: detection in urticarial syndromes and ability to release histamine from basophils, J Allergy Clin Immunol 77:187 (abstract).
6. Kaplan AP, Garofalo J, Sigler R, et al. (1981) Idiopathic cold urticaria: in vitro demonstration of histamine release upon challenge of skin biopsies, N Engl J Med 305:1074.
7. Soter NA, Wasserman SI, and Austen KF (1976) Cold urticaria: release into the circulation of histamine and eosinophil chemotactic factor of anaphylaxis during cold challenge, N Engl J Med 294:687.
8. Wasserman SI, Soter NA, Center DM, et al. (1977) Cold urticaria: recognition and characterization of a neutrophil chemotactic factor which appears in serum during experimental cold challenge, J Clin Invest 60:189.
9. Grandel KE, Farr RS, Wanderer AA, et al. (1985) Association of platelet-activating factor with primary acquired cold urticaria, N Engl J Med 313:405–409.
10. Ormerod AD, Black AK, Dawes J et al. (1988) Prostaglandin D_2 and histamine release in cold urticaria unaccompanied by evidence of platelet activation, J Allergy Clin Immunol 82:586.
11. Weinstock G, Arbeit L, Kaplan AP (1986) Release of prostaglandin D_2 and kinins in cold urticaria and cholinergic urticaria, J Allergy Clin Immunol 77:188 (abstract).
12. Quinti I, Brozek C, Wood N et al. (1986) Circulating IgG autoantibodies to IgE in atopic syndromes, J Allergy Clin Immunol 77:586.
13. Sigler RW, Evans R III, Horakova Z (1980) The role of cyproheptadine in the treatment of cold urticaria, J Allergy Clin Immunol 65:309.
14. Keahey TM, Greaves MW (1980) Cold urticaria: dissociation of cold-evoked histamine release and urticaria following cold challenge, Arch Dermatol 116:174.
15. Petillo JJ, Natbony SK, Zisblatt M et al. (1983) Preliminary report of the effects of tiaramide on the ice cube test in patients with idiopathic cold urticaria, Ann Allergy 51:511.
16. Houston DP, Bressler RB, Kaliner M et al. (1986) Prevention of mast-cell degranulation by ketotifen in patients with physical urticaria, Ann Int Med 204:507.
17. Costanzi JJ, Coltman CA Jr (1967) Kappa chain cold precipitable immunoglobulin (IgG) associated with cold urticaria. I. Clinical observations, Clin Exp Immunol 2:167.
18. Costanzi JJ, Coltman CA Jr, Donaldson VH (1969) Activation of complement by a monoclonal cryoglobulin associated with cold urticaria, J Lab Clin Med 74:902.
19. Eady RA, Greaves MW (1978) Induction of cutaneous vasculitis by repeated cold challenge in cold urticaria, Lancet 1:336.
20. Eady RAJ, Keahey TM, Sibbald RG et al. (1981) Cold urticaria with vasculitis: report of a case with light and electron microscopic, immunofluorescence, and pharmacological studies, Clin Exp Dermatol 6:355.

21. Wanderer AA, Nuss DP, Tormey AD et al. (1983) Urticarial leukocytoclastic vasculitis with cold urticaria: report of a case and review of the literature, Arch Dermatol 119:145.

22. Soter WA, Joski NP, Twarog FJ (1977) Delayed cold-induced urticaria: a dominantly inherited disorder, J Allergy Clin Immunol 54:294.

23. Kaplan AP, Garofalo J (1981) Identification of a new physically induced urticaria: cold induced cholinergic urticaria, J Allergy Clin Immunol 68:438.

24. Ormerod AD, Kobza-Black A, Milford-Ward A et al. (1988) Combined cold urticaria and cholinergic urticaria—clinical characterization and laboratory findings, Br J Dermatol 118:621.

25. Kaplan AP (1984) Unusual cold-induced disorders: cold dependent dermatographism and systemic cold urticaria, J Allergy Clin Immunol 73:453–456.

26. Kalz F, Bower CM, Prichard H (1950) Delayed and persistent dermographia, Arch Dermatol 61:772.

27. Kivity S, Schwartz Y, Wolf R et al. (1989) Systemic cold-induced urticaria—clinical and laboratory characterization, J Allergy Clin Immunol 85:52.

28. Czarnetzki BM, Frosch PJ, Sprekeler R (1981) Localized cold reflex urticaria, Br J Dermatol 104:83.

29. Ting S, Mansfield LE (1985) Localized cold reflex urticaria, J Allergy Clin Immunol 75:421.

30. Grant RT, Pearson RSB, Comeau WJ (1935) Observations on urticaria provoked by emotion, by exercise, and by warming the body, Clin Sci 2:266.

31. Lawrence CM, Jorizzo JL, Kobza-Black A (1981) Cholinergic urticaria with associated angioedema, Br J Dermatol 105:543.

32. Herxheimer A (1956) The nervous pathway mediating cholinergic urticaria, Clin Sci 15:195.

33. Commens CA, Greaves CA (1978) Tests to establish the diagnosis in cholinergic urticaria, Br J Dermatol 98:47.

34. Kaplan AP, Gray L, Snadt RE et al. (1975) In vivo studies of mediator release in cold urticaria and cholinergic urticaria, J Allergy Clin Immunol 55:394–402.

35. Shelley WB, Shelley CD, Ho AKS (1983) Cholinergic urticaria: acetylcholine-receptor dependent immediate-type hypersensitivity reaction to copper, Lancet 1:843.

36. Moore-Robinson M, Warin KP (1968) Some clinical aspects of cholinergic urticaria, Br J Dermatol 80:794.

37. Sigler RW, Levinson AI, Evans R III, et al. (1979) Evaluation of a patient with cold and cholinergic urticaria, J Allergy Clin Immunol 63:35.

38. Soter NA, Wasserman SI, Austen KF et al. (1980) Release of mast-cell mediators and alterations in lung function in patients with cholinergic urticaria, N Engl J Med 302:604.

39. Kaplan AP, Natbony SF, Tawil AP (1981) Exercise-induced anaphylaxis as a manifestation of cholinergic urticaria, J Allergy Clin Immunol 68:319–324.

40. Casale TB, Keahey TM, Kaliner M (1986) Exercise-induced anaphylactic syndromes. Insights into diagnostic and pathophysiologic features, JAMA 255:2049.

41. Sheffer AL, Austen KF (1980) Exercise-induced anaphylaxis, J Allergy Clin Immunol 66:106.

42. Sheffer AL, Soter NA, McFadden ER Jr, et al. (1983) Exercise-induced anaphylaxis: a distinct form of physical allergy, J Allergy Clin Immunol 71:311.

43. Lewis J, Lieberman P, Treadwell G et al. (1981) Exercise-induced urticaria, angioedema, and anaphylactoid episodes, J Allergy Clin Immunol 68:432.

44. Maulitz RM, Pratt DS, Schocket AL (1979) Exercise-induced anaphylactic reaction to shellfish, J Allergy Clin Immunol 63:433.

45. Novey HS, Fairshter RD, Salness K et al. (1983) Postprandial exercise-induced anaphylaxis. J Allergy Clin Immunol 71:498–502.

46. Kidd JM III, Cohen SH, Sosman AJ et al. (1983) Food dependent exercise-induced anaphylaxis. J Allergy Clin Immunol 71:407.

47. Kivity S, Sneh E, Greif J et al. (1987) The effect of food and exercise on the skin response to compound 48/80 in patients with food-associated exercise-induced urticaria-angioedema. J Allergy Clin Immunol 81:1155.

48. Greaves MW (1971) Histamine excretion yand dermographism in urticaria pigmentosa before and after administration of a specific histidine-decarboxylase inhibitor. Br J Dermatol 85:467.

49. Grant JA, Findlay JR, Thueson DO (1981) Local heat urticaria/angioedema: evidence for histamine release without complement activation. J Allergy Clin Immunol 67:75.

50. Atkins PC, Zweiman, B (1981) Mediator release in local heat urticaria. J Allergy Clin Immunol 26:286.

51. Daman L, Lieberman P, Garner M, et al. (1978) Localized heat urticaria. J Allergy Clin Immunol 61:273.

52. Tennenbaum JT, Lowney E (1973) Localized heat and cold urticaria. J Allergy Clin Immunol 51:57.

53. Michaelsson G, Ros A (1971) Familial localized heat urticaria of delayed type. Acta Derm Venereol 51:279.

54. Matthews KP (1983) Urticaria and angioedema. J Allergy Clin Immunol 72:1.

55. Soter NA, Wasserman SI (1980) Physical urticaria/angioedema: an experimental model of mast cell activation in humans. J Allergy Clin Immunol 66:358.

56. Cauna N, Levine MI (1970) The fine morphology of the human skin in dermographism. J Allergy Clin Immunol 45:266.

57. Aoyama H, Katsumata Y, Olzawa J (1970) Dermographism-inducing principle of urticaria factitia. Jpn J Dermatol 80:122.

58. Newcomb RW, Nelson H (1973) Dermographism mediated by IgE. Am J Med 54:174.

59. Rose B (1941) Studies on blood histamine in cases of allergy. I. Blood histamine during wheal formation. J Allergy 12:327.

60. Kaplan AP, Horakova Z, Katz SI (1978) Assessment of tissue fluid histamine levels in patients with urticaria. J Allergy Clin Immunol 61:350–354.

61. Greaves MW, Sundergoard J (1970) Urticaria pigmentosa and factitious urticaria: direct evidence for release of histamine and other smooth muscle-contracting agents in dermographic skin. Arch Dermatol 101:418.

62. Garofalo J, Kaplan AP (1981) Histamine release and therapy of severe dermatographism. J Allergy Clin Immunol 68:103.

63. Mathews KP (1983) Urticaria and angioedema. J Allergy Clin Immunol 72:11.

64. Smith JA, Mansfield LE, Fokakis A, et al. (1983) Dermographism caused by IgE mediated penicillin allergy. Ann Allergy 57:30.

65. Matthews CNA, Kirby JD, James J, et al. (1973) Dermographism: reduction in wheal size by chlorpheniramine and hydroxyzine. Br J Dermatol 88:279.

66. Matthews CNA, Boss JM, Warin RP, et al. (1979) The effect of H_1 and H_2 histamine antagonists on symptomatic dermographism. Br J Dermatol 101:57.

67. Roberts LJ II, Sweetman BJ, Lewis RA (1980) Increased production of prostaglandin D_2 in patients with systemic mastocytosis. N Engl J Med 303:1400.

68. Ryan TJ, Shim-Young N, Turk JL (1968) Delayed pressure urticaria. Br J Dermatol 80:485.

69. Estes SA, Yang CW (1981) Delayed pressure urticaria: An investigation of some parameters of lesion induction. J Am Acad Dermatol 5:25.

70. Davis KC, Mekori YA, Kohler PF, et al. (1984) Possible role of diet in delayed pressure urticaria. J Allergy Clin Immunol 73:183 (abstract).

71. Parrillo JE, Lawley TJ, Frank MM (1979) Immunologic reactivity in the hypereosinophil syndrome. J Allergy Clin Immunol 64:113.

72. Harber LC, Holloway RM, Sheatley VR, et al. (1963) Immunologic and biophysical studies in solar urticaria. J Invest Dermatol 41:439.

73. Horio T (1978) Photoallergic urticaria induced by visible light: additional cases and further studies. Arch Dermatol 114:1761.

74. Sams WM Jr, Epstein JH, Winkelmann RK (1969) Solar urticaria. investigation of pathogenic mechanisms. Arch Dermatol 99:390.

75. Hawk JLM, Eady RAJ, Challiner AVJ (1980) Elevated blood histamine levels and mast cell degranulation in solar urticaria. Br J Clin Pharmacol 9:183.

76. Soter NA, Wasserman SI, Pathak MA (1979) Solar urticaria: release of mast cell mediators into the circulation after experimental challenge. J Invest Dermatol 72:283.

77. Bonkowsky HL, Bloomer JR, Ebert PS, et al. (1975) Heme synthetase deficiency in human protoporphyria: demonstration of the defect in liver and cultured skin fibroblasts. J Clin Invest 56:1139.

78. Bottomley SS, Tanaka M, Everett MA (1975) Diminished erythroid ferrochetalase activity in protoporphyria. J Lab Clin Med 86:126.

79. Lim HW, Perez HD, Poh-Fitzpatrick, M (1981) Generation of chemotactic activity in serum from patients with erythropoietic protoporphyria and porphyria cutanea tarda. N Engl J Med 304:212.

80. Gigli I, Schothorst AA, Soter NA, et al. (1980) Erythropoietic protoporphyria: photoactivation of the complement system. J Clin Invest 66:517.

81. Lim HW, Poh-Fitzpatrick MB, Gigli I (1984) Activation of the complement system in patients with porphyrias after irradiation in vivo. J Clin Invest 74:1961.

82. Baart DLFH, Beerens EGJ, Van Weelden H, et al. (1978) Complement components in blood serum and suction blister fluid in erythropoietic protoporphyria. Br J Dermatol 99:401.

83. Epstein JH, Tuffanelli DL, Epstein WL (1979) Cutaneous changes in the porphyrias: a microscopic study. Arch Dermatol 107:6789.

84. Moshell AN, Bjornson L (1977) Protection in erythropoietic protoporphyria: Mechanism of protection by β carotene. J Invest Dermatol 68:157.

85. Chalamidas SL, Charles CR (1971) Aquagenic urticaria. Arch Dermatol 104:541.

86. Davis RS, Remigio LK, Schocket AL, et al. (1981) Evaluation of a patient with both aquagenic and cholinergic urticaria. J Allergy Clin Immunol 68:479.

87. Patterson R, Mellies CJ, Blankenship ML, et al. (1972) Vibratory angioedema: a hereditary type of physical hypersensitivity. J Allergy Clin Immunol 50:174.

88. Metzger WJ, Kaplan AP, Beaven MA (1976) Hereditary vibratory angioedema: confirmation of histamine release in a type of physical hypersensitivity. J Allergy Clin Immunol 57:605.

89. Kaplan AP (1997) Urticaria and angioedema. In: Kaplan AP ed., Allergy. Second edition, Saunders WB. Philadelphia, PA, pp. 573–592.

90. Dolovich J, Little DC (1972) Correlates of skin test reactions to *Bacillus subtilis* enzyme preparations. J Allergy Clin Immunol 49:43.

91. Dolovich J, Hargreave FE, Chalmers R, et al. (1973) Late cutaneous allergic responses in isolated IgE-dependent reactions. J Allergy Clin Immunol 52:38–46.

92. Solley GO, Gleich GJ, Jordan RE, et al. (1976) The late phase of the immediate wheal and flare skin reaction. Its dependence upon IgE antibodies. J Clin Invest 58:408–420.

93. Durham SR, Lee TH, Cromwell O, et al. (1984) Immunologic studies in allergen-induced late phase asthmatic reactions. J Allergy Clin Immunol 74:49–60.

94. Reshef A, Kagey-Sobotka A, Adkinson NF Jr, et al. (1989) The pattern and kinetics in human skin of erythema and mediators during the acute and late-phase response (LPR). J Allergy Clin Immunol 84:678–687.

95. Dor PJ, Vervloet D, Supene M, et al. (1983) Induction of late cutaneous reaction by kallikrein injection: comparison with allergic-like late response to compound 48/80. J Allergy Clin Immunol 71:363.

96. Koehn GG, Thorne EG (1972) Urticaria and viral hepatitis. Arch Dermatol 106:422.

97. Cowdry SC, Reynolds JS (1969) Acute urticaria in infectious mononucleosis. Ann Allergy 27:182.

98. Arbesman CE, Reisman RE (1971) Serum sickness and human anaphylaxis. In: Samter M ed. Immunologic Diseases. Little Brown, Boston, pp. 495–510.

99. Paver WK (1971) Discoid and subacute systemic lupus erythematosus associated with urticaria. Aust J Dermatol 12:113.

100. Provost TT, Zone JJ, Synkowski D, et al. (1980) Unusual clinical manifestations of systemic lupus erythematosus. I. Urticaria-like lesions: correlations with clinical and serological abnormalities. J Invest Dermatol 75:495.

101. Ghebrehiwet B (1997) The complement system: mechanism of activation, regulation, and biological functions. In: Kaplan AP ed., Allergy. Second edition, Saunders WB. Philadelphia, Pa, pp. 219–234.

102. Atkins PC, Schwartz LB, Adkinson NF, et al. (1990) In vivo antigen-induced cutaneous mediator release: simultaneous comparisons of histamine, tryptase, and prostaglandin D_2 release and the effect of oral corticosteroid administration. J Allergy Clin Immunol 86:360.

103. Soter NA, Austen KF, Gigli I (1974) Urticaria and arthralgias as a manifestation of necrotizing angiitis. J Invest Dermatol 63:489.

104. Soter NA, Mihm MC Jr, Gigli I, et al. (1976) Two distinct cellular patterns in cutaneous necrotizing angiitis. J Invest Dermatol 66:334.

105. Mathison DA, Arroyave CM, Bhat KN, et al. (1977) Hypocomplementemia in chronic idiopathic urticaria. Ann Intern Med 86:534.

106. Monroe EW, Schulz CI, Maize JC, et al. (1981) Vasculitis in chronic urticaria: an immunopathologic study. J Invest Dermatol 76:103.

107. Natbony SF, Phillips ME, Elias JM, et al. (1983) Histologic studies of chronic idiopathic urticaria. J Allergy Clin Immunol 71:177–183.

108. Phanuphak P, Kohler PF, Stanford RE, et al. (1980) Vasculitis in chronic urticaria. J Allergy Clin Immunol 65:436.

109. Kern F, Lichtenstein LM (1977) Defective histamine release in chronic urticaria. J Clin Invest 57:1360.

110. Phanuphak P, Schocket AL, Arroyave CM, et al. (1980) Skin histamine in chronic urticaria. J Allergy Clin Immunol 65:371.

111. Smith CH, Kepley C, Schwartz L, et al. (1995) Mast cell number and phenotype in chronic idiopathic urticaria. J Allergy Clin Immunol 96:360–364.

112. Mekori YA, Giorno RC, Anderson P, et al. (1983) Lymphocyte subpopulations in the skin of patients with chronic urticaria. J Allergy Clin Immunol 72:681.

113. Elias J, Boss E, Kaplan AP (1986) Studies of the cellular infiltrate of chronic idiopathic urticaria: prominence of T-lymphocytes, monocytes, and mast cells. J Allergy Clin Immunol 78:914–918.

114. Peters MS, Schroeter AL, Kephart GM, et al. (1983) Localization of eosinophil granule major basic protein in chronic urticaria. J Invest Dermatol 81:39.

115. Claveau J, Lavoie A, Brunet C, et al. (1993) Chronic idiopathic urticaria: possible contribution of histamine-releasing factor to pathogenesis. J Allergy Clin Immunol 92:132–137.

116. Leznoff A, Josse RG, Denberg J. et al. (1983) Association of chronic urticaria and angioedema with thyroid autoimmunity. Arch Dermatol 119:636–640.

117. Leznoff A, Sussman GL (1989) Syndrome of idiopathic chronic urticaria and angioedema with thyroid autoimmunity: a study of 90 patients. J Allergy Clin Immunol 84:66–71.

118. Gruber BL, Baeza M, Marchese M, et al. (1988) Prevalance and functional role of anti-IgE autoantibodies in urticarial syndromes. J Invest Dermatol 90:213.

119. Hide M, Francis DM, Grattan CEH, et al. (1993) Autoantibodies against the high-affinity IgE receptor as a cause of histamine release in chronic urticaria. N Engl J Med 328:1595–1604.

120. Tong L, Balakrishnan G, Kochan J, et al. (1996) Assessment of autoimmunity in chronic urticaria patients. J All Clin Immunol 97:424 (abstract).

121. Guo C-B, Liu MC, Galli SJ, et al. (1994) Identification of IgE-bearing cells in the late-phase response to antigen in the lung as basophils. Am J Respir Dis 10:384–390.

122. Charlesworth CN, Hood AF, Soter NA, et al. (1989) Cutaneous late-phase response to allergen. Mediator release and inflammatory cell infiltration, J Clin Invest 83:1519–1526.

123. Kaplan AP (1993) Urticaria and angioedema. In: Middleton Jr. E, Reed CE, Ellis EF, Adkinson Jr. NF, Yunginger JW, Busse WW, eds. Allergy—Principles and Practices. Mosby, St. Louis, Mo., pp. 1553–1580.

25 Atopic Eczema

Johannes Ring, PHD, Ulf Darsow, PHD, and Dietrich Abeck, PHD

CONTENTS

INTRODUCTION

Atopic eczema (AE), also called atopic dermatitis, is an inflammatory, chronically relapsing, noncontagious, and extremely pruritic skin disease. With a prevalence of 2–5% in children (young adults approx 10%), it is one of the most commonly seen dermatoses. The discussion about pathogenesis of this disease is mirrored by the different names that it has been given ("prurigo Besnier," "neurodermitis," "endogenous eczema," and so forth). Atopy is a strikingly common finding in these patients *(1)*. It is defined as "familial hypersensitivity of skin and mucous membranes to environmental substances, associated with increased immunoglobulin E (IgE) formation and/or altered nonspecific reactivity" *(2,3)*.

The atopic diseases atopic eczema, allergic bronchial asthma, and allergic rhinoconjunctivitis are genetically linked within families. A multifactorial trait with gene loci on chromosomes 5 and 11 was proposed by different groups involving immunological markers like interleukin (IL)-4 or the high-affinity IgE receptor *(4–6)*. The concordance of atopic eczema in monocygotic twins is 75–85%, and in dizygotic twins 30% *(3,7)*.

CLINICAL AND PATHOLOGICAL FINDINGS

Often beginning with the clinical sign known as "cradle cap" after the first 3 mo of life, the disease spreads to face and extensor sides of arms and legs of toddlers, showing extensive oozing and crusting *(1,2)*. Later on, the typical preferential pattern with eczematous skin lesions of flexures, neck, and hands develops, accompanied by dry skin as a subjective impression and measurable transepidermal water loss (TEWL). Lichenification is a result of scratching and rubbing, and in adults this may also result in excoriated nodules, the "prurigo form" of atopic eczema. New exacerbations often start without obvious symptoms except increased itching (sometimes localized). This is followed by erythema, papules, and infiltration. Acute atopic eczema is histopathologically characterized by acanthosis, hyperkeratosis, parakeratosis, spongiosis, exocytosis, and a sparse lymphohistiocytic infiltrate. Chronic lichenified lesions show acanthosis, hyperkeratosis, parakeratosis, dense dermal mononuclear infiltrate, increase in mast-cell and capillary number, enlargement of capillary walls

From: *Allergy and Allergic Diseases: The New Mechanisms and Therapeutics*
Edited by: J. A. Denburg © Humana Press Inc., Totowa, NJ

with endothelial hyperplasia, and fibrosis *(3)*. However, these features are not specific for atopic eczema. Complement deposits at the basal layer have also been described *(8)*.

As there is no laboratory marker specific for the disease, "stigmata" and minimal manifestations of atopic eczema have been found to have diagnostic significance (Table 1) *(1,3)*. According to our experience, the clinical diagnosis may be established more simply by finding four of the criteria in the third column of Table 1.

Immunoglobulin E Dysregulation

AE is characterized by increased production of IgE, which is a result of the imbalance of T helper (Th) cell subsets 1 and 2 with a predominance of IL-4-secreting Th2 cells with IL-4 as a potent stimulator of IgE synthesis. In addition, IL-4 inhibits the production of interferon (IFN)γ at the level of transcription *(10)*. In vitro addition of IFNγ, which inhibits IL-4-induced IgE expression to cultured mononuclear cells of patients with atopic dermatitis, significantly reduced both IL-4-receptor expression and IL-4 expression *(11)*. These issues are dealt with in greater detail elsewhere in this volume.

Cell-Mediated Dysfunction

As patients with atopic eczema are prone to develop more frequently a variety of infectious diseases of fungal, viral, or bacterial origin like candidosis, eczema herpeticatum (= Kaposi's varicelliform eruption), or staphylococcal impetigo, defective cellular immunity has been suspected in this disease. However, the hypothesis of a lower prevalence of T-cell-mediated contact allergy in atopic eczema has recently been questioned. Rather, these patients have a different allergic spectrum compared with nonatopics. In some clinical syndromes, increased synthesis of IgE is accompanied by impairment of cellular immunity. The inflammatory infiltrate in AE lesions mainly consists of $CD4^+$ T-lymphocytes, and a correlation with disease activity can be shown for the proportion of activated and unactivated $CD4^+$ cells, as well as a decrease in the proportion of $CD8^+$ cells *(12)*.

Autonomic Nervous System Dysregulation

In response to different pharmacological stimuli, a substantial proportion of patients with atopic eczema shows a decreased β-adrenergic and an increased α-adrenergic or cholinergic reactivity. Clinically, white dermatographism and some psychosomatic interactions may partially be explained by this imbalance, giving rise also to altered (enhanced) releasability of vasoactive mediators like histamine and leukotrienes after appropriate stimulation.

Atopic Eczema and the Role of Food Allergy and Food Intolerance

A provocation of AE by foods in sensitive patients has been repeatedly reported, with the vast majority of cases seen in children *(13,14)* and should be considered in the management of AE when there is a history of provocation by food or when conventional treatment measures are ineffective. Whereas IgE-mediated reactions are the most common ones, a non-immunological, pseudo-allergic reaction to food additives can also provoke AE in some cases *(13)*. According to a study by Guillet and Guillet *(15)* the presence of a food allergy is indicative of a prognosis of severe AE and of associated respiratory atopy. Recommendations in children at risk for atopic diseases suggest the avoidance of highly allergic foods in the first months of life owing to priming the immune system of these genetically predisposed individuals *(16)*. The prophylactic effect of breast-feeding in the development of AE has been shown recently in a prospective study closely following up healthy children from infancy until early childhood over a period of 17 years *(17)*.

Table 1
Clinical Signs of Atopy and Diagnostic Clues for Atopic Eczema

"Stigmata" of atopy (1,3)	"Minimal manifestations" of AE (9)	Clinical diagnosis of AE (3) (four criteria are sufficient)
Sebostasis, xerosis	Cheilitis sicca	Eczematous skin lesions (age-dependent)
Hyperlinearity of palms and soles	Perlèche	Early onset and typical localization of skin lesions according to age
Linear grooves of fingertips	Atopic winter feet (pulpitis sicca, also involving fingertips)	Pruritus
Dennie-Morgan fold (atopy fold, doubled infraorbicular fold)	Retroauricular fissuring	Stigmata of atopy
Hertoghe's sign (hypodense lateral eyebrows)	Keratosis pilaris	Personal or family history of atopy
Short distance of scalp hair growth to eyebrows	Pityriasis alba	IgE-mediated sensitization
Periorbital "shadow"		
White dermatographism (sometimes)		
Delayed blanching after intracutaneous injection of acetylcholine		
Increased irritability by wool fabric		

Table 2
Resident Flora of Normal and Atopic Skin

Resident skin flora	Normal	AE
Micrococcaceae		
Coagulase-negative staphylococci	+	++
Staphylococcus aureus	–	++
Coryneform organisms		
Corynebacteria	+	+
Propionibacteria	+	+
Pityrosporum	+	++

Skin Barrier

The clinical appearance of eczematous inflamed lesions emerging on dry, scaling skin is suggestive of an impairment of skin barrier function. An enhanced TEWL and a reduced skin surface water content are physical parameters that directly reflect this impaired barrier function. The barrier function is maintained by the stratum corneum, which forms a continuous sheet of alternating squamae that are protein-enriched corneocytes embedded in an intercellular matrix consisting of mainly nonpolar lipids having developed as lamellar sheets *(18)*. Atopic skin is characterized by distinct differences in skin surface lipid composition, which especially applies to the ceramide fraction *(19)*. In addition, a shift from long saturated fatty acids toward short-chain saturated fatty acids in both lesional and nonlesional skin of AE compared to normal skin has been demonstrated *(20)*. This defective maturation of lipids and fatty acids in atopic skin may lead to an impaired acylceramide synthesis. Decreased levels of ceramides in atopic skin are not caused by enzymatic changes, since the activity of β-glucocerebrosidase, a major enzyme in ceramide production, and ceramidase, an enzyme essential for ceramide degradation, does not differ from those of age-matched healthy controls *(21)*. These findings imply differences in atopic lipid synthesis based on an altered signal transduction. Interestingly, the regeneration of the epidermal barrier function after tape-stripping-induced pertubation in patients with AE was faster as compared with control subjects, suggesting a persisting mild disturbance of barrier function with permanently activated repair mechanisms in patients with AE *(22)*.

Microbial Colonization

Profound changes in cutaneous flora occur in patients with AE (Table 2) *(23)*, and the pathogenetic importance of microbial organisms has already been discussed a long time ago *(23,24)*. Among these, *Staphylococcus aureus* seems to play a major role *(24)*. Not only is this bacterium responsible for a known, very often quite dramatic complication of AE, called "impetiginized AE," requiring systemic antibacterial treatment *(25)*, but *S. aureus* may also act in addition as a persistent allergen or irritant with inflammatous potency when colonizing atopic skin. The inflammatory reaction may be caused by enterotoxin production with possibly superantigen effects. More than 50% of *S. aureus* isolates cultured from patients with AE have the ability to produce these kinds of enterotoxins *(26)*. It is speculated that staphyloccocal superantigens when released within the epidermis cause a marked immune stimulation *(27)*. The ability of staphylococcal enterotoxin B to elict a dermatitis after application on intact normal or intact atopic skin was shown recently *(28)*. Skov and Baadsgaard

(29) reported that ultraviolet B (UVB)-irradiated major histocompatibility complex (MHC) class II$^+$ keratinocytes were able to activate T-cells in the presence of *S. aureus* enterotoxin B and thereby maintain inflammation in spite of UVB treatment; they suggested that UVB treatment would be more effective when supplemented with antimicrobial agents aimed at eliminating staphylococcal colonization.

Atopic Pruritus

Excruciating itch is the most prominent symptom in atopic eczema. New skin lesions often start with itching ("invisible itch"), and when pruritus is controlled by therapy, the lesions gradually subside. It has been stated that "the diagnosis of active atopic dermatitis cannot be made if there is no history of itching" *(29a)*. Itching is usually intermittent, with exacerbations in the evening, and may be precipitated by a number of stimuli such as sweating, contact with wool, psychological stress, or immunological influences (*see* below). The itch of atopic eczema has some uncommon features, among which its limited respon-siveness to antihistamine therapy (when the sedative effects of first-generation H$_1$ blockers are excluded) is most prominent. In contrast, steroids are often able to give instant relief, in addition to physical measures such as cooling or intense heating of the skin (which may, in turn, cause excessive drying, thus perpetuating the itch sensation). Most authors interpret the response of atopic pruritus to steroids and cyclosporine A as proof that mediators other than histamine are important in atopic pruritus. The presumed itch mediator(s) may act directly or indirectly through cascade-like release of other mediators on the itch receptor. This receptor most probably consists of free endings of unmyelinated, slow-conducting C fibers at the dermal-epidermal junction. The C fibers contain neuropeptides (substance P, vasoactive intestinal polypeptide [VIP] neurotensin A, somatostatin, neuropeptide Y, and opioid peptides) that may be released after appropriate stimuli (like scratching) and cause vasodilatation and so-called neurogenic inflammation, thus probably perpetuating the eczema. When injected intradermally in humans, they elicit itching of different degree and a wheal and flare response like histamine (for a review *see* ref. *30*). Therefore, they are thought of as histamine releasers and, indeed, their action is inhibited by antihistamines. Serotonin, especially in combination with prostaglandins, produces itch after intradermal injection; this therefore is theoretically unresponsive to antihistamines and treatable by serotonin antagonists.

Microscopic signs of inflammation can be demonstrated in dry atopic skin, resulting in a high degree of irritability *(35)*. The mechanism of dry-skin itch is still poorly understood; also nonatopic skin does itch when desiccated. Owing to the mononuclear-cell infiltrate consisting mainly of T-lymphocytes near the dermal–epidermal junction that is found in AE and many other pruritic dermatoses, the cytokine IL-2 has been proposed to be a possible pruritogen in a controlled trial *(31)*. We could show a weak itch effect of IL-2 in a randomized crossover trial with 10 healthy volunteers *(37a)* using a well-established skin-prick model *(32)*. Cutaneous reactivity to histamine and vasoactive neuropeptides (substance P) has been reported to be decreased (for a review *see* ref. *33*), unchanged, or increased (for a review *see* ref. *34*) in patients with AE. These contradictory findings may point to a possibly temporary autonomic dysregulation of small skin vessels, probably dependent on the acuity of disease, and variable histamine metabolism. They also shed light on the methodological problems of itch investigations. In summary, several biogenic peptides, enzymes, and synthetic compounds have been described as itch elicitors when injected intradermally; however, most of them are known histamine releasers, and no evidence for a peripherally acting, histamine-independent pruritogenic effect has been demonstrated consistently yet.

Psychosomatic Factors

Pruritus severity of atopic eczema has been described as directly related to severity of depressive symptoms when psychosomatic relations were investigated *(36)*. Increased itch and sweating in lichenified skin areas following emotional stimuli can be recorded by means of psychophysiological methods (for a review *see* refs. *37* and *38*). In addition, some investigations on parent–child relationship showed different emotional impressions of the diseased children as compared to controls *(39,40)*. Increased "fear scores" on personality questionnaires of patients with atopic eczema have been reported by different investigators *(41,42)*. However, the question remains whether these findings have any impact on the etiology of eczema. They may also be results of the prolonged coping process of the patient and his family with the chronic disease. In contrast, emotionally stressful events have been shown to precede the deterioration of eczematous symptoms, not to follow them *(43)*. These findings have been questioned with regard to children by Gil et al. *(44)*. Further investigations in the field of psychoneuroimmunology *(45)* may shed light on the reasons for contradictory results.

Atopy Patch Test with Aeroallergens: A New Diagnostic Tool?

Some patients with atopic eczema suffer from exacerbation of their skin lesions after contact with certain aeroallergens, e.g., house dust mite, pollen, or animal dander, and improve after appropriate avoidance strategies have been applied *(46)*. Immunologic mechanisms may contribute to the phenomenon of itchy skin when clothes are taken off in some patients and their skin comes in contact with air (this has been called "atmoknesis") *(47)*. In an experimental setting, atopic eczema lesions have been induced in nine of 20 patients by bronchial provocation with a standardized house dust mite extract. The nine reacting patients had a history of bronchial asthma *(48)*.

It has been repeatedly shown that in certain patients eczematous skin lesions can be induced by epicutaneous patch testing with aeroallergens, e.g., house dust mite *(49–69)*. For this test procedure, namely, an "epicutaneous patch test using allergens known to induce an IgE-mediated sensitization and the evaluation of an eventually occurring eczematous skin reaction," we have proposed the term "atopy patch test" (APT) *(63)*.

An early study describing patch testing with aeroallergens was published in 1982 by Mitchell and coworkers *(59)*; since then, the methods used show wide variations. Thus, 15–100%-positive APT results in atopic eczema have been reported. Skin abrasion *(56,59,60)*, tape stripping *(51,68)*, and sodium lauryl sulfate application *(66)* were frequently used to enhance allergen penetration. These manipulations were found necessary because protein allergens of high molecular weight and pronounced hydrophility were thought not to pass the skin barrier. However, studies with APT on nonabraded, nonpretreated skin were also performed *(54,63,69)* with different rates of positive reactions. The results are obviously partially related to the allergen content in the preparations used. As an approach for standardization, we performed comparative epicutaneous tests with aeroallergens in different concentrations and vehicles on uninvolved, untreated skin *(54)*:

1. There was a clear dose–response relation between allergen concentration and positive APT reactions. After 48 h, 72% clear-cut positive reactions were provoked with 10,000 protein nitrogen unit (PNU)/g allergen concentration. In addition, twice as many APT reactions occurred with petrolatum compared to hydrogel vehicle. This held true for different reaction intensity and allergen concentration (Table 3). Figure 1 shows an example of dose-dependent APT reactions to an increasing concentration of house dust mite allergen in petrolatum.

Table 3
Number of Positive APT Reactions after 48 h with Different Allergen Concentrations
and Vehicles in 36 Patients with Atopic Eczema (Data from Ref. 54)

	Intensity of reactions				
	(+)	+	++	+++	Total ≥+
Allergen concentration in petrolatum					
1000 PNU/g	19	9	2	0	11 (19.3%)
10,000 PNU/g	12	13	11	3	27 (47.4%)
Total in petrolatum	31	22	13	3	38 (66.7%)
Allergen concentration in hydrogel					
1000 PNU/g	8	2	3	0	5 (8.8%)
10,000 PNU/g	10	5	7	2	14 (24.6%)
Total in hydrogel	18	7	10	2	19 (33.3%)
Total	49	29	23	5	57 (100%)

2. The most frequent clear-cut positive APT reactions were elicited by house dust mite *Dermatophagoides pteronyssinus* (36.1%). Reactions to cat dander and grass pollen were seen in 22.2 and 16.7% of patients. The individual allergen pattern of the patients varied with their skin-prick and radioallergo absorbent test (RAST) results.
3. Only for grass pollen, a significant concordance with a matching history was shown in another study involving 79 patients with atopic eczema *(70)*, suggesting that the patients were able to remember seasonal exacerbations more consistently. In this patient group, the positive predictive value with regard to the individual history of the APT even with crude, unprocessed grass pollen was higher than with the classic tests for IgE-mediated hypersensitivity (Table 4).
4. High allergen-specific IgE is not mandatory for a positive APT since a small subgroup of patients with a positive APT (approx 10%) showed a negative skin prick and RAST. In most APT-positive patients a statistically significantly elevated specific IgE level was found compared to the patients with negative APT results. Thus, an important role for IgE in the reaction mechanism of the APT can be presumed.

In a further study we were able to show that APT was positive in 69% of patients with an air-exposed pattern of skin lesions as compared to 39% of a control group of "inconspicuous" atopic eczema distribution *(55)*. A clear dose-response relationship between allergen concentration and number of patients with positive APT reactions was obtained in both patient groups (Fig. 2). However, the mode of this dose-dependent increase in positive results in group I differed significantly from the APT reactivity of group II; in the investigated dose range from 500 to 10,000 PNU/g, only group II showed a linear dose-response. These results confirm that aeroallergens are able to elicit eczematous skin lesions in a dose-dependent way in different groups of patients with atopic eczema when applied epicutaneously on untreated skin. Patients with predominantly air-exposed lesions of atopic eczema showed a significantly higher frequency of positive APT reactions.

The IgE-dependency of APT reactions has been demonstrated by Langeland and coworkers *(58)*, who were able to transfer APT reactivity by serum in a Prausnitz-Küstner test. As described

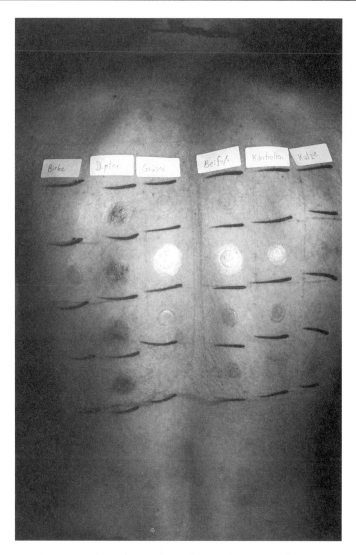

Fig. 1. Dose-response of atopy patch test in a patient with atopic eczema after removal of Finn chambers after 48 h. Allergen concentration increases from top to bottom from 3000 to 10,000 PNU/g.

above, a significant association of positive APT reactions and specific serum IgE exists. Langerhans cells carry IgE receptors of different classes *(66,71,72)*. This might explain IgE-associated activation of allergen-specific T-cells finally leading to eczematous skin lesions in the APT. van Reijsen et al. *(73)* and Sager et al. *(74,75)* characterized allergen-specific T-cell clones derived from skin specimens taken from APT sites. Mite allergen in the epidermis under natural conditions *(76)* as well as in APT sites *(56,66)* has been demonstrated in proximity to Langerhans cells. With this in mind, the relationship between APT and distribution of eczematous skin lesions may lead to the hypothesis that a subgroup of patients with atopic eczema exists with an increased, IgE-mediated aeroallergen-specific cutaneous reactivity leading to eczematous skin changes. This increased reactivity may distinguish the APT-positive patients from others with atopic eczema and specific IgE to aeroallergens. The exact mechanism remains to be elucidated. Recently, increased TEWL in patients with atopic eczema over positive APT

Table 4
Positive Predictive Value of Different Diagnostic Measures
in Patients with Atopic Eczema with Regard to a History
of Grass Pollen-Induced Seasonal Exacerbation, $n = 79$

Test	Positive predictive value[a] with regard to patient's history
APT: grass pollen mixture	0.45
APT: unprocessed *DG* pollen[b]	0.53
Skin prick test	0.21
Specific IgE	0.20

[a]Ratio of true positive compared to all positive.
[b]*DG*, dactylis glomerata.

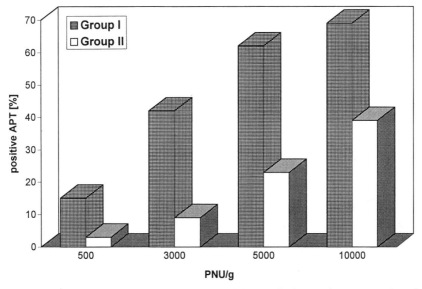

Fig. 2. Dose-response of atopy patch test comparing clinically distinct patient groups ($p = 0.03$). Both groups were best differentiated with an allergen concentration of 5000 PNU/g. Group I: patients with eczematous skin lesions predominantly located in air-exposed areas. Group II: control patients with atopic eczema (data from ref. 55).

reactions compared to classic contact allergic patch test was described *(77)*. Features of the skin barrier may contribute to different epicutaneous reaction patterns.

CONCLUSION

At least in a subgroup of patients with atopic eczema, IgE-mediated allergic reactions play a pathophysiological role. On the other hand, there are many patients in which nonspecific factors such as irritants or psychosomatic influence appear to be of major importance. As with other atopic diseases, atopic eczema may be classified into "extrinsic/allergic" and "intrinsic/cryptogenic" forms. Thus, careful allergy diagnosis is mandatory in patients with atopic eczema not responding to mild topical treatment. Clinical relevance of a given allergic sensitization should be evaluated in each individual patient.

REFERENCES

1. Rajka G (1989) Essential Aspects of Atopic Dermatitis. Springer, Berlin.
2. Ruzicka T, Ring J, Przybilla B, eds (1991) Handbook of Atopic Eczema. Springer, Berlin.
3. Ring J (1990) Angewandte Allergologie. MMV Medizin Verlag, Munich.
4. Cookson WOCM, Sharp PA, Faux JA, Hopkin JM (1989) Linkage between immunoglobulin E responses underlying asthma and rhinitis and chromosome 11q. Lancet 334:1292–1295.
5. Marsh DG, Neely JD, Breazeale DR, Ghosh B, Freidhoff LR, Ehrlich-Kautzky E, Schou C, Krishnaswamy G, Beaty TH (1994) Linkage analysis of IL-4 and other chromosome 5q31.1 markers and total serum IgE concentrations. Science 264:1152–1156.
6. Van Herwerden L, Harrap SB, Wong ZYH, Abramson MJ, Kutin JJ, Forbes AB, Raven J, Lanigan A, Walters EH (1995) Linkage of high-affinity IgE receptor gene with bronchial hyperreactivity, even in absence of atopy. Lancet 346:1262–1265.
7. Schultz-Larsen F, Holm NV, Henningsen K (1986) Atopic dermatitis. A genetic-epidemiologic study in a population-based twin sample. J Am Acad Dermatol 15:487–494.
8. Ring J, Senter T, Cornell RC, Arroyave CM, Tan EM (1978) Complement and immunoglobulin deposits in the skin of patients with atopic dermatitis. Br J Dermatol 99:495–501.
9. Wüthrich B (1991) Minimal forms of atopic eczema. In: Ruzicka T, Ring J, Przybilla B, eds. Handbook of Atopic Eczema. Springer, Berlin, pp. 46–53.
10. Vercelli D, Jabara H, Lauener R, Geha R (1990) IL-4 inhibits the synthesis of INF-gamma and induces the synthesis of IgE in human mixed lymphocyte cultures. J Immunol 144:570–573.
11. Renz H, Jujo K, Bradley K, et al. (1992) Enhanced IL-4 production and IL-4 receptor expression in atopic dermatitis and their modulation by interferon-gamma. J Invest Dermatol 99:403–408.
12. Sowden J, Powell R, Allen B (1992) Selective activation of circulating CD4$^+$ lymphocytes in severe adult atopic dermatitis. Br J Dermatol 127:228–232.
13. Przybilla B, Ring J (1990) Food allergy and atopic eczema. Semin Dermatol 9:220–225.
14. Van Bever HP, Docx M, Stevens WJ (1989) Food and food additives in severe atopic dermatitis. Allergy 44:588–594.
15. Guillet G, Guillet M-H (1992) Natural history of sensitizations in atopic dermatitis: a 3-year follow-up in 250 children. Arch Dermatol 128:187–192.
16. Defaie F, Abeck D, Brockow K, Vieluf D, Hamm M, Behr-Völtzer C, Ring J (1996) Konzept einer altersabhängigen Basis- und Aufbaudiät für Säuglinge und Kleinkinder mit nahrungsmittelassoziiertem atopischem Ekzem. Allergo J 5:231–235.
17. Saarinen UM, Kajosaari M (1995) Breastfeeding as prophylaxis against atopic disease: prospective follow-up study until 17 years old. Lancet 346:1065–1069.
18. Elias PM, Fengold KR (1992) Lipids and the epidermal water barrier: metabolism, regulation and pathophysiology. Semin Dermatol 11:176–182.
19. Imokawa G, Abe A, Jin K, Higaki Y, Kawashima M, Hidano A (1991) Decreased level of ceramides in stratum corneum of atopic dermatitis: an etiologic factor in atopic dry skin? J Invest Dermatol 96:523–526.
20. Schäfer L, Kragballe K (1991) Abnormalities in epidermal lipid metabolism in patients with atopic dermatitis. J Invest Dermatol 96:10–15.
21. Jin K, Higaki Y, Tagaki Y, Higuchi K, Yada Y, Kawashima M, Imokawa G (1994) Analysis of beta-glucocerebrosidase and ceramidase activities in atopic and aged dry skin. Acta Derm Venereol (Stockh) 74:337–340.
22. Gfesser M, Rügemer J, Schreiner V, Stäb F, Disch R, Abeck D, Ring J. Time course of epidermal barrier recovery after acetone- or tape-stripping-induced barrier-perturbation in atopic eczema and normal skin. Contact Dermatitis, submitted.
23. Ring J, Abeck D, Neuber K (1992) Atopic eczema: role of microorganisms on the skin surface. Allergy 47:265–269.
24. Abeck D, Ruzicka T (1991) Bacteria and atopic eczema: merely association or etiologic factor. In: Ruzicka T, Ring J, Przybilla B, eds. Handbook of Atopic Eczema. Springer, Heidelberg, pp. 212–220.
25. Ring J, Brockow K, Abeck D (1996) The therapeutic concept of "patient management" in atopic eczema. Allergy 51:206–215.
26. Akiyama H, Toi Y, Kanzaki H, Tada J, Arata J (1996) Prevalence of producers of enterotoxins and toxic shock syndrome toxin-1 among *Staphylococcus aureus* strains isolated from atopic dermatitis lesions. Arch Dermatol Res 288:418–420.

27. Cooper KD (1994) Atopic dermatitis: recent trends in pathogenesis and therapy. J Invest Dermatol 102:128–137.
28. Strange P, Skov L, Lisby S, Nielsen PL, Baadsgaard O (1996) Staphylococcal enterotoxin B applied on intact normal and intact atopic skin induces dermatitis. Arch Dermatol 132:27–33.
29. Skov L, Baadsgaard O (1996) Ultraviolett B-exposed major histocompatibility complex class II positive keratinocytes and antigen-presenting cells demonstrate a differential capacity to activate T cells in the presence of staphylococcal superantigens. Br J Dermatol 134:824–830.
29a. Hanifin JM, Rajka G (1980) Diagnostic features of atopic dermatitis. Acta Derm Venereol (Suppl)92:44.
30. Hägermark Ö (1992) Peripheral and central mediators of itch. Skin Pharmacol 5:1–8.
31. Wahlgren CF, Linder MT, Hägermark Ö, Scheynius A (1995) Itch and inflammation induced by intra-dermally injected interleukin-2 in atopic dermatitis and healthy subjects. Arch Dermatol Res 287:572–580.
32. Darsow U, Ring J, Scharein E, Bromm B (1996) Correlations between histamine-induced wheal, flare and itch. Arch Dermatol Res 288:436–441.
33. Koppert W, Heyer G, Handwerker HO (1996) Atopic eczema and histamine-induced sensations. Dermatology 192:227–232.
34. Wahlgren CF (1991) Itch and atopic dermatitis: clinical and experimental studies. Acta Derm Venereol (Stockh.) Suppl 165:1–53.
35. Uehara M (1985) Clinical and histological features of dry skin in atopic dermatitis. Acta Derm Venereol (Stockh.) Suppl 114:82–86.
36. Gupta MA, Gupta AK, Schork NJ (1994) Depression modulates pruritus perception: a study of pruritus in psoriasis, atopic dermatitis, and chronic idiopathic urticaria. Psychosom Med 56:36–40.
37. Borelli S (1967) Psyche und Haut. In: Gottron HA, ed. Handbuch der Haut- und Geschlechtskrankheiten, Vol. 8. Springer, Berlin, pp. 264–268.
37a. Darsow U, Scharein E, Bromm B, Ring J (1997) Skin testing of pruritogenic activity of histamine and cytokines at the dermal-epidermal junction level. Br J Dermatol 137:475–477.
38. Whitlock A (1976) Psychophysiologic Aspects of Skin Disease. Saunders, Toronto.
39. Ring J, Palos E, Zimmermann F (1986) Psychosomatische Aspekte der Eltern-Kind-Beziehung bei atopischem Ekzem im Kindesalter. I. Psychodiagnostische Testverfahren bei Eltern und Kindern und Vergleich mit somatischen Befunden. Hautarzt 37:560–567.
40. Ring J, Palos E (1986) Psychosomatische Aspekte der Eltern-Kind-Beziehung bei atopischem Ekzem im Kindesalter. II. Erziehungsstil, Familiensituation im Zeichentest und strukturierte Interviews. Hautarzt 37:609–617.
41. Gieler U, Stangier U, Braehler E (1973) Hauterkrankungen in psychologischer Sicht. Hogrefe, Göttingen.
42. White A, Horn DJ, Varigos GA (1990) Psychological profile of the atopic eczema patient. Australian J Dermatol 31:13–16.
43. Schubert HJ (1989) Psychosoziale Faktoren bei Hautkrankheiten: Empirische Untersuchungen zu diagnostischen und Therapeutischen Fragestellungen mit Hilfe zeitreihenanalytischer Methoden. Vadenoeck und Ruprecht, Göttingen.
44. Gil KM, Sampson HA (1989) Psychological and social factors of atopic dermatitis. Allergy 44:84–89.
45. Panconesi E (1984) Stress and skin diseases: psychosomatic dermatology. In Parish LC, ed. Clinics in Dermatology. Lippincott, Philadelphia.
46. Tan B, Weald D, Strickland I, Friedman P (1996) Double-blind controlled trial of effect of house dust-mite allergen avoidance on atopic dermatitis. Lancet 347:15–18.
47. Bernhard JD (1989) Nonrashes. 5. Atmoknesis: pruritus provoked by contact with air. Cutis 44:143–144.
48. Tupker R, DeMonchy J, Coenraads P, Homan A, van der Meer J (1996) Induction of atopic dermatitis by inhalation of house dust mite. J Allergy Clin Immunol 97:1064–1070.
49. Ring J, Bieber T, Vieluf D, Kunz B, Przybilla B (1991) Atopic eczema, Langerhans cells and allergy. Int Arch Allergy Appl Immunol 94:194–201.
50. Adinoff A, Tellez P, Clark R (1988) Atopic dermatitis and aeroallergen contact sensitivity. J Allergy Clin Immunol 81:736–742.
51. Bruynzeel-Koomen C, van Wichen D, Spry C, Venge P, Bruynzeel P (1988) Active participation of eosinophils in patch test reactions to inhalant allergens in patients with atopic dermatitis. Br J Dermatol 118:229–238.
52. Clark R, Adinoff A (1989) Aeroallergen contact can exacerbate atopic dermatitis: patch test as a diagnostic tool. J Am Acad Dermatol 21:863–869.
53. Darsow U, Vieluf D, Ring J (1993) Concordance of atopy patch test, prick test and specific IgE in patients with atopic eczema. J Derm Sci 6(1):95 (abstract).

54. Darsow U, Vieluf D, Ring J (1995) Atopy patch test with different vehicles and allergen concentrations— an approach to standardization. J Allergy Clin Immunol 95:677–684.
55. Darsow U, Vieluf D, Ring J (1996) The atopy patch test: an increased rate of reactivity in patients who have an air-exposed pattern of atopic eczema. Br J Dermatol 135:182–186.
56. Gondo A, Saeki N, Tokuda Y (1986) Challenge reactions in atopic dermatitis after percutaneous entry of mite antigen. Br J Dermatol 115:485–493.
57. Imayama S, Hashizume T, Miyahara H, Tanahashi T, Takeishi M, Kubota Y, Koga T, Hori Y, Fukuda H (1992) Combination of patch test and IgE for dust mite antigens differentiates 130 patients with atopic dermatitis into four groups. J Am Acad Dermatol 27:531–538.
58. Langeland T, Braathen L, Borch M (1989) Studies of atopic patch tests. Acta Derm Venereol (Stockh) (Suppl)144:105–109.
59. Mitchell E, Chapman M, Pope F, Crow J, Jouhal S, Platts-Mills T (1982) Basophils in allergen-induced patch test sites in atopic dermatitis. Lancet I:127–130.
60. Norris P, Schofield O, Camp R (1988) A study of the role of house dust mite in atopic dermatitis. Br J Dermatol 118:435–440.
61. Platts-Mills T, Mitchell E, Rowntree S, Chapman M, Wilkins S (1983) The role of dust mite allergens in atopic dermatitis. Clin Exp Dermatol 8:233–247.
62. Reitamo S, Visa K, Kaehoenen K, et al. (1989) Patch test reactions to inhalant allergens in atopic dermatitis. Acta Derm Venereol (Stockh) (Suppl 144)11:119–121.
63. Ring J, Kunz B, Bieber T, Vieluf D, Przybilla B (1989) The "atopy patch test" with aeroallergens in atopic eczema. J Allergy Clin Immunol 82:195 (abstract).
64. Seidenari S, Manzini BM, Danese P, Giannetti A (1992) Positive patch tests to whole mite culture and purified mite extracts in patients with atopic dermatitis, asthma and rhinitis. Ann Allergy 69(3):201–206.
65. Seifert H, Wollemann G, Seifert B, Borelli S (1987) Neurodermitis: Eine Protein-Kontaktdermatitis? Dtsch Derm 35:1204–1214.
66. Tanaka Y, Anan S, Yoshida H (1990) Immunohistochemical studies in mite antigen-induced patch test sites in atopic dermatitis. J Derm Sci 1:361–368.
67. Vocks E, Seifert H, Seifert B, Drosner M (1991) Patch test with immediate type allergens in patients with atopic dermatitis. In: Ring J, Przybilla B, eds. New Trends in Allergy, III. Springer, Berlin, pp. 230–233.
68. van Voorst Vader PC, Lier JG, Woest TE, Coenraads PJ, Nater JP (1991) Patch tests with house dust mite antigens in atopic dermatitis patients: methodological problems. Acta Derm Venereol (Stockh) 71(4): 301–305.
69. Vieluf D, Kunz B, Bieber T, Przybilla B, Ring J (1993) "Atopy Patch Test" with aeroallergens in patients with atopic eczema. Allergo J 1:9–12.
70. Darsow U, Behrendt H, Ring J (1997) Gramineae pollen as trigger factors of atopic eczema—evaluation of diagnostic measures using the atopy patch test. Br J Dermatol 137:201–207.
71. Bieber T, Rieger A, Neuchrist C, Prinz JC, Rieber EP, Boltz-Nitulescu G, Scheiner O, Kraft D, Ring J, Stingl G (1989) Induction of FCeR2/CD23 on human epidermal Langerhans cells by human recombinant IL4 and IFN. J Exp Med 170:309–314.
72. Bieber T (1994) FCeRI on human Langerhans cells: a receptor in search of new functions. Immunol Today 15:52–53.
73. van Reijsen FC, Bruynzeel-Koomen CAFM, Kalthoff FS (1992) Skin-derived aeroallergen-specific T-cell clones of Th2 phenotype in patients with atopic dermatitis. J Allergy Clin Immunol 90:184–192.
74. Sager N, Neumann C, Marghescu S (1992) Der Epikutantest auf Inhalationsallergene ist eine immunspezifische Spättypreaktion. Z. Hautkr. 67(5):600–604.
75. Sager N, Feldmann A, Schilling G, Kreitsch P, Neumann C (1992) House dust mite-specific T cells in the skin of subjects with atopic dermatitis: frequency and lymphokine profile in the allergen patch test. J Allergy Clin Immunol 89:801–810.
76. Maeda K, Yamamoto K, Tanaka Y, Anan S, Yoshida H (1992) House dust mite (HDM) antigen in naturally occurring lesions of atopic dermatitis (AD): the relationship between HDM antigen in the skin and HDM antigen-specific IgE antibody. J Derm Science 3:73–77.
77. Giesser M, Rakoski J, Ring J (1996) Disturbance of epidermal barrier function in atopy patch test reactions in atopic eczema. Br J Dermatol 135:560–565.

26 Pathogenesis of Asthma

Paul M. O'Byrne, MB, FRCPI, FRCP(C), FCCP

CONTENTS

INTRODUCTION

Asthma is a common disease, with a prevalence of 5–10% in most countries in which this has been studied. In addition, in some, particularly younger, populations the prevalence of asthma is increasing. This trend has been recognized in children in Australia (1), New Zealand (2), and the United Kingdom (3). These increases may result from changes in diagnostic labeling and subsequent treatment strategies or from a real increase in prevalence due to an increase in exposure to risk factors in a susceptible population. Support for the latter suggestion comes from studies that have described an increase in hospitalizations in children for severe asthma in the United States (4) and the epidemics of asthma deaths that occurred in several countries in the early 1980s (5).

Asthma is currently described clinically by the presence of characteristic symptoms of dyspnea, chest tightness, wheezing, and cough and by the presence of reversible airway narrowing and airway hyperresponsiveness to a variety of inhaled bronchoconstrictor stimuli.

Asthma can be a very mild and intermittent disease in many patients; indeed, it is likely that this is the case in most patients with the disease. However, other patients, perhaps making up 5–10% of all asthmatics, have very severe, occasionally life-threatening, asthma. Others, perhaps 20–25% of all asthmatics, have persistent symptoms, which require regular daily treatment. The reasons for these differences in severity of asthma are poorly understood.

AIRWAY HYPERRESPONSIVENESS IN ASTHMA

Almost all adult patients with current symptomatic asthma have airway hyperresponsiveness to inhaled pharmacological constrictor stimuli (6) (Fig. 1). In unusual circumstances, symptomatic asthma associated with variable airflow obstruction has been demonstrated when airway

From: *Allergy and Allergic Diseases: The New Mechanisms and Therapeutics*
Edited by: J. A. Denburg © Humana Press Inc., Totowa, NJ

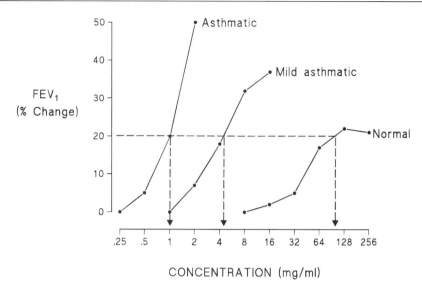

Fig. 1. Dose-response curves to inhaled constrictor agonists in a normal subject and asthmatic subjects with mildly and severely increased airway hyperresponsiveness. The responses are measured as the fall in FEV_1 from baseline values, and in these examples the responses are expressed as the provocative concentrations of the agonist causing a 20% fall in FEV_1. Both the mild asthmatic and normal subjects demonstrate a plateau response, which is lost in the more severe asthmatic subject.

responsiveness has been considered normal *(7)*. It has not been possible to define an exact level of airway responsiveness that would distinguish asthmatic subjects from nonasthmatic subjects. This is because there is a continuous distribution of airway responsiveness in the general population, with asthmatic subjects in one tail of this distribution *(8)*. Thus, the level of airway responsiveness that is chosen to distinguish asthmatics from normals depends not only on the method employed and the degree of standardization used, but also on the degree of sensitivity and specificity of the measurement that is acceptable to an individual investigator.

Airway hyperresponsiveness can be stable over several years in many asthmatic subjects *(9)*. However, there are a number of inhaled stimuli such as allergen *(10,11)* ozone *(12)*, and chemical sensitizers, such as toluene diisocyanate (TDI) *(13)*, or plicatic acid from western red cedar *(14)*, and upper respiratory viral infections *(15)* that can cause airway hyperresponsiveness in human subjects. This exposure and subsequent airway hyperresponsiveness is associated with an increase in symptoms of asthma and an increase in the amount of treatment required to control symptoms *(16)*. Identifying the significance of these stimuli has been important in the management of individual patients with asthma, in that removal of the stimulus can, in some instances, and particularly with occupational sensitizing agents, cure the disease *(14)*. In addition, exposure to a sensitizing agent also means that some patients can have airway hyperresponsiveness and symptomatic asthma at one time but not at another.

Tests of airway hyperresponsiveness can be very sensitive for a diagnosis of asthma in adult patients *(6)*. This is because airway hyperresponsiveness is present in almost all adult patients with asthma, if the measurement is made at the time symptoms are present. However, in studies of children, a rather high prevalence of asymptomatic airway hyperresponsiveness has been described. For example, in New Zealand, 79% of children with symptomatic asthma requiring regular treatment had methacholine airway hyperresponsiveness, whereas 6.7% of children who had never had any respiratory symptoms had demonstrable airway hyperresponsiveness *(17)*. A similar result was found in Australian children *(18)*. Therefore, in children, a single measurement of methacholine airway responsiveness may be neither very sensitive nor specific for a diagnosis of asthma.

In groups of asthmatic subjects, the severity of airway hyperresponsiveness correlates with the severity of asthma and with other important variables present in asthma, such as variations in peak expiratory flow rates (19) and the improvement in forced expired volume in 1 s (FEV_1) after inhaled bronchodilator (20). In addition, the severity of airway hyperresponsiveness is related, in populations of asthmatic subjects, to the amount of treatment needed to optimally control symptoms (16). Lastly, the degree of bronchoconstriction caused by exercise or hyperventilation of cold, dry air in asthmatic subjects, is related to the level of airway hyperresponsiveness (21,22). As these stimuli are considered to act through release of endogenous mediators, it is likely that airway hyperresponsiveness to these endogenous mediators plays a role in causing symptoms after exercise or inhalation of cold dry air in asthmatic patients.

Airway hyperresponsiveness to inhaled agonists such as histamine or methacholine can also be demonstrated in patients with chronic irreversible airflow obstruction (20). The degree of airflow obstruction, as indicated by the reduction on FEV_1 and FEV_1/VC (vital capacity) ratio, correlates with the increase in airway responsiveness (20). This suggests that, in patients with irreversible airflow obstruction, the airway hyperresponsiveness demonstrated is a result of reduced airway caliber. Airway hyperresponsiveness has also been described in patients with atopy, but no symptomatic asthma (23), and in patients with other diseases, such as cystic fibrosis (24) and irritable bowel disease (25). Therefore, although the presence of airway hyperresponsiveness is very sensitive in adult patients, for a diagnosis of asthma, it is not very specific. Thus, the test will have a high negative predictive value, but a lower positive predictive value.

GENETICS OF AIRWAY HYPERRESPONSIVENESS

It has been recognized for many years that familial clustering exists for asthma, and more recently for airway hyperresponsiveness (26–29). This could reflect a genetic predisposition for the development of asthma, shared environmental risk(s), or most likely a combination of both. Several major problems exist for investigators studying the genetics of asthma; these include the fact that asthma is clearly not a single genetic abnormality, but rather a complex multigenic disease, with a very strong environmental component. In addition, researchers have had a lot of difficulty in precisely defining the asthma phenotype to study. This is because there is no acceptable definition of asthma, and the diagnosis is made by a combination of symptoms and the physiological abnormalities of the airways. For this reason, several groups of investigators have focused on the genetic basis of airway hyperresponsiveness. Studies of monozygotic and dizygotic twins have suggested that there is some genetic basis for the development of airway hyperresponsiveness, but that environmental factors are more important (30,31). Also, measurements of airway hyperresponsiveness in young infants (mean age 4.5 wk) have indicated that airway hyperresponsiveness can be present very early in life, and that a family history of asthma and parental smoking are risk factors for its development (32). More recently, reports of genetic linkage of airway hyperresponsiveness have been published. One study has identified genetic linkage between histamine airway hyperresponsiveness and several genetic markers on chromosome 5q, near a locus that regulates serum IgE levels (33). Another study has identified linkage between a highly polymorphic marker of the β-subunit of the high-affinity IgE receptor on chromosome 11q and methacholine airway hyperresponsiveness, even in patients with nonatopic asthma (34). Thus, a genetic basis for airway hyperresponsiveness seems very likely; however, the genetic linkage studies need to be confirmed by other investigators in different patient populations. One specific gene polymorphism (Glu 27) of the nine identified of the B_2-adrenoceptor has also been associated with increased methacholine airway hyperresponsiveness (35), while another polymorphism (Gly 16) was associated with the presence of nocturnal asthma (36).

ENVIRONMENTAL STIMULI AND ASTHMA

Almost all children with asthma, or adult asthmatics whose asthma began in childhood, are atopic, as measured by increased levels of serum IgE and/or by positive skin prick tests to common environmental allergens (37–40), whereas > 50% of patients with adult onset asthma are atopic. The observation that inhalation of an allergen can cause symptoms of asthma was originally made more than 100 yr ago by Blackley, and in 1934, Stevens described symptoms of asthma for several days after inhalation challenges with allergens (41). However, the first thorough description of the response to inhaled allergen was made in 1952 by Herxheimer (42), who identified that there could be two distinct components to the response to inhaled allergen, which he called the immediate and late reactions. In the late 1960s, Altounyan described another important consequence of the inhalation of allergen, in that exposure to grass pollen during the grass pollen season could increase airway responsiveness to inhaled histamine in sensitized subjects (43). Subsequently, Cockcroft and coworkers (44) demonstrated that the increase in histamine and methacholine responsiveness that occurs after inhaled allergen occurs in association with the late asthmatic response after allergen and that subjects who only have an isolated early response after inhaled allergen do not develop airway hyperresponsiveness.

The inhalation of environmental allergens is the most important cause of asthma. Epidemiological studies have demonstrated that close associations exist between the presence of atopy, especially to house dust mite and cat dander, and the presence of airway hyperresponsiveness and symptomatic asthma (37–39). Occupational sensitizing agents, many of which do not act through a classical IgE-mediated allergic reaction, are an important cause of adult onset asthma (45). Thus, it is a plausible hypothesis that all asthma is initiated by inhalation of an environmental stimulus, some of which have been identified and some of which are not yet known.

In many patients, the regular exposure to environmental allergens or occupational sensitizing agents is the cause of persisting asthma. This has been best demonstrated by the studies that have removed allergic asthmatic patients from the regular daily exposure to the offending allergen (most often house dust mite) and have demonstrated improvements in asthma symptoms, amounts of treatment needed to control symptoms, and in physiological abnormalities, such as airway hyperresponsiveness (46). In addition, for asthma caused by exposure to the occupational sensitizing agent plicatic acid from western red cedar, evidence exists that prolonged exposure can result in persisting asthma, even after the exposure is removed (45). It is conceivable that similar effects occur with regular exposure to environmental allergens, although this has not been proven.

AIRWAY INFLAMMATION AND ASTHMA

Over the past 10 years, much of the research focus in asthma has been on the role of airway inflammation in causing symptoms, bronchoconstriction, and airway hyperresponsiveness. However, the concept that airway inflammation is involved in the pathogenesis of asthma is not new. In 1892, William Osler published the medical textbook The Principles and Practice of Medicine. In the chapter on asthma, Osler describes "bronchial asthma ... in many cases is a special form of inflammation of the smaller bronchioles" (47). This reflected the then current descriptions of the pathology of the airways of patients dying of severe, fatal asthma. A more complete description of airway inflammation in patients dying of acute asthma was provided by Dunnill and colleagues *(48)* in the 1960s. Thus, although airway inflammation and its structural consequences had been recognized for more than 100 yr, it was accepted that inflammation was confined to the airways of asthmatic patients with very severe, often fatal, disease. More recently, the importance of airway inflammation in the pathogenesis of asthma, ranging in severity from mild to severe, or in transient asthma after exposure to an inflammatory stimulus has been recognized.

Dorland's Medical Dictionary defines inflammation as the "condition into which tissues enter as a reaction to injury." A common manifestation of inflammation is the presence, at some time in the process, of activated inflammatory cells at the affected tissue site. The type of inflammatory cell varies with the type of inflammation. The most important inflammatory cell at sites of acute inflammation is the neutrophil. However, in other, more chronic inflammatory conditions, eosinophils, lymphocytes, or mast cells appear to be more prominent. For the purposes of this chapter, airway inflammation will be defined as the presence of activated inflammatory cells in the airways. Although this definition is restrictive and excludes other important components of inflammatory events, such as edema and vasodilation, quantifying numbers, and occasionally state of activation, of inflammatory cells it has been the most commonly used index of airway inflammation in studies of asthma to date. It must also be recognized, however, that the structural consequences of persisting airway inflammation in asthma may be as, or more, important than the presence of the activated inflammatory cells.

Environmental Stimuli and Airway Inflammation

The identification of environmental stimuli that can cause asthma has proven to be important in studies of airway inflammation in asthma. This is because the evidence that the presence of inflammatory cells is causally related to the development of airway hyperresponsiveness and asthma in human subjects initially depended on studies that have examined numbers of cells and cellular differentials in bronchoalveolar lavage fluid (BAL) before and after inhalation of ozone *(49)*, the occupational sensitizing agent TDI *(50)*, and allergen *(51)*, all of which are known to cause airway hyperresponsiveness and transient asthma, or exacerbate persisting asthma. These studies have all demonstrated an acute inflammatory response in the airways associated with the development of variable airflow obstruction, airway hyperresponsiveness, and asthma. In addition, the studies have suggested that the stimulus that initiates the airway hyperresponsiveness determines the type of cellular response. For example, a substantial increase in neutrophils and a smaller increase in eosinophils were described in BAL in subjects with airway hyperresponsiveness following TDI *(50)*. In contrast, airway challenge with plicatic acid, which is responsible for western red cedar asthma, a different form of occupational asthma, caused increases in eosinophil numbers but not neutrophils in BAL *(52)*. After allergen challenge, some studies describe increases in eosinophils *(51)*, or eosinophils and neutrophils *(53)*, or eosinophils, lymphocytes, and basophils *(54)*. However, measurements in these studies have been carried out at different time points and with different challenge techniques, which might explain the varied results.

A more recent focus has been the examination of the state of activation of the inflammatory cells after allergen inhalation *(55,56)*. These studies have identified that eosinophils are activated, as indicated by increased levels of eosinophil cationic protein (ECP) and positive staining for the marker for cleaved ECP (EG2), as early as 3 h *(55)* and persisting for more than 24 h in BAL after allergen inhalation *(55,56)* (Fig. 2); in addition there are increased numbers of degranulated eosinophils *(57)*.

More recently, a less invasive method than bronchoscopy has been developed, using sputum induced by the inhalation of hypertonic saline, to quantify and characterize inflammatory

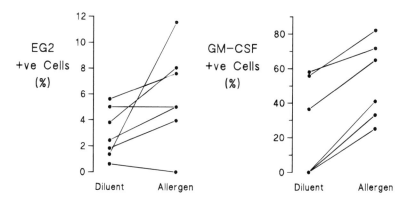

Fig. 2. Percentage of BAL cells positive for EG2 and GM-CSF in asthmatic subjects after allergen or diluent challenge. Allergen challenge significantly increased the number of BAL cells positive for EG2 and GM-CSF. Reproduced with permission from ref. *56.*

cells in asthmatic airways. Studies using this method have demonstrated that eosinophils increase markedly in sputum samples of asthmatics undergoing a naturally occurring exacerbation of their asthma *(58)*, as well as 24 h after allergen inhalation, which persists for 3 d after allergen *(59)*. Increases in circulating eosinophils and basophils have also been documented 24 h after allergen inhalation, as have increased numbers of circulating progenitors of eosinophils and basophils (Eo/B), but not for granulocytes or macrophages *(60)* (Fig. 3). These results suggest that there is a selective stimulation of the bone marrow to produce progenitors following allergen challenge. This has been studied in allergic dogs, who do develop an increase in bone marrow progenitors 24 h after allergen inhalation, an effect that is abolished by pretreating the airways with the inhaled glucocorticosteroid budesonide *(61)*.

Persisting Asthma and Airway Inflammation

There have been a number of studies that have provided information on cell populations in BAL fluid in mild stable asthmatics with persistent airway hyperresponsiveness and asthma *(62–64)*. Common findings in all of these studies as well as in examinations of bronchial mucosal biopsies *(65–69)* are the presence of increased numbers of inflammatory cells such as eosinophils, lymphocytes, and mast cells compared with normal control subjects with normal airway responsiveness. The eosinophils have shown signs of activation, as indicated by increased levels of granular proteins, major basic protein (MBP) *(63)*, and ECP *(64,65)*. In the bronchial mucosa, the eosinophils have shown morphological features of activation, as indicated by heterogeneity of the granular structure *(66)* or as eosinophil granules lying free in the mucosal interstitium *(67)*. Azzawi and colleagues *(68)* and Poston et al. *(69)* have also demonstrated increased numbers of EG2 positive cells, as well as significant increases in numbers of activated T-lymphocytes *(68)*. Mast cells in the airway mucosa have exhibited various stages of degranulation *(67)*, suggesting that mediator release is an ongoing process in the airways of stable asthmatics with persistent airway hyperresponsiveness.

Some studies have correlated numbers of inflammatory cells in BAL with the severity of methacholine airway hyperresponsiveness or clinical severity in stable asthmatics. Kirby et al. *(62)* demonstrated close correlations between degree of airway hyperresponsiveness in subjects with mild asthma and number of mast cells and eosinophils, respectively, in lavage fluid. Kelly and coworkers *(70)* showed correlations between numbers of neutrophils and airway hyperresponsiveness. Bousquet et al. *(64)* have demonstrated that the numbers of eosinophils

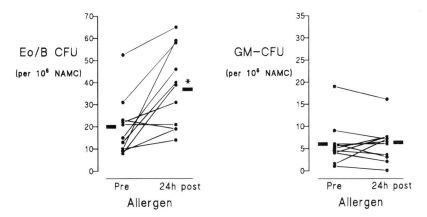

Fig. 3. Numbers of circulating progenitors for Eo/B measured 24 h after diluent and allergen in stable atopic asthmatics. Allergen challenge increased the numbers of circulating Eo/B progenitors. Reproduced with permission from ref. *60*.

and levels of ECP in BAL correlated with the severity of asthma as measured by an asthma severity score, and with pulmonary function (Fig. 4).

These studies can be summarized as demonstrating the presence of activated inflammatory cells, eosinophils, neutrophils, lymphocytes, and mast cells in the airways of asthmatics even at a time when they are considered stable and asymptomatic. The numbers of cells increase following a stimulus that causes airway hyperresponsiveness, as well as in natural exacerbations of asthma. The presence of activated eosinophils appears to be the best correlated with the presence of pulmonary function abnormalities, airway hyperresponsiveness, and asthma severity. However, the precise role that eosinophils and the other cells demonstrated to be increased in asthma are playing in the pathogenesis is still under very active investigation.

MECHANISMS OF PERSISTING AIRWAY INFLAMMATION

The mechanisms by which the direct effector cells in asthma, most likely eosinophils and mast cells, are recruited into the airways and persist and are activated in the airways very likely involve an important role for cytokines. There are now more than 30 different protein mediators that are classed as cytokines. Some of these have been implicated in the pathogenesis of asthma, mainly because of their ability to promote inflammatory cell growth and differentiation, or inflammatory cell migration and activation, or cause changes in the structural cells of the airways. The study of the cytokines in asthma is not yet as developed as for other mediators, such as the leukotrienes, mainly because of the lack of specific antagonists that can be studied in humans. However, the cytokines interleukin (IL)-3, IL-5, and granulocyte-macrophage colony-stimulating factor (GM-CSF) may be important because of their ability to promote eosinophil and mast cell differentiation, recruitment and activation into the airways, and prolong the survival of these cells once in the airways. All of these cytokines, as well as IL-4, which is necessary for immunoglobulin E (IgE) production, are produced by one type of helper T-cell, the Th2 cell, which is present in asthmatic airways *(71)*. In addition, other airway cells may be responsible for the production of these cytokines *(72,73)*. Increased amounts of GM-CSF *(61,71,74,75)*, IL-5 *(75,76)*, but not IL-3 *(77)*, are present in airway biopsies from mild asthmatics, and the levels increase after allergen challenge *(56,74)* (Fig. 2). It would appear very likely that these, as well as other, cytokines are responsible for the presence of persisting activated eosinophils and mast cells in asthmatic airways; however, further studies

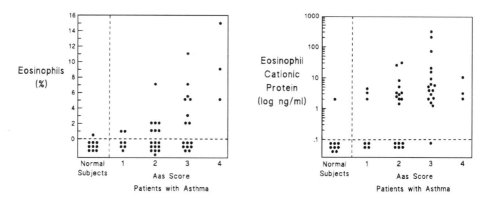

Fig. 4. Percentage of eosinophils (left figure) and levels of ECP (right figure) in BAL from normal subjects and patients with asthma of increasing severity, as indicated by increasing Aas score. Reproduced with permission from ref. *64.*

with drugs that block the action of specific cytokines will be needed to precisely establish their role in asthma.

AIRWAY STRUCTURAL CHANGES IN MILD ASTHMA

A number of structural changes have been described in asthmatic airways that appear to be characteristic of the disease, even in patients with mild persisting asthma, and that may be responsible for the presence of persisting airway hyperresponsiveness in asthma. These changes include patchy desquamated epithelium, thickening of the reticular collagen layer below the basement membrane, and airway smooth muscle hypertrophy. Both epithelial damage and smooth muscle hypertrophy have been implicated in the pathogenesis of airway hyperresponsiveness in asthma.

Epithelial damage and desquamation are present in airways of patients with asthma *(78)*. One hypothesis to explain epithelial damage and desquamation in asthmatic airways is that basic proteins released from activated eosinophils damage the epithelium. Levels of MBP have been shown to be increased in BAL from asthmatic patients *(63)*. MBP has also been identified in tissue sections from airways of patients dying from severe asthma by means of immuno-fluorescence *(79)*. Even in sections where identifiable eosinophils could not be seen, evidence showed MBP to be present in epithelium and submucosa, giving signs of tissue damage.

Several hypotheses have been proposed to explain how epithelial damage may result in airway hyperresponsiveness in asthma. These have included increased permeability of the airway epithelium, loss of inhibitory mediators generated by the airway epithelium, and loss of neutral endopeptidase. Several studies have compared the permeability of the respiratory epithelium in normal subjects, asthmatics, and asymptomatic smokers. These studies demonstrated that the clearance of inhaled radiolabeled aerosols from the lung into the blood was much faster in the asymptomatic smokers with normal airway responsiveness than in either the normal subjects with normal airway responsiveness or the asthmatic subjects with airway hyperresponsiveness *(80)*. These results make it very unlikely that an increase in airway epithelial permeability is the cause of airway hyperresponsiveness in asthma.

The epithelium has been reported to release a factor that reduces the airway smooth muscle contractile responses to agonists such as histamine and acetylcholine *(81)*. This mediator has been called epithelium-derived relaxing factor (EpDRF). The hypothesis that loss of an inhibitory EpDRF may be responsible for airway hyperresponsiveness in asthma has not been possible to test in human subjects. Airway epithelial cells are known to release prostaglandin E2 (PGE_2) *(82)*, which has potent inhibitory effects in the airways, such as presynaptic modulation and inhibition of acetylcholine release from muscarinic nerves *(83)*. In addition, PGE_2 is able to reduce contractile responses to inhaled histamine, acetylcholine, and methacholine *(84)* and bronchoconstrictor responses to exercise *(85)* and allergen inhalation *(86)* in asthmatics. The airway epithelium also contains enzymes, neutral endopeptidases, capable of metabolizing tachykinins, such as substance P *(87)*, which are bronchoconstrictor and proinflammatory mediators. Loss of these inhibitory mediators may have important results in asthmatic airways; however, this hypothesis has not yet been tested in asthmatic subjects.

Airway hyperresponsiveness in asthma is nonspecific. This means that asthmatic airways are more responsive to all bronchoconstrictor mediators acting on airway smooth muscle receptors. One explanation for the lack of specificity is that the underlying abnormality in asthmatic airways resides in the smooth muscle. The increase in airway smooth muscle volume in asthmatics causing airway hyperresponsiveness may be directly related to thickening of asthmatic airways. James et al. *(88)* have, by using modeling studies, demonstrated that a small increase in the thickness of the airway wall, which is not possible to demonstrate by changes in spirometric indices, could result in airway hyperresponsiveness in asthma.

MECHANISMS OF BRONCHOCONSTRICTION IN ASTHMA

Bronchoconstriction is the cause of almost all of the symptoms in asthma, with the possible exception being cough. The mechanism of bronchoconstriction is not fully understood, but involves airway smooth muscle constriction, airway edema, increased secretions in the airways, and possibly vascular engorgement. The airway smooth muscle constriction and possibly the airway edema can be rapidly and often completely reversed by inhaled B_2-agonists, whereas the increased secretions and vascular engorgement are not, and indeed may even be made worse by B_2-agonists. Most bronchoconstriction that occurs in asthmatics occurs spontaneously, without any obvious initiating cause. However, many irritants and environmental stimuli can cause bronchoconstriction, including pollutants, such as cigarette smoke *(89)*, SO_2 *(90)*, and NO_2 *(91)*, cold dry air *(92)*, and exercise *(93)*. Other, more specific, stimuli cause bronchoconstriction only in subsets of asthmatics. These include environmental allergens in sensitized subjects (discussed above) and nonsteroidal anti-inflammatory drugs in "aspirin-sensitive" asthmatics *(94)*.

The mediators possibly responsible for bronchoconstriction in asthma have been extensively studied. These studies have been greatly aided by the availability of selective and potent mediator antagonists and synthetase inhibitors to study in asthmatic subjects. It is now clear that the most important mediators of bronchoconstriction in asthma are the cysteinyl leukotrienes (LTs) C_4, D_4, and E_4.

The cysteinyl LTs are products of the action of the enzyme 5-lipoxygenase (5-LO) on arachidonic acid. The biosynthesis likely occurs at or near the nuclear membrane and requires that 5-LO associate with an 18-kDa protein, 5-lipoxygenase-activating protein (FLAP). This interaction produces LTA_4, which is an intermediate in the synthesis of LTC_4, which is metabolized to an equieffective metabolite LTD_4 and finally to a less potent, stable excretory product LTE_4. These products are known together as the cysteinyl LTs, to distinguish them from another 5-LO product, LTB_4, which has a different range of biological activities. In the airways, the cysteinyl LTs activate a single type of receptor, the cys LT_1 receptor. A different receptor subtype, the cys LT_2 receptor, exists in pulmonary blood vessels.

The cysteinyl LTs are the most potent constrictors of human airways yet discovered, being 10^3–10^4 times more potent than histamine *(95,96)* (Fig. 5). They are released in asthmatic air-

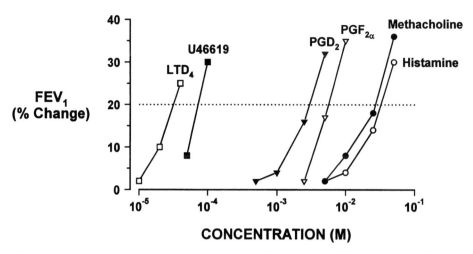

Fig. 5. Airway responsiveness as measured by the % change in FEV_1 to a variety of bronchoconstrictor mediators (histamine, methacholine, PGD_2 and PGF_{2a}, the thromboxane mimetic U46619, and LTD_4) expressed as molar concentrations, in one stable asthmatic subject. The subject has airway hyperresponsiveness to all the mediators studied; however, LTD_4 is the most potent.

ways after inhalation of allergens or aspirin, as measured by increases in urinary LTE_4 production *(97–99)*. A number of compounds have been developed that can inhibit the action of LTs, either by antagonizing the cys LT_1 receptor, or by inhibiting their production by a direct action on 5-LO, or by inhibiting FLAP. These compounds have undergone clinical trials in asthma. They antagonize bronchoconstriction caused by exercise *(100)*, allergen *(101)*, cold air *(102)*, and aspirin *(103)*; they partially reverse spontaneous bronchoconstriction, an effect that appears additive to the effects of inhaled B_2-agonists *(104,105)*; and they improve asthma symptoms and reduce B_2-agonist use *(106,107)*. LTE_4 may also be involved in the recruitment of airway inflammatory cells in asthma *(108)*.

In contrast to the activity and efficacy of the anti-LT drugs in clinical models of asthma, as well as in persisting asthma, no other mediator antagonist or inhibitor has shown efficacy in both the clinical models and persisting asthma. Anticholinergics do slightly improve resting airway caliber in both asthmatics and normals, suggesting that persisting tone in the airways is cholinergically mediated *(109)*. Anticholinergics are also somewhat effective bronchodilators in asthmatics *(109)*, but do not improve the other clinical manifestations of asthma. Antihistamines partially attenuate exercise-induced bronchoconstriction *(110)*, but are ineffective in treating asthma *(111)*. Antagonists to thromboxane and platelet-activating factor (PAF) are also ineffective in the clinical models *(112,113)* and in treating asthma *(114,115)*.

CONCLUSIONS

Airway inflammation appears to be central to the pathogenesis of all of the clinical manifestations of asthma. Many studies have now demonstrated the presence of activated eosinophils and of mast cells in the airway lumen and airway wall of patients with asthma, even those with mild disease. The presence and survival of these inflammatory cells may be promoted by the presence of an increased level of proinflammatory cytokines, such as GM-CSF and IL-5, in asthmatic airways. These cells also have the capacity to release potent bronchoconstrictor mediators such as the cysteinyl LTs, which are responsible, in part at least, for airway narrowing in asthma and for allergen-, exercise-, and aspirin-induced asthma. Other cells, such as a subset of helper T-lymphocytes (Th2), may also be important in maintaining the inflammatory cascade. Airway structural changes caused by the persisting inflammation, such as airway epithelial damage or altered smooth muscle function or volume, are likely important in the pathogenesis of stable, longstanding airway hyperresponsiveness. Mediators released from the inflammatory cells may be responsible for these changes; the cysteinyl LTs are the most important mediators of bronchoconstriction identified to date. Despite the great increase in knowledge about the importance of airway inflammation in the pathogenesis of asthma, the precise sequence of events that leads to the presence of persisting airway inflammatory cells, airway structural changes, and airway hyperresponsiveness in asthma remains to be clarified.

ACKNOWLEDGMENTS

The author is the recipient of a Medical Research Council of Canada Senior Scientist Award.

REFERENCES

1. Robertson CF, Heycock E, Bishop J, Nolan T, Olinsky A, Phelan P (1991) Prevalence of asthma in Melbourne schoolchildren: changes over 26 years. Br Med J 302:1116–1118.
2. Burrows B, Sears MR, Flannery EM, Herbison GP, Holdaway MD (1995) Relations of bronchial responsiveness to allergy skin test reactivity, lung function, respiratory symptoms, and diagnoses in thirteen-year-old New Zealand children. J Allergy Clin Immunol 95:548–556.
3. Burney PGJ, Chinn S, Rona RJ (1990) Has the prevalence of asthma increased in childhood? Evidence from the national study of health and growth 1973–86. Br Med J 300:1306–1310.
4. Gerstman BB, Bosco LA, Tomita DK (1993) Trends in the prevalence of asthma hospitalization in the 5- to 14-year-old Michigan Medicaid population, 1980 to 1986. J Allergy Clin Immunol 91:838–843.
5. Sears MR, Rea HH, Rothwell RPG, O'Donnell TV, Holst PE, Gillies AJD, Beaglehole R (1986) Asthma mortality: comparison between New Zealand and England. Br Med J 293:1342–1345.
6. Cockcroft DW, Killian DN, Mellon JJA, Hargreave FE (1977) Bronchial reactivity of inhaled histamine: a method and clinical survey. Clin Allergy 7:235–243.
7. Hargreave FE, Ramsdale EH, Pugsley SO (1984) Occupational asthma without bronchial hyperresponsiveness. Am Rev Respir Dis 130:513–515.
8. Cockcroft DW, Berscheid BA, Murdock KY (1983) Unimodal distribution of bronchial responsiveness to inhaled histamine in a random human population. Chest 83:751–754.
9. Juniper EF, Frith PA, Hargreave FE (1982) Long term stability of bronchial responsiveness to histamine. Thorax 37:288–291.
10. Cartier A, Thomson NC, Frith PA, Roberts R, Hargreave FE (1982) Allergen-induced increase in bronchial responsiveness to histamine: relationship to the late asthmatic response and change in airway caliber. J Allergy Clin Immunol 70:170–177.
11. Boulet LP, Cartier A, Thomson NC, Roberts RS, Dolovich J, Hargreave FE (1983) Asthma and increases in nonallergic bronchial responsiveness from seasonal pollen exposure. J Allergy Clin Immunol 71:399–406.
12. Golden JA, Nadel JA, Boushey HA (1978) Bronchial hyperirritability in healthy subjects after exposure to ozone. Am Rev Respir Dis 118:287–294.
13. Fabbri LM, Boschetto P, Zocca E, Milani G, Pivirotto F, Plebani M, Burlina A, Licata B, Mapp CE (1987) Bronchoalveolar neutrophilia during late asthmatic reactions induced by toluene diisocyanate. Am Rev Respir Dis 136:36–42.
14. Chan-Yeung M, Lam S, Koener S (1982) Clinical features and natural history of occupational asthma due to western red cedar (Thuja plicata). Am J Med 72:411–415.
15. Empey DW, Laitinen LA, Jacobs L, Gold WM, Nadel JA (1976) Mechanisms of bronchial hyperreactivity in normal subjects after upper respiratory tract infections. Am Rev Respir Dis 113:131–139.
16. Juniper EF, Frith PA, Hargreave FE (1981) Airway responsiveness to histamine and methacholine: relationship to minimum treatment to control symptoms of asthma. Thorax 36:575–579.
17. Sears MR, Jones DT, Holdaway MD, Hewitt CJ, Flannery EM, Herbison GP, Silva PA (1986) Prevalence of bronchial reactivity to inhaled methacholine in New Zealand children. Thorax 41:283–289.

18. Salome CM, Peat J, Britton WJ, Woolcock AJ (1987) Bronchial hyperresponsiveness in two populations of Australian schoolchildren. Clin Allergy 17:271–281.
19. Ryan G, Latimer KM, Dolovich J, Hargreave FE (1982) Bronchial responsiveness to histamine: relationship to diurnal variation of peak flow rates and improvement after bronchodilators. Thorax 37:423–429.
20. Ramsdale EH, Morris MM, Roberts RS, Hargreave FE (1984) Bronchial responsiveness to methacholine in chronic bronchitis: relationship to airflow obstruction and cold air responsiveness. Thorax 39:912–918.
21. Anderton RC, Cuff MT, Frith PA, Cockcroft DW, Morse JLC, Jones NL, Hargreave FE (1979) Bronchial responsiveness to inhaled histamine and exercise. J Allergy Clin Immunol 63:315–320.
22. O'Byrne PM, Ryan G, Morris M, McCormack D, Jones NL, Morse JLC, Hargreave FE (1982) Asthma induced by cold air and its relation to nonspecific bronchial responsiveness to methacholine. Am Rev Respir Dis 125:281–285.
23. Brand PL, Rijcken B, Schouten JP, Koeter GH, Weiss ST, Postma DS (1992) Perception of airway obstruction in a random population sample. Relationship to airway hyperresponsiveness in the absence of respiratory symptoms. Am Rev Respir Dis 146:396–401.
24. van Haren EH, Lammers JW, Festen J, Heijerman HG, Groot CA, van Herwaarden L (1995) The effects of the inhaled corticosteroid budesonide on lung function and bronchial hyperresponsiveness in adult patients with cystic fibrosis. Respir Med 89:209–214.
25. White AM, Stevens WH, Upton AR, O'Byrne PM, Collins SM (1991) Airway responsiveness to inhaled methacholine in patients with irritable bowel syndrome. Gastroentrology 100:68–74.
26. Longo G, Strinati R, Poli F, Fumi F (1987) Genetic factors in nonspecific bronchial hyperreactivity. An epidemiologic study. Am J Dis Child 141:331–334.
27. Hopp RJ, Bewtra AK, Biven R, Nair NM, Townley RG (1988) Bronchial reactivity pattern in nonasthmatic parents of asthmatics. Ann Allergy 61:184–186.
28. Clifford RD, Pugsley A, Radford M, Holgate ST (1987) Symptoms, atopy, and bronchial response to methacholine in parents with asthma and their children. Arch Dis Child 62:66–73.
29. Peat JK, Britton WJ, Salome CM, Woolcock AJ (1987) Bronchial hyperresponsiveness in two populations of Australian schoolchildren. II. Relative importance of associated factors. Clin Allergy 17:283–290.
30. Zamel N, Leroux M, Vanderdoelen JL (1984) Airway response to inhaled methacholine in healthy nonsmoking twins. J Appl Physiol 56:936–939.
31. Nieminen MM, Kaprio J, Koskenvuo M (1991) A population-based study of bronchial asthma in adult twin pairs. Chest 100:70–75.
32. Young S, Le Souef PN, Geelhoed GC, Stick SM, Turner KJ, Landau LI (1991) The influence of a family history of asthma and parental smoking on airway responsiveness in early infancy. N Engl J Med 324:1168–1173.
33. Postma DS, Bleecker ER, Amelung PJ, Holroyd KJ, Xu J, Panhuysen CI, Meyers DA, Levitt RC (1995) Genetic susceptibility to asthma—bronchial hyperresponsiveness coinherited with a major gene for atopy. N Engl J Med 333:894–900.
34. van Herwerden L, Harrap SB, Wong ZYH, Abramson MJ, Kutin JJ, Forbes AB, Raven J, Lanigan A, Walters EH (1995) Linkage of high-affinity IgE receptor gene with bronchial hyperreactivity, even in absence of atopy. Lancet 346:1262–1265.
35. Hall IP, Wheatley A, Wilding P, Liggett SB (1995) Association of Glu 27 beta 2-adrenoceptor polymorphism with lower airway reactivity in asthmatic subjects. Lancet 345:1213–1214.
36. Turki J, Pak J, Green SA, Martin RJ, Liggett SB (1995) Genetic polymorphisms of the beta 2-adrenergic receptor in nocturnal and nonnocturnal asthma. Evidence that Gly 16 correlates with the nocturnal phenotype. J Clin Invest 95:1635–1641.
37. Peat JK, Tovey E, Gray EJ, Mellis CM, Woolcock AJ (1994) Asthma severity and morbidity in a population sample of Sydney schoolchildren: Part II—Importance of house dust mite allergens. Aust NZ J Med 24:270–276.
38. Peat JK, Salome CM, Woolcock AJ (1990) Longitudinal changes in atopy during a 4-year period: relation to bronchial hyperresponsiveness and respiratory symptoms in a population sample of Australian schoolchildren. J Allergy Clin Immunol 85:65–74.
39. Sherrill D, Sears MR, Lebowitz MD, Holdaway MD, Hewitt CJ, Flannery EM, Herbison GP, Silva PA (1992) The effects of airway hyperresponsiveness, wheezing, and atopy on longitudinal pulmonary function in children: a 6-year follow-up study. Pediatr Pulmonol 13:78–85.

40. Sporik R, Holgate ST, Platts-Mills TA, Cogswell JJ (1990) Exposure to house-dust mite allergen (Der p I) and the development of asthma in childhood. A prospective study. N Engl J Med 323:502–507.

41. Stevens FA (1934) A comparison of pulmonary and dermal sensitivity to inhaled substances. J Allergy 5:285–288.

42. Herxheimer H (1952) The late bronchial reaction in induced asthma. Int Arch Allergy 3:323–328.

43. Altounyan REC (1970) Changes in histamine and atropine responsiveness as a guide to diagnosis and evaluation of therapy in obstructive airways disease. In: Pepys J, Frankland AW, eds. Disodium Cromoglycate in Allergic Airways Disease. Butterworth, London, pp. 47–53.

44. Cockcroft DW, Ruffin RE, Dolovich J, Hargreave FE (1977) Allergen-induced increase in non-allergic bronchial reactivity. Clin Allergy 7:503–513.

45. Chan-Yeung M, Lam S (1986) Occupational asthma: state of the art. Am Rev Respir Dis 133:686–703.

46. Platts-Mills TA, Mitchell EB, Nock P, Tovey ER, Moszor H, Wilkins S (1982) Reduction of bronchial hyperreactivity during prolonged allergen avoidance. Lancet 2:675–678.

47. Osler W (1892) The Principle and Practice of Medicine. Appleton, New York, p. 497.

48. Dunnill MS, Massarell GR, Anderson JA (1969) A comparison of the quantitive anatomy of the bronchi in normal subjects, in status asthmaticus, in chronic bronchitis and in emphysema. Thorax 24:176–179.

49. Stelzer J, Bigby BG, Stulbarg M, Holtzman MJ, Nadel JA, Ueki IF, Leikauf GD, Goetzl EJ, Boushey HA (1986) Ozone-induced changes in bronchial reactivity to methacholine and airway inflammation in humans. J Appl Physiol 60:1231–1326.

50. Fabbri LM, Boschetto P, Zocca E, Milani G, Pivirotto F, Plebani M, Burlina A, Licata B, Mapp CE (1987) Bronchoalveolar neutrophilia during late asthmatic reactions induced by toluene diisocyanate. Am Rev Respir Dis 136:36–42.

51. DeMonchy JGR, Kauffman HF, Venge P, Koeter GH, Jansen HM, Sluiter HJ, DeVries K (1985) Bronchoalveolar eosinophilia during allergen-induced late asthmatic reaction. Am Rev Respir Dis 131:373–376.

52. Lam S, LeRiche J, Phillips D, Chan-Yeung M (1987) Cellular and protein changes in bronchial lavage fluid after late asthmatic reaction in patients with red cedar asthma. J Allergy Clin Immunol 80:44–50.

53. Metzger WJ, Zavala D, Richerson HB, Moseley P, Iwamota P, Monick M, Sjoerdsma K, Hunnunghake GW (1987) Local allergen challenge and bronchoalveolar lavage of allergic asthmatic lungs. Am Rev Respir Dis 135:433–440.

54. Diaz P, Gonzalez MC, Galleguillos FR, Ancic P, Cromwell O, Shepherd D, Durham SR, Gleich GJ, Kay AB (1989) Leucocytes and mediators in bronchoalveolar lavage during allergen-induced late-phase asthmatic reactions. Am Rev Respir Dis 139:1383–1389.

55. Aalbers R, Kauffman HK, Vrugt B, Smith M, Koeter G, Timens W, De Monchy JGR (1993) Bronchial lavage and bronchoalveolar lavage in allergen-induced single early and dual asthmatic responses. Am Rev Respir Dis 147:76–81.

56. Woolley KL, Adelroth E, Woolley MJ, Ellis R, Jordana M, O'Byrne PM (1995) Effects of allergen challenge on eosinophils, eosinophil cationic protein and granulocyte-macrophage colony-stimulating factor in mild asthma. Am J Respir Crit Care Med 151:1915–1924.

57. Gizycki M, Ädelroth E, Rogers A, O'Byrne PM, Jeffery PK (1997) Myofibroblast involvement in the allergen-induced late response in mild atopic asthma. Am J Respir Cell Mol Biol 16:664–673.

58. Gibson PG, Girgis-Gabardo A, Hargreave FE, Morris MM, Mattoli S, Kay JM, Dolovich J, Denberg J (1989) Cellular characteristics of sputum from patients with asthma and chronic bronchitis. Thorax 44:693–699.

59. Pin I, Freitag AP, O'Byrne PM, Girgis-Gabardo A, Watson RM, Dolovich J, Denberg JA, Hargreave FE (1992) Changes in the cellular profile of induced sputum after allergen-induced asthmatic responses. Am Rev Respir Dis 145:1265–1269.

60. Gibson PG, Manning PJ, O'Byrne PM, Girgis-Gabardo A, Denburg JA, Hargreave FE (1991) Allergen-induced asthmatic responses: relationship between increases in airway responsiveness and increases in circulating eosinophils, basophils and their progenitors. Am Rev Respir Dis 143:331–335.

61. Woolley MJ, Denburg JA, Ellis R, Dahlback M, O'Byrne PM (1994) Allergen-induced changes in bone marrow progenitors and airway responsiveness in dogs and the effect of inhaled budesonide on these parameters. Am J Respir Cell Mol Biol 11:600–606.

62. Kirby JG, Hargreave FE, Gleich GJ, O'Byrne PM (1987) Bronchoalveolar cell profiles of asthmatic and nonasthmatic subjects. Am Rev Respir Dis 136:379–383.

63. Wardlaw AJ, Dunnette S, Gleich GJ, Collins JV, Kay AB (1988) Eosinophils and mast cells in bronchoalveolar lavage in subjects with mild asthma. Am Rev Respir Dis 137:62–69.

64. Bousquet J, Chanez P, Lacoste JY, Barneon G, Ghavanian N, Enander I, Venge P, Ahlstedt S, Simony Lafontaine J, Godard P, et al. (1990) Eosinophilic inflammation in asthma. N Engl J Med 323:1033–1039.
65. Woolley KL, Adelroth E, Woolley MJ, Ellis R, Jordana M, O'Byrne PM (1994) Granulocyte-macrophage colony-stimulating factor, eosinophils and eosinophil cationic protein in mild asthmatics and non-asthmatics. Eur Respir J 7:1576–1584.
66. Beasley R, Roche WR, Roberts JA, Holgate ST (1989) Cellular events in the bronchi in mild asthma and after bronchial provocation. Am Rev Respir Dis 139:806–817.
67. Jeffery PK, Wardlaw AJ, Nelson F, Collins JV, Kay AB (1989) Bronchial biopsies in asthma. An ultra-structural, quantitative study and correlation with hyperreactivity. Am Rev Respir Dis 140:1745–1753.
68. Azzawi M, Bradley B, Jeffery PK, et al. (1990) Identification of activated T-lymphocytes and eosinophils in bronchial biopsies in stable atopic asthma. Am Rev Respir Dis 142:1407–1413.
69. Poston RN, Chanez P, Lacoste JY, Litchfield T, Lee TH, Bousquet J (1992) Immunohistochemical characterization of the cellular infiltration in asthmatic bronchi. Am Rev Respir Dis 145:918–921.
70. Kelly C, Ward C, Stenton CS, Bird G, Hendrick PJ, Walters EH (1988) Number and activity of inflammatory cells in bronchoalveolar lavage fluid in asthma and their relation to airway hyperresponsiveness. Thorax 43:684–692.
71. Robinson DS, Hamid Q, Ying S, Tsicopoulos A, Barkans J, Bentley AM, Corrigan C, Durham SR, Kay AB (1992) Predominant T_{H2}-like bronchoalveolar T-lymphocyte populations in atopic asthma. N Engl J Med 326:298–304.
72. Takanashi S, Nonaka R, Xing Z, O'Byrne PM, Dolovich J, Jordana M (1994) Interleukin 10 inhibits LPS-induced survival and cytokine production by human peripheral blood eosinophils. J Exp Med 180:711–715.
73. Nonaka M, Nonaka R, Woolley K, Adelroth E, Miura K, O'Byrne PM, Dolovich J, Jordana M (1995) Distinct immunohistochemical localization of IL-4 in human inflamed airway tissues. J Immunol 155:3234–3244.
74. Bentley AM, Meng Q, Robinson DS, Hamid Q, Kay AB, Durham SR (1993) Increases in activated T-lymphocytes, eosinophils, and cytokine mRNA expression for interleukin-5 and granulocyte/macrophage colony-stimulating factor in bronchial biopsies after allergen inhalation challenge in atopic asthmatics. Am J Respir Cell Mol Biol 8:35–42.
75. Broide DH, Paine MM, Firestein GS (1992) Eosinophils express interleukin 5 and granulocyte-macrophage colony-stimulating factor mRNA at sites of allergic inflammation in asthmatics. J Clin Invest 90:1414–24.
76. Hamid Q, Azzawi M, Ying S, Moqbel R, Wardlaw AJ, Corrigan CJ, Bradley B, Durham SR, Collins JV, Jeffery PK, et al. (1991) Expression of mRNA for interleukin-5 in mucosal bronchial biopsies from asthma. J Clin Invest 87:1541–1546.
77. Woolley KL, Adelroth E, Woolley MJ, Ramis I, Abrams JS, Jordana M, O'Byrne PM (1996) Interleukin-3 in bronchial biopsies from non-asthmatics and patients with mild and allergen-induced asthma. Am J Resp Crit Care Med 153:350–355.
78. Laitinen LA, Heino M, Laitinen A, Kava T, Haahtela T (1985) Damage of the airway epithelium and bronchial reactivity in patients with asthma. Am Rev Resp Dis 131:599–606.
79. Gleich GJ, Frigas E, Loegering DA, et al. (1979) Cytotoxic properties of the eosinophil major basic protein. J Immunol 123:2925–2927.
80. O'Byrne PM, Dolovich M, Dirks R, Roberts RS, Newhouse MT (1984) Lung epithelial permeability: Relation to nonspecific airway responsiveness. J Appl Physiol 57(1):77–84.
81. Flavahan NA, Aarhuus LL, Rimele TJ, Vanhoutte PM (1985) Respiratory epithelium inhibits bronchial smooth muscle tone. J Appl Physiol 58:834–838.
82. Leikauf GD, Ueki IF, Nadel JA, Widdicombe JH (1985) Bradykinin stimulates CI secretion and prostaglandin E_2 release by canine tracheal epithelium. Am J Physiol 248:F48–F55.
83. Walters EH, O'Byrne PM, Fabbri LM, Graf PD, Holtzman MJ, Nadel JA (1984) Control of neurotransmission by prostaglandins in canine trachealis smooth muscle. J Appl Physiol 57:129–134.
84. Manning PJ, Lane CG, O'Byrne PM (1989) The effect of oral prostaglandin E_1 on airway responsiveness in asthmatic subjects. Pulmonary Pharmacol 2:121–124.
85. Melillo E, Woolley KL, Manning PJ, Watson RM, O'Byrne PM (1994) Effect of inhaled PGE_2 on exercise-induced bronchoconstriction in asthmatic subjects. Am J Respir Crit Care Med 149:1138–1141.
86. Pavord ID, Wong CS, Williams J, Tattersfield AE (1993) Effect of inhaled prostaglandin E2 on allergen-induced asthma. Am Rev Respir Dis 148:87–90.

87. Dusser DJ, Jacoby DB, Djokic TD, Rubinstein I, Borson DB, Nadel JA (1989) Virus induces airway hyperresponsiveness to tachykinins: role of neutral endopeptidase. J Appl Physiol 67:1504–1511.
88. James Al, Pare PD, Hogg JC (1989) The mechanics of airway narrowing in asthma. Am Rev Respir Dis 139:242–246.
89. Menon PK, Stankus RP, Rando RJ, Salvaggio JE, Lehrer SB (1991) Asthmatic responses to passive cigarette smoke: persistence of reactivity and effect of medications. J Allergy Clin Immunol 88:861–869.
90. Higgins BG, Francis HC, Yates CJ, Warburton CJ, Fletcher AM, Reid JA, Pickering CA, Woodcock AA (1995) Effects of air pollution on symptoms and peak expiratory flow measurements in subjects with obstructive airways disease. Thorax 50:149–155.
91. Moseler M, Hendel Kramer A, Karmaus W, Forster J, Weiss K, Urbanek R, Kuehr J (1994) Effect of moderate NO_2 air pollution on the lung function of children with asthmatic symptoms. Environ Res 67:109–124.
92. Chandler-Deal E Jr, McFadden ER Jr, Ingram RH Jr, Breslin FJ, Jaegar JJ (1980) Airways responsiveness to cold air and hyperventilation in normal subjects and in those with hayfever and asthma. Am Rev Respir Dis 121:621–628.
93. Anderson SD (1985) Exercise-induced asthma. The state of the art. Chest 87S:191–195.
94. Stevenson DD (1984) Diagnosis, prevention and treatment of adverse reactions to aspirin and non-steroidal anti-inflammatory drugs. J Allergy Clin Immunol 74:617–622.
95. Dahlen SE, Hedqvist P, Hammarstrom S, Samuelsson B (1980) Leukotrienes are potent constrictors of human bronchi. Nature 288:484–486.
96. Adelroth E, Morris MM, Hargreave FE, O'Byrne PM (1986) Airway responsiveness to leukotrienes C_4 and D_4 and to methacholine in patients with asthma and normal controls. N Engl J Med 315:480–484.
97. Manning PJ, Rokach J, Malo JL, Ethier D, Cartier A, Girard Y, Charleson S, O'Byrne PM (1990) Urinary leukotriene E_4 levels during early and late asthmatic responses. J Allergy Clin Immunol 86:211–20
98. Taylor GW, Black P, Turner N, Taylor I, Maltby NH, Fuller RW, Dollery CT (1989) Urinary leukotriene E_4 after antigen challenge and in acute asthma and allergic rhinitis. Lancet i:584–587.
99. Kumlin M, Dahlen B, Bjorck T, Zetterstrom O, Granstrom E, Dahlen S-E (1992) Urinary excretion of leukotriene E_4 and 11-dehydro-thromboxane B_2 in response to bronchial provocations with allergen, aspirin, leukotriene D_4 and histamine in asthmatics. Am Rev Respir Dis 146:96–103.
100. Manning PJ, Watson RM, Margolskee DJ, Williams V, Schartz JI, O'Byrne PM (1990) Inhibition of exercise-induced bronchoconstriction by MK-571, a potent leukotriene D_4 receptor antagonist. N Engl J Med 323:1736–1739.
101. Taylor IK, O'Shaughnessy KM, Fuller RW, Dollery CT (1991) Effect of a cysteinyl leukotriene receptor antagonist, ICI 204–219, on allergen-induced bronchoconstriction and airway hyperreactivity in atopic subjects. Lancet 337:690–694.
102. Israel E, Dermarkarian R, Rosenberg M, et al. (1990) The effects of a 5-lipoxygenase inhibitor on asthma induced by cold, dry air. N Engl J Med 323:1740–1744.
103. Israel E, Fischer AR, Rosenburg MA, Lilly CM, Callery JC, Shapiro J, Cohn J, Rubin R, Drazen JM (1993) The pivitol role of 5-lipoxygenase products in the reaction of aspirin-sensitive asthmatics to aspirin. Am Rev Respir Dis 148:1447–1451.
104. Gaddy J, Bush RK, Margolskee D, Williams VC, Busse W (1992) The effects of a leukotriene D_4 (LTD_4) antagonist (MK-571) in mild to moderate asthma. Am Rev Respir Dis 146:358–363.
105. Hui KP, Barnes NC (1991) Lung function improvement in asthma with a cysteinyl-leukotriene receptor antagonist. Lancet 337:1062–1063.
106. Israel E, Rubin P, Kemp JP, et al. (1993) The effect of inhibition of 5-lipoxygenase by Zileuton in mild-to-moderate asthma. Ann Intern Med 119:1059–1066.
107. Spector SL, Smith LJ, Glass M (1994) Effects of 6 weeks of therapy with oral doses of ICI 204,219, a leukotriene D_4 receptor antagonist, in subjects with bronchial asthma. Am J Respir Crit Care Med 150:618–623.
108. Laitinen LA, Laitinen A, Haahtela T, Vilkka V, Spur BW, Lee TH (1993) Leukotriene E_4 and granulocytic infiltration into asthmatic airways. Lancet 341:989–990.
109. Barnes PJ (1986) State of the art: neural control of human airways in health and disease. Am Rev Respir Dis 134:1289–1314.
110. Hartley JPR, Nogrady SG (1980) Effect of an inhaled antihistamine on exercise-induced asthma. Thorax 35:675–679.

111. Bousquet J, Godard P, Michel FB (1992) Antihistamines in the treatment of asthma. Eur Respir J 5:1137–1142.

112. Manning PJ, Stevens WH, Cockcroft DW, O'Byrne PM (1991) The role of thromboxane in allergen-induced asthmatic responses. Eur Respir J 4:667–672.

113. Freitag A, Watson RW, Matsos G, Eastwood C, O'Byrne PM (1993) The effect of a platelet activating factor antagonist, WEB 2086, on allergen-induced asthmatic responses. Thorax 48:594–598.

114. Kuitert LM, Angus RM, Barnes NC, Barnes PJ, Bone MF, Chung KF, Fairfax AJ, Higenbotham TW, O'Connor BJ, Piotrowska B, et al. (1994) Effect of a novel potent platelet-activating factor antagonist, modipafant, in clinical asthma. Am J Respir Crit Care Med 149:1142–1148.

115. Gardiner PV, Young CL, Holmes K, Hendrick DJ, Walters EH (1993) Lack of short-term effect of the thromboxane synthetase inhibitor UK-38,485 on airway reactivity to methacholine in asthmatic subjects. Eur Respir J 6:1027–1030.

27

Pathogenesis of Allergic Conjunctivitis

Sergio Bonini, MD, PhD and Stefano Bonini, MD

CONTENTS

INTRODUCTION

In recent years, tremendous progress in the understanding of allergic mechanisms has brought new insights into the pathophysiology and clinical aspects of several allergic diseases, as clearly documented by the previous chapters in this section of the book.

On the contrary, from several—even recent—reviews on the pathogenesis of allergic conjunctivitis it appears that the eye has been considered a "segregated organ," without taking full advantage of the flowering of information on allergic mechanisms. Accordingly, the pathogenesis and clinical management of allergic eye diseases are still often referred to by older concepts of allergy, and solely considered as an example of a type I immediate hypersensitivity mechanism.

In fact, under the term "allergic conjunctivitis" are commonly grouped heterogeneous entities that differ in their clinical manifestations, mainly seasonal allergic conjunctivitis (SAC), perennial allergic conjunctivits (PAC), atopic keratoconjunctivitis (AKC), vernal keratoconjunctivitis (VKC), and giant-papillary conjunctivitis (GPC) or contact-lens conjunctivitis (CLC) *(1–6)* (Table 1). The rationale for including these entities under the umbrella of "allergic conjunctivitis" is based on the assumption that a common type I hypersensitivity mechanism according to Gell and Coombs *(7)* plays a central role in causing the clinical signs and symptoms of all forms of allergic involvement. In other words, it has long been believed that the immunoglobulin E (IgE)–allergen interaction at the mast cell and basophil surface triggers the release of mediators, which in turn cause the clinical reactions observed in allergic conjunctivitis. Vasodilation is reflected by redness of the eye, exudation by edema and chemosis, hypersecretion by tearing and excess mucus, and stimulation of nerve endings by itching and burning.

However, several clinical observations cannot be explained by this conventional view of ocular allergy. In fact, many patients with a "red allergic eye" (particularly those with VKC or GPC) have no family or personal history of atopy. Moreover, clinical sensitization to com-

From: *Allergy and Allergic Diseases: The New Mechanisms and Therapeutics*
Edited by: J. A. Denburg © Humana Press Inc., Totowa, NJ

Table 1
Symptoms and Signs of Allergic Eye Diseases

Disease Symptoms	Signs
Seasonal and perennial allergic conjunctivitis	
Tearing	Mild hyperemia
Burning	Mild eczema
Mild itching	Mild papillary reaction (often absent)
Vernal keratoconjunctivitis	
Intense itching	Cobblestone papillae
Tearing	Intense hyperemia
Photophobia	Mucus discharge
Sensation of foreign body	Milky conjunctiva
	Punctate keratopathy
	Trantas dots
	Togby's ulcer
Atopic keratoconjunctivitis	
Itching	Hyperemia
Burning	Eczematous lesions of eyelids
Tearing	Corneal ulcers
	Cataracts
	Pannus
	Keratoconus
	Retinal Detachment
Contact-lens conjunctivitis	
Itching	Giant papillae
Pain	Excessive mucus production
Sensation of foreign body	Corneal lesions
Lens intolerance	

mon allergen cannot be detected by skin tests or immunoassays for IgE antibodies in many cases of "allergic" eye patients.

Finally, the severe inflammatory and proliferative lesions of some forms of "allergic conjunctivitis" do not resemble the typical type I hypersensitivity reaction and do not improve with conventional antiallergic treatments.

On the basis of these considerations, this chapter will be aimed at presenting a revised model of pathogenesis of allergic conjunctivitis that is much more in line with that which is current for other allergic diseases. In particular, we shall present data supporting the occurrence in the eye, too, of mechanisms other than the typical type I immediate hypersensitivity followed by a unitary hypothesis of the pathogenesis of allergic eye diseases in which we posit preferential involvement of different pathophysiological abnormalities in the varying clinical manifestations of ocular allergy.

RECENT ADVANCES IN UNDERSTANDING
ALLERGIC MECHANISMS IN THE EYE

Recent data from several groups, including our own, indicate that at least three additional mechanisms can be involved in causing a "red allergic eye" apart from the classical IgE–allergen interaction.

Non-IgE Activation of Mast Cells and Basophils

Mast cells containing both tryptase and chymase represent a typical finding in biopsies from allergic conjunctivitis patients. They are increased in number and show an abnormal intraepithelial distribution in different forms of allergic conjunctivitis, including those without evidence of sensitization to common allergens (8–10).

Mast cell activation and mediator release can be documented in allergic conjunctivitis by increased levels of tryptase in tears (11). In fact in SAC, in which tryptase values are often normal in basal conditions, allergen challenge induces a significant increase of lacrimal tryptase. However, 6 h after allergen provocation, when histamine and other mediators are still present in increased amounts in tears but allergen is no longer present at the tissue level, tryptase in tears returns to normal values, thus suggesting a trigger effect on tissue basophils mediated by substances other than allergen. Accordingly, passive transfer of ocular late-phase reaction through tears obtained before and after allergen challenge suggests that neither allergen nor IgE is responsible for the mast cell/basophil activation observed during transfer experiments (12). Finally, lacrimal tryptase values are also increased in VKC, even in skin test-negative forms (11).

All the above reported data clearly suggest that mast cell/basophil activation in human allergic diseases of the external eye is not necessarily triggered by an allergen–IgE-dependent pathway, but that other mechanisms can be operating, as has clearly been shown in other organs and tissues. It is, for instance, conceivable that in the eye, histamine releasing factors mainly released by mononuclear cells following allergen (but also viral, bacterial, or other antigenic) provocation can induce mast cell and basophil activation and mediator release without an allergen–IgE interaction.

Late-Phase Inflammatory Ocular Reaction

Extensive evidence has accumulated indicating that a late-phase allergic reaction, sustained by a complex network of inflammatory cells and mediators, can also occur in the eye, as previously shown in other allergic target organs. The late-phase ocular reaction to allergen challenge was first demonstrated in an experimental model involving rats challenged topically with di-dinitrophenylated *bis*-lysine (13). Tears collected from these animals showed cells and mediators typical of an early-phase immunological reaction, followed by a long-standing inflammatory phase, during which there was a statistically significant increase in neutrophil, eosinophil, lymphocyte, and atypical epithelial cell levels in the antigen-treated eyes versus the control eyes.

Similar results were then obtained in man, using allergen for conjunctival provocation of allergic subjects (14). Allergen challenge caused the typical early-phase reaction within 20 min. This initial reaction was dose-dependent (15). When a small dose of allergen was used, the reaction was not so pronounced, and recovery occurred spontaneously within a brief period. With larger allergen doses, the reaction persisted and progressed to a late-phase reaction. Typically, high doses of allergen induced a continuous reaction manifested by burning, redness, itching, tearing, and a foreign-body sensation that began 4–8 h after challenge and persisted for up to 24 h (16). As seen in the earlier animal models, this clinical reaction was accompanied by a significant recruitment of inflammatory cells in tears. Twenty minutes after challenge, these cells consisted principally of neutrophils. Mediators of allergic inflammation, such as histamine and leukotrienes B_4 and C_4, were also released during this early reaction phase (17). Eosinophils and lymphocytes increased in prominence 6–24 h after challenge. Eosinophils predominated in the late-phase reaction, and eosinophil peroxidase as well as eosinophil cationic protein (ECP), which are not found in the eyes of normal subjects, were detected in the tears of allergic subjects and increased dramatically after provocation with allergen *(18)*.

Interestingly enough, the increase of eosinophils and eosinophil products observed in SAC or PAC during the late-phase allergic reaction is also present in both skin-test positive and skin-test negative VKC and is not confined to ocular tissues. In fact, activated peripheral eosinophils *(19)* as well as increased serum levels of ECP and EDN/EPX (eosinophil-derived neurotoxin/eosinophil protein X) *(20)* are also present in VKC patients. These data therefore suggest that, at least in some forms of allergic conjunctivitis such as VKC, eosinophilic inflammation—but not IgE sensitization—is the more relevant feature of the disease and is associated with signs of systemic activation of eosinophils.

Nonspecific Conjunctival Hyperreactivity

Target organ hyperreactivity to nonspecific stimuli is known to occur in several allergic diseases, including bronchial asthma. We have shown that nonspecific hyperreactivity may also play a role in allergic diseases of the eye *(21)*. In 24 asymptomatic patients with a previous diagnosis of vernal conjunctivitis and 10 healthy volunteers, one eye was challenged with increasing doses of histamine diphosphate, and the other eye was challenged with phosphate-buffered saline. Dose-dependent ocular redness was seen in both patients and controls 2–5 min after histamine, but not saline, challenge. At the two lowest doses (0.01 and 0.05 mg/mL), redness was significantly more intense in the patients than in controls. In addition, the mean concentration of histamine required to cause a significant reaction was significantly lower for patients than for controls ($p < 0.02$).

These results suggest that "nonspecific conjunctival hyperreactivity" can represent a distinct pathophysiological abnormality in allergic eye diseases. This nonspecific hyperreactivity might well explain the ocular reaction induced by nonsensitizing stimuli as well as the variability of symptoms in allergic conjunctivitis, which does not necessarily correlate with environmental changes such as levels of the sensitizing allergens. Accordingly, natural nonspecific stimulation with agents such as wind, dust, and sunlight may act only as triggers of an abnormal nonspecific reactivity of the conjunctiva in allergic patients.

THE PATHOGENETIC SPECTRUM OF ALLERGIC CONJUNCTIVITIS

The above-reported progress in understanding mechanisms of allergic conjunctivitis indicates that the pathogenesis of these diseases is much more complex than previously believed and that additional mechanisms other than a type I immediate hypersensitivity reaction can be involved in the distinct pathophysiological entities of a "red allergic eye." A simplified schematization of the main abnormalities occurring in allergic conjunctivitis is shown in Fig. 1. The clinical spectrum depends on the pathophysiological abnormality that is prevalent in different forms of a "red allergic eye." These occur in four major pathophysiological forms: increased allergen recognition and specific IgE response; exaggerated polyclonal total IgE (and IgG$_4$) production; allergic inflammation with prevalence of mast cells and eosinophils; increased responsiveness of the target organ.

Increased Allergen Recognition and Specific IgE Response

The ability to respond to substances (such as pollen or dust allergens) that do not elicit a clinically relevant specific IgE response in the majority of subjects is a typical feature of allergic patients. The molecular mechanisms for allergen recognition and response at the level of the T-cell receptor/major histocompatibility complex (MHC) is at present largely clarified

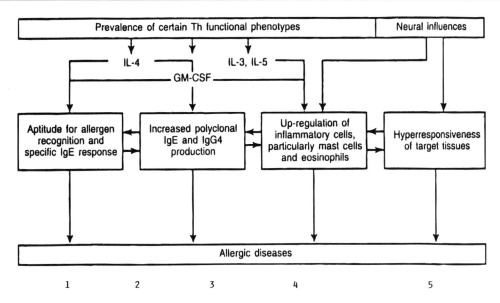

Fig. 1. Schematic and didactic representation of the four major abnormalities leading to the heterogenous groups of allergic diseases of the eye. Numbers refer to different forms of allergic conjunctivitis (*see* Table 2) located along the pathophysiological spectrum of allergic conjunctivitis in relation to their prevalent pathophysiological abnormality.

(22). Ongoing research is leading to better understanding, including manipulation of relevant epitopes involved in allergen recognition with reference to different allergens and human leukocyte antigen (HLA) specifics *(23,24).*

Studies of associations between HLA antigens and specific IgE response in allergic conjunctivitis are limited and do not allow definite conclusions. There is no reason, however, to think that susceptibility to sensitization to purified allergens in relation to given HLA haplotypes has, in the eye, peculiarities different from those of other allergic diseases. On the contrary, in view of its anatomical position, the allergic conjunctiva undergoes a higher exposure to sensitizing airborne allergens. Therefore, in spite of a lower sensitivity of the allergic conjunctiva compared to that of the allergic skin *(14)* and despite the cleaning function of tears, eye symptoms and a clinically relevant IgE response are particularly frequent in subjects with sensitization to airborne allergens. In fact in an epidemiological survey of 898 consecutive allergic patients *(25),* a "red allergic eye" was found in 40 percent of cases. In the same survey IgE antibodies to airborne allergens were found in 68% of patients with allergic conjunctivitis, ranging from 99.6% (in SAC) to 18% (in GPC). In our experience, the isolation of a specific IgE response to the eye (with tear IgE antibodies in subjects with negative skin tests), although possible in theory, was very difficult to confirm.

Polyclonal Total IgE (and IgG₄) Overproduction

It is well known that allergic patients are high total IgE (and IgG_4) responders and that increased levels of total IgE (and IgG_4) are present in both serum and tears of various forms of allergic conjunctivitis *(26,27).* This increased polyclonal IgE activation seems, at least in part, to be independent of the presence of a specific IgE response. In fact, high total serum and tear IgE are detectable also in forms of AKC or VKC without clinical evidence of sensitization *(25).* Moreover, it is also possible to speculate that sensitization to multiple allergens in subjects with high total IgE is not the cause for this last abnormality but rather the result of a widespread tendency to form IgE antibodies to many potential sensitizing substances in those subjects, i.e., an exaggerated polyclonal total IgE response.

It is widely accepted that Ig isotype switching to IgE and IgG_4 as well as the synthesis of these Ig isotypes is mainly under the control of interleukin (IL)-4 and IL-13, and therefore of a predominant T-helper 2 (Th2)-functional, CD4 T-cell response *(28)*. Therefore, MHC-linked susceptibility to a specific IgE response and a Th2-driven polyclonal total IgE overproduction can represent distinct abnormalities in allergic subjects, undergoing different genetic and environmental control and occurring isolated or in combination in different allergic subjects.

Upregulation of Inflammatory Cells (Mast Cells and Eosinophils)

Studies of late-phase reactions following conjunctival allergen challenge as well as bioptic and mediator studies of the allergic conjunctiva clearly indicate that allergic conjunctivitis is characterized by different degrees of an allergic eosinophilic inflammation similar to that observed in other allergic diseases such as asthma and rhinitis. Mast cells, activated eosinophils, and $CD4^+$ cells with a Th2 functional phenotype are increased in number, altered in distribution between subepithelium and epithelium, and show increased mediator releasability in the allergic conjunctiva *(10,29,30)*. Although it is conceivable that within the concept of "upregulation of inflammatory cells" are subsumed several pathophysiological abnormalities that undergo different genetic and environmental control, there is no doubt that an overexpression of the cytokine gene cluster located on chromosome 5q *(31)* and leading to a Th2 functional phenotype represents a peculiar feature of allergic eye diseases *(28)*. In VKC, for instance, we recently presented evidence that the major pathophysiological abnormalities of the disease might well represent the phenotypic outcome of the upregulation of the 5q-cytokine gene cluster, in which IL-3 influences the maturation and priming of mast cells and basophils, IL-4, IL-13, and IL-9 the IgE response, and IL-5 the differentiation, activation, accumulation, degranulation, and survival of eosinophils *(29)*.

Hyperresponsiveness of Target Tissues

Studies of conjunctival hyperreactivity to histamine previously reported (and possibly to other nonspecific stimuli) suggest that an increased responsiveness of human conjunctiva, independent of that induced by allergic inflammation, can represent a distinct basic abnormality in allergic eye diseases as it does for bronchial hyperreactivity in bronchial asthma.

The mechanisms leading to basal tissue hyperreactivity are still largely unexplored. Neural influences might certainly be relevant in this area. Nerve–mast cell interactions *(32)*, neuropeptides *(33)*, as well as the complex neuroendocrine immune network *(34)* represent fascinating new fields of investigation that might open new approaches for pharmacological control of allergic eye diseases.

Pathophysiological Features of Different Forms of Allergic Conjunctivitis

It is quite evident that close relationships do exist between the four major pathophysiological abnormalities just described. For instance, specific and total IgE response can influence each other, a higher degree of IgE sensitization more easily leads to long-standing eosinophilic inflammation, or IgE responses and eosinophil inflammation increase responsiveness of target organs. A revised nosology of the different forms of allergic conjunctivitis is presented in Table 2 describing a spectrum of pathophysiological abnormalities on the basis of their relative prevalence in different individual cases *(25,35)*.

SEASONAL ALLERGIC CONJUNCTIVITIS

SAC in some patients sensitive to grass allergens can be considered at one end of the pathogenetic spectrum of allergic conjunctivitis. In these cases, a typical type I immediate

Table 2
Pathophysiological Features of Different Forms of Allergic Conjunctivitis

Allergic conjunctivitis (seasonal)	Allergic conjunctivitis (seasonal/perennial)	Atopic keratoconjunctivitis	Vernal keratoconjunctivitis	Contact-lens conjunctivitis
Familial and personal history of atopy	Familial and personal history of atopy	Familial and personal history of atopy	Familial and personal history of atopy possible	No familial or personal history of atopy
Low total IgE	High total IgE	High total IgE	High total IgE	Low total IgE
Monosensitization to seasonal (grass) allergens	High sensitization to seasonal allergens or sensitization to perennial (*Parietaria*, HDM) or multiple allergens	Sensitization to multiple allergens not always detectable (food, mites)	Sensitization to one or several allergens in 50% of cases	No evidence of sensitization to common allergens
No eosinophilic inflammation out of season	Persistent minimal allergic inflammation	Severe allergic inflammation	Eosinophilic inflammation and nonspecific conjunctival hyperreactivity	Allergic inflammation /conjunctival hyperreactivity
EPR following allergen challenge	LPR following allergen challenge	Diagnostic tests: unsatisfactory	Inflammatory markers needed	No usefulness of allergy tests
Usefulness of specific IgE tests	Usefulness of specific IgE test	Allergen avoidance, if possible. Steroids often required	Steroids often required. No efficacy of hyposensitization	No contact lenses
Efficacy of antihistamines, cromones. No need of hyposensitization	Antihistamines, cromones, hyposensitization			

hypersensitivity mechanism appears to be operating. Due to genetic (HLA) and environmental influences, these patients develop sensitization to grass. Family and personal history of atopy are often present. Eye symptoms are modest, often associated with allergic rhinitis. No symptoms or signs of eye involvement are present out of the pollen season, when eosinophils and eosinophil products are not detectable. Total IgE level is low. Conjunctival provocation tests usually elicit a typical early-phase reaction, except when large allergen doses are used. In these SAC patients, therefore, IgE measurement can fulfill diagnostic aims. Hyposensitization is usually not necessary, in view of the complete effectiveness of common antiallergic drugs (antihistamines, cromones).

SEASONAL AND PERENNIAL ALLERGIC CONJUNCTIVITIS

Along the pathogenetic spectrum of allergic conjunctivitis there are some patients with clinically seasonal allergic conjunctivitis with a high degree of sensitization to grass or more long-lasting pollen allergens (for instance *Parietaria officinalis* in Mediterranean areas), as well as patients sensitive to perennial allergens (*Dermatophagoides pterouyssinus*) or those with multiple sensitivities. In these patients, susceptibility to atopy—shown by a family history of atopy and by association with other allergic diseases such as rhinitis or asthma—is associated with an upregulation of the total IgE response (high total serum IgE). Conjunctival provocation tests often induce both an intense early and a late-phase allergic response. Eosinophil and eosinophil products can often be increased both in tears and serum even during clinical remission (persistent minimal allergic inflammation). The high level of sensitization shown by IgE tests (highly positive skin tests and/or IgE antibody immunoassays, high total IgE, LPR following allergen challenge) is complemented, at a diagnostic level, by detection of inflammatory markers in tears and serum (eosinophils, ECP). Antihistamines and cromones are usually effective therapies, but hyposensitization may be required, especially in monosensitive patients with conjunctivitis associated with severe rhinitis and asthma.

ATOPIC KERATOCONJUNCTIVITIS

In this more severe form of allergic conjunctivitis, a high "atopic tone" is marked by a positive family and personal history of atopy, high total IgE, and signs of eosinophilic inflammation often involving not only the conjunctiva but also the cornea. Clinical sensitization to common allergens is not always detectable by skin tests and IgE immunoassays. In some cases, multiple sensitivities are present but their relationship to clinical symptoms is questionable. Accordingly, specific IgE tests are only of limited value, and possibly other tests to document the high level of atopy and the severity of eosinophilic inflammation might be more useful. Common antiallergic treatments (including hyposensitization in patients with a documented sensitization) are not satisfactory, and often steroids are required to control the symptoms and signs of the conjunctival inflammation.

VERNAL KERATOCONJUNCTIVITIS

This rare form of allergic conjunctivitis can be considered a suitable model of Th2 disease and overexpression of the 5q cytokine gene cluster *(29,36)*.

In fact, mast cells, activated eosinophils, and CD4[+] cells (with a Th2 functional phenotype) are the prominent histopathological feature. Tear tryptase levels are increased, showing an ongoing mast cell degranulation. Skin tests and immunoassays for IgE antibodies are positive in approx 50% of patients, especially in those with family and personal history of atopy. Total tear and serum IgE, however, is usually high and activated eosinophil and eosinophil products are detectable at both tissue and peripheral level, independent of the presence of clinical sen-

Clinical form of conjunctivitis	IgE antibodies	IgE total	Allergen challenge	Eosinophilic inflammation	Conjunctival hyperreactivity
1. SAC	+ (grass)	Low	EPR	-	-
2. SAC/PAC	+++ (seasonal) (perennial or multiple)	High	LPR	+	+/-
3. AKC	+/- foods, multiple	High	=	++	+
4. VKC	+/-	High	=	+++	++
5. CLC	-	Low	=	+	++

Fig. 2. Pathophysiological features of allergic conjunctivitis.

sitization to single or multiple allergens. Nonspecific conjunctival hyperreactivity to histamine is present, and this can possibly explain the hyperresponsiveness of VKC patients to non-specific stimuli such as light, wind, or dust.

Antiallergic drugs are often of limited efficacy. However, their use can reduce the need for steroids, which are the only really effective treatment at present but also the major iatrogenic cause for severe side effects and complications of the disease.

CONTACT-LENS CONJUNCTIVITIS

Although CLC is usually included in the spectrum of allergic conjunctivitis, in our experience the occurrence of a personal and family history of atopy, association with other allergic diseases, and the presence of sensitization to common allergens are, in CLC, not more frequent than in a control population. In this case, as in other cases of "red eye" induced by stimulation with nonspecific substances, the major pathophysiological abnormality seems to be an abnormal reactivity of local tissues. Since the mechanisms underlying this abnormal hyperresponsiveness are obscure, the diagnostic tools for its evaluation and drugs for its modulation still represent an unexplored area. However, IgE tests in these cases are of limited value. Conjunctival hyperresponsiveness to histamine or other nonspecific stimuli can represent a better tool to investigate one of the basic tissue abnormalities (Fig. 2).

CONCLUDING REMARKS

Allergic conjunctivitis and "red eye" represent a heterogeneous group of diseases. The classical type I immediate hypersensitivity mechanism, which has long been invoked as a unifying hypothesis to explain the pathogenesis of allergic conjunctivitis, is not sufficient to explain the pathophysiological abnormalities present in a large proportion of patients with allergic conjunctivitis. Accordingly, currently available diagnostic tests are often unsatisfactory, and therapeutic approaches not always effective.

Recent advances derived from studies of patients with different forms of allergic conjunctivitis suggest a more complex pathogenesis in which a Th2-type allergic inflammation with mast cells and eosinophils as well as a nonspecific conjunctival hyperreactivity can play roles of equal importance to that of allergen-IgE-induced mast cell and basophil mediator release. The pathophysiological approach suggested here can represent a scheme to be tested in clinical practice in individual cases of allergic conjunctivitis, with the aim of improving its diagnosis and optimizing a more selective treatment in the single patient with "red allergic eye."

REFERENCES

1. Allansmith MR (1982) The Eye and Immunology. Mosby, St. Louis.
2. Easty DL (1987) Allergy and the eye. In: Allergy—An International Textbook. (Lessof, MH, Lee TH, Kemeny, DM eds) John Wiley, New York, pp. 513–528.
3. Bonini Se, Bonini St, Tomassini M (1992) Les allergies oculaires. In: Traite d'Allergologie (Charpin J, Vervloet D, eds) Flammarion, Paris, Chapter 52.
4. Bielory L, Frohman L (1992) Allergic and immunologic disorders of the eye. J Allergy Clin Immunol 86:1–20.
5. Abelson MB, Schaefer K (1993) Conjunctivitis of allergic origin: immunologic mechanisms and current approaches to therapy. Surv Ophthalmol 38(Suppl):115–132.
6. Friedlander MH (1993) Conjunctivitis of allergic origin: clinical presentation and differential diagnosis. Surv Ophthalmol 38(Suppl):105–114.
7. Coombs RRA, Gell PGH (1975) Classification of allergic reactions responsible for clinical hypersensitivity and disease. In: Gell PGH, Coombs RRA, Lachmann PJ, Clinical aspects of immunology, third edn. Oxford: Blackwell, pp. 761–882.
8. Irani AM, Butrus SI, Tabbara KF, et al. (1990) Human conjunctival mast cells: distribution of MCT and MCTC in vernal conjunctivitis and giant papillary conjunctivitis. J Allergy Clin Immunol. 86:34–40.
9. Morgan SJ, Williams JH, Walls AF, et al. (1991) Mast cell numbers and staining characteristics in the normal and allergic human conjunctiva. J Allergy Clin Immunol 87:111–116.
10. Magrini L, Metz D, Bacon A, et al. (1993) Immunohistochemistry and inflammation of vernal keratoconjunctivitis. Invest Ophthalmol Vis Sci ARVO Suppl 34:857.
11. Magrini L, Centofanti M, Schiavone M, et al. (1992) Increased tryptase tear levels in allergic conjunctivitis. In: XVth Europ. Congress Allergology and Clin. Immunol. Paris, p. 254.
12. Bonini St, Centofanti M, Schiavone M, et al. (1993) Passive transfer of the ocular late phase reaction. Ocular Immunol Inflamm 1:323–325.
13. Bonini Se, Trocme SD, Barney NP, et al. (1987) Late-phase reaction and tear fluid cytology in the rat ocular anaphylaxis. Curr Eye Res 6:659–665.
14. Bonini Se, Bonini St, Vecchione A, et al. (1988) Inflammatory changes in conjunctival scrapings after allergen provocation in humans. J Allergy Clin Immunol 82:462–469.
15. Bonini St, Bonini Se, Bucci MG, et al. (1990) Allergen dose response and late symptoms in a human model of ocular allergy. J Allergy Clin Immunol 86:869–876.
16. Bonini St, Centofanti M, Schiavone M, et al. (1994) The pattern of ocular late phase reaction induced by allergen challenge in hay fever conjunctivitis. Ocular Immunol Inflamm 2:195–97.
17. Bonini Se, Bonini St, Berruto A, et al. (1989) Conjunctival provocation test as a model for the study of allergy and inflammation in humans. Int Arch Allergy Appl Immunol 88:144–148.
18. Bonini Se, Tomassini M, Bonini St, et al. (1992) The eosinophil has a pivotal role in allergic inflammation of the eye. Int Arch Allergy Appl Immunol 99:354–358.
19. Rutella S, Bonini St, Rumi C, et al. (1995) Flow cytometry of peripheral blood leucocytes in vernal keratoconjunctivitis. J Allergy Clin Immunol 95:376 (abstract).
20. Tomassini M, Magrini L, Bonini St, et al. (1994) Increased serum levels of eosinophil cationic protein and eosinophil derived neurotoxin (protein X) in vernal keratoconjunctivitis. Ophthalmology 101:1808–1811.
21. Bonini St, Bonini Se, Schiavone M, et al. (1992) Conjunctival hyperresponsiveness to ocular histamine challenge in patients with vernal conjunctivitis. J Allergy Clin Immunol 89:103–107.
22. Blumenthal M, Bonini S (1990) Immunogenetics of specific immune responses to allergens in twins and families. In: Marsh DG, Blumenthal M, eds. Genetic and Environmental Factors in Clinical Allergy. University of Minnesota Press, Minneapolis, pp. 132–142.
23. Bonini S, Rasi G, Trilló ME, et al. (1983) Atopy in twins. J Allergy Clin Immunol. pp. 71–100.
24. Bonini S, Trilló ME, Rasi G, et al. (1982) IgE and IgG serum levels in twins. In: Abs. XI Inter. Congress of Allergology and Clinical Immunology. London: Macmillan, p. 817.
25. Bonini Se, Bonini St (1987) Studies of allergic conjunctivitis. Chibret Int J 5:12–22.
26. Marsh DG (1990) Immunogenetic and immunochemical factors determining imune responsiveness to allergens: studies in unrelated subjects. In: Marsh DG, Blumenthal M, eds. Genetics and environmental factors in clincal allergy. Minneapolis: University of Minnesota Press. pp. 97–122.
27. Bonini S, Adorno D, Piazza M, et al. (1980) Allergic diseases and HLA antigens. In: Oehling A et al., eds. Advances in allergology and clinical immunology. Oxford: Pergamon, p. 778.

28. Del Prete, G (1992) Human Th1 and Th2 lymphocytes: their role in the pathophysiology of atopy. Allergy 47:450–455.
29. Bonini Se, Bonini St, and Lambiase A (1995) Vernal keratoconjunctivitis: a model of C5q cytokine gene cluster disease. Int Arch Allergy Appl Immunol. 107:95–98.
30. Trocme SD, Aldave AJ (1994) The eye and eosinophil. Surv Ophthalmol. 39:251–252.
31. van Leeuwen Bh, Martinson ME, Webb CG, et al. (1989) Molecular organization of the cytokine gene cluster, involving the human IL-3, IL-4, IL-5 and GM-CSF genes on human chromosome 5. Blood. 73:1142–1148.
32. Marshall JS, Stread RH, Macsciarri C, et al. (1990) The role of mast cell degranulation products in mast cell hyperplasia. 1. Mechanisms of action of nerve growth factor. J Immunol. 144:1885–1892.
33. Foreman JC (1987) Neuropeptides and pathogenesis of allergy. Allergy 42:1–11.
34. Bonini Se, Bonini St, Lambiase A, et al. (1995) Immune, endocrine and neural aspects of allergic inflammation. In: Proceedings 1, XVI European Congress of Allergology and Clinical Immunology (A. Basomba and J Sastre eds) Monduzzi, Bologna, pp. 475–480.
35. Bonini Se, Bonini St (1993) IgE and non-IgE mechanisms in ocular allergy. Ann Allergy. 71:296–298.
36. Maggi E, Biswas P, Del Prete G, et al. (1991) Accumulation of Th2-like helper T cells in the conjunctiva of patients with vernal conjunctivitis. J Immunol 146:1169–1174.

VI   THERAPEUTICS

28 Glucocorticoids (Corticosteroids)

Christopher J. Corrigan, MD, PhD

CONTENTS

INTRODUCTION

Inhaled glucocorticoids (GC) suppress the bronchial inflammation that is thought to underlie asthma and now form the mainstay of current antiasthma drug therapy *(1)*. For the vast majority of patients with asthma, both adults and children, the benefits of this therapy substantially outweigh the risks. This chapter will consider clinical aspects of GC therapy, particularly inhaled therapy, for asthma, patterns of clinical response to GC therapy, GC-resistant asthma, and a summary of some of the mechanisms by which GC may exert their therapeutic effects.

AEROSOLIZED GC THERAPY FOR ASTHMA

Aerosol therapy for asthma allows a favorable benefit-to-risk ratio to be achieved, because very small doses of inhaled medication may provide optimal therapy with minimal unwanted effects. The therapeutic efficacy of drugs administered by aerosolization depends, however, not only on the pharmacological properties of the inhaled drug but also on the characteristics of the delivery device, which influences the amount of drug deposited in the lung and the pattern of drug distribution in the airways.

Aerosols consist of airborne suspensions of fine particles, which may be solid or liquid, of a range of sizes whose distribution approximates that of a log-normal distribution. The size of an aerosol particle and respiratory variables influence the deposition of inhaled aerosols in the airways. Particles >10 μm in diameter are unlikely to deposit in the lungs, whereas particles < 0.5 μm are likely to reach the alveoli without deposition and subsequently be exhaled. Particles of size 1–5 μm are therefore most likely to be deposited in the lower respiratory tract.

The proportion of an inhaled, aerosolized dose of drug reaching the lungs is small (typically < 20% of the total dose). The remainder of the dose is swallowed and absorbed from the gastrointestinal tract. The small fraction of the dose reaching the airways is absorbed into the bloodstream. Thus, the swallowed fraction of the dose is absorbed and metabolized as for an oral formulation, whereas the fraction reaching the airways is absorbed into the bloodstream

From: *Allergy and Allergic Diseases: The New Mechanisms and Therapeutics*
Edited by: J. A. Denburg © Humana Press Inc., Totowa, NJ

and metabolized in the same way as an intravenous dose. The extent of the desired therapeutic effect depends on local tissue concentrations. These observations have several implications for the optimal characteristics of topically administered drugs such as those administered by aerosol. They should combine high intrinsic activity within the target organ with rapid inactivation of the systemically absorbed drug. Fewer unwanted systemic effects should be expected with drugs having a low oral bioavailability (whether due to poor gastrointestinal absorption or high first-pass hepatic metabolism). In addition, disease states may influence the degree of pulmonary absorption *(2)*.

GC Aerosol Delivery Systems

Glucocorticoids are commonly administered as preformed aerosols in metered dose inhalers (MDIs) or dry powder devices. Whichever device is used, it should be ensured that the patient knows how to use it correctly. Most MDIs contain suspensions of drug in propellant, typically a mixture of chlorofluorocarbons designed to achieve the vapor pressure and spray characteristics for optimal drug delivery. Finely divided particles (usually <1 µm) of the drug are suspended in the pressurised liquid propellant. Metering chambers typically contain 25–100 µL of propellant, which is released when the canister is depressed into the actuator. The size of the initial droplets formed is approx 30 µm, but this is rapidly reduced by evaporation so that the inhaled particles have a size closer to the ideal 5 µm. MDIs deliver only a small proportion of the dose of the drug (approx 20%) *(3)* to the lungs, mainly because of impaction in the oropharynx. For optimal pulmonary drug deposition the medication should be released at the beginning of a slow inspiration lasting about 5 s that is followed by 10 s of breath-holding *(4)*. There are two principal problems that limit the use of MDIs. First, many patients, particularly the very young, very old, and disabled, cannot use the inhaler satisfactorily because of poor coordination between activating the inhaler and inhaling. Secondly, they contain chlorofluorocarbon propellants, which are thought to damage the ozone layer. Future legislation makes it likely that the use of such propellants will be limited. Several inhalation aids or "spacer" devices have been developed to improve the deficiency of MDIs. These not only help patients with poor hand-to-mouth coordination, but also reduce drug deposition in the oropharynx (which may be as little as 5% of the inhaled dose with some spacer devices, compared with 80% or more of the dose with MDIs). Because they decrease aerosol velocity, however, spacer devices tend to reduce drug availability in the lungs *(2,3)*.

Dry powder inhalers have also been devised to deliver GC to patients who have difficulty in using an MDI. The appropriate dosage is placed in a capsule along with a filler such as lactose or glucose. In use, the capsule is pierced or sheared. Inhalation results in rotation of the capsule itself or a propeller, resulting in the contents of the capsule becoming broken up and entering the inspired air. The energy required is derived from the patients' inspiratory effort, and the need for coordination between inhalation and activation is obviated. Inhalation should be as fast as possible for optimal drug deposition, but even with good inspiratory flow rates, only approx 6% of drug is deposited in the airways *(5)*, mainly because the drug particles are larger than the optimal size required for pulmonary deposition. Recently, more convenient multidose dry powder inhalers have been introduced. Potential problems with dry powder inhalers include esophageal irritation and consequent cough. The drug may also stick to the capsule or fail to disperse, resulting in deposition of most of the drug in the mouth.

Inhaled GC in Asthma

GC administered by inhalation have proved to be a great advance in the management of asthma, combining efficacy with reduction of systemic unwanted effects that may be associated with long-term systemic therapy *(6)*.

Topically active GC used for asthma therapy include beclomethasone dipropionate, betamethasone valerate, budesonide, triamcinolone, fluticasone 17α-propionate, and flunisolide. Of these, beclomethasone and budesonide are by far the most extensively used, although the use of fluticasone is increasing in the UK. Budesonide, beclomethasone dipropionate, and fluticasone 17α-propionate are structural analogs of the basic GC structure that have been designed to combine the properties of high topical potency with rapid systemic clearance. Beclomethasone dipropionate acts, in part, as a pro-drug. When incubated with human lung tissue in vitro the drug is rapidly hydrolyzed to beclomethasone 17- and 21-monopropionate *(7)*. Beclomethasone 17-monopropionate has approx 30-fold greater affinity for human lung cytosolic glucocorticoid receptors than beclomethasone dipropionate *(7)*. Extensive hydrolysis of the swallowed fraction of the drug also occurs in the intestine, and both monopropionates undergo rapid metabolism in the liver by oxidative and reductive pathways to produce inactive metabolites that are subsequently secreted into the bile. The elimination half-lives of beclomethasone dipropionate and 17-monopriopionate are very rapid (30 and 37 min, respectively), ensuring a favorable ratio of topical to systemic effects. Budesonide is an equal mixture of two epimers designated 22R and 22S. 22R-budesonide is 2–3 times more potent in a human skin vasoconstrictor assay than the 22S form, although the pharmacokinetics of the two compounds are similar. The affinity of budesonide for human lung GC receptors is roughly equivalent to that of beclomethasone 17-monopropionate. Budesonide, which is swallowed, has 7–13% bioavailability and is 90% metabolized during the first pass through the liver by the cytochrome P450 oxidation system to inactive metabolites (6β-hydroxy-budesonide and 16α-hydroxy-prednisolone from the 22S and 22R epimers respectively) *(8)*. The elimination half-time is rapid (120–180 min). Fluticasone 17α-propionate has marked topical activity and a very favorable pharmacokinetic profile, with high plasma clearance, oral bioavailability <1%, and almost complete first-pass hepatic metabolism of absorbed drug *(9)*, although the bioavailability has been based on theoretical calculations that presuppose no distribution of fluticasone into erythrocytes, which is observed with all other GC. Owing to its high intrinsic potency, fluticasone 17α-propionate can be used at a low dose, and clinical tests suggest antiasthmatic equipotency of fluticasone and beclomethasone dipropionate in the dose ratio of 1:2 *(10)*. The main metabolite is 17β-carboxylic acid, which is thought to be inactive *(9)*.

Oropharyngeal deposition, and thereby systemic absorption of inhaled GC, is reduced by the use of a spacing device, and the development of candidiasis can be prevented by mouth rinsing.

Comparison of Beclomethasone, Budesonide, and Fluticasone

Inhaled GC generally provide a local therapeutic effect at dosages insufficient to elicit systemic effects, although these may occur when very high inhaled dosages are employed. It has been demonstrated that inhaled GC do indeed act locally *(11)*, and it has been emphasized that the degree of local activity relative to the potential for systemic effects is a critical determinant of the therapeutic value of any inhaled GC.

THERAPEUTIC EFFICACY

Numerous studies conducted over the last decade have compared the therapeutic efficacy of beclomethasone dipropionate and budesonide in adults and children with asthma. In adults, the majority of studies comparing the effects of standard dosages of beclomethasone dipropionate (400–800 μg/d) and budesonide (200–800 μg/d) in improving lung function and symptom scores and reducing the use of β$_2$-agonists indicate that, at these dosages, beclomethasone dipropionate and budesonide are of equivalent efficacy *(12–14)*. The same general conclusions were reached in trials comparing higher dosages of these drugs (beclomethasone dipropionate up to 1500 μg/d and budesonide up to 1600 μg/d) *(15,16)*. Short-term comparisons of equal daily dosages of beclomethasone dipropionate and budesonide in children with asthma have also demonstrated the therapeutic equivalence of the two inhaled GC *(17,18)*.

Several recent studies have compared the therapeutic efficacy of inhaled fluticasone 17α-propionate with that of budesonide *(19,20)* and beclomethasone dipropionate *(21)* in adults and children with mild to moderate asthma. When administered at half the daily dosage of budesonide or beclomethasone, in accordance with its greater potency, fluticasone was at least as effective as the other drugs in improving subjective and objective measurements of asthma severity. Of two studies addressing the therapy of severe asthma in adults, one short-term study *(10)* showed equivalent therapeutic efficacy of inhaled fluticasone (1 mg/d) and beclomethasone dipropionate (2 mg/d), whereas a long-term study *(22)* comparing 1 yr of therapy with inhaled beclomethasone dipropionate and fluticasone (both 1.5 mg/d) suggested a significantly greater objective improvement in asthma severity and a reduction in disease exacerbations with fluticasone. It should be noted, however, that the fluticasone in this study was administered at twice the dosage shown to exhibit equivalent potency to that of beclomethasone.

ADRENAL SUPPRESSION

At dosages of up to 400 µg/d (or fluticasone propionate at the equivalent dosage of 200 µg/d) neither beclomethasone dipropionate, budesonide, nor fluticasone generally cause significant adrenal suppression in adults *(14,19,20)* or children *(18)*. Higher-dose therapy (≥1500 µg/d) is associated with some suppression of adrenal function (as measured by depression of morning and nocturnal plasma cortisol concentrations) in some *(15)* but not all *(16)* studies in adults and children. One short-term study *(10)* suggested that inhaled fluticasone propionate (1 mg/d) causes less suppression of plasma cortisol concentrations than beclomethasone dipropionate (2 mg/d). The clinical significance, if any, of these observations, which have been made in short-term studies, is not, however, clear. Furthermore, there is considerable variability in these measurements between the different studies and a wide range of response to inhaled GC within each study population.

BONE METABOLISM

Several recent studies in adults suggest that normal dosages of inhaled GC have no effect on bone formation, as measured by bone mass and bone density and biochemical markers *(23,24)*. Collation of short-term studies with inhaled beclomethasone and budesonide suggests that these drugs cause a dose-dependent reduction in serum osteocalcin concentrations *(25–28)*. Unfortunately, these studies in treated asthmatics have in general been retrospective analyses in which confounding factors such as previous oral GC therapy and the natural reduction in bone density that occurs with ageing make the data difficult to interpret. Only large-scale, prospective studies will properly enable comparative tolerability to be evaluated in this context.

In children, long-term studies *(29,30)* suggest that inhaled GC do not significantly affect growth. Although recent knemometry studies have demonstrated short-term effects on bone growth velocity in children receiving inhaled GC *(31)*, these studies, if extrapolated to a period of usage of inhaled GC of five years, suggest that the leg length of the children would be 5 cm shorter than is the case in practice. It seems more likely that these short-term changes in growth velocity are corrected spontaneously in the longer term. Furthermore, it is possible that poorly controlled asthma has a greater bearing on the long-term growth of children than inhaled GC therapy *(29)*.

OTHER UNWANTED EFFECTS

Inhaled GC therapy has been incriminated in some uncontrolled studies in the development of cataracts *(32)*. Again, analysis of such studies has been confounded by factors such as the additional use of oral GC, age effects, and problems of cataract classification. There have been no prospective studies of the instance of cataract formation in asthmatics receiving inhaled GC. Thus, there remains no firm evidence of a direct causal link between the use of these agents and cataract formation.

PATTERNS OF CLINICAL RESPONSE TO GC THERAPY

Patterns of Asthma

Turner-Warwick (33) identified a number of clinical patterns of asthma based on individual patients' variability in lung function tests and response to therapy as follows:

1. The "brittle" asthmatic (intractable, persistent asthma with wide variability in peak expiratory flow rate (PEFR) and a poor response to all conventional therapy).
2. The "morning dipper" (worsening of asthma during the night and early morning, with spontaneous improvement during the day). Clinical studies on such patients (34) showed that this pattern was not attributable to recumbency or house dust mite allergy and that circadian variability of airways obstruction in asthmatic shift workers was intimately related to sleep and virtually independent of solar time.
3. The "irreversible" asthmatic (patients never achieving a predicted normal PEFR, but showing a reversible component, or showing reversibility of forced vital capacity (FVC) but not forced expiratory volume in 1 (FEV_1)/PEFR, or "drifters" showing "irreversible" obstruction over hours or days that gradually improves with weeks of intensive therapy).

These observations were important, since they highlighted the variability of asthma patterns and responsiveness to drugs within and between patients. On the other hand, in defining "patterns of asthma" it is important to recognize that the pattern of airways obstruction may be independent of the response to GC therapy. The pattern of GC responsiveness may also be influenced by the presence of "aggravating factors" (see below) as well as the duration of onset and severity of disease exacerbation in individual patients.

Patterns of Response to GC

Three examples of individual patterns of response to oral GC are shown in Fig. 1. All patients had asthma with marked diurnal variability and a clear response to inhaled bronchodilator therapy. There were no identifiable "aggravating factors." Patients were treated with oral prednisolone 20 mg once daily in the morning for a week followed by 40 mg daily for a second week. The first patient showed a prompt response to prednisolone within 2 d, with minimal further improvement even with the higher prednisolone dosage. The second patient had comparable airways obstruction and bronchodilator responsiveness that improved more gradually. In contrast, the third patient demonstrated marked airways obstruction and bronchodilator responsiveness with virtually no response to oral prednisolone even at high dosage for 14 d.

In assessing GC responsiveness, the optimal time of therapy and drug dosage remains ill defined. Webb (35) investigated the time course and dose-response relationship of the clinical response to oral GC therapy in a double-blind, controlled trial in 10 adult asthmatics. Patients were followed for a 2-yr period, and sequential exacerbations of their disease were treated in random order with 0.2, 0.4, or 0.6 mg/kg prednisolone daily for a 10-d period. Within individual subjects a dose-response relationship was observed, with higher prednisolone dosages resulting in greater improvements in PEFR. Importantly, however, it was observed that a

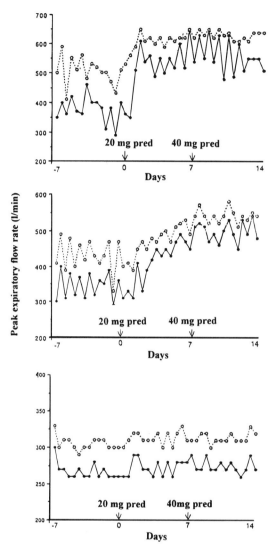

Fig. 1. Patterns of PEFR response of three asthmatic individuals to oral GC therapy. Recordings show 7 d without therapy, then 7 d of therapy with prednisolone 20 mg/d followed by 7 d at 40 mg/d. Closed and open circles refer to PEFR measurements before and after (respectively) inhaled salbutamol 400 µg administered by metered dose inhaler.

"plateau" of response was not achieved within 10 d of therapy, neither was there a "plateau" of response at the highest dosage of prednisolone employed. Thus, although important considerations in trials of GC therapy include limitation of dosages because of potential unwanted effects, these data suggest that in doubtful responders, a higher, more prolonged course of GC therapy may be required to assess GC responsiveness. This may not be the case in children, in whom the response may be complete within 3–4 d *(36)*.

Clinical Assessment of GC Responsiveness

There are many possible causes for poor asthma control and an apparent lack of responsiveness to oral or inhaled GC therapy, as has recently been emphasized *(37)*. The pattern and magnitude of the response of asthmatics to GC therapy may be influenced by the following:

1. Patient compliance (understanding of the disease and its therapy, regular dosing, correct inhaler technique);
2. Incorrect or additional diagnosis (pulmonary emboli, bronchiectasis, cardiac failure, endobronchial lesions, hyperventilation, underlying systemic disease such as vasculitis);
3. Environmental provoking factors (allergens, occupational agents, nonsteroidal anti-inflammatory drugs, β_2-adrenergic blockers, coloring agents, preservatives);
4. Esophageal reflux (may be asymptomatic);
5. Upper respiratory tract disease (rhinitis and/or sinusitis with postnasal drip);
6. Laryngeal spasm (characteristically this occurs in young women; at endoscopy there is "paradoxical" adduction of the vocal cords on inspiration during attacks, with normal specific airways conductance and a flow-volume loop suggestive of upper airways obstruction), and
7. Hormonal abnormalities (exacerbations of asthma in pregnancy, pre- and postmenopause, hyper- and hypothyroidism).

Finally, there exists a group of patients with clear-cut asthma and bronchodilator responsiveness who show no response to high dosages of either inhaled or oral GC (GC-resistant asthma, *see* GC-Resistant Asthma). It is in this group of patients that alternative anti-inflammatory therapy may be considered.

MECHANISMS OF ANTIASTHMA ACTIVITY OF GC

Despite several decades of usage of GC as anti-inflammatory agents, in general very little is known about the precise mechanisms by which they ameliorate inflammatory diseases. GC exert a number of generalized anti-inflammatory activities, such as capillary vasoconstriction and reduction of vascular permeability, that may be relevant to suppression of inflammation however caused. In the case of asthma, it is now generally accepted that bronchial mucosal inflammation, with selective local accumulation of eosinophils, is a fundamental feature of disease pathogenesis. In this scenario, eosinophils are regarded as proinflammatory effector cells whose products damage the bronchial mucosa, causing variable airways obstruction and bronchial hyperresponsiveness. Selective eosinophil accumulation and activation in asthma is in turn brought about by the release of eosinophil-active cytokines, particularly interleukin (IL)-3, IL-5, and granulocyte-macrophage colony-stimulating factor (GM-CSF), principally from activated T-cells but also partly from other inflammatory cells, including mast cells and eosinophils themselves *(38)*.

Immunocytochemical studies of bronchial biopsies taken from patients with asthma *(39–43)* have shown that activated (CD25[+]) T-cells can be detected in the bronchial mucosa and that their numbers can be correlated both with the numbers of local activated eosinophils and with disease severity. Activated (CD25[+], HLA-DR[+]) CD4 but not CD8 T-cells were also detected in the peripheral blood of patients with severe asthma *(45–57)*, and their numbers were reduced following GC therapy to a degree that correlated with the degree of clinical improvement. In one of these studies *(46)*, elevated serum concentrations of IL-5 were also detected in a proportion of the asthmatics, but not in nonasthmatic controls, and again concentrations were reduced in association with GC therapy. Elevated serum concentrations of IL-5 were also seen in a proportion of patients with severe, GC-dependent asthma *(47)*. As shown *(48)* by semiquantitative polymerase chain amplification of reverse transcribed cytokine-specific messenger ribonucleic acid (mRNA), peripheral blood T-cells from both atopic and nonatopic severe asthmatics contained elevated quantities (relative to β-actin) of mRNA encoding IL-5 as compared with controls, although elevated quantities of IL-4 mRNA in these cells were seen in all atopic subjects as compared with nonatopic controls regardless of their asthmatic status. The quantities of IL-5 mRNA were reduced in association with oral GC therapy of the asthmatics and clinical improvement.

Measurement of cytokines in vivo is problematical because of their low concentrations, rapid metabolism, and unquantifiable degree of dilution. Furthermore, "physiological" concentrations of cytokines have in general not been defined, and so it is often unknown whether a specific assay, such as enzyme-linked immunosorbent assay (ELISA) is sufficiently sensitive. One alternative to the direct measurement of cytokines is the detection of their mRNA using the technique of *in situ* hybridization with cytokine-specific complementary ribonucleic acid (cRNA) probes or riboprobes. Although this is not a strictly quantitative technique, and with the proviso that mRNA synthesis does not necessarily equate with secretion of the corresponding protein, it does have the advantage that it can localize the secretion of cytokines within cells and tissues. Using this technique, it was demonstrated that IL-5 mRNA was elaborated by cells in bronchial biopsies from a majority of mild asthmatics but not normal controls *(49)*. The amount of mRNA correlated broadly with the numbers of activated T-cells and eosinophils in biopsies from the same subjects. In another study *(50)*, it was shown that significantly elevated percentages of bronchoalveolar lavage (BAL) cells expressed mRNA encoding IL-2, IL-3, IL-4, IL-5, and GM-CSF but not interferon (IFN)γ in mild atopic asthmatics as compared with nonatopic normal controls. Separation of $CD2^+$ T-cells from the remainder of the BAL cells showed that the majority (>90%) of the cells expressing IL-5 and IL-4 mRNA were T-cells. Similarly, using sequential *in situ* hybridization and immunocytochemistry, the majority of cells expressing mRNA encoding IL-5 and IL-4 in asthmatic bronchial biopsies were shown to be T-cells, with a lesser but significant contribution from mast cells and eosinophils *(51)*. Over a broad range of asthma severity, the percentages of BAL fluid cells from atopic asthmatics expressing mRNA encoding IL-5, IL-4, IL-3, and GM-CSF, but not IL-2 and IFNγ, could be correlated with the severity of asthma symptoms and bronchial hyperresponsiveness *(52)*. Elevated percentages of peripheral-blood CD4 but not CD8 T-cells from patients with exacerbation of asthma expressed mRNA encoding IL-3, IL-4, IL-5, and GM-CSF but not IL-2 and IFNγ as compared with controls *(53)*. Elevated spontaneous secretion of IL-3, IL-5, and GM-CSF was also demonstrable in these patients using an eosinophil survival-prolonging assay. Again, the percentages of CD4 T-cells expressing mRNA encoding IL-3, IL-5, and GM-CSF, as well as spontaneous secretion of these cytokines by the CD4 T-cells, were reduced in association with GC therapy and clinical improvement. In a double-blind, parallel group study, therapy of mild atopic asthmatics with oral prednisolone, but not placebo, resulted in clinical improvement associated with a reduction in the percentages of BAL fluid cells expressing IL-5 and IL-4 and an increase of those expressing IFNγ *(54)*. Conversely, artificial exacerbation of asthma by allergen bronchial challenge of sensitized atopic asthmatics was associated with increased numbers of activated T-cells and eosinophils and increased expression of mRNA encoding IL-5 and GM-CSF in the bronchial mucosa *(55)*.

Taken together, these studies provide overwhelming evidence in support of the general hypothesis that, in asthma, activated CD4 T-cells secrete cytokines that are relevant to the accumulation and activation of eosinophils in the bronchial mucosa and that GC exert their antiasthma effect at least partly by reducing the synthesis of cytokines by these cells.

GC-RESISTANT ASTHMA

Introduction

Although GC are effective for asthma therapy in the majority of patients, the concept that not all asthmatic patients respond to oral GC was first proposed nearly thirty years ago *(56)*.

In this study, the authors described asthmatic patients in whom disease was poorly controlled, and the typical peripheral-blood eosinopenic response diminished, on large oral dosages of GC. These patients nevertheless developed Cushingoid facies. Later, it was recognized that there are some asthmatics in whom the diurnal pattern of airways obstruction is little altered by GC therapy *(34)* *(see* also the Clinical Assessment of GC Responsiveness subsection above). The first attempt to define GC-resistant (GR) asthma in objective terms *(57)* was based on changes in baseline FEV_1 following a 14-d course of oral prednisolone (40 mg/d). Patients showing improvements of <15% of baseline were classified as resistant, whereas those showing improvements of 30% or more were considered GC-sensitive (GS). All patients, in contrast, showed marked improvements in FEV_1 in response to inhaled β_2-agonists, indicating that, in both GS and GR asthmatics, airways obstruction is potentially reversible. Clearly, these FEV_1 responses represent opposite ends of a continuum of clinical response. Most subsequent studies have employed definitions of GR and GS asthma similar or identical to the above, in both adults and children *(58,59)*. The possibility that "GR" asthmatics who show no clinical response after 2 wk of oral GC therapy might nevertheless respond following more protracted therapy has never been addressed *(see* also the Patterns of Response to GC subsection above), although it was shown *(37,60)* that 90% of severe asthmatic children who showed an improvement in FEV_1 >15% of baseline on high-dose oral GC therapy did so within 10 d. The possibility that GR asthmatics might be identified by a diminished peripheral-blood eosinopenic response to GC therapy has never been systematically pursued. Here we will focus on the evidence that clinically GR asthma may be attributable at least in part to resistance of T-cells to inhibition by GC, and on what information is available regarding the mechanism of this resistance.

Functional T-Cell Abnormalities in GR Asthma

A pioneering study in this field showed *(61)* that there were no differences in the total numbers of peripheral-blood monocytes, CD4/8 T-cells, and Ia-positive cells in GS and GR asthmatics. When peripheral-blood mononuclear cells from the GS and GR asthmatics were cultured with the T-cell mitogen phytohemagglutinin (PHA) in soft agar in vitro, similar numbers of T-cell colonies were observed. Coincubation with methylprednisolone (10^{-8} mol/L), however, produced a lesser degree of inhibition of colony formation by the cells from the GR asthmatics, suggesting impaired T-cell inhibition by GC in these patients. This observation was followed up with two reports *(62,63)* characterizing peripheral-blood T-cells of GS and GR asthmatics. In summary, it was demonstrated in these reports that PHA-induced proliferation of peripheral-blood T-cells was inhibited by dexamethasone at therapeutic concentrations in GS, but not GR, asthmatics. This resistance was not absolute but relative, reflecting a shift in the dose-response curve. In other words, T-cells from GR asthmatics can be inhibited by GC, but only at concentrations requiring GC dosages that most physicians would not contemplate using for protracted periods in clinical practice. Taking the GS and GR asthmatics together, a significant correlation was observed between the clinical (FEV_1) response to oral prednisolone therapy and the degree of inhibition of T-cell proliferation by dexamethasone in vitro. These data not only confirm that T-cells from GR asthmatics are refractory to inhibition by GC, but are also consistent with the hypothesis that GC ameliorate asthma at least partly through T-cell inhibition, with the corollary that GR asthma arises at least partly from T-cell refractoriness to this inhibition. Consistent with this, it was demonstrated *(63)* that elevated percentages of peripheral-blood T-cells expressed the activation markers CD25 and HLA-DR in GR, as compared to GS asthmatics, with no differences in the total cell numbers, suggesting persistent T-cell activation in the GR patients despite GC therapy. It was also shown that dexamethasone at therapeutic concentrations inhibited

PHA-induced secretion of IL-2 and IFNγ by T-cells of GS, but not GR, asthmatics. In the GR asthmatics, clinical resistance to therapy could not be accounted for by differences in absorption and clearance of plasma prednisolone derived from orally administered prednisone. Although the GC receptors in peripheral-blood T-cells from the GR asthmatics showed a reduced binding affinity for dexamethasone as compared to those from GS patients (mean dissociation constant $[K_d]$ 9.0 vs 3.4 nM), this difference was not considered sufficient to account fully for the profound differences in GC sensitivity exhibited by these cells in vitro. These findings have been generally confirmed, although it has been suggested that, in individual patients, borderline-abnormal GC clearance and receptor abnormalities may contribute to a poor clinical response *(64)*.

It has subsequently been shown *(65)* that the inhibition of PHA-induced proliferation of peripheral-blood T-cells from asthmatics by dexamethasone in vitro is reproducible both in the short term and when patients are retested after intervals of several months. This suggests that the degree of GC sensitivity of peripheral-blood T-cells from asthmatics, and by inference their clinical sensitivity to GC therapy, remains relatively constant, although it remains possible that sensitivity in individual patients might vary to some degree according to the severity of their disease *(see* the next subsection).

These data also suggest that other drugs that inhibit T-cells might be useful for asthma therapy, and in particular that drugs that inhibit T-cells by mechanisms distinct from those of GC might be useful for the therapy of GR asthma. It has been shown *(63,65)* that the immunosuppressive drugs cyclosporin A and rapamycin inhibit T-cells by mechanisms distinct from those of GC and that these drugs inhibit proliferation of T-cells from GS and GR asthmatics to an equivalent extent. Clinical studies to evaluate the efficacy of drugs such as these for therapy of GR asthma are urgently required. The therapeutic efficacy of cyclosporin A in chronic, severe, oral GC-dependent asthma has recently been demonstrated in a controlled trial *(66)*, although it was not possible formally to identify these patients as GS or GR by the above criteria.

Finally, there exists evidence for a differential effect of GC on T-cells from GS and GR asthmatics in vivo *(67)*. In this study, BAL was performed in GS and GR asthmatics before and after a course of oral prednisone, and expression by BAL cells of mRNA encoding cytokines was measured by *in situ* hybridization. Whereas prednisone therapy of the GS asthmatics was associated with reductions in the percentages of BAL cells expressing mRNA encoding IL-4 and IL-5 and elevation of the percentages of cells expressing mRNA encoding IFNγ, only a decrease in the percentages of cells expressing mRNA encoding IFNγ was observed in association with prednisone therapy of the GR asthmatics. In addition, compared with the GS asthmatics, the GR patients had elevated percentages of BAL cells expressing mRNA encoding IL-2 and IL-4 at baseline. These data are compatible with the hypothesis that GC exert differential effects on cytokine mRNA expression in T-cells from GS and GR asthmatics. The authors also speculated that the elevated expression of IL-2 and IL-4, at least at the level of mRNA, in the GR asthmatics might have been responsible, at least in part, for the impaired GC responsiveness of these cells *(see* T-Cell Abnormalities in GR Asthma: Inherent or Induced?).

T-Cell Abnormalities in GR Asthma: Inherent or Induced?

In general, GR asthmatics are not Addisonian and do not have elevated plasma cortisol concentrations *(62)*, suggesting that the impaired GC responsiveness observed in their peripheral-blood T-cells is not a generalized phenomenon. One attractive possibility is that impaired T-cell GC responsiveness in asthma may be induced by the action of pro-inflammatory cytokines within the local environment of the inflammatory process. In this regard, there exists evidence that the GC receptor ligand binding affinity of peripheral-blood T-cells in asthmatics may be altered in the short term according to disease severity in vivo and by exposure to cytokines in vitro. The GC receptor ligand binding affinities of peripheral-blood T-cells from a group of poorly controlled asthmatics were reduced as compared with normal controls (median K_d 29.0 vs 8.0 nM). GC therapy of these asthmatics, which was accompanied by clinical improvement and reduced indices of T-cell activation, was associated with a significantly increased affinity of the T-cell GC receptors (68). In a detailed study of GC receptor binding in peripheral-blood mononuclear cells from GS and GR asthmatics, two distinct abnormalities were observed (69). A majority of GR asthmatics (15 out of 17) demonstrated a significantly reduced receptor binding affinity (mean K_d 42.1 nM) as compared with GS patients (mean K_d 21.6 nM) and normal controls (mean K_d 7.9 nM). This abnormality was confined to T-cells, reverted to normal after culture of the T-cells in vitro for 48 h, but could be sustained by culture in the simultaneous presence of high concentrations of IL-2 and IL-4. The remaining two GR asthmatics had abnormally low numbers of nuclear GC receptors with normal binding affinity. This abnormality was not confined to T-cells and was not influenced by the presence of exogenous cytokines. It was further shown (70) that this abnormality could be induced by culture of peripheral-blood T-cells from normal donors with IL-2 and IL-4 in vitro (mean K_d 36.1 nM with IL-2/4 vs 6.7 nM with medium alone) and that induction was associated with a reduced inhibitory effect of methylprednisolone on the proliferation of the T-cells induced by phorbol ester and ionomycin. The physiological significance of these relatively small differences in ligand binding affinity in T-cells is difficult to assess, and mechanisms whereby short-term, reversible variability in this affinity could occur have not been identified. There is no evidence for polymorphism of the gene encoding the GC receptor in GS and GR asthmatics that could account for variability in ligand binding affinity (71). Nevertheless, it is clear that cytokine-induced changes in GC receptor binding affinity might contribute to the genesis of glucocorticoid resistance in T-cells. Cytokine exposure might also modify the responsiveness of T-cells to GC in other ways. For example, it was shown that activated GC receptors from T-cells of GR asthmatics showed impaired binding to their specific response elements as compared with those from T-cells of GS patients (72). Scatchard analysis suggested that this was attributable to reduced numbers of activated receptors available for binding to the response elements, but not a reduced affinity for binding. One interpretation of these observations is that interactions of the GC receptor with other transcriptional regulatory elements induced in T-cells by exposure to cytokines or otherwise might inhibit the binding of this receptor to its response element, resulting in refractoriness to GC-mediated effects (see also GC Actions: The New). Whether this is indeed the case, and how far such mechanisms explain differences in the GC responsiveness of T-cells from GS and GR asthmatics, remains to be determined. Finally, the possibility that exogenous cytokines might induce abnormalities in T-cell GC sensitivity still cannot fully explain why these abnormalities differ in cells from GS and GR asthmatics. It would seem necessary to postulate further that T-cells from GR asthmatics are for some reason hypersensitive to cytokines, or that GR asthma is associated with overproduction of cytokines in the context of disease of equivalent severity, or both. With the exception of one study, mentioned above, showing elevated percentages of BAL cells expressing mRNA encoding IL-2 and IL-4 in GR as compared with GS asthmatics with disease of equivalent severity (67), there are no studies suggesting that T-cells from GR asthmatics secrete greater quantities of, or are more sensitive to, cytokines in vivo. Furthermore, the fact that cutaneous vasoconstrictor responses to topical GC are impaired in GR as compared with GS asthmatics (73) suggests that this phenomenon may not always be manifest only in the context of ongoing inflammation.

Summary

In summary, there is adequate evidence that clinical GC resistance in asthma can be attributed at least partly to a relative resistance of T-cells to inhibition by GC. Although GR asthma defined according to the present criteria represents one end of a spectrum of clinical response, in clinical practice these patients would not be exposed for prolonged periods to dosages of GC sufficient to inhibit significantly their T-cells in vivo. A more rational approach to the selection of alternative therapy for such patients might be possible when the mechanisms of this resistance are identified. In the meantime, there is some justification for assessing other drugs that inhibit T-cells from GR asthmatics at therapeutic concentrations for their efficacy and risk/benefit ratios in clinical practice.

ANTI-INFLAMMATORY ACTIONS OF GC
AT THE MOLECULAR LEVEL

GC Actions: The Old Model

The present model of GC action proposes the existence of an "activated" GC receptor protein that is found within the cytoplasm of all human cells. The "inactivated" form of the protein is associated with two molecules of a 90-kDa heat shock protein (hsp90). GC enter cells apparently by simple diffusion and bind to the receptor, leading to its "activation," which involves dephosphorylation and dissociation from hsp90, with subsequent rapid translocation of the GC/receptor complex to the nucleus. Within the nucleus, the complex binds as a dimer to specific sites in the genome, termed GC response elements (GRE), situated upstream of the promoter regions of GC-responsive genes. Binding of the complex to the GRE modulates expression of the target gene *(74)*.

GC Actions: The New Model

This rather simple model (Fig. 2) of GC action does not readily explain the wide variety of effects of GC on different cells according to their state of differentiation. Although there is some variability in the precise nucleotide sequences of GREs *(74)*, this is not so extensive as to account for the unique patterns of gene expression imposed by GC on cells of various end-differentiated phenotypes. In the case of inflammation, GC act in general to dampen the response of cells and tissues to changes in their homeostasis brought about by exposure to proinflammatory stimuli. For example, exposure of both inflammatory and tissue structural cells (such as endothelial cells, epithelial cells and fibroblasts) to the proinflammatory cytokines IL-1, IL-6, and tumor necrosis factor (TNF)α initiates a whole cascade of proinflammatory events involving increased gene transcription, including synthesis of new cytokines and other inflammatory mediators, expression of new surface proteins, and enhanced secretion of extracellular matrix proteins. These effects are mediated through the activation of transcriptional regulatory proteins distinct from the GC receptor, often in association with increased intracellular concentrations of protein kinase C (PKC). Two important examples of such proteins include activating protein-1 (AP-1), itself a heterodimer of two proteins termed Fos and Jun, and NFκB *(75)*. These proteins also bind to specific regulatory elements in the promoter regions of genes, including cytokine genes, thereby enhancing gene expression. It is now clear that activated transcriptional regulatory proteins may interact with each other directly within the nucleus or cytoplasm of cells, thereby modulating the effects that each would otherwise exert on gene transcription *(76)*. For example, direct protein–protein interaction between the activated GC receptor and AP-1 has been demonstrated in cultured cells *(77)*. Thus, the induction of activated GC receptors following exposure of cells

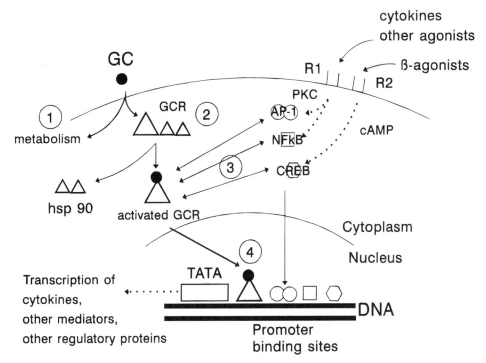

Fig. 2. Possible mechanisms of GC resistance. GC enter cells by passive diffusion and bind to the GC receptor (GCR) with dissociation of the hsp90 dimer. The activated GCR then enters the nucleus and binds to specific regulatory elements within the promoter regions of regulated genes, thus modulating transcription. Other transcriptional regulatory proteins (such as AP-1 and NFκB, induced by cytokines and other agonists through PKC-dependent pathways, and CREB, induced by β-agonists and other agonists through cAMP-dependent pathways) may interact with the activated GCR, thus preventing it from exerting its modulatory activity on regulated genes. GC resistance might arise from: (1) enhanced GC metabolism by resistant cells (theoretical); (2) reduced binding of the GC to its receptor (some evidence); (3) functional inactivation of the GCR in the presence of elevated concentrations of other transcriptional activating proteins (some evidence); (4) reduced binding of the activated GCR to its regulatory element, owing to either an abnormality of the GCR or to an abnormality of the regulatory element (theoretical). Confirmation or refutation of these and other possible mechanisms of GC resistance will require further studies.

to GC may antagonize the activities of proinflammatory transcriptional regulators such as AP-1, and this may be an important aspect of the anti-inflammatory actions of GC *(78)*. There is some evidence that GC resistance in T-cells from GR asthmatics might be mediated by enhanced expression of transcriptional activator proteins that bind to and inactivate the GC receptor (*see* the T-Cell Abnormalities in GR Asthma: Inherent or Induced subsection above).

β₂-agonists may also influence gene transcription through elevation of intracellular cyclic 3′, 5′-adenosine monophosphate (cAMP), which in turn activates protein kinase A (PKA) *(79)*. Within the nucleus, PKA phosphorylates the transcriptional regulatory protein termed cAMP response element binding protein (CREB), thereby enhancing its deoxyribonucleic acid (DNA) binding activity. CREB is known to interact with AP-1 *(80)* and might therefore inhibit some of its proinflammatory activities. Alternatively, CREB might interact with the activated GC receptor, thereby inhibiting the anti-inflammatory actions of GC.

Summary

These exciting advances suggest that the activities of GC on particular cells result from a complex interaction between the activated GC receptor and other transcriptional regulatory elements, which upsets the equilibrium of overall gene expression in these cells according to their state of differentiation and exposure to environmental factors such as cytokines. Although the net effect of GC exposure in many cells is a downmodulation of expression of inflammatory mediators, it is possible that this effect might be overcome in certain inflammatory environments or that defects may exist in cells of certain individuals that limit the ability of GC to exert these activities. A better understanding of these processes might pave the way for more rational approaches to anti-inflammatory therapy in the future.

REFERENCES

1. National Heart & Lung and Blood Institute, National Institute of Health (1992) International consensus report on diagnosis and treatment of asthma. (Publication no. 92-3091). Eur Respir J 5:601–641.
2. Summers QA (1991) Inhaled drugs and the lung. Clin Exp Allergy 21:259–268.
3. Newman SP, Moren F, Pavia D, Little F, Clarke SW (1981) Deposition of pressurized suspension aerosols inhaled through extension devices. Am Rev Respir Dis 124:317–320.
4. Newhouse MT, Dolovich MB (1986) Control of asthma by aerosols. N Engl J Med 315:870–874.
5. Vidgren M, Paronen P, Vidgren P, Vainio P, Nuutinen J (1990) In vivo evaluation of the new multiple dose powder inhaler and the Rotahaler using gamma scintigraphy. Acta Pharm Nord 2:3–10.
6. Barnes PJ (1989) A new approach to the treatment of asthma. N Engl J Med 321:1517–1527.
7. Wurthwein G, Rohdewald P (1990) Activation of beclomethasone dipropionate by hydrolysis to beclomethasone 17-monopropionate Biopharm Drug Dispos 11:381–394.
8. Edsbacker S, Andersson P, Lindberg C, Ryrfeldt A, Thalen A (1987) Metabolic acetal splitting of budesonide. A novel inactivation pathway for topical glucocorticoids. Drug Metab Dispos 15:412–417.
9. Harding SM (1990) The human pharmacology of fluticasone propionate. Respir Med 84 (Suppl A):25–29.
10. Barnes NC, Marone G, Di Maria GU, Visser S, Utama I, Payne SL (1993) A comparison of fluticasone propionate, 1 mg daily, with beclomethasone dipropionate, 2 mg daily, in the treatment of severe asthma. International study group. Eur Respir J 6:877–885.
11. Toogood JH, Frankish CW, Jennings BH, Baskerville JC, Borga O, Lefcoe NM, Johansson SA (1990) A study of the mechanism of the antiasthmatic action of inhaled budesonide. J Allergy Clin Immunol 85:872–880.
12. Rafferty P, Tucker LG, Frame MH, Fergusson RJ, Biggs BA, Crompton GK (1985) Comparison of budesonide and beclomethasone dipropionate in patients with severe chronic asthma: assessment of relative prednisolone-sparing effects. Br J Dis Chest 79:244–250.
13. Rosenhall L, Lundqvist G, Adelroth E, Glennow C (1982) Comparison between inhaled and oral corticosteroids in patients with chronic asthma. Eur J Respir Dis Suppl 122:154–162.
14. Stiksa G, Glennow C (1985) Once daily inhalation of budesonide in the treatment of chronic asthma: a clinical comparison. Ann Allergy 55:49–51.
15. Selroos O, Halme M (1991) Effect of a volumatic spacer and mouth rinsing on systemic absorption of inhaled corticosteroids from a metered dose inhaler and dry powder inhaler. Thorax 46:891–894.
16. Svendsen UG, Frolund L, Heinig JH, Madsen F, Nielsen NH, Weeke B (1992) High-dose inhaled steroids in the management of asthma. A comparison of the effects of budesonide and beclomethasone dipropionate on pulmonary function, symptoms, bronchial responsiveness and the adrenal function. Allergy 47 (2 pt 2):174–180.
17. Field HV, Jenkinson PM, Frame MH, Warner JO (1982) Asthma treatment with a new corticosteroid aerosol, budesonide, administered twice daily by spacer inhaler. Arch Dis Child 57:864–866.
18. Springer C, Avital A, Maayan C, Rosler A, Godfrey S (1987) Comparison of budesonide and beclomethasone dipropionate for treatment of asthma. Arch Dis Child 62:815–819.
19. Langdon CG, Capsey LJ (1994) Fluticasone propionate and budesonide in adult asthmatics: a comparison using dry-powder inhaler devices. Br J Clin Res 5:85–99.
20. Langdon CG, Thompson J (1994) A multicentre study to compare the efficacy and safety of inhaled fluticasone propionate and budesonide via metered-dose inhalers in adults with mild to moderate asthma. Br J Clin Res 5:73–84.

21. Leblanc P, Mink S, Keistinen T, Saarelainen PA, Ringdal N, Payne SL (1994) A comparison of fluticasone propionate 200 µg/day with beclomethasone 400 µg/day in adult asthma. Allergy 49:380–385.
22. Fabbri L, Burge PS, Croonenborgh L, Warlies F, Weeke B, Ciaccia A, Parker C (1993) Comparison of fluticasone propionate with beclomethasone dipropionate in moderate to severe asthma treated for one year. Thorax 48:817–823.
23. Mackenzie CA, Tsanakas J, Tabachnik E, Radford M, Berdel D, Gotz MH, Parker C (1994) An open study to assess the long term safety of fluticasone propionate in asthmatic children. Br J Clin Pract 48:15–18.
24. Peretz A, Bourdoux PP (1991) Inhaled corticosteroids, bone formation, and osteocalcin. Lancet 338:1340.
25. Sorva R, Turpeinen M, Juntunen-Backman K, Karonen SL, Sorva A (1992) Effects of inhaled budesonide on serum markers of bone metabolism in children with asthma. J Allergy Clin Immunol 90:808–815.
26. Jennings BH, Andersson KE, Johansson SA (1991) The assessment of the systemic effects of inhaled glucocorticoids. The effects of inhaled budesonide vs oral prednisolone on calcium metabolism Eur J Clin Pharmacol 41:11–16.
27. Toogood JH, Jennings B, Hodsman AB, Baskerville J, Fraher LJ (1991) Effects of dose and dosing schedule of inhaled budesonide on bone turnover. J Allergy Clin Immunol 88:572–580.
28. Leech JA, Hodder RV, Ooi DS, Gay J (1993) Effects of short-term inhaled budesonide and beclomethasone dipropionate on serum osteocalcin in premenopausal women. Am Rev Respir Dis 148:113–115.
29. Balfour-Lynn L (1986) Growth and childhood asthma. Arch Dis Child 61:1049–1055.
30. Varsano I, Volovitz B, Malik H, Amir Y (1990) Safety of 1 year of treatment with budesonide in young children with asthma. J Allergy Clin Immunol 85:914–920.
31. Wolthers OD, Pedersen S (1992) Controlled study of linear growth in asthmatic children during treatment with inhaled glucocorticosteroids. Paediatrics 89:839–842.
32. Nassif E, Weinberger M, Sherman B, Brown K (1987) Extrapulmonary effects of maintenance corticosteroid therapy with alternate-day prednisone and inhaled beclomethasone in children with chronic asthma. J Allergy Clin Immunol 80:518–529.
33. Turner-Warwick M (1977) On observing patterns of airflow obstruction in chronic asthma. Br J Dis Chest 71:73–86.
34. Clark TJH, Hetzel MR (1977) Diurnal variation of asthma. Br J Dis Chest 71:87–92.
35. Webb JR (1986) Dose response of patients to oral corticosteroid treatment during exacerbations of asthma. Br Med J 292:1045–1047.
36. Kamada AK, Leung DYM, Gleason MC, Hill MR, Stefler SJ (1992) High dose systemic glucocorticoid therapy in the treatment of asthma: a case of resistance and patterns. J Allergy Clin Immunol 90:685–687.
37. Woolcock AJ (1993) Steroid resistant asthma: what is the clinical definition? Eur Respir J 6:743–747.
38. Corrigan CJ, Kay AB (1992) The role of T lymphocytes and eosinophils in the pathogenesis of asthma. Immunol Today 13:501–507.
39. Azzawi M, Bradley B, Jeffery PK, Frew AJ, Wardlaw AJ, Knowles G, Assoufi B, Collins JV, Durham SR, Kay AB (1990) Identification of activated T lymphocytes and eosinophils in bronchial biopsies in stable atopic asthma. Am Rev Respir Dis 142:1410–1413.
40. Jeffery PK, Wardlaw AJ, Nelson FC, Collins JV, Kay AB (1989) Bronchial biopsies in asthma: an ultrastructural, quantitative study and correlation with hyperreactivity. Am Rev Respir Dis 140:1745–1753.
41. Bradley BL, Azzawi M, Assoufi B, Jacobson M, Collins JV, Irani A, Schwartz LB, Durham SR, Jeffery PK, Kay AB. (1991) Eosinophils, T-lymphocytes, mast cells, neutrophils and macrophages in bronchial biopsies from atopic asthmatics: comparison with atopic non-asthma and normal controls and relationship to bronchial hyperresponsiveness. J Allergy Clin Immunol 88:661–674.
42. Bentley AM, Maestrelli P, Saetta M, Fabbri LM, Robinson DR, Bradley BL, Jeffery PK, Durham SR, Kay AB (1992) Activated T-lymphocytes and eosinophils in the bronchial mucosa in isocyanate-induced asthma. J Allergy Clin Immunol 89:821–829.
43. Bentley AM, Menz G, Storz C, Robinson DR, Bradley B, Jeffery PK, Durham SR, Kay AB (1992) Identification of T-lymphocytes, macrophages and activated eosinophils in the bronchial mucosa in intrinsic asthma relationship to symptoms and bronchial responsiveness. Am Rev Respir Dis 146:500–506.
44. Corrigan CJ, Hartnell A, Kay AB (1988) T-lymphocyte activation in acute severe asthma. Lancet i:1129–1131.
45. Corrigan CJ, Kay AB (1990) CD4 T-lymphocyte activation in acute severe asthma. Relationship to disease severity and atopic status. Am Rev Respir Dis 141:970–977.
46. Corrigan CJ, Haczku A, Gemou-Engesaeth V, Doi S, Kikuchi Y, Takatsu K, Durham SR, Kay AB (1993) CD4 T-lymphocyte activation in asthma is accompanied by increased concentrations of interleukin-5: effect of glucocorticoid therapy. Am Rev Respir Dis 147:540–547.

47. Alexander AG, Barkans J, Moqbel R, Barnes NC, Kay AB, Corrigan CJ (1994) Serum interleukin-5 concentrations in atopic and non-atopic patients with glucocorticoid-dependent chronic severe asthma. Thorax 49:1231–1233.

48. Doi S, Gemou-Engesaeth V, Kay AB, Corrigan CJ (1994) Polymerase chain reaction quantification of cytokine messenger RNA expression in peripheral blood mononuclear cells of patients with severe asthma: effect of glucocorticoid therapy. Clin Exp Allergy 24:854–687.

49. Hamid Q, Azzawi M, Ying S, Moqbel R, Wardlaw AJ, Corrigan CJ, Bradley B, Durham SR, Collins JV, Jeffery PK, Quint DJ, Kay AB (1991) Expression of mRNA for interleukin-5 in mucosal bronchial biopsies from asthma. J Clin Invest 87:1541–1546.

50. Robinson DS, Hamid Q, Ying S, Tsicopoulos A, Barkans J, Bentley AM, Corrigan C, Durham SR, Kay AB (1992) Evidence for a predominant "Th2-type" bronchoalveolar lavage T-lymphocyte population in atopic asthma. N Engl J Med 326:298–304.

51. Ying S, Durham SR, Corrigan CJ, Hamid Q, Kay AB (1995) Phenotype of cells expressing mRNA for Th2-type (interleukin-4 and interleukin-5) and Th1-type (interleukin-2 and interferon-gamma) cytokines in bronchoalveolar lavage and bronchial biopsies from atopic asthmatics and normal control subjects. Am J Respir Cell Mol Biol 12:477–487.

52. Robinson DS, Ying S, Bentley AM, Meng Q, North J, Durham SR, Kay AB (1993) Relationships among numbers of bronchoalveolar lavage cells expressing messenger ribonucleic acid for cytokines, asthma symptoms, and airway methacholine responsiveness in atopic asthma. J Allergy Clin Immunol 92:397–403.

53. Corrigan CJ, Hamid Q, North J, Barkans J, Moqbel R, Durham SR, Kay AB (1995) Peripheral blood CD4, but not CD8 T-lymphocytes in patients with exacerbation of asthma transcribe and translate messenger RNA encoding cytokines which prolong eosinophil survival in the context of a TH2-type pattern: effect of glucocorticoid therapy. Am J Respir Cell Mol Biol 12:567–578.

54. Robinson DS, Hamid Q, Ying S, Bentley AM, Assoufi B, North J, Meng Q, Durham SR, Kay AB (1993) Prednisolone treatment in asthma is associated with modulation of bronchoalveolar lavage cell interleukin-4, interleukin-5 and interferon-gamma cytokine gene expression. Am Rev Respir Dis 148:420–406.

55. Bentley AM, Meng Q, Robinson DS, Hamid Q, Kay AB, Durham SR (1993) Increases in activated T-lymphocytes, eosinophils and cytokine messenger RNA for IL-5 and GM-CSF in bronchial biopsies after allergen inhalation challenge in atopic asthmatics. Am J Respir Cell Mol Biol 8:35–42.

56. Schwartz HL, Lowell FC, Melby JC (1968) Steroid resistance in bronchial asthma. Ann Intern Med 69:493–499.

57. Carmichael J, Paterson IC, Diaz P, Crompton GK, Kay AB, Grant IWB (1981) Corticosteroid resistance in chronic asthma. Br Med J 282:1419–1422.

58. Kamada AK, Leung DY, Szefler SJ (1992) Steroid resistance in asthma: our current understanding. Pediatr Pulmonol 14:180–186.

59. Alvarez J, Surs W, Leung DYM, Iklé D, Gelfand EW, Szefler SJ (1992) Steroid resistant asthma: immunologic and pharmacologic features. J Allergy Clin Immunol 89:714–721.

60. Kamada AK, Szefler SJ, Leung DYM (1993) The growing problem of steroid resistant asthma. Drug Ther 23:55–68.

61. Poznansky MC, Gordon ACH, Douglas JG, Krajewski AS, Wyllie AH, Grant IWB (1984) Resistance to methylprednisolone in cultures of blood mononuclear cells from glucocorticoid-resistant asthmatic patients. Clin Sci 67:639–645.

62. Corrigan CJ, Brown PH, Barnes NC, Szefler SJ, Tsai JJ, Frew AJ, Kay AB (1991) Glucocorticoid resistance in chronic asthma: glucocorticoid pharmacokinetics, glucocorticoid receptor characteristics and inhibition of peripheral blood T-cell proliferation by glucocorticoids *in vitro*. Am Rev Respir Dis 144:1016–1025.

63. Corrigan CJ, Brown PH, Barnes NC, Tsai JJ, Kay AB (1991) Glucocorticoid resistance in chronic asthma: peripheral blood T-lymphocyte activation and a comparison of the T-lymphocyte inhibitory effects of glucocorticoids and cyclosporin A. Am Rev Respir Dis 144:1026–1032.

64. Kamada AK, Spahn JD, Surs W, Brown E, Leung DY, Szefler SJ (1994) Coexistence of glucocorticoid receptor and pharmacokinetic abnormalities: factors that contribute to a poor response to treatment with glucocorticoids in children with asthma. J Pediatr 124:984–986.

65. Haczku A, Alexander A, Brown P, Assoufi B, Li B, Kay AB, Corrigan C (1994) The effect of dexamethasone, cyclosporine and rapamycin on T-lymphocyte proliferation *in vitro*: comparison of cells from patients with glucocorticoid-sensitive and glucocorticoid-resistant chronic asthma. J Allergy Clin Immunol 93:510–519.

66. Alexander AG, Barnes NC, Kay AB (1992) Trial of cyclosporin in corticosteroid-dependent chronic severe asthma. Lancet 339:324–328.
67. Leung DY, Martin RJ, Szefler SJ, Sher ER, Ying S, Kay AB, Hamid Q (1995) Dysregulation of inter-leukin 4, interleukin 5 and interferon gamma gene expression in steroid-resistant asthma. J Exp Med 181:33–40.
68. Spahn JD, Leung DY, Surs W, Harbeck RJ, Nimmagadda S, Szefler SJ (1995) Reduced glucocorticoid binding affinity in asthma is related to ongoing allergic inflammation. Am J Respir Crit Care Med 151:1709–1714.
69. Sher ER, Leung DM, Surs W, Kam JC, Zieg G, Kamada AK, Szefler SJ (1994) Steroid-resistant asthma cellular mechanisms contributing to inadequate response to glucocorticoid therapy. J Clin Invest 93:33–39.
70. Kam JC, Szefler SJ, Surs W, Sher ER, Leung DY (1993) Combination IL-2 and IL-4 reduces glucocorti-coid receptor-binding affinity and T cell response to glucocorticoids. J Immunol 151:3460–3466.
71. Lane SJ, Arm JP, Staynov DZ, Lee TH (1994) Chemical mutational analysis of the human glucocorticoid receptor cDNA in glucocorticoid-resistant bronchial asthma. Am J Respir Cell Mol Biol 11:42–48.
72. Adcock IM, Lane SJ, Brown CR, Peters MJ, Lee TH, Barnes PJ (1995) Differences in binding of gluco-corticoid receptor to DNA in steroid-resistant asthma. J Immunol 154:3500–3505.
73. Brown PH, Teelucksingh S, Matusiewicz SP, Greening AP, Crompton GK, Edwards CR (1991) Cutaneous vasoconstrictor response to glucocorticoids in asthma. Lancet 337:576–580.
74. Beato M (1989) Gene regulation by steroid hormones. Cell 56:335–344.
75. Kishimoto T, Taga T, Akira S (1994) Cytokine signal transduction. Cell 76:253–262.
76. Latchman DS (1990) Eukaryotic transcription factors. Biochem J 270:281–289.
77. Yang-Yen HF, Chambard JC, Sun Y-L, Smeal T, Schmidt TJ, Drouin J, Karin M (1990) Transcriptional interference between c-Jun and the glucocorticoid receptor: mutual inhibition of DNA binding due to direct protein-protein interaction. Cell 62:1205–1215.
78. Barnes PJ, Adcock IM (1993) Anti-inflammatory actions of steroids: molecular mechanisms. Trends Pharmacol Sci 14:436–441.
79. Yamamoto KK, Gonzalez GA, Biggs WH, Montminy MR (1989) Phosphorylation-induced binding and transcriptional efficacy of nuclear factor CREB. Nature 334:494–498.
80. Masquilier D, Sassone-Corsi P (1992) Transcriptional cross-talk: nuclear factors CREM and CREB bind to AP-1 sites and inhibit activation by Jun. J Biol Chem 267:22,460–22,466.

29 Beta-Agonists

Harold S. Nelson, MD

CONTENTS

INTRODUCTION

The β$_2$-adrenergic agonists are the most effective bronchodilators for patients with bronchial asthma. They have been demonstrated to be superior to theophylline and anticholinergic agents for producing immediate bronchodilation *(1)*, to sustained-release theophylline for maintenance therapy *(2)* and for treatment of acute severe episodes of asthma *(3)*, and to anticholinergics, methylxanthines, and cromolyn for prevention of exercise-induced bronchoconstriction *(4)*. Despite this impressive evidence for their effectiveness in controlling the symptoms of bronchial asthma, avoidance of the use of the β-agonist except for very occasional treatment of acute symptoms has been advocated, owing to concerns regarding their safety when employed on a regular basis *(5–9)*. These reservations regarding the use of β-agonists stem from a number of observations of undesired consequences that have been reported with their regular use (Table 1).

THE β-ADRENERGIC RECEPTOR AND ITS REGULATION

The β-agonists react with specific receptors that are found on the surface of many cells *(10)*. Occupation of the receptor initiates a response that includes activation of the α subunit of a guanine nucleotide-binding regulatory protein (Gs). This α subunit then activates the surface-associated enzyme adenylyl cyclase, resulting in conversion of adenosine triphosphate (ATP) to cyclic adenosine monophosphate (cAMP). cAMP, in turn, activates protein kinase A, which phosphorylates certain key proteins in the cell, leading to the characteristic β-adrenergic responses *(10)*. However β$_2$-agonists may relax airway smooth muscles in part by activating membrane potassium channels through the activated α subunits of the Gs protein, independent of cAMP, resulting in inhibition of calcium influx *(11)*.

Of more immediate interest are the control mechanisms that provide regulation of the activity and number of the β-receptors. Continuous stimulation of the β$_2$-adrenergic receptor leads to a rapid waning of receptor-mediated adenylyl cyclase responses (desensitization). This involves phosphorylation of the receptor and its uncoupling from adenylyl cyclase *(12)*. In

From: *Allergy and Allergic Diseases: The New Mechanisms and Therapeutics*
Edited by: J. A. Denburg © Humana Press Inc., Totowa, NJ

Table 1
Adverse Effects Reported with Use of β-Agonists

1. Systemic side effects
   Hypokalemia, hyperglycemia, tremor

2. Cardiovascular
   Inotropy, chronotropy, ectopy, decreased diastolic blood pressure, decreased arterial oxygen saturation

3. Bronchodilator
   Decline in baseline pulmonary function, decline in bronchodilator response

4. Bronchoprotection
   Increased bronchial hyperresponsivness to specific and nonspecific stimuli, decreased protection against nonspecific bronchial challenge, decreased protection against specific challenge—allergen and exercise

5. Worsening of asthma control
   Increased symptoms, increased requirement for rescue bronchodilators, increased exacerbations, increased asthma deaths

addition, internalization of the receptor may occur (sequestration). Both processes can occur within minutes and are as rapidly terminated with removal of β_2-agonist stimulation *(12)*. Longer exposure to β_2-agonist stimulation results in diminished β_2-receptor synthesis. β_2-receptor messenger ribonucleic acid (mRNA) is decreased owing to either inhibition of gene transcription or increased posttransciptional processing of the mRNA. The resulting downregulation of the number of β-receptors can explain most of the phenonema that have been observed with the regular use of the β_2-agonists.

In vitro corticosteroids increase both β_2-receptor mRNA and receptor numbers *(13)*. Corresponding clinical observations include both reversal of β_2-agonist-induced downregulation of receptor number on peripheral leukocytes *(14)* and restoration of bronchodilator response to inhaled β_2-agonist in patients who were unresponsive *(15)*. However, recent studies have been unable to demonstrate a protective effect of inhaled or oral corticosteroids against diminished β-agonist bronchoprotection to methacholine challenge or decreased in vitro alveolar macrophage response to β_2-agonist stimulation resulting from previous β_2-agonist therapy *(16,17)*.

THE ROLE OF β_2-AGONISTS IN THE TREATMENT OF ASTHMA

β_2-agonists, particularly the long-acting agents, can be shown both in vitro and in vivo to have actions in addition to bronchial smooth muscle relaxation that could be useful and could be termed "anti-inflammatory" *(18)*. These include decreased vascular permeability, increased chloride and water secretion by bronchial epithelial cells, increased ciliary function, and suppression of secretion of proinflammatory mediators by mast cells and eosinophils. β_2-agonists may also inhibit cholinergic neurotransmission by prejunctional β_2-receptors *(19)*. They have been shown in vitro to have potentially deleterious effects for asthma, as well, including increasing immunoglobulin E (IgE) secretion by B-lymphocytes *(20)* and, at high doses, interference with corticosteroid-receptor deoxyribonucleic acid (DNA) binding in human lung tissue *(21)*. A separate issue that has been raised is that of β_2-agonist enantiomers. Commercially available β_2-agonists are racemic mixtures of equal parts of R- and S-enantiomers, of which only the R configurations react with the β_2-receptors *(22)*. Studies in guinea pigs have suggested that the S-enantiomer, rather than being inert, can induce bronchial hyperresponsiveness *(22)*. Further studies will determine the relevance of these studies to humans.

Long-acting β_2-agonists have been shown to reduce serum levels of eosinophil granular proteins when given prior to allergen challenge *(23,24)*. Both bronchoalveolar lavage fluid levels of eosinophil cationic protein (ECP) and evidence of oxidative metabolism by alveolar macrophages were reduced after 4 wk of regular salmeterol treatment *(25)*. However, bronchoalveolar lavage before and after long-term administration of salmeterol has shown no effect on the levels of eosinophils or epithelial cells *(26)* or on the numbers of lymphocytes or markers of lymphocyte activation *(26,27)*. Therefore, in the absence of clear-cut reduction in the chronic inflammation of asthma, the β_2-agonists should be considered drugs that relieve symptoms, but that do not modify the disease, either favorably or adversely. When viewed in this manner, the appropriate role of β-agonists in asthma therapy becomes more clearly defined.

Short-Acting β_2-Agonists

All patients with asthma should have available a metered dose inhaler containing a short-acting β-agonist. The short-acting β_2-agonists are the drugs of choice for relief of acute symptoms of asthma, both the occasional breakthrough symptoms during the day and acute exacerbations requiring emergency care *(3)*. The short-acting β_2-agonists are also preferred for pretreatment to prevent exercise-induced bronchospasm (EIB) because of their rapid onset of action and effectiveness over a period up to 2 h. With more prolonged, repetitive activity, use of a long-acting β-agonist may be preferred for prevention of EIB.

Inhaled short-acting β_2-agonists are sufficient treatment by themselves for patients who have mild asthma. The indication for proceeding to the next step, the introduction of regular anti-inflammatory therapy, varies among the guidelines that have been developed *(28–30)*. The revised NHLBI Guidelines *(28)* recommend anti-inflammatory therapy for those patients whose asthma symptoms occur more than twice weekly or who have evidence of reversible airflow obstruction during asymptomatic periods.

The short-acting β_2-agonists are available in a variety of preparations. For most indications the metered dose inhaler is to be preferred because of its efficiency and lower cost. Even for treatment of acute severe asthma, administration of a short-acting β-agonist by metered dose inhaler used with a spacer device has been found to be as effective as by nebulizer *(31)*. There is very little role in asthma treatment for oral or injected preparations of the short-acting β_2-agonists.

Long-Acting β_2-Agonists

The long-acting β_2-agonists salmeterol and formoterol are the logical choice for maintenance bronchodilator therapy of asthma. These drugs, by virtue of extended side chains, are very lipophilic, a property that may in part account for their long duration of action *(18,32)*. However, it appears that the long side chain of salmeterol, in addition, binds to a site within the β_2-receptor apart from the region that activates adenylyl cyclase, the so-called exo-site, which accounts for many of its unique properties *(18)*. Both salmeterol and formoterol have been shown to produce bronchodilation that is still detectable at 24 h *(33)*, thus allowing for 12-h dosing *(34–36)*. Studies up to 1 yr have shown that the bronchodilation initially produced by salmeterol was sustained *(37,38)*, as was the bronchodilator response to albuterol administered periodically during the course of a year's treatment with salmeterol *(39)*.

Use of the long-acting β_2-agonists should be considered in patients whose symptoms are not adequately controlled by the use of anti-inflammatory therapy, which the long-acting agents should supplement, not replace. The guidelines *(28–30)* (Table 2) are ambiguous regarding the

Table 2
Guidelines to the Pharmacologic Therapy of Asthma

Expert Panel (1997) (28)

Mild/Intermittent	Mild/Persistent	Moderate/Persistent	Severe/Persistent
Short-acting inhaled β-agonists PRN up to 2 times weekly plus pretreatment	Short-acting inhaled β-agonists as needed for symptoms	Short-acting inhaled β-agonists as needed for symptoms	Short-acting inhaled β-agonists as needed for symptoms
	Anti-inflammatory: Cromolyn/nedocromil or low-medium-dose inhaled corticosteroids Alternative but not preferred: sustained-release theophylline leukotriene pathway modifiers	Anti-inflammatory: Inhaled corticosteroids (medium dose) or Inhaled corticosteroids and Long-acting bronchodilator: long-acting inhaled β-agonist, sustained-release theophylline or long-acting β-agonist tablets	Anti-inflammatory: high-dose inhaled corticosteroids Long-acting bronchodilators: long-acting inhaled β-agonist Sustained-release theophylline and/or oral β-agonists If required: Oral corticosteroids daily or alternate days

International Consensus (1992) (29)

Mild—Step 1	Moderate—Step 2	Moderate—Step 3	Severe—Step 4
Short-acting inhaled β-agonists up to 3 times weekly plus pretreatment	Short-acting inhaled β-agonists up to 3–4 times per day	Short-acting inhaled β-agonists up to 3–4 times per day	Short-acting inhaled β-agonists up to 3–4 times per day
	Anti-inflammatory: Cromolyn/nedocromil or low-dose inhaled corticosteroids	Anti-inflammatory: Medium-dose inhaled corticosteroids	Anti-inflammatory Medium-high-dose inhaled corticosteroids and oral corticosteroids

preference between moderate-to-high-dose inhaled steroids and the addition of a sustained acting bronchodilator as the next step if symptoms are not controlled by low-dose inhaled corticosteroids *(29)*. This issue was addressed in a study in England in which 426 adults still symptomatic despite treatment with beclomethasone 200 µg twice daily were randomized to either the addition of salmeterol 50 µg bid to the existing beclomethasone dose, or an increase of beclomethasone to 500 µg bid *(40)*. The results of this study greatly favored the combination of low-dose beclomethasone and salmeterol. Symptoms and pulmonary function were better controlled and exacerbations were not higher on the combined therapy. Nevertheless, many feel uncomfortable that they may be leaving airway inflammation untreated in using this approach. This quandary may be avoided if steroids are initially introduced in the form of an oral preparation or at moderately high inhaled doses so that the degree to which the symptoms are responsive to corticosteroid therapy may be assessed. Sustained bronchodilators, usually the long-acting β_2-agonists, may then be added if continuing symptoms warrant, followed by gradually tapering of the corticosteroids to the minimal effective level.

UNDESIRED CONSEQUENCES OF β_2-AGONIST THERAPY

Systemic Side Effects Associated with Use of β_2-Agonists

The β_2-agonists most widely employed (albuterol *[41]*, terbutaline *[42]*, pirbuterol *[43]*, bitolterol *[44]*, formoterol *[41]*, and salmeterol *[18]*) are all selective agonists for the β_2-adrenergic receptor. Except with use of excessive doses, both their pulmonary and extrapulmonary actions are largely limited to the actions of these receptors. Several β_2-agonists that are still occasionally employed clinically, including isoproterenol *(45)*, fenoterol *(41,46)*, and metaproterenol *(47)*, are less selective for β_2-adrenergic receptors. However, even selective β_2-adrenergic agonists cause hypokalemia, which is of some potential concern *(46)*, and hyperglycemia, which is of little consequence *(48)*. Muscle tremor is also mediated by β_2-receptors and is potentially a problem with oral administration, but with inhalation it is not a problem for most patients.

A portion of the adrenergic receptors in cardiac tissue are β_2 in type *(49)*. The cardiac β_2-receptors predominantly subserve chronotropic responses (increase in heart rate); however, all β-agonists appear to have some potential to produce inotropic effects (increased force of contraction). Inotropic stimulation increases myocardial oxygen consumption, which is potentially harmful in the presence of hypoxemia caused by severe asthma *(46)*. All of the β_2-agonists increase the QT_c interval *(41,50)*, prolongation of which has been a predictor of sudden death in patients with cirrhosis and ischemic heart disease as well as in apparently normal individuals *(51)*. This effect is probably also enhanced in the presence of hypoxia *(51)*. Nevertheless, cardiac arrhythmias have only rarely been reported with regularly prescribed β-agonists, usually in predisposed individuals *(52)*. Specific β-agonists also act on the vascular system, leading to vasodilation of peripheral vessels and a fall in diastolic blood pressure *(53)*. Compensatory vascontriction of pulmonary vessels in areas of decreased ventilation together with the increased cardiac output can result in a transient fall in arterial oxygen tension that may exceed 5 mmHg *(54)*.

In addition to being less β_2-selective, fenoterol and isoproterenol are also complete β-agonists, whereas albuterol, terbutaline, and salmeterol are only partial agonists *(18,46)*. Maximum stimulation with the complete agonist fenoterol produced greater cardiac inotropic changes and hypokalemia than maximal stimulation with the partial agonist albuterol and did this at approximately half the dose employed with albuterol *(46)*. Thus, in the setting of excessive use, potentially harmful extrapulmonary responses are more likely with a complete agonist *(46)*.

Rapid development of tolerance with regular therapy has been reported for many of the systemic effects of β-agonist stimulation, including hypokalemia *(48)*, chronotropy *(48,55)*, inotropy *(55,56)*, tremor *(55,56)*, and fall in diastolic blood pressure *(57)*. Evaluation of patients during regular use and 2 mo after stopping long-acting oral β_2-agonists revealed no difference in potassium levels, which were low in the serum and normal in the muscles both while taking and after discontinuation of the β_2-agonist *(58)*. Skeletal muscle magnesium was also unaffected, being reduced both while taking and after stopping therapy *(58)*.

Decreased Bronchodilator Action by β_2-Agonists

Two observed results of regular use of β_2-agonists, a decline in the duration of the bronchodilator response and a fall in pulmonary function in the absence of exogenous β-agonist stimulation, are probably closely related.

Decreased sensitivity to the bronchodilator action of β-agonists with regular use (termed subsensitivity) was first reported nearly two decades ago *(59)* and repeatedly confirmed *(55,60–65)*. Failure to observe this phenomenon more consistently can be traced to a failure to appreciate two facts. First, downregulation of the bronchodilator response is not agonist-specific and occurs during the course of β_2-agonist therapy of asthma. There is a decline in bronchodilator response observed only with β_2-agonist-naive subjects or when there is a β_2-agonist-free washout period, usually accomplished by the use of ipratropium as an alternative bronchodilator before the first dose of β_2-agonist *(55,64,65)*. Second, although there is often a trend toward reduction in the maximum bronchodilator response *(60–62)*, bronchodilator subsensitivity is consistently demonstrated only if observations are extended to the duration of bronchodilation *(55,63,65)*. The dynamics of the development of bronchodilator "subsensitivity" were clearly demonstrated in the study reported by Repsher *(63)*. Fifty-four patients had avoided β_2-agonists for 4 wk prior to the first measurement of the bronchodilator response to two inhalations of albuterol. The patients then employed albuterol two inhalations four times daily for 12 wk, coming to the clinic every 4 wk to have their bronchodilator response to albuterol recorded. Over the course of 12 wk there was a statistically insignificant decrease in the absolute peak forced expiratory volume in 1 s (FEV_1) achieved. On the other hand, by wk 8 and 13 the absolute levels of FEV_1 were lower 3–6 h after dosing, and the duration of significant elevation of the FEV_1 decreased from an initial 240 min to 168 min (30%). Most of the decrease occurred in the first 4 wk, but there was a further decrease after 8 wk. It is clear from this study why "subsensitivity" is the more appropriate term for this gradual reduction in bronchodilation, rather than tachyphylaxis, which denotes a rapid change in responsiveness.

That a decline in baseline pulmonary function can occur when exogenous β_2-agonists are withheld has also been known for nearly two decades *(62)*. It is likely that this reflects downregulation of the β_2-adrenergic receptors produced by regular use *(10,12)*. As long as β_2-agonists are administered, bronchodilation continues, but in their absence a diminished number of receptors is available for binding by the circulating endogenous catecholamines, resulting in reduced β_2-adrenergic bronchodilation. Reviewing the studies in which a decline in baseline pulmonary function has been reported, it is evident that this is always in the setting of regular administration of the β_2-agonist, followed by overnight withholding of the drug before the pulmonary function is measured *(8,18,66–70)*. Indeed, in those studies in which serial measurements of pulmonary function have been performed the maximum fall in FEV_1 has been documented from 10 h *(70)* to 23 h *(67)* following the last dose of the β_2-agonist. There is then return to the original level of pulmonary function *(66,69)*. To place this decline in pulmonary function in proper perspective, it has never been observed during the effective period of bronchodilation, which is about 3 h for short-acting β-agonists *(62,63)* or 12 h for the long-acting agonists *(55,65,71)*. Furthermore, a decline in pulmonary function to below the control level has not been observed on discontinuing the long-acting β-agonists salmeterol *(72)* and formoterol *(73)*.

Decreased Protection Against Bronchial Challenge

β-agonists are very effective at protecting against bronchoconstriction produced by histamine or methacholine. If there has been a suitable β-agonist washout, the initial degree of protection may be as much as 10 doubling dilutions *(74)*. With regular administration of the β-agonist there is a rapid but only partial loss of this protection *(74–76)*. This partial loss of protection has been shown to develop in only a few days and then to remain stable for months *(74)*. It is notable, however, that there always remains some degree of protection; usually the provocative dose is still increased by greater than two doubling doses *(6,16,67,74,75,77)*.

It is very likely that challenges with exercise and AMP, as well as with allergen, involve release of mediators, probably from mast cells in the airways. β_2-agonists exert a considerable degree of protection against challenges with exercise, allergen, and AMP. It has been suggested that this protection includes reduction of mast cell mediator release in addition to functional antagonism of bronchial smooth muscle contraction *(3)*. With regular administration of β_2-agonists the loss of protection against these challenges may be greater than the loss of protection against methacholine or histamine *(6,8,75,78)*. However, although reduced, there is not complete loss of protection within the effective duration of action of the β-agonist.

Increased Nonspecific Bronchial Hyperresponsiveness

Just as withholding of exogenous short-acting β_2-agonists can often be shown to result in a decline in pulmonary function to below the control value, so too, removal of exogenous β_2-adrenergic stimulation frequently results in a period of increased susceptibility to non-specific bronchoconstrictor stimuli *(18,66,67,79–81)*. This, too, is a transient phenomenon. When multiple measurements have been made following the termination of exogenous β_2-agonists, the maximum sensitivity to histamine or methacholine challenge has been recorded at 23 h *(67)* to 59 h *(66)*.

Since the β-agonists may counter the bronchoconstrictive effect of exercise or allergen inhalation by suppression of mast cell mediator release through receptors on the mast cells, as well as by functional antagonism to airway smooth muscle contraction, regular administration of β_2-agonists may be expected to result in downregulation of both of these actions *(82)*. Therefore it is not surprising that withholding of exogenous β_2-agonists results in increased sensitivity to allergen challenge *(6)*. There is, however, evidence, as noted above, that this increased sensitivity to allergen is seen only when β-agonist therapy is withheld beyond its duration of pharmacological effect, which for albuterol is only a few hours.

Of more relevance to current asthma therapy is the question whether increased bronchial responsiveness follows administration of the long-acting β_2-agonists salmeterol and formoterol. The effect of withdrawing both of these drugs on bronchial responsiveness to histamine and methacholine has been examined. Discontinuing chronic treatment with salmeterol *(74,83,84)* and formoterol *(73)* has not been followed by any rebound bronchial hyperresponsivness, just as there has been no decline in pulmonary function below the baseline on stopping these drugs *(72,73)*.

Worsening of Asthma

The proposition that regular use of β_2-agonists could make asthma control worse was made most forcefully by the study conducted in New Zealand and reported by Sears and coworkers *(85)*. In this study, 89 patients with stable asthma were treated for 6 mo each with four times

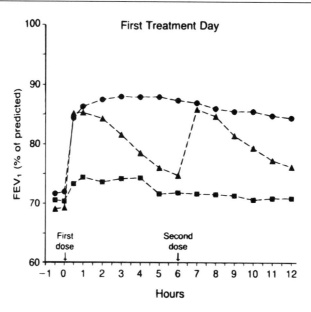

Fig. 1. Bronchodilator response to salmeterol, albuterol, and placebo. Mean FEV_1 as a percentage of predicted value. The salmeterol and placebo groups received placebo as their second dose, and the albuterol group received albuterol. ● Salmetrol ($n = 75$); ▲, albuterol ($n = 73$); ■, placebo ($n = 77$). (Reproduced from ref. *34*.)

daily inhaled fenoterol or placebo, and β_2-agonist rescue treatment was allowed with both regiments. Many of these patients were taking inhaled corticosteroids, but no other asthma medication was allowed. Based on a hierarchy of signs and symptoms, asthma was judged to be better controlled in 70% on as-needed β_2-agonists whereas only 30% were judged better controlled with regular administration of fenoterol. Subsequent publications have provided more details from this study *(7,86)*. For the most part, the differences between the groups were small and often not significant *(86)*. As a whole, the differences noted with regular fenoterol reflected those that would be anticipated when regular treatment with a short-acting β-agonist produces receptor downregulation and the treatment is then withheld for a number of hours before observations are made. As noted above, under these conditions the anticipated findings include a decline in pulmonary function and an increase in bronchial sensitivity to methacholine. It is noteworthy that this study was conducted with fenoterol, which was dispensed in an effective dose at least twice that of albuterol or terbutaline *(87)*. It would be anticipated that fenoterol would produce greater downregulation of receptors than would albuterol or terbutaline and hence, would be more apt to demonstrate clinical evidence of subsensitivity. Studies comparing regular to as-need-only inhaled albuterol have failed to reproduce the findings with fenoterol *(34–36)*.

It has become apparent, from the longer-term studies comparing asthma control while patients are using short-acting β-agonists on a regular or on an only-as-needed schedule, that regular, short-acting β-agonists are not an effective maintenance therapy for asthma *(18,85,34,35)*. As demonstrated in Fig. 1 *(34)*, the bronchodilator response to albuterol is rapid but not sustained, and its duration of protection against bronchoconstrictor stimuli is even shorter. Albuterol is a drug suitable for relief of acute symptoms and short-term prophylaxis, but does not provide sustained symptom relief during the day and is particularly ineffective in preventing bronchoconstriction during the night *(88)*. It is also apparent from Fig. 1 that the long-acting β_2-agonists, here represented by salmeterol, provide sustained

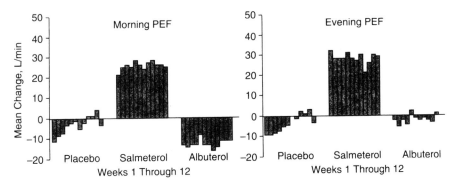

Fig. 2. Peak expiratory flows (PEFs) during treatment with salmeterol, albuterol, and placebo. Change in PEF from prerandomization period (week-to-week mean). Values were recorded daily for 12 wk after randomization. The difference in mean change is significant for salmeterol vs placebo or albuterol for both morning and evening PEF values ($p < 0.001$). (Reproduced from ref. *35*.)

bronchodilation, suggesting they should provide effective control of asthma symptoms and maintenance of bronchodilation with twice daily dosing. This effectiveness of salmeterol was confirmed in the same studies *(34,35)* in which reduced asthma symptoms and requirements for rescue bronchodilator and improvement in morning peak flows were sustained throughout the study (Fig. 2) *(35)*. Similar results have been reported with regular use of the other long-acting β-agonist, formoterol, when compared to placebo *(89)*. The greater suitability of the long-acting β-agonists for maintenance treatment of asthma was demonstrated in an asthma-specific quality-of-life study of 141 subjects who received treatment for 1 mo each with placebo, albuterol four times daily, and salmeterol twice daily *(90)*. Although conventional measurements of asthma signs and symptoms were significantly improved with albuterol, only salmeterol produced clinically meaningful improvement in the subjects' quality of life.

A widely expressed concern is that the consequences of receptor downregulation with regular use of β_2-agonists could translate into long-term deterioration of asthma *(5–9)*. Exacerbations occurred earlier and more often with regular fenoterol in the New Zealand study *(7)*. A similar increase in the rate of exacerbations has been sought in long-term studies with other short-acting and with the long-acting β_2-agonists. In placebo-controlled studies conducted in the United States comparing regular albuterol to regular salmeterol there was no significant difference in the rate of exacerbations in the three treatment groups *(34,35)*. A compilation of exacerbations requiring hospitalization was made from a number of controlled studies conducted during the development of salmeterol *(91)*. The rate of hospitalization in 4,658 subjects receiving salmeterol was 1.2% compared to 2.0% in 3,466 subjects receiving placebo or comparator drugs, including albuterol and theophylline.

β_2-Agonists and Asthma Deaths

Use of particular β-agonists has been implicated in two epidemics of asthma deaths *(92)*. The first of these occurred in several countries, including the United Kingdom, New Zealand, and Australia, in the 1960s. The rise in asthma deaths followed shortly the introduction of β_2-agonists dispensed from pressurized metered dose inhalers. Retrospective analysis has suggested a connection between this epidemic and sales of an inhaler delivering high doses of isoproterenol *(11)*. A second epidemic increase in asthma deaths occurred in New Zealand in the late 1970s. Again respective analysis appeared to establish a relationship between patients being prescribed a particular β_2-agonist inhaler and an increased risk of death. The inhaler in this instance, fenoterol, shared features with the high-dose isoproterenol inhaler in being less β_2-selective than other commonly employed β_2-agonists such as albuterol and terbutaline *(73)*, in functioning as a complete agonist of the β_2-receptors and hence being capable of producing a greater maximum degree of receptor stimulation *(46)*, and finally in delivering a relatively larger amount of drug per actuation *(92)*. Three case control studies from New Zealand of subjects dying from asthma each found an increased relative risk of dying if the asthmatic had been prescribed fenoterol *(92)*. The risk was even greater if only subjects with severe asthma were included *(92)*. The results of these case control studies appear to have been confirmed in a separate study conducted in Canada *(93)*. Although the unique characteristics of fenoterol provide a plausible explanation for the increased deaths in New Zealand, there may be other factors contributing *(94)*. It is impossible to rule our a prescribing bias that patients with more severe asthma were preferentially prescribed fenoterol, although no evidence to support that has been presented. On the other hand, many of New Zealand deaths were in patients who did not receive medical attention in their final attack *(93)*. Deaths also occurred selectively in the economically less privileged portion of the New Zealand population, in which access to medical care may have been limited by economics and availability *(94)*. This may have led to delayed use of corticosteroids, progressively worsening airway obstruction, hypoxia, and increasing susceptibility to cardiac side effects of fenoterol *(87)*. The epidemic of asthma deaths in New Zealand began to abate when increasing attention was given to prompt and adequate treatment of exacerbations *(94)*, but the most precipitous decline in mortality followed shortly publicity regarding possible dangers of fenoterol and a resulting marked decline in use of that drug *(92)*.

The pattern of deaths in New Zealand differed from that which was observed in a study of asthma mortality and drug use based on data from the province of Saskatchewan in Canada *(95)*. In this study, among 12,301 individuals who had received ten or more prescriptions for asthma drugs over the period of 1978 to 1987, there were 44 deaths and 85 near-fatal episodes of asthma recorded. Deaths occurred suddenly only 16% of the time, the others were documented as resulting from progressive respiratory failure *(95)*. The initial analysis of these 129 deaths and near-deaths compared to matched controls revealed an increased risk of death or near-death associated not only with the use of β_2-agonists, but also with theophylline and oral steroids *(95)*, suggesting that the cases had had more severe asthma. Reanalysis of the data has indeed resulted in a revision of the original conclusion that β-agonists were contributing to the deaths from asthma *(77)*. Rather, the excessive use of β_2-agonists appears to be primarily a marker of severe asthma, which itself is a cause of fatal asthma. However, a pattern of increasing use of β_2-agonists places the patient at increased risk of death and should alert their physician to the need for a reassessment of their overall treatment *(96)*.

Concerns have been expressed regarding deaths associated with the use of salmeterol *(97,98)*. Two letters addressed the results of a surveillance study that was undertaken in England shortly after the introduction of salmeterol *(99,100)*. In this study of 16-wk duration, 16,787 patients received salmeterol twice daily and 8,393 albuterol four times daily *(101)*. Withdrawals owing to asthma were significantly more common in subjects on albuterol (3.8 vs 2.9%), and hospitalization for asthma occurred in 1.22% of subjects receiving albuterol and 1.15% of those receiving salmeterol. However, there were 12 deaths in patients receiving salmeterol and only 2 in those on albuterol. This difference is not significant by conventional standards ($p = 0.105$), but that has not stilled the debate regarding what conclusions should be drawn from this study.

A retrospective study of the safety of salmeterol was undertaken by the Drug Safety Research Unit of the University of Southampton *(102)*. One year following approval of salmeterol in the United Kingdom, a list of patients and prescribing physicians was obtained from governmental records. Questionnaires were mailed to each prescribing physician, and information was returned on 15,407 patients, approximately half those originally identified. By the time of response these patients had been prescribed salmeterol up to 2 yr earlier. Seventy-three deaths from asthma had occurred in these patients. Thirty-nine had taken salmeterol in the last month before their death. These 39 patients were older and had more severe asthma than the average patient with asthma. Their mean age was 57.9 yr, 59.0% had been hospitalized, and 84.6% had received some oral glucocorticosteroids in the year prior to their death. Twenty of the 39 deaths occurred in the first 4 mo after beginning salmeterol. However, review of patient records identified only four in whom either acute or progressive deterioration of asthma was temporally related to the introduction of salmeterol. Even in these four, a definite relationship to salmeterol could not be established.

A similar survey was conducted by the same unit 1 yr following the introduction of nedocromil *(103)*. During the first year following the introduction of nedocromil there were 39 deaths in 12,307 patients, for a rate of 0.00317, compared to 56 deaths in 15,407 patients receiving salmeterol, for a rate of 0.00363.

USE OF OTHER BRONCHODILATORS IN ASTHMA

Theophylline

Theophylline is effective in relieving residual asthma symptoms when added to inhaled or alternate-day oral corticosteroids *(104)*. Asthma control in patients on long-term theophylline therapy has been reported to deteriorate with discontinuation of theophylline *(103,105,106)*. Theophylline has been shown to blunt the late bronchoconstrictive phase following allergen challenge *(107)*. Bronchial biopsies performed while patients were and were not employing theophylline revealed that theophylline decreases the number of lymphocytes *(106,108)* as well as the number of cells containing the proinflammatory cytokines interleukin-4 (IL4) and interleukin-5 (IL-5) *(108)*. Thus, in addition to controlling symptoms, theophylline has anti-inflammatory properties, the importance of which, however, has not been determined by long-term studies. These anti-inflammatory effects have been observed at serum levels between 5 and 10 µg/mL, which is within the targeted therapeutic range *(106–108)*.

The guidelines (Table 2) list sustained-release theophylline as an alternative to long-acting β-agonists for treatment of symptoms not controlled by inhaled corticosteroids. A direct comparison of sustained-release theophylline and salmeterol has been conducted *(2)*. Despite individual titration of theophylline dose to achieve blood levels between 10 and 15 µg/mL, only half the subjects were found to have levels that high during the trial. Salmeterol proved to be more effective in controlling the symptoms of asthma, including nocturnal awakening, as well as in producing higher peak flow levels. Theophylline, on the other hand, produced more side effects. Thus the first choice for sustained bronchodilator therapy for most persons would appear to be the long-acting β-agonists.

Anticholinergic Agents

Ipratropium is a quaternary ammonium anticholinergic compound that is remarkably free of side effects. Although the quaternary ammonium anticholinergics are inherently longer acting than the short-acting β-agonists, their action does not last nearly as long as that of the long-acting β_2-agonists. Furthermore, they are slower in onset of action and less effective than the short-acting β_2-agonists *(109)*. They appear to exert their bronchodilator effect predominantly in the large, central airways, whereas β_2-agonists dilate both central and peripheral airways *(110)*. Therefore use of the anticholinergic agents would appear not to be indicated for maintenance therapy of asthma.

Ipratropium has been reported to provide a small amount of additional bronchodilation in children with acute asthma who have received maximum β_2-agonist therapy *(111)*. Nebulized ipratropium may therefore have occasional use in the setting of acute refractory asthma.

CONCLUSIONS

The β_2-adrenergic agonists are the most effective bronchodilators for patients with bronchial asthma *(1)*. The short-acting agents are appropriate for relief of symptoms and short-term prevention of induced bronchoconstriction, especially caused by exercise. They are not appropriate or effective for maintenance bronchodilation *(34,35)*. The long-acting, inhaled β_2-agonist salmeterol, on the other hand, is an effective maintenance bronchodilator but is not appropriate for treatment of acute symptoms *(18)*. Formoterol, the other long-acting β_2-agonist, also provides effective maintenance bronchodilation with twice daily dosing. Formoterol's potential role in treating acute episodes is not clear, since it, unlike salmeterol, has a rapid onset of action *(32)*. The inhaled β_2-agonists, short- or long-acting, have not been demonstrated to have clinically useful anti-inflammatory actions. Therefore they are indicated only for symptom relief and not as a substitute for anti-inflammatory or disease-modifying agents.

There have been concerns expressed about the potential harmful effects of β_2-agonist therapy for bronchial asthma *(see* Table 1). When given by inhalation the systemic side effects are rarely a problem to the patient. The suggestion that regular use of β_2-agonists may make asthma worse gains support largely from findings on discontinuing a course of treatment with the short-acting agonists. Shortly after the last dose there is often a period of decreased lung function and increased bronchial hyperresponsiveness that persists only a few hours *(66,67,69)*. Deterioration of asthma has never been demonstrated during the duration of action of the short-acting agonists, only following their discontinuation. Similar declines in pulmonary function and increases in bronchial hyperresponsiveness have not been demonstrated with termination of treatment with either salmeterol *(72)* or formoterol *(73)*. Therefore, since only the long-acting β_2-agonists are appropriately used for maintenance therapy, the rebound previously reported with short-acting agents is of no clinical consequence.

The final concern, that use of β_2-agonists contributes to asthma deaths, has support only for two agents, isoproterenol and fenoterol, which appear to have shared the features of excessive dosing, β_2-nonselectivity, and complete agonism for the β_2-receptor *(93)*. Any relation of the commonly employed β_2-agonists to asthma deaths appears to relate to their increased use with severe asthma, which itself is likely to be the cause of the increased deaths *(96)*.

Thus, β_2-agonists, properly used, appear to be safe and effective agents for the treatment of bronchial asthma. Patients should not be denied the benefits that they offer owing to poorly supported concerns regarding their safety.

REFERENCES

1. Chaieb J, Belcher N, Rees PJ (1989) Maximum achievable bronchodilatation in asthma. Respir Med 83:497–502.
2. Fjellbirkeland L, Gulsvik A, Palmer JBD (1994) The efficacy and tolerability of inhaled salmeterol and individually dose-titrated, sustained-release theophylline in patients with reversible airways disease. Respir Med 88:599–607.
3. Siegel D, Sheppard D, Gelb A, Weinberg PF (1985) Aminophylline increases the toxicity but not the efficacy of an inhaled beta-adrenergic agonist in the treatment of acute exacerbations of asthma. Am Rev Respir Dis 132:283–286.
4. Godfrey S, Konig P (1976) Inhibition of exercise-induced asthma by different pharmacological pathways. Thorax 31:137–143.

5. Page C, Costello J (1992) Controversies in respiratory medicine: regular inhaled beta-agonists—clear clinical benefit or a hazard to health? (2) Why β-agonists should not be used regularly. Respir Med 86:477–479.

6. Cockcroft DW, McParland CP, Britto SA, Swystun VA, Rutherford BC (1993) Regular inhaled salbutamol and airway responsiveness to allergen. Lancet 342:883–837.

7. Sears MR (1995) Is the routine use of inhaled β-adrenergic agonists appropriate in asthma treatment? No. Am J Respir Crit Care Med 151:600–601.

8. Inman MD, O'Byrne PM (1996) The effect of regular inhaled albuterol on exercise-induced bronchoconstriction. Am J Respir Crit Care Med 153:65–69.

9. Adcock IM, Stevens DA, Barnes PJ (1996) Interactions of glucocorticoids and β_2-agonists. Eur Respir J 9:160–168.

10. Barnes PJ (1995) Beta-adrenergic receptors and their regulation. Am J Respir Crit Care Med 152:838–860.

11. Small RC, Chiu P, Cook SJ, Cook R, Foster RW, Isaac L (1993) β-Adrenoceptor agonists in bronchial asthma: role of K^+-channel opening in mediating their bronchodilator effects. Clin Exp Allergy 23:802–811.

12. Yu SS, Lefkowitz RJ, Hausdorff WP (1993) β-adrenergic receptor sequestration. A potential mechanism of receptor resensitization. J Biol Chem 268:337–341.

13. Mak JCW, Nishikawa M, Barnes PJ (1995) Glucocorticosteroids increase β_2-adrenergic receptor transcription in human lung. Am J Physiol 268:L41–L46.

14. Hui KK, Conolly ME, Tashkin DP (1982) Reversal of human lymphocyte β-adrenoceptor desensitization by glucocorticoids. Clin Pharmacol Ther 32:566–571.

15. Ellul-Micallef R, Fenech FF (1975) Effect of intravenous prednisolone in asthmatics with diminished adrenergic responsiveness. Lancet ii:1269–1271.

16. Cockcroft DW, Swystun VA, Bhagat R (1995) Interaction of inhaled β_2-agonist and inhaled corticosteroid on airway responsiveness to allergen and methacholine. Am J Respir Crit Care Med 152:1485–1489.

17. Hjemdahl P, Zetterllund A, Larsson K (1996) β_2-agonist treatment reduces β_2-sensitivity in alveolar macrophages despite corticosteroid treatment. Am J Respir Crit Care Med 153:573–581.

18. Johnson M, Butchers PR, Coleman RA, Nials AT, Strong P, Sumner MJ, Vardey CJ, Whelan CJ (1993) The pharmacology of salmeterol. Life Sci 52:2131–2143.

19. Rhoden KJ, Meldrum LA, Barnes PJ (1988) Inhibition of cholinergic neurotransmission in human airways by β_2-adrenoceptors. J Appl Physiol 65:700–705.

20. Coqueret O, Dugas B, Mencia-Huerta JM, Braquet P (1995) Regulation of IgE production from human mononuclear cells by β_2-adrenoceptor agonists. Clin Exp Allergy 25:304–311.

21. Peters MJ, Adcock IM, Brown CR, Barnes PJ (1995) Beta-adrenoceptor agonists interfere with glucocorticoid receptor DNA-binding in rat lung. Eur J Pharmacol (Mol Pharmacol) 289:275–281.

22. Morley J (1992) Beta agonists and asthma mortality: *deja vu*. Clin Exp Allergy 22:724–725.

23. Pedersen B, Dahl R, Larsen BB, Venge P (1993) The effect of salmeterol on the early- and late-phase reaction to bronchial allergen and postchallenge variation in bronchial reactivity, blood eosinophils, serum eosinophil cationic protein and serum eosinophil protein X. Allergy 48:377–382.

24. Wong BJ, Dolovich J, Ramsdale H, O'Byrne P, Gontovnick L, Denburg JA, Hargreave FE (1992) Formoterol compared with beclomethasone and placebo on allergen-induced asthmatic responses. Am Rev Respir Dis 146:1156–1160.

25. Dahl R, Pedersen B, Venge P (1991) Bronchoalveolar lavage studies. Eur Respir Rev 1:272–275.

26. Gardiner PV, Ward C, Booth H, Allison A, Hendrick DJ, Walters EH (1994) Effect of eight weeks of treatment with salmeterol on bronchoalveolar lavage inflammatory indices in asthmatics. Am J Respir Crit Care Med 150:1006–1011.

27. Gratziou C, Roberts JA, Walls A, Holgate ST, Howarth P (1992) Lymphocyte population in BAL of asthmatics after salmeterol treatment. Eur Respir J 5:207s (abstract).

28. National Heart, Lung and Blood Institute (1997) National Asthma Education and Prevention Program Expert Panel Report 2. Guidelines for the diagnosis and management of asthma. NIH Publication no. 97-4051, US Government, Bethesda, MD.

29. Sheffer AL (1992) International consensus report on the diagnosis and management of asthma. Clin Exp Allergy 22(Suppl):1–72.

30. National Institutes of Health, National Heart, Lung and Blood Institute (1995) Global Initiatives for Asthma. Global Strategy for Asthma Management and Prevention. NHLBI/WHO Workshop Report. Publication no. 95-3659, US Government, Bethesda, MD.

31. Colacone A, Afilalo M, Wolkove N, Kreisman H (1993) A comparison of albuterol administered by metered dose inhaler (and holding chamber) or wet nebulizer in acute asthma. Chest 104:835–841.
32. Anderson GP, Linden A, Rabe KF (1994) Why are long-acting beta-adrenoceptor agonists long-acting? Eur Respir J 7:569–578.
33. Rabe KF, Jorres R, Nowak D, Behr N, Magnussen H (1993) Comparison of the effects of salmeterol and formoterol on airway tone and responsiveness over 24 hours in bronchial asthma. Am Rev Respir Dis 147:1436–1441.
34. Pearlman DS, Chervinsky P, LaForce C, Seltzer JM, Southern DL, Kemp JP, Dockhorn RJ, Grossman J, Liddle RF, Yancey SW, Cocchetto DM, Alexander WJ, van As A (1992) A comparison of salmeterol with albuterol in the treatment of mild-to-moderate asthma. N Engl J Med 327:1420–1450.
35. D'Alonzo GE, Nathan RA, Henochowicz S, Morris RJ, Ratner P, Rennard SI (1994) Salmeterol xinafoate as maintenance therapy compared with albuterol in patients with asthma. JAMA 271:1412–1416.
36. Chapman KR, Kesten S, Szalai JP (1994) Regular vs as-needed inhaled salbutamol in asthma control. Lancet 343:1379–1382.
37. Britton MG, Earnshaw JS, Palmer JB (1992) A twelve month comparison of salmeterol with salbutamol in asthmatic patients. Eur Respir J 5:1062–1067.
38. Lundback B, Rawlinson DW, Palmer JBD (1993) Twelve month comparison of salmeterol and salbutamol as dry powder formulations in asthmatic patients. Thorax 48:148–153.
39. Lotvall J, Lunde H, Ullman A, Tornqvist H, Svedmyr N (1992) Twelve months treatment with inhaled salmeterol in asthmatic patients. Effects on β_2-receptor function and inflammatory cells. Allergy 47:477–483.
40. Greening AP, Ind PW, Northfield M, Shaw G (1994) Added salmeterol versus higher-dose corticosteroid in asthma patients with symptoms on existing inhaled corticosteroid. Lancet 344:219–224.
41. Bremner P, Woodman K, Burgess C, Crane J, Purdie G, Pearce N, Beasley R (1993) A comparison of the cardiovascular and metabolic effects of formoterol, salbutamol and fenoterol. Eur Respir J 6:204–210.
42. Westling H (1979) Circulatory effects of β_2-receptor agonists in man. Acta Pharacol Toxicol 44 (Suppl 11):36–40.
43. Willey RF, Grant IWB, Pocock SJ (1976) Effects of oral salbutamol and pirbuterol on FEV_1, heart rate and blood pressure in asthmatics. Br J Clin Pharmacol 3:595–600.
44. Kass I, Mingo TS (1980) Bitolterol mesylate (WIN 32784) aerosol: a new long-acting bronchodilator with reduced chronotrophic effects. Chest 78:283–287.
45. Choo-Kang YFJ, Simpson WT, Grant IWB (1969) Controlled comparison of bronchodilator effect of three beta-adrenergic stimulant drugs administered by inhalation to patients with asthma. Br Med J 2:287–289.
46. Bremner P, Siebers R, Crane J, Beasley R (1996) Partial vs full β-receptor agonism. A clinical study of inhaled albuterol and fenoterol. Chest 109:957–962.
47. McEvoy JDS, Vall-Spinosa A, Paterson JW (1973) Assessment of orciprenaline and isoproterenol infusions in asthmatic patients. Am Rev Respir Dis 108:490–500.
48. Lipworth BJ, Struthers AD, McDevitt DG (1989) Tachyphylaxis to systemic but not to airway responses during prolonged therapy with high dose inhaled salbutamol in asthmatics. Am Rev Respir Dis 140:586–592.
49. Stiles GL, Taylor S, Lefkowitz RJ (1983) Human cardiac beta-adrenergic receptors: subtype heterogeneity delineated by direct radioligand binding. Life Sci 33:467–473.
50. Clifton GD, Hunt BA, Patel RC, Burki NK (1990) Effect of sequential doses of parenteral terbutaline on plasma levels of potassium and related cardiopulmonary responses. Am Rev Respir Dis 141:575–579.
51. Kiely DG, Cargill RI, Grove A, Struthers AD, Lipworth BJ (1995) Abnormal myocardial repolarisation in response to hypoxaemia and fenoterol. Thorax 50:1062–1066.
52. Higgins RM, Cookson WOCM, Lane DJ, John SM, McCarthy GL, McCarthy ST (1987) Cardiac arrhythmias caused by nebulised beta-agonist therapy. Lancet ii:863–864.
53. Teule GJJ, Majid PA (1980) Haemodynamic effects of terbutaline in chronic obstructive airways disease. Thorax 35:536–542.
54. Williams AJ, Weiner C, Reiff D, Swenson ER, Fuller RW, Hughes JM (1994) Comparison of the effect of inhaled selective and non-selective adrenergic agonists on cardiorespiratory parameters in chronic stable asthma. Pulmon Pharmacol 7:235–241.

55. Newnham DM, McDevitt DG, Lipworth BJ (1994) Bronchodilator subsensitivity after chronic dosing with eformoterol in patients with asthma. Am J Med 97:29–37.

56. Maconochie JG, Minton NA, Chilton JE, Keene ON (1994) Does tachyphylaxis occur to the non-pulmonary effects of salmeterol? Br J Clin Pharmacol 37:199–204.

57. Nelson HS, Branch LB, Raine D, Spaulding H, Black JW, Pfeutze B, Wood D (1977) β-adrenergic subsensitivity induced by chronic administration of terbutaline. Int Arch Allergy Appl Immunol 55:362–373.

58. Gustafson T, Boman K, Rosenhall L, Sandstrom T, Wester PO (1996) Skeletal muscle magnesium and potassium in asthmatics treated with oral beta2-agonists. Eur Respir J 9:237–240.

59. Nelson HS, Raine D Jr, Doner HC, Posey WC (1977) Subsensitivity to the bronchodilator action of albuterol produced by chronic administration. Am Rev Respir Dis 116:871–878.

60. Branscomb BV (1978) Efficacy and side effects of fenoterol compared with isoproterenol administered by metered-dose inhalers in asthma. Chest 73(Suppl 6):1002–1004.

61. Plummer AI (1978) The development of drug tolerance to beta2 adrenergic agents. Chest 73(Suppl 6):949–957.

62. Weber RW, Smith JA, Nelson HS (1982) Aerosolized terbutaline in asthmatics: development of subsensitivity with long-term administration. J Allergy Clin Immunol 70:417.

63. Repsher LH, Anderson JA, Bush RK, Falliers CJ, Kass I, Kemp JP, Reed C, Siegel S, Webb DR (1984) Assessment of tachyphylaxis following prolonged therapy of asthma with inhaled albuterol aerosol. Chest 85:34–38.

64. Georgopoulos D, Wong D, Anthonisen NR (1990) Tolerance to β2-agonists in patients with chronic obstructive pulmonary disease. Chest 97:280–284.

65. Newnham DM, Grove A, McDevitt DG, Lipworth BJ (1995) Subsensitivity of bronchodilator and systemic β2-adrenoceptor responses after regular twice daily treatment with eformoterol dry powder in asthmatic patients. Thorax 50:497–504.

66. Wahedna I, Wong CS, Wisniewski AF, Pavord ID, Tattersfield AE (1993) Asthma control during and after cessation of regular beta2-agonist treatment. Am Rev Respir Dis 148:707–12.

67. Vathenen AS, Knox AJ, Higgins BG, Britton JR, Tattersfield AS (1988) Rebound increase in bronchial responsiveness after treatment with inhaled terbutaline. Lancet i:554–557.

68. Trembath PW, Greenacre JK, Anderson M, Dimmock S, Mansfield L, Wadsworth J, Green M (1979) Comparison of four weeks treatment with fenoterol and terbutaline aerosols in adult asthamtics. A double-blind, cross-over study. J Allergy Clin Immunol 63:395–400.

69. de Jong W, van der Mark TW, Koeter GH, Postma DS (1996) Rebound airway obstruction and responsiveness after cessation of terbutaline: effects of budesonide. Am J Respir Crit Care Med 153:70–75.

70. Van Schayck CP, Dompeling E, van Herwaarden CL, Folgering H, Verbeeck AL, Henk JM, van der Hoogen HJ, van Weel C (1991) Bronchodilator treatment in moderate asthma or chronic bronchitis: continuous or on demand? A randomized controlled study. Br Med J 303:1426–1431.

71. Grove A, Lipworth BJ (1995) Bronchodilator subsensitivity to salbutalmol after twice daily salmeterol in asthmatic patients Lancet 346:201–206.

72. Ullman A, Hedner J, Svedmyr N (1990) Inhaled salmeterol and salbutamol in asthmatic patients. An evaluation of asthma symptoms and the possible development of tachyphylaxis. Am Rev Respir Dis 142:571–575.

73. Yates DH, Sussman HS, Shaw MJ, Barnes PJ, Chung KF (1995) Regular formoterol treatment in mild asthma. Effect on bronchial responsiveness during and after treatment. Am J Respir Crit Care Med 152:1170–1174.

74. Cheung D, Timmers MC, Zwinderman AH, Bel EH, Dijkman JH, Sterk PJ (1992) Long-term effects of a long-acting β2-adrenoreceptor agonist, salmeterol, on airway hyperresponsiveness in patients with mild asthma. N Engl J Med 327:1198–1203.

75. O'Connor BJ, Aikman SL, Barnes PJ (1992) Tolerance to the non-bronchodilator effects of inhaled β2-agonists in asthma. N Engl J Med 327:1204–1208.

76. Bhagat R, Kalra S, Swystun VA, Cockcroft DW (1995) Rapid onset of tolerance to the bronchoprotective effect of salmeterol. Chest 108:1235–1239.

77. Bhagat R, Swystun VA, Cockcroft DW (1996) Salbutamol-induced increased airways responsiveness to allergen and reduced protection versus methacholine: dose response. J Allergy Clin Immunol 97:47–52.

78. Ramage L, Lipworth BJ, Ingram CG, Cree IA, Dhillon DP (1994) Reduced protection against exercise induced bronchoconstriction after chronic dosing with salmeterol. Respir Med 88:363–368.

79. Kraan J, Koeter GH, van der Mark TW, Sluiter HJ, de Vries K (1985) Changes in bronchial hyperreactivity induced by 4 weeks of treatment with antiasthmatic drugs in patients with allergic asthma: A comparison between budesonide and terbutaline. J Allergy Clin Immunol 76:628–636.

80. Kerrebijn KF, van Essen-Zandvliet EE, Neijens HJ (1988) Effect of long-term treatment with inhaled corticosteroids and beta-agonists on the bronchial responsiveness in children with asthma. J Allergy Clin Immunol 79:653–659.

81. van Schayck CP, Graafsma SJ, Visch MB, Dompeling E, van Weel C, van Herwaarden CL (1990) Increased bronchial hyperresponsivness after inhaling salbutamol during 1 year is not caused by subsensitization to salbutamol. J Allergy Clin Immunol 86:793–800.

82. Chong LK, Morice AH, Yeo WW, Schleirmer RP, Pachell PT (1995) Functional desensitization of β-agonist responses in human lung mast cells. Am J Respir Cell Mol Biol 13:540–546.

83. Booth HJ, Fishwick K, Harkawat R, Devereux G, Hendrick DJ, Walters EH (1993) Changes in methacholine induced bronchoconstriction with the long acting β_2-agonist salmeterol in mild to moderate asthmatic patients. Thorax 48:1121–1124.

84. Meijer GG, Postma DS, Mulder PGH, van Aalderen WM (1995) Long-term circadian effects of salmeterol in asthmatic children treated with inhaled corticosteroids. Am J Respir Crit Care Med 52:1887–1892.

85. Sears MR, Taylor DR, Print CG, Lake DC, Li Q, Flannery EM, Yates DM, Lucas MK, Herbison GP (1990) Regular inhaled beta-agonist treatment in bronchial asthma. Lancet 336:1391–1396.

86. Sears MR, Taylor DR, Print CG, Lake DC, Herbison GP, Flannery EM (1992) Increased inhaled bronchodilator vs increased inhaled corticosteroid in the control of moderate asthma. Chest 102:1709–1715.

87. Beasley R, Windom H, Pearce N, Burgess C, Crane J (1991) Asthma mortality and inhaled beta agonist therapy. Aust NZ J Med 21:753–763.

88. Joad JP, Ahrens RC, Lindgren SD, Weinberger MM (1987) Relative efficacy of maintenance therapy with theophylline, inhaled albuterol, and the combination for chronic asthma. J Allergy Clin Immunol 79:78–85.

89. Kesten S, Chapman KR, Broder I, Cartier A, Hyland RH, Knight A, Malo JL, Mazza JA, Moote DW, Small P, Tarlo S, Gontovnick L, Rebuck AJ (1991) A three-month comparison of twice daily inhaled formoterol versus four times daily inhaled albuterol in the management of stable asthma. Am Rev Respir Dis 144:622–625.

90. Juniper EF, Johnston PR, Borkhoff CM, Guyatt GH, Boulet LP, Haukioja A (1995) Quality of life in asthma clinical trials: comparison of salmeterol and sal butamol. Am J Respir Crit Care Med 151:66–70.

91. Palmer JBD (1991) Salmeterol in clinical practice. Eur Respir Rev 1:297–300.

92. Beasley R, Pearce N, Crane J, Burgess C (1992) Fenoterol and death from asthma in New Zealand. Int Arch Allergy Immunol 99:302–305.

93. Crane J, Pearce N, Burgess C, Beasley R (1995) Asthma and the β-agonist debate. Thorax 50(Suppl 1):s5–s10.

94. Garrett J, Kolbe J, Richard G, Whitlock T, Rea H (1995) Major reduction in asthma morbidity and continued reduction in asthma mortality in New Zealand: What lessons have we learned? Thorax 50:303–11.

95. Spitzer WO, Suissa S, Ernst P, Horwitz RI, Habbick B, Cockcroft D, Boivin J-F, McNutt M, Buist AS, Rebuck AS (1992) The use of beta-agonists and the risk of death and near death from asthma. N Engl J Med 326:501–506.

96. Suissa S, Blais L, Ernst P (1994) Patterns of increasing β-agonist use and the risk of fatal or near-fatal asthma. Eur Respir J 7:1602–1609.

97. Clark CE, Ferguson AD, Siddorn JA (1993) Respiratory arrests in young asthmatics on salmeterol. Respir Med 87:227–228.

98. Finkelstein FN (1994) Risks of salmeterol? N Engl J Med 331:1314.

99. Crompton GK (1993) Bronchodilator treatment in asthma. Regular treatment with beta agonists remains unevaluated. Br Med J 306:1611.

100. Sears MR, Taylor DR (1993) Bronchodilator treatment in asthma. Increase in deaths during salmeterol treatment unexplained. Br Med J 306:1610–1611.

101. Castle W, Fuller R, Hall J, Palmer J (1993) Serevent nationwide surveillance study: comparison of salmeterol with salbutamol in asthmatic patients who require regular bronchodilator treatment. Br Med J 306:1034–1037.

102. Mann RD (1994) Results of prescription event monitoring study of salmeterol. Br Med J 309:1018.

103. Drug Surveillance Research Unit, University of Southampton, Southampton, England. (1990) Prescription Event Monitoring News 7:41–42.

104. Nassif EG, Weinburger M, Thompson R, Huntley W (1981) The value of maintenance theophylline in steroid-dependent asthma. N Engl J Med 304:71–75.

105. Brenner MR, Berkowitz R, Marshall N, Struck RC (1988) Need for theophylline in severe steroid-requiring asthmatics. Clin Allergy 18:143–150.

106. Kidney J, Dominquez M, Taylor PM, Rose M, Chung KF, Barnes PJ (1995) Immunomodulation by theophylline in asthma. Demonstration by withdrawal of therapy. Am J Respir Crit Care Med 151:1907–14.

107. Ward AJ, McKenniff M, Evans JM, Page CP, Costello JF (1993) Theophylline—an immunomodulatory role in asthma? Am Rev Respir Dis 147:518–523.

108. Djukanovic R, Finnerty JP, Lee C, Wilson S, Madden J, Holgate ST (1995) The effects of theophylline on mucosal inflammation in asthmatic airways: biopsy result. Eur Respir J 8:831–833.

109. Vichyanond P, Sladek WA, Sur S, Hill MR, Szefler SJ, Nelson HS (1990) Efficacy of atropine methylnitrate alone and in combination with albuterol in children with asthma. Chest 98:637–642.

110. Ohrui T, Yanai M, Sekizawa K, Morikawa M, Sasaki H, Takishima T (1992) Effective site of bronchodilation by beta-adrenergic and anticholinergic agents in patients with chronic obstructive pulmonary disease; direct measurement of intrabronchial pressure with a new catheter. Am Rev Respir Dis 146:88–91.

111. Schuh S, Johnson DW, Callahan S, Canny G, Levison H (1995) Efficacy of frequent nebulized ipratropium bromide added to frequent high-dose albuterol therapy in severe childhood asthma. J Pediatr 126:639–645.

30

Sodium Cromoglycate and Nedocromil Sodium

Alan M. Edwards, MRCGP,
Alexis E. Harper, MSc, D. Ken Rainey, PhD,
and Alan A. Norris, PhD

INTRODUCTION

The major allergic diseases are all inflammatory diseases of body surfaces, namely the bronchial mucosa, the nasal mucosa, the conjunctiva, the skin, and the gastrointestinal mucosa. The pathological changes and inflammatory mechanisms in allergic disease are common to the different tissues, involving tissue damage, tissue restructure, and the presence of activated inflammatory cells, particularly eosinophils, mast cells, lymphocytes, and macrophages.

The primary factor that leads to the development of allergic disease is exposure to the relevant allergens with the probable involvement of genetic predisposition, reinforced by a number of adjuvant factors, including maternal smoking and nutrition during pregnancy, and infections during infancy, and possibly exposure to atmospheric pollutants.

Sodium cromoglycate and nedocromil sodium are drugs with anti-inflammatory and anti-allergic properties. In clinical use, they are applied topically to, and have their primary effect on, the body surface that is affected by the allergic inflammation and have little or no effect on other sites and no systemic effects. Both drugs were developed originally as inhaled formulations for the treatment of asthma, and most of the knowledge about their mechanisms of action has been derived from models of asthma.

INFLAMMATORY BASIS OF ASTHMA

The inflammatory basis of asthma was first described over 30 yr ago *(1)*. Since then, similar markers of inflammation have been described in bronchial biopsies taken from asthmatic

From: *Allergy and Allergic Diseases: The New Mechanisms and Therapeutics*
Edited by: J. A. Denburg © Humana Press Inc., Totowa, NJ

patients *(2)*. Even in mild disease, the airways are infiltrated with activated mast cells, eosinophils, and T-lymphocytes *(3)*.

It is believed that airway inflammation results from exposure to allergens and manifests clinically as a variable obstruction and increased reactivity. Although allergen exposure is considered the main driving force for this inflammation, the airways react abnormally to allergic and nonallergic stimuli. Exposure of sensitized airways to allergens causes a bronchoconstriction that develops, in chronic form, into a combination of inflammation and bronchoconstriction. Antigen-induced airway obstruction comprises early and late bronchoconstrictive phases *(4)*. The early reaction results from bronchial mucosal mast cell mediator release, and during the late reaction there is an influx of activated neutrophils followed by eosinophils, T-lymphocytes, and mast cells *(5)*. This cellular response is accompanied by an increase in bronchial reactivity. To date, the only agents that have been shown to prevent the late reaction and the increase in reactivity are sodium cromoglycate and nedocromil sodium (the chromones) and oral and inhaled corticosteroids *(6)*.

The recruitment of inflammatory cells into the bronchial mucosa results from the expression of adhesion cell molecules, intercellular adhesion molecule (ICAM-1), vascular cell adhesion molecule (VCAM)-1, and the selections on the surface of vascular endothelial cells *(7)*. The increased expression of these adhesion molecules probably results from the action of cytokines, particularly interleukin-1, tumor necrosis factor-α (TNFα), interferon (IFNγ), and interleukin-4 (IL-4). The source of these cytokines remains speculative but is likely to be mast cells, T-lymphocytes, or macrophages *(8)*.

EFFECTS ON INFLAMMATORY CELLS

The mast cell is the primary triggering cell in allergic inflammation *(9)*. Studies with the chromones have demonstrated similar inhibition in classic in vivo antiallergy models based on rat connective tissue mast cells *(10)* and, in vitro, of anti-immunglobotin (anti-IgE)-induced release of histamine from rat peritoneal mast cells *(11)* and human mast cells derived from bronchoalveolar lavage (BAL) and enzymatic dispersion of lung (DL) parenchyma *(12)*. In the latter model, both compounds were more effective against BAL than DL cells, with nedocromil sodium more potent than sodium cromoglycate. In clinical practice it is likely that it is the mast cells near to the bronchial lumen that trigger the events in allergic asthma.

Sodium cromoglycate and nedocromil sodium have also been shown to inhibit the release of the cytokine TNFα from rat peritoneal mast cells *(13,14)*. TNFα is one of the cytokines involved in the upregulation of adhesion molecules on endothelial and epithelial cells. The expression of the adhesion molecules ICAM-1 and VCAM-1 is significantly reduced by treatment of asthmatics with sodium cromoglycate *(15)*, the inhibition of the expression of VCAM-1 correlates with the reduction of activated eosinophils (EG2$^+$ cells) in the bronchial mucosa, and the inhibition of ICAM-1 correlates with the reduction of T lymphocytes, particularly CD4$^+$ cells. In vivo, a biopsy study has shown that the number of EG2$^+$ cells in the bronchial submucosa was reduced significantly after 16 wk of treatment with nedocromil sodium compared with regularly administered salbutamol *(16)*.

Sodium cromoglycate and nedocromil sodium have been shown to inhibit antibody-dependent cytotoxicity of neutrophils to granulocyte-macrophage colony-stimulating factor (GM-CSF) and TNFα *(17)*. Nedocromil sodium was more effective than sodium cromoglycate in assays of neutrophil and eosinophil activation (enhancement of complement [C3b] and Fc [IgG] membrane receptor expression and death of *Schistosomula mansoni* larvae) *(18)*. The compounds display similar inhibition of neutrophil chemotaxis but a differential inhibitory effect, according to stimulus, on eosinophil chemotaxis *(19,20)*.

Nedocromil sodium has been shown to reduce the release of TNFα, IL-8, and ICAM-1 from cultured human bronchial epithelial cells exposed to ozone and to inhibit the recruitment and activation of eosinophils mediated by these epithelial cell cytokines. In addition, nedocromil sodium reduced the eosinophil-mediated dysfunction of epithelial cell ciliary motility *(21)*. Other studies with cultured human bronchial epithelial cells have shown nedocromil sodium to inhibit production of GM-CSF *(22)* and IL-8 *(23)* following challenge of the cells with IL-1 and an inhibition of cell surface ICAM-1 expression induced by challenge with histamine *(24)*. Nedocromil sodium inhibited IL-6 production from human airway macrophages following challenge with specific antigen or with anti-IgE *(25)*. Immunologically induced lysosomal enzyme release from human alveolar macrophages and oxygen radical release from human monocytes are also reduced by treatment of the cells with nedocromil sodium *(26)*. Sodium cromoglycate has shown inhibition of IgE-mediated release of human alveolar macrophage neutrophil chemotactic factor and β-glucuronidase *(27)*.

The initial stimulus for allergic inflammatory events is the reaction between antigen and IgE antibodies attached to mast cells. In addition to the direct effects on inflammatory cells and the recruitment of these cells, sodium cromoglycate and nedocromil sodium have been shown to inhibit the synthesis of IgE antibodies by human B lymphocytes (as demonstrated by the inhibition of IgE messenger rionucleic nucleic acid [mRNA] production) when these cells are stimulated with IL-4 and B-cell activating agents such as T cells, a monoclonal antibody (MAb) to the B-cell antigen, CD40, or hydrocortisone *(28–30)*. Specifically, the chromones inhibited the Sμ-to-Sε switch recombination mechanism in response to B cell activating stimuli in IL-4-treated cells and had no effect on the induction of ε germline transcripts induced by IL-4 alone. No inhibitory effects were observed on IgM or IgA formation by B-cells, although IgG$_4$ production was also suppressed *(28,30)*.

The relevance of this finding in clinical usage still needs to be determined but does indicate a fundamental effect on the allergic process not shared by other classes of drugs. In a study in children with atopic dermatitis in whom an aqueous solution of sodium cromoglycate was applied to the skin, there was a reduction in the amount of IgE synthesized by isolated purified B-lymphocytes after treatment, but no reduction in serum IgE levels *(31)*. In a clinical study in which two-thirds of the patients demonstrated a good clinical response to treatment with inhaled sodium cromoglycate, these patients also demonstrated a significant reduction in BAL-fluid house-dust mite specific IgE antibodies *(32)*. Similar clinical research has yet to be conducted with nedocromil sodium.

The bronchospasm induced by administration of aspirin or other nonsteroidal anti-inflammatory agents to aspirin-sensitive asthmatics (ASA) is thought to be mediated by the activation of circulating blood cells, in particular, platelets. In the presence of aspirin, platelets from ASA generate cytotoxic mediators capable of killing *S. mansoni* larvae. Despite its specificity, this test is considered representative of disease activity. Platelet activity was inhibited ex vivo within 15 min of pretreatment of ASA with 4 mg inhaled nedocromil sodium. There was no effect with 5 mg or 20 mg sodium cromoglycate *(33)*. Furthermore, nedocromil sodium can inhibit IgE-mediated activation of passively sensitized human blood platelets following exposure to *Schistosomula* antigen *(26)* and the generation of thromboxane B$_2$ and intracellular messengers (e.g., inositol 1,4,5-triphosphate) from thrombin-stimulated platelets *(34)*.

Both nedocromil sodium and sodium cromoglycate were without effect on an assay of CD4$^+$ (helper) T-lymphocyte proliferation. The corticosteroid dexamethasone inhibited T-cell proliferation *(35)*. As these cells are implicated in the late-phase reaction, through release of neutrophil chemotactic factor and leukotriene B$_4$ release-enhancing factors, the inhibitory effect of the chromones on this reaction may not be mediated via T-lymphocytes.

NEURAL EFFECTS

Neural mechanisms in asthma mediate the symptomatic consequences of airway inflammation, such as coughing and wheezing, and potentiate inflammation through control of smooth muscle tone, secretions, blood flow, and microvascular permeability. In addition to the cholinergic and adrenergic neural pathways, epithelial damage may expose vagal, nonmyelinated, afferent C-fibers to inflammatory mediators and results in local reflex release of neurally derived mediators, thereby contributing to the inflammation and the symptoms.

The ability of sodium cromoglycate and nedocromil sodium to modulate reflex effects may be inferred from the reduction by sodium cromoglycate of capsaicin-induced stimulation of anesthetized dog pulmonary C-fiber endings *(36)* and of the enhanced response to capsaicin and the severity of cough in patients taking angiotensin-converting enzyme (ACE) inhibitors *(37)*. The activation by nedocromil sodium of a population of bronchial C-fibers in the dog lung may contribute to its ability to inhibit reflex responses such as cough, which is mediated largely by myelinated Aδ-fibers, by interfering with or blocking neuronal transmission *(38)*.

Nedocromil sodium inhibits substance P-induced histamine release from human lung mast cells *(39)* and substance P-induced potentiation of contraction of the isolated innervated rabbit trachea preparation, when stimulated preganglionically *(40)*. It also inhibits nonadrenergic, noncholinergic contraction of the isolated guinea pig bronchus *(41)* although sodium cromoglycate is without effect in this model. These drugs can therefore have a direct effect on some of the neural mechanisms associated with allergic disease as well as an indirect effect by reducing upregulated neural reflexes.

ANIMAL PHARMACOLOGY

Despite the lack of truly predictive animal models of asthma, it is possible to mimic many of the acute inflammatory components of asthma in a variety of models. Given the relative newness of these models, more data are available for nedocromil sodium.

Nedocromil sodium has been shown to inhibit cell infiltration in the lungs of several species, including sheep *(42)*, guinea pigs *(43,44)*, and dogs *(45)*, induced by antigen and noxious gases (ozone and SO_2), in addition to blocking the acute bronchospasm in sheep *(46)*, monkeys *(47)*, and guinea pigs *(44)*.

Specifically, the allergic sheep and guinea pig models responded to *Ascaris suum* antigen and ovalbumin challenge, respectively, with early and late phases of bronchoconstriction and associated late increases in BAL neutrophils (guinea pig) and/or eosinophils. Both sodium cromoglycate and nedocromil sodium inhibited the pulmonary and cellular changes *(42,44,46,48)*.

Marked differences between nedocromil sodium and sodium cromoglycate were demonstrated when studies were carried out in a primate model of lung inflammation that was induced by infecting *Macaca arctoides* monkeys with *Ascaris suum* ova *(47)*. Bronchoalveolar lavage cells containing up to 20% mast cells released histamine and the newly formed mediators leukotriene C_4 and prostaglandin D_2 when stimulated with *Ascaris* antigen or antibody to human IgE. Addition of nedocromil sodium to the cells prior to challenge suppressed the release of mediators. Sodium cromoglycate was virtually inactive over the same concentration range *(11)*. The differential effects of nedocromil sodium and sodium cromoglycate were confirmed in vivo from measurements of bronchospasm (total lung resistance and dynamic lung compliance) using anesthetized infected monkeys challenged with aerosolized *Ascaris* antigen. The bronchospasm was significantly inhibited by pretreating animals with an aerosol of 2% nedocromil sodium, whereas sodium cromoglycate had no significant effects.

Nedocromil sodium has been shown to possess antitussive properties in conscious dogs trained to inhale an aerosol of 1% citric acid. Pretreatment with 2% nebulized sodium cromoglycate had little effect on the onset time to the first cough, whereas 2% nedocromil sodium produced a significant delay in time to cough *(49)*. A positive control response to codeine phosphate (5 mg/kg iv) was achieved in this model. These data provide in vivo evidence for an effect of nedocromil sodium on neuronal mechanisms, and this finding has been confirmed in clinical studies.

BIOCHEMICAL MECHANISM OF ACTION

It is likely that the effects of nedocromil sodium and sodium cromoglycate on the events described in the different cell types are mediated through common biochemical pathways and a common receptor. As it is unlikely that the drug enters the cell, this receptor is probably within the cell membrane. This probable similarity in mechanism of action has been linked to the inhibition of chloride transport in a variety of cells *(50)*.

The secretion of mediators from mast cells is dependent on an increase in intracellular calcium. An initial rise is due to the release from intracellular stores, and a secondary influx maintains the raised levels *(51)*. The secondary influx is through a calcium-specific channel that requires membrane hyperpolarization to support calcium influx. This membrane hyperpolarization is probably provided by a specific chloride current *(52)*.

Both agents reduce the open channel probability of single chloride channels isolated from sheep airway epithelial cells *(53)* and inhibit the whole cell chloride current activated in pulmonary endothelial cells by exposure to hypotonic saline *(54)*. It is uncertain whether the biophysical properties of each of the chloride channels is the same; functionally, the difference may be regulation of cell volume rather than the secretion of mediators. In addition, changes in chloride flux have been shown in nedocromil sodium-treated isolated rabbit vagal nerves, which contain predominantly nonmyelinated sensory fibers *(55)*.

Early studies showed that sodium cromoglycate inhibited the influx of calcium ions *(56)* and also phosphorylated a 78-kDA protein in rat peritoneal mast cells *(57)*. These findings were associated with an inhibition of histamine release following antigen challenge *(58)*. A similar phosphorylation can be induced with cyclic guanosine monophosphate (cGMP). Although the relationship between the effects of sodium cromoglycate on chloride channels and on cGMP-dependent phosphorylation of this 78-kDA protein remains to be elucidated *(59)*, an effect on chloride currents is observed on key inflammatory cells modulated by sodium cromoglycate and nedocromil sodium.

CONSIDERATIONS FOR THERAPEUTIC USE

The presence of airway inflammation has been confirmed in even the mildest forms of asthma. It is characterized by the identification of activated inflammatory cells in the bronchial mucosa and lumen, and in alterations in tissue structure (edema, loss of bronchial epithelium and neural involvement). The pathophysiological function and interaction of the plethora of cell- and neurally derived mediators are gradually being defined. It is likely that, through the inhibition of mast cell activation and mediator release, sodium cromoglycate and nedocromil sodium can reduce the presence and activation of secondary, key effector inflammatory cells (eosinophils, macrophages and bronchial epithelial cells). Direct effects of the chromones on these cells have also been observed. Many of these in vitro anti-inflammatory effects have been translated into observations from animal models and from clinical research, and more recent research in vitro has identified-two unique features of these drugs: inhibition of IgE synthesis and a unifying extracellular, biochemical mechanism of action on cell chloride channels. The effect on lgE synthesis suggests that these drugs may have a role during the development of allergic disease. Although such a proposal awaits better identification of candidate patients, the excellent tolerability of sodium cromoglycate and nedocromil sodium supports their suitability for early intervention studies. The hypothesis for a chloride channel-based mechanism of action may provide a single explanation for the activity of these drugs on a range of inflammatory cells, and the likely extracellular mode of action supports the lack of toxicity of these agents.

Current therapeutic guidelines *(60,61)* indicate the chromones for the maintenance treatment of mild persistent to moderately severe asthma, both preceding and alongside standard doses of inhaled corticosteroids. Our current understanding of the effects of these drugs and of the mechanism of action supports this early and well-tolerated chronic use.

REFERENCES

1. Dunnil MS (1960) The pathology of asthma with special reference to changes in the bronchial mucosa. J Clin Pathol 13:27–33.
2. Beasley R, Roche WR, Roberts JA, Holgate ST (1989) Cellular events in the bronchi in mild asthma and after bronchial provocation. Am Rev Respir Dis 139:806–817.
3. Djukanovic R, Lai CKW, Wilson JW, Britten KM, Wilson SJ, Roche WR, Howarth PH, Holgate ST (1992) Bronchial mucosal manifestations of atopy: a comparison of markers of inflammation between atopic asthmatics, atopic nonasthmatics and healthy control. Eur Respir J 5:538–544.
4. Pepys J (1973) Disodium cromoglycate in clinical and experimental asthma. In: Austen KF, Lichtenstein CM, eds. Asthma: Physiology, Immunopharmacology and Treatment Academic, London, Press, pp. 279–294.
5. Montefort S, Gratizou C, Goulding D, Polosa R, Haskard DO, Howarth PH, Holgate ST, Carroll MP (1994) Bronchial biopsy evidence for leukocyte infiltration and upregulation of leukocyte-endothelial cell adhesion molecules 6 hours after local allergen challenge of sensitised asthmatic airways. J Clin Invest 93:1411–1421.
6. Cockcroft DW, Murdock KY (1987) Comparative effects of inhaled salbutamol, sodium cromoglycate, and beclomethasone dipropionate on allergen-induced early asthmatic responses, late asthmatic responses, and increased bronchial responsiveness to histamine. J Allergy Clin Immunol, 79:734–740.
7. Springer TA (1990) Adhesion receptors of the immune system. Nature 346:425–434.
8. Gordon JR, Galli SJ (1991) Release of both preformed and newly synthesised tumour necrosis factor-α (TNFα)/cachetin by mouse mast cells stimulated with Fc$_\epsilon$R1. A mechanism for sustained action of mast cell derived TNFα during IgE-dependent biological responses. J Exp Med 174:103–107.
9. Liu MC, Bleecker ER, Lichtenstein LM, Kagey-Sobotka A, Nic Y, McLemore TL, Permutt S, Proud D, Hubbard WC (1990) Evidence for elevated levels of histamine, prostaglandin D$_2$, and other bronchoconstricting prostaglandins in the airways of subjects with mild asthma. Am Rev Respir Dis 142:126–132.
10. Riley PA, Mather ME, Keogh RW, Eady RP (1987) Activity of nedocromil sodium in mast-cell-dependent reactions in the rat. Int Arch Allergy Appl Immunol 82:108–110.
11. Wells E, Jackson CG, Harper ST, Mann J, Eady RP (1986) Characterization of primate bronchoalveolar mast cells. II. Inhibition of histamine, LTC$_4$ and PGD$_2$ release from primate bronchoalveolar mast cells and a comparison with rat peritoneal mast cells. J Immunol 137:3941–3945.
12. Leung KBP, Flint KC, Brostoff J, Hudspith BN, Johnson NM, Lau HYA, Liu WL, Pearce FL (1988) Effects of sodium cromoglycate and nedocromil sodium on histamine secretion from human lung mast cells. Thorax 43:756–761.
13. Bissonnette EY, Enciso JA, Befus AD (1995) Interferon and antiallergic regulation of histamine and tumour necrosis factor-alpha in rat mast cell subsets. Int Arch Allergy Immunol 107:156–157.
14. Bissonnette EY, Befus AD (1993) Modulation of mast cell function in the gastrointestinal tract. In: Willace JL, The Handbook of Immunopharmacology: Immunopharmacology of the Gastrointestinal System, Academic, London, pp. 95–103.
15. Hoshino M, Nakamura Y (1995) The effect of disodium cromoglycate on infiltration of inflammatory cells into bronchial mucosa and on expression of adhesion molecules in asthmatics. Jpn J Allergol 44:593–601.

16. Manolitsas ND, Wang J, Devalia JL, Trigg CJ, McAulay AE, Davies RJ (1995) Regular albuterol, nedocromil sodium, and bronchial inflammation in asthma. Am J Respir Crit Care Med 151:1925–1930.
17. Rand TH, Lopez AF, Gamble JR, Vadas MA (1988) Nedocromil sodium and cromolyn (sodium cromoglycate) selectively inhibit antibody-dependent granulocyte-mediated cytotoxicity. Int Arch Allergy Appl Immunol 87:151–158.
18. Moqbel R, Cromwell O, Walsh GM, Wardlaw AJ, Kurlak L, Kay AB (1988) Effects of nedocromil sodium (Tilade) on the activation of human eosinophils and neutrophils and the release of histamine from mast cells. Allergy 43:268–276.
19. Bruijnzeel PLB, Warringa RAJ, Kok PTM (1989) Inhibition of platelet-activating factor- and zymosan-activated serum-induced chemotaxis of human neutrophils by nedocromil sodium, BN 52021 and sodium cromoglycate. Br J Pharmacol 97:1251–1257.
20. Bruijnzeel PLB, Warringa RAJ, Kok PTM, Kreukniet J (1990) Inhibition of neutrophil and eosinophil induced chemotaxis by nedocromil sodium and sodium cromoglycate. Br J Pharmacol 99:798–802.
21. Devalia JL, Rusznak C, Abdelaziz MM, Davies RJ (1996) Nedocromil sodium and airway inflammation in vivo and in vitro. J Allergy Clin Immunol 98:S51–57.
22. Marini M, Soloperto M, Zheng Y, Mezzetti M, Mattoli S (1992) Protective effect of nedocromil sodium on the IL1-induced release of GM-CSF from cultured human bronchial epithelial cells. Pulmonary Pharmacol 5:61–65.
23. Vittori E, Sciacca F, Colotta F, Mantovani A, Mattoli S (1992) Protective effect of nedocromil sodium on the interleukin-1-induced production of interleukin-8 in human bronchial epithelial cells. J Allergy Clin Immunol 90:76–84.
24. Vignola AM, Chanez P, Lacoste P, Campbell AM, Norris A, Michel FB, Bousquet J, Godard P (1993) Nedocromil modulates the histamine induced expression of ICAM-1 and HLA DR molecules on bronchial epithelial cells. Am Rev Respir Dis 147(4):A45.
25. Borish L, Williams J, Johnson S, Mascali JJ, Miller R, Rosenwasser LJ (1992) Anti-inflammatory effects of nedocromil sodium: inhibition of alveolar macrophage function. Clin Exp Allergy 22:984–990.
26. Thorel T, Joseph M, Vorng H, Capron A (1988) Regulation of IgE-dependent antiparasite functions of rat macrophages and platelets by nedocromil sodium. Int Arch Allergy Appl Immunol 85:227–231.
27. Tsicopoulos A, Lassalle P, Joseph M, Tonnell AB, Thorel T, Dessaint JP, Capron A (1988) Effect of disodium cromoglycate on the inflammatory cells bearing the Fc epilson receptor Type II (Fc$_\varepsilon$RII). Int J Immunopharmacol 10:227–236.
28. Loh RKS, Jabara HH, Geha RS (1994) Disodium cromoglycate inhibits Sμ to Sε deletional switch recombination and IgE synthesis in human B cells. J Exp Med 180:663–671.
29. Kimata H, Yoshida A, Ishioka C, Mikawa H (1991) Disodium cromoglycate (DSCG) selectively inhibits IgE production and enhances IgG$_4$ production by human B cells in vitro. Clin Exp Immunol 84:395–399.
30. Loh RKS, Jabara HH, Geha RF (1996) Mechanisms of inhibition of IgE synthesis by nedocromil sodium: nedocromil sodium inhibits deletional switch recombination in human B cells. J Allergy Clin Immunol 97:1141–1150.
31. Kimata H, Hiratsuka S (1994) Effect of topical sodium cromoglycate solution on atopic dermatitis: combined treatment of sodium cromoglycate solution with the oral anti-allergic medication, oxatomide. Eur J Pediatr 153:66–71.
32. Diaz P, Galleguillos FR, Cristina Gonzalez M, Pantin CFA, Kay AB (1984) Bronchoalveolar lavage in asthma: The effect of disodium cromoglycate (cromolyn) on leukocyte counts, immunoglobulins, and complement. J Allergy Clin Immunol 74:41–48.
33. Marquette CH, Joseph M, Tonnel AB, Vorng H, Lassalle P, Tsicopoulos A, Capron A, Tsicopoulos A, Capron A (1990) The abnormal in vitro response to aspirin of platelets from aspirin-sensitive asthmatics is inhibited after inhalation of nedocromil sodium but not of sodium cromoglycate. Br J Clin Pharmacol 29:525–531.
34. Roth M, Soler M, Lefkowitz H, Chem I, Emmons LR, Anstine D, Hornung M, Perruchoud AP (1993) Inhibition of receptor-mediated platelet activation by nedocromil sodium. J Allergy Clin Immunol 91:1217–1225.
35. O'Hehir RE, Moqbel R (1989) Action of nedocromil sodium and sodium cromoglycate on cloned human allergen-specific CD4$^+$ T lymphocytes. Drugs 37(Suppl 1):23–25.
36. Dixon M, Jackson DM, Richards IM (1980) The action of sodium cromoglycate on 'C' fibre endings in the dog lung. Br J Pharmacol 70:11–13.
37. Hargreaves MR, Benson MK (1995) Inhaled sodium cromoglycate in angiotensin-converting enzyme inhibitor cough. Lancet 45:13–16.

38. Jackson DM, Norris AA, Eady RP (1989) Nedocromil sodium and sensory nerves in the dog lung. Pulmonary Pharmacol 2:179–184.

39. Louis RE, Radermecker MF (1990) Substance P-induced histamine release from human basophils, skin and lung fragments: effect of nedocromil sodium and theophylline. Int Arch Allergy Appl Immunol 92:329–333.

40. Armour CL, Johnson PRA, Black JL (1991) Nedocromil sodium inhibits substance P-induced potentiation of cholinergic neural responses in the isolated innervated rabbit trachea. J Auton Pharmacol 11:167–172.

41. Verleden GM, Belvisi MG, Stretton CD, Barnes PJ (1991) Nedocromil sodium modulates nonadrenergic, noncholinergic bronchoconstrictor nerves in guinea pig airways in vitro. Am Rev Respir Dis 143:114–118.

42. Abraham WM, Sielczak MW, Wanner A, Perruchoud AP, Blinder L, Stevenson JS, Ahmed A, Yerger LD (1988) Cellular markers of inflammation in the airways of allergic sheep with and without allergen-induced late responses. Am Rev Respir Dis 138:1565–1571.

43. Pretolani M, Lefort J, Silva P, Malanchere E, Dumarey C, Bachelet M, Vargaftig BB (1990) Protection by nedocromil sodium of active immunization-induced bronchopulmonary alterations in the guinea pig. Am Rev Respir Dis 141:1259–1265.

44. Hutson PA, Holgate ST, Church MK (1988) Inhibition by nedocromil sodium of early and late phase bronchoconstriction and airway cellular infiltration provoked by ovalbumin inhalation in conscious sensitized guinea-pigs. Br J Pharmacol 94:6–8.

45. Jackson DM, Eady RP (1988) Acute transient SO_2-induced airway hyperreactivity: effects of nedocromil sodium. J Appl Physiol 65:1119–1124.

46. Abraham WM, Stevenson JS, Chapman GA, Tallent MW, Jackowski J (1987) The effect of nedocromil sodium and cromolyn sodium on antigen-induced responses in allergic sheep in vivo and in vitro. Chest 92:913–917.

47. Eady RP, Greenwood B, Jackson DM, Orr TSC, Wells E (1985) The effect of nedocromil sodium and sodium cromoglycate on antigen-induced bronchoconstriction in the Ascaris-sensitive monkey. Br J Pharmacol 85:323–325.

48. Hutson PA, Holgate ST, Church MK (1988) The effect of cromolyn sodium and albuterol on early and late phase bronchoconstriction and airway leukocyte infiltration after allergen challenge of non-anesthetized guinea pigs. Am Rev Respir Dis 138:1157–1163.

49. Jackson DM (1988) The effect of nedocromil sodium, sodium cromoglycate and codeine phosphate on citric acid-induced cough in dogs. Br J Pharmacol 93:609–612.

50. Norris AA, Alton EWFW (1996) Chloride transport and the action of sodium cromoglycate and nedocromil sodium in asthma. Clin Exp Allergy 26:250–253.

51. Beaven MA, Rogers J, Moore JP, Hesketh TR, Smith GA, Metcalfe JC (1984) The mechanism of the calcium signal and correlation with histamine release in 2H3 cells. J Biol Chem 259:129–136.

52. Penner R, Matthews G, Neher E (1988) Regulation of calcium influx by second messengers in rat mast cells. Nature 334:499–504.

53. Alton EWFW, Kingsleigh-Smith DJ, Munkonge FM, Smith SN, Lindsay ARG, Gruenert DC, Jeffery PK, Norris AA, Geddes DM, Williams AJ (1996) Asthma prophylaxis agents alter the function of an airway epithelial chloride channel. Am J Respir Cell Mol Biol 14:380–387.

54. Heinke S, Szucs G, Norris A, Droogmans G, Nilius B (1995) Inhibition of volume-activated chloride currents in endothelial cells by chromones. Br J Pharmacol 115:1393–1398.

55. Jackson DM, Pollard CE, Roberts SM (1992) The effect of nedocromil sodium on the isolated rabbit vagus nerve. Eur J Pharmacol 221:175–177.

56. Foreman JC, Hallet MB, Mongar JL (1977) Site of action of the antiallergic drugs cromoglycate and doxantrazole. Br J Pharmacol 59:473P.

57. Theoharides TC, Sieghart W, Greengard P, Douglas WW (1980) Antiallergic drug cromolyn may inhibit secretion by regulating phosphorylation of a mast cell protein. Science 207:80–82.

58. Wells E, Mann J (1983) Phosphorylation of a mast cell protein in response to treatment with anti-allergic compounds. Biochem Pharmacol 32:837–842.

59. Mackay G, Pearce F (1993) Extracellular cGMP has a spectrum of activity in rodent isolated mast cells similar to that of sodium cromoglycate. Br J Pharmacol 109:65P.

60. National Institutes of Health (NIH), NHLBI (1995) Global Strategy for Asthma Management and Prevention. National Heart, Lung, and Blood Institute (NHLBI)/World Health Organization (WHO) Workshop Report, March 1993. Publication no. 95-3659, National Institutes of Health, Bethesda, MD.

61. National Heart, Lung, and Blood Institute, National Institutes of Health (1992) International Consensus Report on Diagnosis and Treatment of Asthma. Publication no. 92-3091, National Institutes of Health, Bethesda, MD.

31

Airway Remodeling and Repair

Peter M. Hockey, MBBCH, MRCP,
Ratko Djukanović, MD, MSC, DM,
William R. Roche, MSC, MD, FRCPATH,
and Steven T. Holgate, MD, DSC, FRCP

CONTENTS

INTRODUCTION

It is now universally accepted that asthma is a disease process revolving around inflammation and its effects on airway pathophysiology. The inflammatory features of asthma are characterized by immunohistological and cytokine profiles that appear to be specific for asthma and, importantly, are not demonstrable in the nonatopic, nonasthmatic, normal individual. They have been shown to include edema, hyperplasia of mucus-secreting cells, hypertrophy of smooth muscle, collagen deposition beneath the epithelial basement membrane, intraluminal cellular and mucus debris, cellular infiltration of the epithelium, and sloughing of the epithelial cell layer with subsequent denudation of the normal air–tissue interface. These changes have been shown to be present to a varying degree in patients with mild, asymptomatic disease right through to those dying in status asthmaticus. Although considerable attention has focused on the documentation of morphological abnormalities, especially by means of bronchial biopsy studies, to date comparatively little attention has been paid to the healing process. As with inflammatory processes in other tissues, chronic insult to the airways is likely to lead to a cycle of inflammation and repair, although the factors that determine the balance between the two remain largely unknown *(1)*.

There have been few long-term studies of the pathology of asthma, but what evidence does exist suggests that severe and poorly controlled asthma progresses to an increasingly irreversible state *(2)*. Severe and prolonged inflammation in any organ is almost always accompanied by tissue remodeling, and the airways are no exception. Although previously limited to histological examination, a better anatomical view of gross airway changes has added considerably to the phenotypic features of chronic asthma. The recent advances in radiological imaging techniques and, in particular, high resolution spiral computerized tomography have added more information to our knowledge of structural airway changes. However, the clinical correlates of airway remodeling remain undetermined in terms of the rate and time of onset and reversibility by anti-inflammatory agents or allergy avoidance *(3)*.

From: *Allergy and Allergic Diseases: The New Mechanisms and Therapeutics*
Edited by: J. A. Denburg © Humana Press Inc., Totowa, NJ

It is reasonable to hypothesize that the severity and chronicity of asthma may result from the dysregulation of cytokine networks, leading to persistent inflammation in structurally altered airways, which, in the extreme, may become refractory to treatment. The responsibility for disease progression probably does not lie with any single cellular element but embraces T- and B-cells, mast cells, eosinophils, endothelial cells, epithelial cells, and myofibroblasts acting cooperatively with each other and with the formed elements of the airways, including smooth muscle and nerves, leading to the phenotype that is characteristic of severe disease. This integrated view of asthma as a chronic disease of ongoing inflammation and repair leads us to incriminate a number of effector cells, although emerging evidence points to a shift from mast cells and eosinophil to T-lymphocytes as disease becomes more severe. Continuous T-cell activation leads to their oligoclonal expansion and activation, with a mixed pattern of cytokine expression and failure of the normal counter-regulatory mechanisms. T-cells drive the ongoing inflammatory process not only with regard to eosinophil recruitment and activation, but a cytokine shift can be demonstrated with allergen instillation away from interleukin (IL)-2, IL-12, and interferon-γ (IFNγ) favoring production of IL-3, IL-4, IL-5, and IL-13 *(1)*. The ensuing recruitment of mast cells and eosinophils by this process contributes to the maintenance of mucosal inflammation through their release of proinflammatory cytokines and proteases. Cytokine-induced immunoglobulin E (IgE) production may lead to disease progression by shifting specificity from external to other antigens, including autoantigens, and through the formation of autoantibodies against IgE *(1)*. These cellular processes occur in addition to the microvasculature activation and proinflammatory active participation of the epithelium, which will be described subsequently.

THE CONCEPT OF REPAIR AND REMODELING

The ideal outcome of any physiological repair process is the restitution of tissue integrity. When this is not achieved, scarring follows injury. Commonly, the attempt at repair is followed by a residual marker of inflammation or damage. A typical marker of the asthmatic form of inflammation is the thickening of the bronchial "basement membrane," which was originally felt to be an epithelial response to damage and subsequently a cause of airway dysfunction. Further gross anatomical abnormalities are increasingly being recognized by the application of high-resolution computerized tomography to varying degrees of asthma severity. A recent study has demonstrated a number of irreversible abnormalities in a group of randomly chosen nonsmoking asthmatics with varying disease severity. These changes include bronchiectasis, emphysema, bronchial thickening, and linear shadows, which were found to be more extensive in severe than in mild disease and in nonallergic rather than allergic subjects *(4)*. Although the demonstration of bronchiectasis does not necessarily imply clinical significance, it does provide evidence for the presence of airway remodeling *(5)*. Despite considerable progress in the understanding of initiating factors of the inflammatory cycle occurring in the epithelial and subepithelial microcosm (such as allergens, viruses, and air pollutants), the mechanisms of signaling that are at work to regulate the inflammation–repair cycle remain poorly understood and probably vary from individual to individual. Although it is increasingly appreciated that both the inflammatory leukocytes and structural cells participate in the inflammatory response, for the purpose of clarity this review will address the epithelium and subepithelial compartments separately and point to interactions as appropriate.

The Epithelium

The bronchial epithelium of the respiratory tract has as its ultimate aim protection from the external environment. Although once viewed as a passive barrier serving as a target for the inflammatory response, it is now increasingly realized that the epithelium is an important

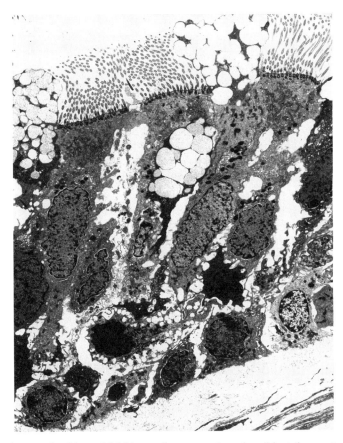

Fig. 1. Electron micrograph of bronchial biopsy from an asthmatic subject demonstrating loss of intercellular adhesion (uranyl acetate/lead citrate, ×2000).

source of inflammatory products *(6)*. Much of our current information is gained from direct examination of bronchial biopsy material. The site of bronchial epithelial cell damage has been demonstrated to occur along a suprabasal plane of cleavage between the suprabasal and basal cell layers *(7)*, suggesting that the adhesion molecules anchoring the columnar ciliated cells are the target of the inflammatory insult either because they are closest to the source of inflammation or because these links are weaker than those between the individual epithelial cells. Indeed, analysis of epithelial cells recovered by bronchoalveolar lavage (BAL) and embedded into spur resin for electron microscopy shows that, in asthma, a greater proportion of epithelial cells can be found in clumps as opposed to single cells when compared with healthy nonasthmatic individuals *(8)* (Fig. 1). As part of, or perhaps in reaction to, this damage the epithelium produces a host of inflammatory products with potential roles in asthma, including arachidonic acid products, endothelin, nitric oxide (NO), and cytokines. In addition in asthma the increased expression intercellular adhesion molecule (ICAM)-1, HLA-DR, and CD44 demonstrates the capacity of the epithelium to participate directly in inflammatory cell recruitment and activation.

ARACHIDONIC ACID METABOLISM

In terms of arachidonic acid metabolism, the epithelium is a major source of 15-hydroxyeicosatetraenoic acid (15-HETE). Although 15-HETE and 15-dihydroxy acids exhibit some mediator functions, more active oxidative products of arachidonic acid are prostaglandin E2 (PGE_2) and $PGF_{2\alpha}$ with their opposing actions on bronchial smooth muscle tone. The demonstration of epithelial expression of the inducible form of cyclo-oxygenase (COX2) over the constitutive form (COX1) is evidence of epithelial modification in asthma (9–11). This change is suppressed by corticosteroid treatment in parallel with their clinical efficacy, and in asthma poorly controlled with corticosteroids, COX2 upregulation might be expected to persist.

ENDOTHELIN

A further powerful and active epithelially derived compound is endothelin. The finding that cultured human airway epithelial cells from asthmatics secrete increased amounts of endothelin suggests increased production by the epithelium with endothelin levels in BAL from asthmatics being increased (12,13). Human endothelin is comprised of three structurally distinct 21-amino-acid peptides (ET-1, ET-2, ET-3) encoded by separate genes. In addition to its potent vasoconstrictor property ET-1 is a powerful airway smooth muscle constrictor mediated through the ET_B receptor subtype. Importantly, ET-1 is a mitogen for airway smooth muscle and is chemoattractant and mitogenic for fibroblasts and provides an activating signal for collagen synthesis largely mediated through ET_B receptors (1). This provides a good example of the direct interaction between, and a possible role for, the epithelium and subepithelium in remodeling of the airway.

CYTOKINES

Human bronchial epithelial cells in vitro constitutively synthesize and release a range of interleukins (IL-1β, IL-6, IL-8) and granulocyte-macrophage colony-stimulating factor (GM-CSF), with greatly enhanced production occurring on exposure to IL-1β or tumor necrosis factor (TNF)-α, the early-acting cytokines from lung inflammatory cells (14). GM-CSF is produced by the airway epithelium under basal conditions and may be induced by treatment with histamine and IL-1. In asthmatics the production of GM-CSF is increased compared with normals (15). In addition, in vitro experiments have shown that myofibroblasts from human airways cultured in the presence of GM-CSF prolong eosinophil survival (16). The evidence for the effects of these growth factors and fibrogenic cytokines comes predominantly from studies of patients with pulmonary fibrosis, and there have been few studies exploring this topic in asthma (14).

It has been suggested that the proliferative response of columnar epithelial cells following injury is likely to result from release of autocrine growth factors. These could include the epidermal growth factor receptor stimulants, transforming growth factor-α (TGFα), and epidermal growth factor itself, in addition to endothelin (3,17). The proliferation of tracheal epithelial cultures from rats is reduced following exposure to neutralizing antisera to TGFα, and the production of TGFα is increased in growing cells compared with those at confluent density, indicating an autocrine action of this growth factor. Excessive production of growth factors, including endothelin, may stimulate proliferation of underlying fibroblasts and airway smooth muscle cells in the subepithelium.

The Subepithelium

The subepithelial airway compartment plays a key role in the propagation and continuation of airway inflammation, especially in terms of cellular recruitment from the vasculature. Inflammatory cell migration from the bloodstream into the tissues is critical to the genesis of an inflammatory response. The initial step must be adherence of the leukocyte to an endothelial cell. This is achieved by the interaction of adhesion molecules expressed on the cell surfaces of endothelial cells and their ligands present on the circulating leukocytes. The principal recognized adhesion molecules are ICAM-1, vascular cell adhesion molecule-1 (VCAM-1),

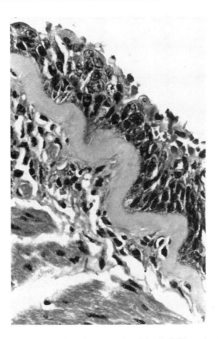

Fig. 2. Postmortem bronchial mucosa showing dense subepithelial fibrosis (hematoxylin and eosin, ×240).

endothelial-leukocyte adhesion molecule-1 (ELAM-1), and granule-associated membrane protein-140 (GMP-140). During inflammation adhesion molecule expression is upregulated, leading to enhanced recruitment of inflammatory cells from the vascular compartment. Increased adhesion molecule expression on the epithelium associated with allergen exposure in the laboratory leads to the recruitment of cells, especially eosinophils, to the epithelial surface, where activation, degranulation, and release of cytotoxic products will result in further epithelial damage.

THE BASEMENT MEMBRANE

This is a thin layer of specialized extracellular matrix that in addition to providing mechanical support may influence cellular behavior *(18)*. A number of subepithelial abnormalities in the asthmatic airway have been described. One of the first described abnormalities was the observation of extensive subepithelial collagen deposition, which has been shown to consist of crosslinked, banded collagen types I, III, and V along with fibronectin *(19,20)*. This thickening of the subbasement membrane is seen even in mild disease and appears to persist despite anti-inflammatory therapy *(21)*. The extracellular matrix in the basement membrane comprises glycosaminoglycan and proteoglycan macromolecules, which form a highly hydrated, gel-like substance in which fibrous proteins are embedded. These fibrous proteins may be structural (collagen and elastin) or adhesive (fibronectin and laminin). Type IV collagen, fibronectin, and laminin are produced by bronchial epithelial cells. Fibronectin and tenascin, (a further glycoprotein), are considered transitional components of the basement membrane, because their expression in adult lung is sparse or absent. However, tenascin is re-expressed in the basement membrane of asthmatic patients, possibly as a result of increased turnover of the airway epithelium *(22)*. Recent work has shown that tenascin in the basement membrane is significantly decreased by inhaled steroid therapy, in spite of the absence of change in the thickness of the collagen band *(21)*. This suggests that inflammation but not fibrosis is prevented by inhaled steroids, although there is some evidence to the contrary *(23)* (Fig. 2–4).

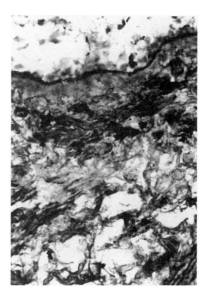

Fig. 3. Fibronectin staining in basement membrane and underlying lamina reticularis (immunoperoxidase ×300).

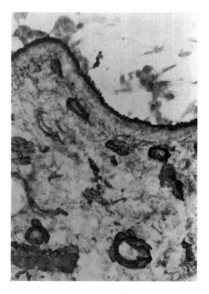

Fig. 4. Collagen IV staining demonstrating true epithelial basement membrane and vascular basement membranes (immunoperoxidase, ×300).

SUBEPITHELIAL MYOFIBROBLASTS

In addition to their capacity to secrete matrix proteins, it has recently been shown that cultures of human bronchial subepithelial myofibroblasts produce GM-CSF, IL-6, IL-8, and stem cell factor (SCF) constitutively and that the supernatant from cultures can greatly extend eosinophil survival *(24)*. An excess of myofibroblasts beneath the bronchial epithelium is demonstrable in asthmatic subjects, with a close correlation between the myofibroblast numbers and the depth of the collagen layer, suggesting that myofibroblasts lying beneath the

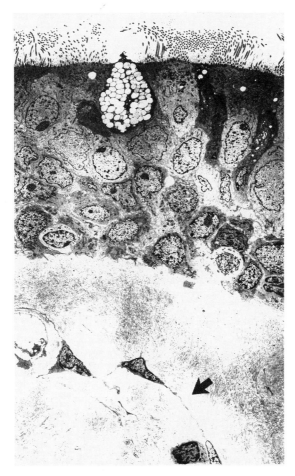

Fig. 5. Electron micrograph demonstrating myofibroblasts (arrow) within the interstitial collagen of the lamina reticularis (×2000).

epithelium are the main source of deposited collagen *(25)* (Figs. 5 and 6). There is a significant correlation between the number of epithelial cells expressing TGFβ and the number of vimentin-positive cells as well as the thickness of the basement membrane, suggesting an interaction between epithelial cells, fibroblasts, and collagen deposition *(14)*. Following epithelial damage there may be large areas of denuded basement membrane, and this results in exposure of the lung parenchyma not only to inflammatory mediators but also to pulmonary surfactant. Recent evidence suggests that surfactant may modify pulmonary fibroblast participation in inflammation-associated cascade effects by inhibiting deoxyribonucleic acid (DNA) synthesis and secondary inflammatory mediator production such as IL-6 and PGE$_2$ *(26)*.

Mast Cells

The mast cell, too, has come under increasing scrutiny and appears to play a significant role in airway remodeling. In addition to being a source of cytokines with central roles in allergic responses (including IL-4, IL-5, IL-6, and IL-8) the mast cell, stimulated by stromal cells, is able to produce and release TNFα *(27–29)*. TNFα has powerful growth promoting activity on the fibroblast *(30)*, and in vitro experiments have shown that myofibroblasts from human airways cultured in the presence of TNF produce significant amounts of GM-CSF, which

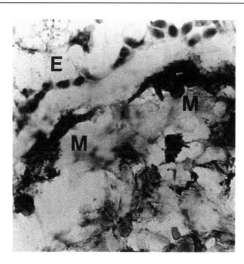

Fig. 6. Immunohistochemical demonstration of myofibroblasts (M) beneath the bronchial epithelium (E) in an asthmatic subject demonstrated by monoclonal antibody PR2D3 (×400).

prolongs eosinophil survival *(16)*. Eosinophils in turn contain TGFβ and platelet-derived growth factor (PDGF), which are profibrotic cytokines contained in eosinophil granules. Mast cell tryptase is able to upregulate the cell surface expression of ICAM-1 to an extent similar to TNFα. These findings suggest an important role for the mast cell in epithelial repair, in the recruitment of granulocytes, and in rendering the lower respiratory tract vulnerable to human rhinovirus (HRV) infection, since the major type of HRV utilizes ICAM-1 to gain access to epithelial cells and upregulate cytokine production.

Summary

It has been suggested that the mechanisms of airway repair recapitulate the main events associated with embryonic lung development *(31)*. However, these developmental equivalents in asthma are occurring in concert with the inflammatory process, which includes the release of numerous cytokines and TGFβ. It has been suggested that communication between cell types and the extracellular matrix proteins may be a central determinant of the disease process. The changes occurring in all parts of the airway, e.g., greater than normal ratio of goblet to ciliated epithelial cells, thickened basement membrane, and increased inflammatory cell numbers, may result in altered communication between epithelial cells and the lamina propria. The increased tenascin, collagens, and fibronectin with resultant thickening of the basement membrane may further alter cellular communication. Corticosteroids, although having a normalizing effect on epithelial cell type and alteration in basement membrane composition, may improve cellular communication and subsequently the clinical expression of asthma *(31)*.

EPITHELIAL DAMAGE AND REPAIR CYCLE

Epithelial damage results in persistent activation of repair mechanisms, abnormal epithelial–mesenchymal interactions, and detrimental remodelling of the airway. We propose the following steps in epithelial damage and repair in asthmatic airways.

Immediate Damage and Effects

The cellular recruitment to the epithelium in asthma results in an influx of a number of cell types, of which eosinophils play a key role. Since the arginine-rich eosinophil granule proteins can destroy the bronchial epithelium in vitro, it is plausible that infiltrated eosinophils in asthmatic epithelium may be responsible for cell damage in vivo. It has been shown that epithelial damage at an ultrastructural level correlates directly with the degree of eosinophil infiltration and bronchial hyperresponsiveness *(1)*. Based on findings in a bovine epithelial explant model, we suggest that activated eosinophils mediate epithelial detachment via a cognate interaction involving ICAM-1 and the subsequent release of metalloendoproteases, oxidants, and arginine-rich proteins.

METALLOENDPROTEASES

Asthmatic BAL has been shown to contain increased concentrations of the 92-kDa gelatinase metalloproteinase along with other metalloendoproteases. Eosinophils are an important source of the 92-kDa gelatinase, which has a broad substrate specificity in being able to degrade both basement membrane collagen type IV and interstitial matrix molecules *(32)*. This enzyme is likely to be importance both in cell migration and tissue remodeling.

OXIDANTS

Eosinophil peroxidase is a highly charged, largely cell-associated protein that is released asynchronously with eosinophil cationic protein (ECP) and major basic protein (MBP). Antioxidants have been shown to inhibit the tissue damaging effects of eosinophil-mediated lung injury that are mediated through the products of eosinophil peroxidase.

BASIC PROTEINS

There is a large body of evidence implicating the disruptive effects of eosinophil basic proteins (MBP, ECP, EDN) on epithelial integrity in asthma. Their extreme cationicity renders matrix proteoglycans as susceptible targets. A number of proinflammatory cytokines, including IL-4, IL-8, IFNγ, and basic fibroblast growth factor (b-FGF), are tightly bound to GAG side-chains of highly O-sulfated proteoglycans, an association that stabilizes the cytokine, localizes its activity, and determines its specificity. We suggest that an interaction of the eosinophil basic proteins with cytokine binding sites on matrix molecules results in release of free cytokine, so that a wider range of activity is achieved in severe disease *(33–35)*.

Tryptase comprises in excess of 20% of the total granule content of protein and is the major secretory component of mast cells. It is uniquely stabilized in its action by its being bound to heparin, which serves to preserve its integrity and direct specificity of the enzyme. Tryptase is capable of cleaving several components of the extracellular matrix (e.g., collagen VI, fibronectin) and can activate matrix metalloproteases (stromelysin). This provides more evidence for the role of the mast cell, and in particular tryptase, in airway remodeling *(36–38)*.

The mechanisms referred to above result in immediate damage and selective cell loss owing to injury with loss of barrier function.

Immediate Response

During this phase of cellular injury epithelial cells adjacent to areas of damage are believed to reduce cell–substrate adhesion and migrate to form a temporary squamous barrier. Detailed examination of bronchial biopsies via electron microscopy has led to a greater knowledge of cell adhesion and its breakdown in asthma. The columnar cell bears the brunt of the cellular damage, and this requires the cleavage of desmosomal linkages. The remaining basal cells remain attached to the basement membrane through their hemidesmosomes containing the integrin α6β4. Upregulation of the adhesion protein CD44 involving >70% of the epithelium in asthma provides evidence for the importance of CD44 in inflammation and in modulating the adhesive behavior of epithelial cells *(39)*. Rickard et al. *(40)* have demonstrated migration of bovine bronchial epithelial cells. A number of stimuli to cell migration have been identified—fibronectin being one of the first inflammatory glycoproteins to be identified as a chemotactic factor. Extracellular matrix components such as laminin and type IV collagen were shown to support epithelial cell chemotaxis. Airway epithelial cells have been demonstrated to produce TGFβ *(41)*, which is itself a weak epithelial cell chemoattractant. TGFβ is, however, a potent stimulus of epithelial cell production of fibronectin, which is a powerful epithelial cell chemoattractant. This autocrine or paracrine mediator production may be important in regulating epithelial response to injury *(42)*. Recent evidence also suggests a role for additional cytokines (epidermal growth factor [EGF], TGFα, acidic fibroblast growth factor [a-FGF], hepatocyte growth factor [HGF]) in the chemotaxis and growth-promoting activity on type II cells following acute lung injury *(43)*.

The migration of epithelial cells to an area of injury requires interaction with the underlying connective tissue substrate. This relies in part on the expression of cell surface integrin receptors, which can be regulated by inflammatory components *(40,44,45)*. Cells interact with matrix proteins through specific cell surface receptors. Some fibronectin receptors are members of the integrin family of receptors. Laminin and type IV collagen have multiple domains that are though to interact with integrin receptors, but the recognition sites in the matrix proteins are not completely described *(13)*.

Although much of the focus so far has been on the epithelial cell participation in the cycle of inflammation and repair, there is involvement, too, of the underlying mesenchymal cells in terms of the collagen band formation and smooth muscle hypertrophy. Together with their connective tissue matrix products they may play an important role in the development of fixed airway obstruction and airway remodeling.

Proliferative Response

The apparent thickening of the subepithelial basement membrane in asthma results from the deposition of collagen types I, III, and V and fibronectin *(25)* and that produced by proliferating myofibroblasts. It is of interest that airway epithelial cells are capable of driving fibroblast recruitment *(46)*, proliferation *(47)*, and connective tissue matrix production *(48)*. As in most biological systems there appears to be a feedback mechanism, and besides releasing stimulatory mediators, airway epithelial cells release inhibitory factors to inhibit fibroblast responses. PGE appears to be most potent in this regard *(49,50)*. The presence of tenascin in the lamina *reticularis* indicates that this is a site of high matrix turnover and cell migration, toward which both epithelial cells and myofibroblasts contribute. In addition to their capacity to secrete matrix proteins, we have recently shown that cultures of human bronchial subepithelial myofibroblasts produce GM-CSF, IL-6, IL-8, and SCF constitutively and that the supernatant from cultures could greatly extend eosinophil survival *(51)*. GM-CSF transcription, demonstrated by ribonuclease (RNase) protection assay, was greatly upregulated in the presence of TNFα and was accompanied by secretion of GM-CSF, which accounted for the majority of the eosinophil survival capacity of the supernatants. The enhancement of GM-CSF production by TNFα was inhibited in a dose-dependent manner by prednisolone, but maximum inhibition was not achieved until 1 mM, a concentration far beyond that achieved therapeutically. These findings suggest that human myofibroblasts located beneath the bronchial epithelium establish close contact with eosinophils and mast cell and, as such, play a critical role in upregulating mucosal inflammation, especially in chronic disease. Thus, there may be an interplay between the inflammatory response and normal epithelial repair at the expense of abnormal subepithelial remodelling leading to functional limitation in airway disease *(52)*. We have also shown that mast cell tryptase can enhance proliferation of epithelial cells, fibroblasts, and smooth muscle cells, upregulate expression of ICAM-1, stimulate IL-8 release, and induce eosinophil chemotaxis and activation, all of which are dependent on preservation of the enzyme's catalytic site *(36–38)*. This provides yet more evidence for the role of the mast cell not only in remodeling but also in repair.

Ongoing Damage

The continuous cycle of the aforementioned processes may further compromise epithelial and subepithelial integrity. Lack of appropriate downregulation of the normal response may produce a similar effect.

CONCLUSION

The airway is a dynamic system responding continuously to physiological demands and the external environment. Dysregulation of control mechanisms in this system may lead to the phenotypic expression of disease. The occurrence in asthma of disordered cytokine and cellular responses lends support to the concept of altered regulation of repair mechanisms. In an attempt to minimize structural pulmonary damage, repair mechanisms are invoked, and in this attempt to diminish ongoing damage abnormal repair and subsequent remodeling occurs. The continuous interaction between epithelial cell damage and subsequent inflammatory cell recruitment results in a cycle of repair and remodeling involving all cells in the airway and is not localized only to the epithelium. It is speculated that ongoing and unchecked inflammation, repair, and remodeling results in chronicity of disease with further functional impairment. The challenge lies in further identification of the pathways responsible and identification of areas for possible therapeutic intervention.

REFERENCES

1. Holgate ST. The inflammation-repair cycle in asthma. Eur Respir Rev, in press.
2. Burrows B, Lebowitz MD, Barbee RA, Cline MG (1991) Findings before diagnoses of asthma among the elderly in a longitudinal study of a general population sample. J Allergy Clin Immunol 88:870–877.
3. Stewart AG, Tomlinson PR, Wilson J (1993) Airway wall remodelling in asthma: a novel target for the development of anti-asthma drugs. Trends Pharmacol Sci 14:275–279.
4. Paganin F, Seneterre E, Chanez P, Daures JP, Bruel JM, Michel FB, Bousquet J (1996) Computed tomography of the lungs in asthma: influence of disease severity and etiology. Am J Respir Crit Care Med 153:110–114.
5. Lynch DA, Newell JD, Tschomper BA, Cink TM, Newman LS, Bethel R (1994) Uncomplicated asthma in adults: comparison of CT appearance of the lungs in asthmatic and healthy subjects. Radiology 188:829–833.
6. Raeburn D, Webber SE (1994) Proinflammatory potential of the airway epithelium in bronchial asthma. Eur Respir J 7:2226–2233.
7. Montefort S, Roberts JA, Beasley R, Holgate ST, Roche W (1992) The site of disruption of the bronchial epithelium in asthmatic and non-asthmatic subjects. Thorax 47:499–503.
8. Montefort S, Roche WR, Holgate ST (1993) Bronchial epithelial shedding in asthmatics and non-asthmatics. Respir Med 87:S9–S11.
9. Bradding P, Redington AE, Djukanovic R, Conrad DJ, Holgate ST (1995) 15-1 ipoxygenase immunoreactivity in normal and asthmatic airways. Am J Respir Crit Care Med 151:1201–1204.
10. Shannon VR, Chanez P, Bousquet J, Holtzman MJ (1993) Histochemical evidence for induction of arachidonate 15-lipoxygenase in airway disease. Am Rev Respir Dis 147:1024–1028.
11. Springall DR, Meng Q-H, Redington AE, Howarth PH, Polak JM (1995) Inflammatory genes in asthmatic airway epithelium: suppression by corticosteroids. Eur Respir J 8:445 (abstract).
12. Springall DR, Howarth PH, Counihan H, Djukanovic R, Holgate ST, Polak JM (1991) Endothelin immunoreactivity of airway epithelium in asthmatic patients. Lancet 337:697–701.
13. Albelda SM (1991) Endothelial and epithelial cell adhesion molecules. Am J Respir Cell Mol Biol 4:195–203.
14. Bousquet J, Vignola AM, Chanez P, Campbell AM, Bonsignore G, Michel F-B (1995) Airways remodelling in asthma: no doubt, no more? Int Arch Allergy Immunol 107:211–214.

15. Marini M, Vittori E, Hollemborg J, Mattoli S (1992) Expression of the potent inflammatory cytokines, granulocyte colony-stimulating factor and interleukin-6 and interleukin-8, in bronchial epithelial cells of patients with asthma. J Allergy Clin Immunol 89:1001–1009.
16. Zhang S, Mohammed Q, Burbidge A, Morland CM, Roche WR (1996) Cell cultures from bronchial subepithelial myofibroblasts enhance eosinophil survival in vitro. Eur Respir J 9:1839–1846.
17. Pons F, Boichot E, Lagente V, Touvay C, Mencia-Huerta JM, Braquet P (1991) Role of endothelin in pulmonary function. Pulmon Pharmacol 5:213–219.
18. Raghow R (1994) The role of extracellular matrix in post inflammatory wound healing and fibrosis. FASEB J 8:823–831.
19. Holgate ST, Wilson JR, Howarth PH (1992) New insights into airway inflammation by endobronchial biopsy. Am Rev Respir Dis 145:S2–S6.
20. Roche WR, Beasley R, Williams JH, Holgate ST (1989) Subepithelial fibrosis in the bronchi of asthmatics. Lancet 1:5520–5524.
21. Laitinen LA, Laitinen A (1995) Inhaled corticosteroid treatment and extracellular matrix in the airways in asthma. Int Arch Allergy Immunol 107:215–216.
22. Laitinen A, Altraja A, Linden M, Stallenheim G, Venge P, Hakansson L, Virtanen I, Laitinen LA (1994) Treatment with inhaled budesonide and tenascin expression in bronchial mucosa of allergic asthmatics. Am J Respir Crit Care Med 149:A942.
23. Trigg CJ, Manolitsas ND, Wang J, Calderon MA, McAulay A, Jordan SE, Herdman MJ, Jhalli N, Duddle JM, Hamilton SA, Devalia JL, Davies RJ (1994) Placebo-controlled immunopathologic study of four months of inhaled corticosteroids in asthma. Am J Respir Crit Care Med 150:17–22.
24. Zhang S, Howarth PH, Roche WR (1996) Cytokine production by bronchial myofibroblasts. J Pathol 180:95–101.
25. Brewster CEP, Howarth PH, Djukanovic R, Wilson J, Holgate ST, Roche WR (1990) Myofibroblasts and subepithelial fibrosis in bronchial asthma. Am J Respir Cell Mol Biol 3:507–511.
26. Thomassen MJ, Antal JM, Barna B, Divis LT, Meeker DP, Wiedemann HP (1996) Surfactant down regulates synthesis of DNA and inflammatory mediators in normal human lung fibroblasts. Am J Physiol (Lung Cell Mol Physiol 14) 270:L159–L163.
27. Shah A, Church MK, Holgate ST (1995) Tumour necrosis factor alpha: a potential mediator of asthma. Clin Exp Allergy 25:1038–1044.
28. Bradding P, Feather IH, Wilson S, Bardin PG, Heusser CH, Holgate ST, Howarth PH (1993) Immunolocalisation of cytokines in the nasal mucosa of normal and perennial rhinitic subjects: The mast cell as a source of IL-4, IL-5 and IL-6 in human allergic mucosal inflammation. J Immunol 151: 3853–3865.
29. Bradding P, Roberts JA, Britten KM, Montefort S, Djukanovic R, Heusser C, Howarth PH, Holgate ST (1994) Interleukin-4, -5, -6 and TNFα in normal and asthmatic airways: evidence for the human mast cell as a source of these cytokines. Am J Respir Cell Mol Biol 10:471–480.
30. Piguet PF, Grau GE, Vassalli P (1990) Subcutaneous perfusion of tumour necrosis factor induces local proliferation of fibroblasts, capillaries, and epidermal cells or massive tissue necrosis. Am J Pathol 136:103–110.
31. Laitinen LA, Laitinen A (1996) Remodeling of asthmatic airways by glucocorticosteroids. J Allergy Clin Immunol 97:153–158.
32. Stahle-Backdahl M, Parks WC (1993) 92-Kd gelatinase is actively expressed by eosinophils and stored by neutrophils in squamous cell carcinoma. Am J Pathol 142:995–1000.
33. Teran LM, Carroll M, Frew AJ, Redington AE, Davies DE, Lindley I, Howarth PH, Church MK, Holgate ST (1996) Leukocyte recruitment following local endobronchial allergen challenge in asthma: its relationship to procedure and to airway interleukin-8 release. Am J Respir Crit Care Med 154:496.
34. Redington AE, Madden J, Djukanovic R, Roche WR, Howarth PH, Holgate ST (1995) Transforming growth factor-beta levels in bronchoalveolar lavage are increased in asthma. J Allergy Clin Immunol 95(ii):377 (abstract).
35. Redington AE, Roche WR, Madden J, Frew AJ, Djukanovic R, Holgate ST, Howarth PH (1995) Basic fibroblast growth factor in asthma: immunolocalisation in bronchial biopsies and measurement in bronchoalveolar lavage fluid at baseline and following allergen challenge. Am J Respir Crit Care Med (abstract) 151:A702.
36. Walls AF, He S, Teran L, Buckley MG, Hung KS, Holgate ST, Shute JK, Cairns JA (1995) Granulocyte recruitment by human mast cell tryptase. Int Arch Allergy Immunol 107:372–373.

37. Cairns JA, Walls AF (1996) Mast cell tryptase is a mitogen for epithelial cells. Stimulation of IL-8 production and ICAM-1 expression. J Immunol 156:275–283.

38. Walls AF, He S, Teran L, Holgate ST (1993) Mast cell proteases as mediators of vascular leakage and cell accumulation. J Allergy Clin Immunol 91:256.

39. Lackie PM, Baker JE, Gunthert U, Holgate ST (1997) Expression of CD44 isoforms is increased in the airway epithelium of asthmatic subjects. Amer J Respir Cell Mol Biol 16:14–22.

40. Rickard KA, Taylor J, Rennard SI, Spurzem JR (1993) Migration of bovine bronchial epithelial cells to extracellular matrix components. Am J Respir Cell Mol Biol 8:63–68.

41. Sacco O, Romberger D, Rizzino A, Beckmann J, Rennard SI, Spurzem JR (1992) Spontaneous production of TGF-Beta 2 by primary cultures of bronchial epithelial cells: effects on cell behavior in vitro. J Clin Invest 90:1379–1385.

42. Romberger DJ, Beckmann JD, Claassen L, Ertl RF, Rennard SI (1992) Modulation of fibronectin production of bovine bronchial epithelial cells by transforming growth factor-beta. Am J Respir Cell Mol Biol 7:149–155.

43. Lesur O, Arsalane K, Lane D (1996) Lung alveolar epithelial cell migration in vitro: modulators and regulation processes. Am J Physiol (Lung Cell Mol Biol 14) 270:L311–L319.

44. Rickard KA, Shoji S, Spurzem JR, Rennard SI (1991) Migration of bovine bronchial epithelial cells to extracellular matrix components. Am J Respir Cell Mol Biol 4:440–448.

45. Spurzem JR, Sacco O, Veys T, Rickard K, Rennard SI (1992) TFF-beta increases expression of extracellular matrix receptors on cultured bovine bronchial epithelial cells. Am Rev Respir Dis 145:A668.

46. Shoji S, Rickard KA, Ertl RF, Robbins RA, Linder J, Rennard SI (1989) Bronchial epithelial cells produce lung fibroblast chemotactic factor: fibronectin. Am J Respir Cell Mol Biol 1:13–20.

47. Koizumi S, Ertl R, Rennard S (1991) Bronchial epithelial cells stimulate fibroblast proliferation. Am Rev Respir Dis 143:A526.

48. Kawamoto M, Nakamura Y, Tate L, Ertl RF, Romberger DJ, Rennard SI (1992) Modulation of fibroblast type I collagen and fibronectin production by bronchial epithelial cells. Am Rev Respir Dis 145:A842.

49. Nakamura Y, Ertl RF, Kawamoto M, Tate L, Romberger D, Grossman G, Robbins RA, Rennard SI (1992) Bronchial epithelial cells modulate fibroblast proliferation: role of prostaglandin E2. Am Rev Respir Dis 145:A827.

50. Ertl RF, Valenti V, Spurzem JR, Kawamoto M, Nakamura Y, Veys T, Allegra L, Romberger DJ, Rennard SI (1992) Prostaglandin E inhibits fibroblast recruitment. Am Rev Respir Dis 145:A19.

51. Bradley KH, Kawanami O, Ferrans VJ, Crystal RG (1980) The fibroblast of human lung alveolar structures: a differentiated cell with a major role in lung structure and function. Methods Cell Biol 21A:37–64.

52. Rennard SI, Romberger DJ, Sisson JH, Von Essen SG, Rubinstein I, Robbins RA, Spurzem JR (1994) Airway epithelial cells: functional roles in airway disease. Am J Respir Crit Care Med 150:S27–S30.

INDEX